Nutrition, Diet and Cancer

Sharmila Shankar • Rakesh K. Srivastava
Editors

Nutrition, Diet and Cancer

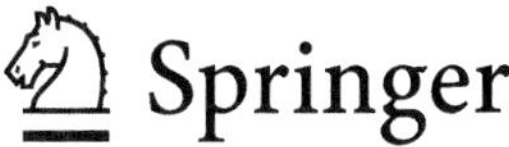

Editors
Assoc. Prof. Sharmila Shankar
Pathology and Laboratory Medicine
University of Kansas Medical Center
Rainbow Blvd 3901
Kansas City, Kansas
USA

Prof. Dr. Rakesh K. Srivastava
Pharmacology and Toxicology
Therapeutics Medicine
University of Kansas Medical Center
Rainbow Blvd 3901
Kansas City, Kansas
USA

ISBN 978-94-007-2922-3 e-ISBN 978-94-007-2923-0
DOI 10.1007/978-94-007-2923-0
Springer Dordrecht Heidelberg London New York

Library of Congress Control Number: 2012934829

Printed on acid-free paper

Springer is part of Springer Science+Business Media (www.springer.com)

Preface

Based on a thorough review of the scientific evidence, this book provides the most authoritative assessment of the relationship between dietary and nutritional factors and the incidence of cancer. It highlights interim dietary guidelines that are likely to reduce the risk of cancer as well as ensure good nutrition. The relationships among nutrition, diet and cancer have advanced in recent years, but much remains to be understood with respect to diet and dietary components in cancer risk and prevention. Continuing accumulation of scientific evidence provides clues about that nutrition is one of the most important determinants of health for the individual, and that specific nutrition habits of various populations can significantly decrease the overall risk of cancer. Sequencing of the human genome has opened the door to an exciting new phase for nutritional science. Unraveling the effects of dietary components on genes and their encoded proteins as well as identifying genetic influences on dietary factors is essential for identifying those who will and will not benefit from intervention strategies for cancer prevention. Other emerging areas that require greater attention include understanding the link between obesity, diet and cancer, the interaction between diet and the microbiome, as well as how dietary agents modulate inflammatory processes. Importantly, nutrigenomics approach may provide useful biomarkers of cancer prevention, early disease, or nutritional status, as well as identify potential molecular targets in cancer processes that are modulated by dietary constituents and/or dietary patterns.

Scientific literature on nutrition for the cancer prevention is inadequate. Whilst the implications of reduced performance status and poor nutritional status on cancer outcomes are documented, there is still a lack of conclusive research data on the potential effect of improvement in nutrition. Our goal is provide the most accurate, up-to-date, and useful textbook possible. These ambitious goals would not be possible without contribution of the authors which represent a diverse group of experts who have endeavored to provide a comprehensive perspective on the dietary agents with nutrigenetics, nutritional epigenomics, nutritional transcriptomics, proteomics, and metabolomics, to allow researchers and dieticians to assimilate these facts into cancer prevention and therapy algorithms. Evidence continues to mount that dietary components are important determinants of cancer risk and tumor behavior. As the era of molecular nutrition grows, a greater understanding about the role of foods and their components on cancer risk and tumor behavior will surely unfold. Such information will provide a new way of understanding of the role of diet and nutrition in the development of effective preemptive approaches to reduce the cancer burden.

We would like to greatly appreciate and sincerely thank for the exceptional contributions of the authors, each of which reflects their commitment to the field of nutrition, diet and cancer.

The University of Kansas Cancer Center
The University of Kansas Medical Center
Kansas City, Kansas

Sharmila Shankar, Ph.D
Rakesh K. Srivastava, Ph.D

Contents

Contributors

Bharat B. Aggarwal Cytokine Research Laboratory, Department of Experimental Therapeutics, The University of Texas MD Anderson Cancer Center, Houston, TX, USA

Amir Ahmad Ph.D. Department of Pathology, Barbara Ann Karmanos Cancer Institute, Wayne State University School of Medicine, Detroit, MI, USA

C. M. Ajila Institut national de la recherche scientifique, Centre Eau, Terre and Environnement/Centre for Water, Earth and Environment, Université du Québec, Québec (QC), Canada

O.I. Aruoma School of Biomedical Sciences and School of Pharmacy, American University of Health Sciences, Signal Hill, USA

M. Mura Assifi Department of Surgery, UCLA David Geffen School of Medicine, UCLA Center for Excellence in Pancreatic Diseases, Hirschberg Laboratory for Pancreatic Cancer Research, Los Angeles, CA, USA

Azfar S. Azmi Ph.D. Department of Pathology, Barbara Ann Karmanos Cancer Institute, Wayne State University School of Medicine, Detroit, MI, USA

T. Bahorun ANDI Centre of Excellence for Biomedical and Biomaterials Research, CBBR Building, MSIRI, University of Mauritius, Réduit, Republic of Mauritius

Sanjeev Banerjee Ph.D. Department of Pathology and Internal Medicine, School of Medicine, Barbara Ann Karmanos Cancer Institute, Wayne State University, Detroit, MI, USA

Bin Bao M.D., Ph.D. Department of Pathology, Barbara Ann Karmanos Cancer Institute, Wayne State University School of Medicine, Detroit, MI, USA

Laura M. Beaver Linus Pauling Institute, Oregon State University, Corvallis, OR, USA

Department of Nutrition and Exercise Sciences, Oregon State University, Corvallis, OR, USA

Anupam Bishayee M. Pharm., Ph.D. Department of Pharmaceutical and Administrative Sciences, School of Pharmacy, American University of Health Sciences, Signal Hill, CA, USA

Goran Bjelakovic Department of Internal Medicine – Gastroenterology and Hepatology, Medical Faculty, University of Nis, Nis, Serbia

The Cochrane Hepato-Biliary Group, Copenhagen Trial Unit, Centre for Clinical Intervention Research, Rigshospitalet, Copenhagen University Hospital, Copenhagen, Denmark

S.K. Brar Institut national de la recherche scientifique, Centre Eau, Terre and Environnement/Centre for Water, Earth and Environment, Université du Québec, Québec (QC), Canada

Malay Chatterjee Department of Pharmaceutical Technology, Jadavpur University, Kolkata, West Bengal, India

Mary Chatterjee Department of Pharmaceutical Technology, Jadavpur University, Kolkata, West Bengal, India

Shyam Sunder Chatterjee Retired Head of Pharmacology Research Laboratories, Dr. Willmar Schwabe GmbH & Co. KG, Karlsruhe, Germany

Gaurav Chaturvedi Department of Molecular and Integrative physiology, University of Kansas Medical Center, Kansas City, KS, USA

Altaf S. Darvesh Department of Pharmaceutical Sciences, College of Pharmacy, Northeast Ohio Medical University, Rootstown, OH, USA

Hiranmoy Das Cardiovascular Stem Cell Research Laboratory, The Dorothy M. Davis Heart and Lung Research Institute, The Ohio State University Medical Center, Columbus, OH, USA

Subhadeep Das Department of Pharmaceutical Technology, Jadavpur University, Kolkata, West Bengal, India

Roderick H. Dashwood Linus Pauling Institute, Oregon State University, Corvallis, OR, USA

Department of Environmental and Molecular Toxicology, Oregon State University, Corvallis, OR, USA

Zora Djuric Ph.D. Departments of Family Medicine and Environmental Health Sciences (Nutrition Program), University of Michigan, Ann Arbor, MI, USA

Q. Ping Dou The Developmental Therapeutics Program, Barbara Ann Karmanos Cancer Institute, and Departments of Oncology, Pharmacology and Pathology, School of Medicine, Wayne State University, Detroit, MI, USA

Guido Eibl M.D. Department of Surgery, UCLA David Geffen School of Medicine, UCLA Center for Excellence in Pancreatic Diseases, Hirschberg Laboratory for Pancreatic Cancer Research, Los Angeles, CA, USA

Christian Gluud Department of Internal Medicine – Gastroenterology and Hepatology, Medical Faculty, University of Nis, Nis, Serbia

The Cochrane Hepato-Biliary Group, Copenhagen Trial Unit, Centre for Clinical Intervention Research, Rigshospitalet, Copenhagen University Hospital, Copenhagen, Denmark

Ajay Goel Ph.D. Gastrointestinal Cancer Research Laboratory, Division of Gastroenterology, Baylor Research Institute and Charles A Sammons Cancer Center, Baylor University Medical Center, Dallas, TX, USA

Sanjay Gupta Ph.D. Department of Urology and Nutrition, Case Western Reserve University, Cleveland, OH, USA

University Hospitals Case Medical Center, Cleveland, OH, USA

Case Comprehensive Cancer Center, Cleveland, OH, USA

Subash C. Gupta Cytokine Research Laboratory, Department of Experimental Therapeutics, The University of Texas MD Anderson Cancer Center, Houston, TX, USA

Emily Ho Linus Pauling Institute, Oregon State University, Corvallis, OR, USA

Department of Nutrition and Exercise Sciences, Oregon State University, Corvallis, OR, USA

Akansha Jain Centre of Advanced Studies, Faculty of Sciences, Banaras Hindu University, Varanasi, Uttar Pradesh, India

Alok Jha Centre of Food Science and Technology, Institute of Agricultural Sciences, Banaras Hindu University, Varanasi, Uttar Pradesh, India

K.S. Kang Adult Stem Cell Research Center, Laboratory of Stem Cell and Tumor Biology, Department of Veterinary Public Health College of Veterinary Medicine, Seoul National University, Sillim-Dong, Seoul, Korea

Vikas Kumar Neuropharmacology Research Laboratory, Department of Pharmaceutics, Institute of Technology, Banaras Hindu University, Varanasi, Uttar Pradesh, India

Kristin Landis-Piwowar Biomedical Diagnostic and Therapeutic Sciences, School of Health Sciences, Oakland University, Rochester, MI, USA

Jingwei Lu Cardiovascular Stem Cell Research Laboratory, The Dorothy M. Davis Heart and Lung Research Institute, The Ohio State University Medical Center, Columbus, OH, USA

Ramzi M. Mohammad Department of Pathology and Internal Medicine, School of Medicine, Barbara Ann Karmanos Cancer Institute, Wayne State University, Detroit, MI, USA

Siddavaram Nagini Department of Biochemistry and Biotechnology, Faculty of Science, Annamalai University, Chidambaram, Tamil Nadu, India

Vidushi S. Neergheen-Bhujun Department of Health Sciences, Faculty of Science and ANDI Centre of Excellence for Biomedical and Biomaterials Research, CBBR Building. MSIRI, University of Mauritius, Réduit, Republic of Mauritius

Dimitrinka Nikolova Department of Internal Medicine – Gastroenterology and Hepatology, Medical Faculty, University of Nis, Nis, Serbia

The Cochrane Hepato-Biliary Group, Copenhagen Trial Unit, Centre for Clinical Intervention Research, Rigshospitalet, Copenhagen University Hospital, Copenhagen, Denmark

Mansi Parasramka Department of Pathology and Internal Medicine, School of Medicine, Barbara Ann Karmanos Cancer Institute, Wayne State University, Detroit, MI, USA

Vincent J. Pompili Cardiovascular Stem Cell Research Laboratory, The Dorothy M. Davis Heart and Lung Research Institute, The Ohio State University Medical Center, Columbus, OH, USA

Sahdeo Prasad Cytokine Research Laboratory, Department of Experimental Therapeutics, The University of Texas MD Anderson Cancer Center, Houston, TX, USA

Ramamurthi Vidya Priyadarsini Department of Biochemistry and Biotechnology, Faculty of Science, Annamalai University, Chidambaram, Tamil Nadu, India

Kaushik Roy Department of Pharmaceutical Technology, Jadavpur University, Kolkata, West Bengal, India

Latha Sabikhi National Dairy Research Institute, Karnal, India

Fazlul H. Sarkar Ph.D. Department of Pathology, Barbara Ann Karmanos Cancer Institute, Wayne State University School of Medicine, Detroit, MI, USA

Birinchi Kumar Sarma Department of Mycology and Plant Pathology, Institute of Agricultural Sciences, Banaras Hindu University, Varanasi, Uttar Pradesh, India

Sharmila Shankar Department of Pathology and Laboratory Medicine, The University of Kansas Cancer Center, The University of Kansas Medical Center, Kansas City, KS, USA

Akanksha Singh Centre of Advanced Studies, Faculty of Sciences, Banaras Hindu University, Varanasi, Uttar Pradesh, India

Ashish Kumar Singh National Dairy Research Institute, Karnal, India

Brahma N. Singh Department of Pharmacology, Toxicology and Therapeutics, and Medicine, The University of Kansas Cancer Center, The University of Kansas Medical Center, Kansas City, KS, USA

H.B. Singh Department of Mycology and Plant Pathology, Institute of Agricultural Sciences, Banaras Hindu University, Varanasi, Uttar Pradesh, India

Rana P. Singh Ph.D. School of Life Sciences, Central University of Gujarat, Gandhinagar, Gujarat, India

Cancer Biology Laboratory, School of Life Sciences, Jawaharlal Nehru University, New Delhi, India

Elizabeth Smerczak Biomedical Diagnostic and Therapeutic Sciences, School of Health Sciences, Oakland University, Rochester, MI, USA

Rakesh K. Srivastava Department of Pharmacology, Toxicology and Therapeutics, and Medicine, The University of Kansas Cancer Center, The University of Kansas Medical Center, Kansas City, KS, USA

Dhanir Tailor School of Life Sciences, Central University of Gujarat, Gandhinagar, Gujarat, India

Su-Ni Tang Department of Pharmacology, Toxicology and Therapeutics, and Medicine, The University of Kansas Cancer Center, The University of Kansas Medical Center, Kansas City, KS, USA

Ajith Kumar Thakur Neuropharmacology Research Laboratory, Department of Pharmaceutics, Institute of Technology, Banaras Hindu University, Varanasi, Uttar Pradesh, India

Vijay S. Thakur Department of Urology and Nutrition, Case Western Reserve University, Cleveland, OH, USA

Sudhir Kumar Tomer National Dairy Research Institute, Karnal, India

Zhiwei Wang Ph.D. Department of Pathology, Barbara Ann Karmanos Cancer Institute, Wayne State University School of Medicine, Detroit, MI, USA

David E. Williams Linus Pauling Institute, Oregon State University, Corvallis, OR, USA

Department of Environmental and Molecular Toxicology, Oregon State University, Corvallis, OR, USA

Jian Zuo The Developmental Therapeutics Program, Barbara Ann Karmanos Cancer Institute, and Departments of Oncology, Pharmacology and Pathology, School of Medicine, Wayne State University, Detroit, MI, USA

Chapter 1
Aberrant Signaling Pathways in Cancer: Modulation by the Dietary Flavonoid, Quercetin

Ramamurthi Vidya Priyadarsini and Siddavaram Nagini

Contents

Abstract Of late, flavonoids, a class of polyphenolic compounds ubiquitously present in the human diet have gained increasing attention in cancer prevention. Defining the anti-cancer mechanisms of quercetin, a major dietary flavonoid has

R.V. Priyadarsini • S. Nagini (✉)
Department of Biochemistry and Biotechnology, Faculty of Science,
Annamalai University, Annamalainagar 608 002, Tamil Nadu, India
e-mail: s_nagini@yahoo.com; snlabau@gmail.com

S. Shankar and R.K. Srivastava (eds.), *Nutrition, Diet and Cancer*,
DOI 10.1007/978-94-007-2923-0_1, © Springer Science+Business Media B.V. 2012

been the topic of intense research over the last two decades. Evidences from experimental studies have shown that quercetin not only offers protection against chemically induced cancers but also suppresses the growth of cancer cells *in vitro* and *in vivo* by enhancing carcinogen detoxification and antioxidant defences, inducing cell cycle arrest and apoptosis, inhibiting matrix invasion and angiogenesis, and modulating intracellular signalling circuits. Epidemiological studies across different populations have also indicated that quercetin intake is associated with reduced risk of various cancers. This review summarizes the preclinical and clinical data on the anti-cancer effects of quercetin, the key molecular mechanisms of action, its synergistic interactions, and adverse side effects to warrant further clinical evaluation of quercetin for cancer prevention and therapy.

Introduction

Cancer, a multifactorial heterogeneous disease, is a major cause of morbidity and mortality worldwide (Jemal et al. 2011). Carcinogenesis, the process of tumor development is a multistep process involving three distinct stages namely initiation, promotion, and progression (Oliveira et al. 2007). The dysregulated cellular evolution during carcinogenesis drives cells to acquire six phenotypic hallmarks of cancer- the ability to proliferate and replicate autonomously, resist cytostatic and apoptotic signals, and induce tissue invasion, metastasis, and angiogenesis thereby initiating the transformation of a normal cell to a malignant phenotype (Hanahan and Weinberg 2011). Thus targeting multiple molecular pathways that are prone to deregulation during carcinogenesis is the major focus in cancer prevention and treatment.

Cancer chemoprevention as defined by Sporn et al. (1976) refers to the use of natural or synthetic agents to reverse, suppress, or prevent either the initiation phase of carcinogenesis, or the progression of neoplastic cells to cancer. In particular, dietary chemoprevention by plant-derived phytochemicals has assumed significance over the last few decades for cancer prevention and therapy due to their safety, affordability, long-term use and ability to target multiple aberrant cellular signalling circuits (Amin et al. 2009). A large number of dietary constituents including flavonoids, isothiocyanates, allyl sulfur compounds, dithiolthiones, phytoestrogens, glucosinolates and indoles from fruits, vegetables, spices, legumes and cereals have been shown to possess promising anticancer properties (Gupta et al. 2010). In particular flavonoids, a group of polyphenolic compounds have gained consideration as potential chemopreventive agents.

Flavonoids

Flavonoids are a class of naturally occurring polyphenolic compounds, ubiquitously present in fruits, vegetables, nuts, and in beverages such as tea, coffee, and wine.

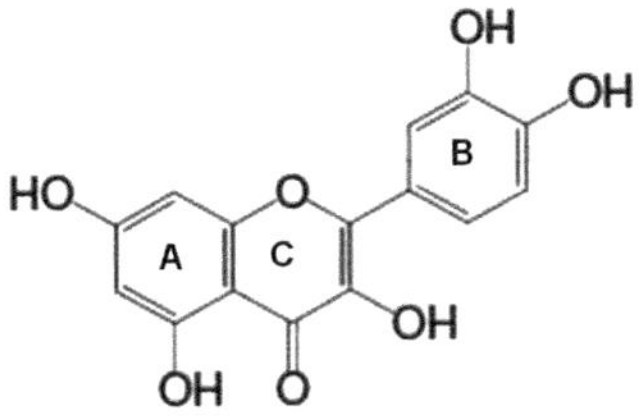

Fig. 1.1 Chemical structure of quercetin. Quercetin consists of a basic flavonoid structure with three rings – *A*, *B* and *C* and 5 hydroxyl groups. The rings *A* and *B* are aromatic, and ring *C* is heterocyclic. The hydroxyl groups are found at 3, 3′, 4′, 5 and 7 positions

Over 5,000 different flavonoids have been identified so far. Most flavonoids possess a common phenylbenzopyrone structure (C6–C3–C6) and are sub-divided into various classes such as flavones, isoflavones, flavonols, flavanols, and flavanone based on the saturation level and opening of the central pyran ring. Human dietary intake of flavonoids is estimated to be around few hundreds of mg/day. Despite their poor solubility in water and rapid rate of metabolism and degradation, the flavonoids are recognized to confer a myriad health benefits (Ren et al. 2003; Clere et al. 2011; Nishiumi et al. 2011). Of the various flavonoids in the diet, quercetin, a member of the flavonol subclass constitutes 70% of the daily dietary intake and has thus attracted substantial research attention as promising anticarcinogenic and chemopreventive agent (de Vries et al. 1997).

Quercetin

Quercetin (3,3′,4′,5,7-pentahydroxyflavone), commonly found in apples, onions and green tea occurs mainly as a glycoside bound to one of the hydroxyl groups of the flavonol. Structurally, quercetin consists of two aromatic and one heterocyclic ring (Fig. 1.1). The position and number of hydroxyl groups attached to the basic ring structure is largely responsible for the biological activity of quercetin. While the physical properties are chiefly attributed to its hydrophobic, co-planar structure, the chemical activities are ascribed to its electron donating property (Boots et al. 2008; Murakami et al. 2008).

Evidence of Anticancer Effects

Accumulating data from various experimental and epidemiological studies have provided substantial proof for the anticancer effects of quercetin.

In vitro

Numerous studies have demonstrated the anti-cancer effects of quercetin on diverse cell systems. Quercetin was shown to inhibit the growth of human cervical cancer (HeLa) cells, and human leukemia HL-60 cells by inducing apoptosis (Vidya Priyadarsini et al. 2010; Lee et al. 2011). Nutritionally relevant concentrations of quercetin are reported to inhibit the growth of estrogen receptor β1-transfected HeLa and DLD-1 colon cancer cells (Bulzomi et al. 2011). Luo et al. (2008) demonstrated that quercetin strongly inhibits the growth of human ovarian cancer cells, OVCAR-3 in a dose-dependent manner. Quercetin was also documented to inhibit the proliferation of CO115, LS180 and CaCo-2 colon adenocarcinoma, A549 lung carcinoma and non-small cell lung cancer (NSCLC) cells by triggering apoptosis (Pawlikowska-Pawlega et al. 2001; Dihal et al. 2006; Murtaza et al. 2006; Chen et al. 2007; Hung 2007).

In vivo

A substantial number of *in vivo* studies on various animal tumor models has provided evidence that quercetin inhibits carcinogenesis by interfering with the initiation, promotion, as well as progression stages of carcinogenesis (Akagi et al. 1995; Pereira et al. 1996; Kamaraj et al. 2007; Priyadarsini et al. 2011). Quercetin administration was shown to inhibit dimethylbenz[a]anthracene (DMBA)-induced hamster buccal pouch as well as rat mammary gland carcinogenesis (Pereira et al. 1996; Priyadarsini et al. 2011). Akagi et al. (1995) demonstrated that dietary administration of quercetin inhibited tumour promotion in the small intestine in a medium-term multi-organ carcinogenesis model.

An analogue of quercetin was shown to interfere with tumor development in Apc (Min) mice and human-derived HCT116 adenocarcinoma-bearing nude mice models of colorectal carcinogenesis (Howells et al. 2010). Quercetin administration was also documented to inhibit the development of experimental lung and liver carcinogenesis (Kamaraj et al. 2007; Oi et al. 2008). Oi et al. (2008) reported that quercetin suppressed tumour formation in a two-stage hepatocarcinogenesis model using N-diethylnitrosamine (DEN) as an initiator and phenobarbital as a promoter in Fisher 344 rats. Seufi et al. (2009) demonstrated the protective effects of quercetin against N-nitrosodiethylamine (NDEA)-induced rat hepatocellular carcinogenesis. Quercetin also suppressed the formation of early preneoplastic lesions in azoxymethane induced rat colon carcinogenesis (Warren et al. 2009). More recently quercetin was shown to inhibit tumor growth and increase survival in rats bearing Walker 256 carcinosarcoma (W256) (Camargo et al. 2011). Table 1.1 summarizes the anticancer effects of quercetin *in vitro* and *in vivo*.

Table 1.1 Summary of the anticancer effects of quercetin *in vitro* and *in vivo*

Type of study	Cell line/Animal tumor model	Mechanisms	Reference(s)
In vitro	Human breast cancer cells, MDA-MB-231	• Increasing cytosolic Ca^{2+} levels • Reducing mitochondrial transmembrane potential • Activation of caspase-3, -8 and −9 • Upregulation of Bax and AIF • Downregulation of Bcl-2	Choi et al. (2008)
	Human cervical cancer cells, HeLa	• Modulation of cell cycle regulatory proteins • Inhibition of NF-κB activation • Induction of G2/M cell cycle arrest • Upregulation of bax, cytochrome C, Apaf-1 and caspases • Downregulation of Bcl-2 and survivin	Vidya Priyadarsini et al. (2010)
	Human colon adenocarcinoma cells (CO115, CaCo-2)	• Induction of cell cycle arrest • Modulation of β-catenin and MAPK signaling • Downregulation of cell cycle associated genes • Upregulation of tumor suppressor genes	Dihal et al. (2006) and Murtaza et al. (2006)
	Human leukemia cells, HL-60	• Upregulation of FasL through activation of ERK and JNK • Activation of caspase-8 and Bid cleavage • Induction of extrinsic apoptosis • Promotion of histone H3 acetylation	Lee et al. (2011)
	Human lung cancer cells, NCI-H209	• Induction of G2/M phase cell cycle arrest • Upregulation of cyclin B, Cdc25c-ser-216-p and Wee1 • Induction of apoptosis via caspase-3 cascade	Hung (2007)
	Human non-small cell lung cancer cells, NSCLC	• Upregulation of death receptor-5 expression • Suppression of survivin expression • Blockade of serine/threonine kinase Akt activity	Chen et al. (2007)
	Human ovarian cancer cells, OVCAR-3	• Inhibition of cell proliferation • Decreased VEGF expression	Luo et al. (2008)

(continued)

Table 1.1 (continued)

Type of study	Cell line/Animal tumor model	Mechanisms	Reference(s)
In vivo	Benzopyrene induced lung carcinogenesis	• Upregulation of antioxidant enzymes • Suppression of oxidant induced damage to cellular biomolecules	Oi et al. (2008)
	DMBA-induced rat mammary carcinogenesis	• Downregulation of t-PA and u-PA enzymes	Pereira et al. (1996)
	DMBA-induced hamster buccal pouch carcinogenesis	• Downregulation of cell proliferation and survival • Upregulation of extrinsic and intrinsic apoptosis • Inhibition of tumour invasion and angiogenesis • Modulation of epigenetic remodelling enzymes	Priyadarsini et al. (2011)
	Colorectal models of carcinogenesis	• Inhibition of cell proliferation • Induction of intrinsic apoptosis • Suppression of β-catenin accumulated crypt formation	Warren et al. (2009) and Howells et al. (2010)
	N-nitrosodiethylamine induced rat hepato-carcinogenesis	• Modulation of oxidant/antioxidant status	Oi et al. (2008)

Epidemiological Studies

Although several epidemiological studies have found an inverse correlation between quercetin consumption and the risk of cancer, few studies did not support a major role for quercetin intake and cancer prevention (Garcia-Closas et al. 1999; Nothlings et al. 2007, 2008; Cui et al. 2008; Gates et al. 2009; Wang et al. 2009; Kyle et al. 2010; Lam et al. 2010; Ekström et al. 2011). A large Swedish population-based case-control study of gastric cancer involving 505 cases and 1,116 controls demonstrated a strong inverse association between high dietary quercetin intake and the risk of noncardia gastric adenocarcinoma, especially in women exposed to smoking-induced oxidative stress (Ekström et al. 2011). Another case-control study carried out in Spain documented a lower risk of gastric cancer with higher intake of quercetin (Garcia-Closas et al. 1999). A case-control study conducted to analyze the effect of flavonoid intake and the risk of developing colorectal cancer in a tea-drinking population with a high colorectal cancer incidence showed that flavonols, in particular quercetin, obtained from non-tea components of the diet was associated with reduced risk of developing colon cancer (Kyle et al. 2010). A lung cancer etiology study conducted by Lam et al. (2010) indicated an inverse correlation between the intake of quercetin-rich foods and lung cancer risk. A population-based case-control study designed by Cui et al. in 2008 also found that quercetin intake

Table 1.2 Summary of the epidemiological data on quercetin intake and risk of human cancers

Type of cancer	Cohort study		Case-control study		References
	Risk reduction	No association	Risk reduction	No association	
Breast cancer	–	1	–	–	Nothlings et al. (2007)
Colorectal cancer	–	1	1	–	Nothlings et al. (2007) and Kyle et al. (2010)
Endometrial cancer	–	1	–	–	Nothlings et al. (2007)
Gastric cancer	–	–	2	–	Garcia-Closas et al. (1999) and Ekström et al. (2011)
Lung cancer	–	–	2	–	Cui et al. (2008) and Lam et al. (2010)
Ovarian cancer	–	1	–	1	Gates et al. (2009) and Wang et al. (2009)
Pancreatic cancer	–	2	–	–	Nothlings et al. (2007 and 2008)

was inversely associated with lung cancer among tobacco smokers. Multiethnic cohort (MEC) studies conducted by Nothlings et al. (2007, 2008) revealed a lower risk for pancreatic cancer, particularly in current smokers with quercetin intake. Some of the epidemiological studies conducted on quercetin are summarized in Table 1.2.

Molecular Mechanisms Underlying Chemoprevention

Carcinogen Activation/Detoxification Enzymes

Inhibition of phase I carcinogen activation enzymes with simultaneous stimulation of phase II carcinogen detoxification enzymes has evolved as a paradigm for testing dietary chemopreventive agents. While phase I metabolic oxidation of carcinogens by cytochrome P450 enzymes generates highly reactive electrophilic intermediates that attack cellular macromolecules, phase II detoxification reactions catalysed by glutathione *S*-transferases (GSTs), uridine diphosphate-glucuronosyl transferases (UGTs), and NAD(P)H quinine oxidoreductase (NQO1) neutralize electrophilic intermediates resulting in a reduction of chemical reactivity and toxicity (Tan and Spivack 2009; Rodriguez-Antona et al. 2010). Based on their hydroxyl and methoxy groups, dietary flavonoids exhibit three distinct modes of action with reference to cancer chemprevention: (1) inhibitors of CYP1 enzyme activity, (2) CYP1 substrates and (3) substrates and inhibitors of CYP1 enzymes. Recently Androutsopoulos et al. (2011) showed that quercetin is a potent inhibitor of CYP1B1 activity. In HepG2 cells, quercetin was found to upregulate the expression of the phase II enzyme, NQO1 by activating Nrf2 (nuclear factor-eythroid2-related factor-2), a nuclear transcription factor that regulates the expression of various cytoprotective enzymes via evoking the antioxidant-responsive element (ARE) (Tanigawa et al. 2007). Quercetin also acts as a potent antagonist of the aryl hydrocarbon receptor (AhR), a ligand-dependent transcription factor that regulates the expression of CYP1 family members including CYP1A1, CYP1A2, and CYP1B1 (Fukuda et al. 2007). Ashida et al. (2000) reported that quercetin antagonises 2,3,7,8-tetrachlorodibenzo-p-dioxin (TCDD)-induced AhR transformation in a cell-free system. Quercetin was also shown to suppress AhR transformation in primary cultured rat hepatocytes (Ashida et al. 2000). The mechanism underlying AhR inactivation by quercetin primarily involved competitive inhibition with dioxins (Fukuda and Ashida 2008).

Cell Proliferation and Cell Cycle Arrest

Deregulated cell cycle progression and cell proliferation is a key trait of cancer. The cell cycle phase transition through S, G2, and M phase is facilitated by the action of cyclin and cyclin-dependent protein kinase (CDK) complexes (Malumbres 2007). Studies on various human cancer cell lines have indicated that quercetin perturbs cell cycle progression by inducing cell cycle arrest at the G1/S or G2/M phase of the cell cycle (G1/S in leukemic cancer cells; G2/M in breast, cervical, HCT116 colon, lung, and laryngeal cancer cells) (Ferrandina et al. 1998; Mertens-Talcott and Percival 2005; Yang et al. 2006; Choi et al. 2008; Samuel et al. 2010; Vidya Priyadarsini et al. 2010). The antiproliferative effects of quercetin are predominantly mediated via its ability to upregulate the expression of various oncosuppressor proteins and cell cycle regulatory molecules such as PTEN, p53, Msh2, $p21^{Cip1/waf1}$, Gadd45, and wee1, and downregulate the expression of cyclins, CDKs, and cell division cycle (CDC) protein phosphatases (Ferrandina et al. 1998; Mertens-Talcott and Percival 2005; Yang et al. 2006; Choi et al. 2008; Samuel et al. 2010). Furthermore, quercetin is also shown to inhibit a wide variety of kinases including phosphoinositide 3-kinase (PI3K), serine/threonine kinase Akt, extracellular signal-regulated protein kinases (ERKs), and Janus kinases (JAK) that play a crucial role in mammalian cell survival signalling (Boly et al. 2011). A study from this laboratory has revealed that quercetin induces cell cycle arrest in HeLa cells by targeting p53, p21, and cyclin D1 (Vidya Priyadarsini et al. 2010). We have also demonstrated that quercetin inhibits cell proliferation in the DMBA-induced hamster buccal pouch carcinogenesis model by upregulating the expression of p21 and p53, and downregulating proliferating cell nuclear antigen (PCNA), GST-P, and cyclin D1 (Priyadarsini et al. 2011).

Apoptosis Induction

Evasion of apoptosis, a hallmark of cancer, contributes to increased survival of cells that have acquired oncogenic mutations. Apoptosis, a form of programmed cell death is initiated by alterations in the mitochondrial outer membrane potential, an event stringently regulated by various protein-protein and protein-membrane interactions of the Bcl-2 family proteins (Llambi and Green 2011). While anti-apoptotic members such as Bcl-2, Bcl-xl, and Bcl-w preserve the integrity of the outer mitochondrial membrane, proapoptotic members such as Bax, Bak, Bad, Bcl-xs, Bik, Bim, and Bid promote membrane permeabilization, allowing efflux of cytochrome *c*, Smac/DIABLO, AIF and EndoG from the mitochondria into the cytosol. Cytosolic release of these proteins in turn facilitates activation of caspases through the formation of the apoptosome complex consisting of cytochrome *c*/Apaf-1/pro-caspase-9. The caspases then carry out the controlled demise of the cell through cleavage of structural proteins, kinases, transcriptional proteins and other molecules essential for cell survival (Danial 2007; Llambi and Green 2011) (Fig. 1.2).

Quercetin was shown to specifically induce apoptosis in various cancer cells while sparing normal cells (Siegelin et al. 2009; Samanta et al. 2010; Seo et al. 2011). The molecular mechanism underlying apoptosis induction by quercetin includes upregulation of the death receptor Fas and its ligand FasL, downregulation of the expression of antiapoptotic Bcl-2 and inhibitor of apoptosis proteins (IAPs), induction of conformational changes in Bax, release of apoptosis-inducing factor (AIF) and cytochrome *c* from the mitochondria to the cytosol, formation of the apoptosome complex, activation of the caspase cascade and cleavage of the DNA repair enzyme poly(ADP-ribose) polymerase (PARP) (Pawlikowska-Pawlega et al. 2001; Mertens-Talcott and Percival 2005; Dihal et al. 2006; Yang et al. 2006; Warren et al. 2009; Vidya Priyadarsini et al. 2010; Bulzomi et al. 2011; Lee et al. 2011). Quercetin was also found to enhance TRAIL (tumor necrosis factor-related apoptosis-inducing ligand)-induced apoptotic cell death in a process involving simultaneous stimulation of death receptor-5 (DR5) expression and suppression of survivin expression by blocking serine/threonine kinase Akt activity (Chen et al. 2007). Quercetin was also shown to target AMP-activated protein kinase (AMPK) and apoptosis signal-regulating kinase (ASK)-1 signaling pathways to induce apoptosis in cancer cells (Lee et al. 2010). Our own work on the inhibitory effects of quercetin on HeLa cells has revealed that quercetin targets Bcl-2 family proteins (Bcl-2, Bcl-xL, Mcl1, Bax, Bad, p-Bad), cytochrome C, Apaf-1, caspases, and survivin to induce intrinsic apoptosis (Vidya Priyadarsini et al. 2010). Furthermore, our investigation on the apoptosis inducing effect of quercetin in an animal model of oral oncogenesis has

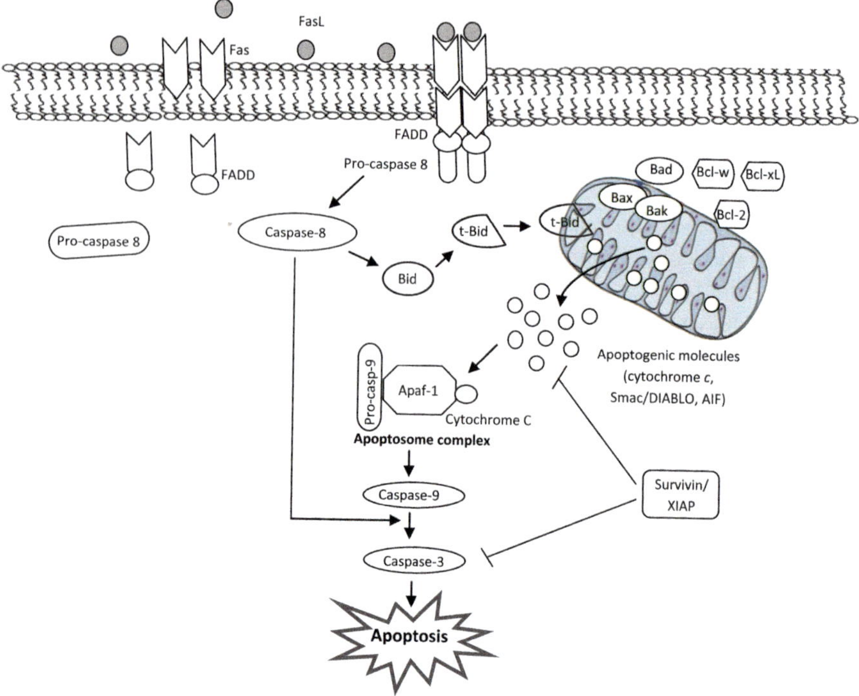

Fig. 1.2 Summary of intrinsic and extrinsic apoptotic signalling pathways. Death receptor-mediated signalling of apoptosis occurs as a result of the binding of Fas ligand to the Fas receptor. Subsequent recruitment of the adaptor FADD results in the activation of pro-caspase-8 and downstream caspase-3 activation. Mitochondria mediated apoptotic signalling occurs as a result of the binding of the proapoptotic proteins to the outer mitochondrial membrane. This results in the release of several apoptogenic molecules from the mitochondria into the cytosol. Cytochrome c released into the cytosol forms a apoptosome complex with Apaf1 and procaspase-9, resulting in the activation of procaspase-9. Active caspase-9 eventually activates caspase-3 resulting in the cleavage of molecules vital for cell survival thereby leading to cell death

demonstrated that quercetin induces apoptosis via both the extrinsic and intrinsic pathways by increasing the expression of Fas, Fas-L, Bax, cytochrome-C, Apaf-1, caspases (-2L-6, -8, -9 and -3), PARP cleavage and decreasing Bcl-2, Mcl-1, survivin, cFLIP, and API1 expression to inhibit the development of HBP carcinomas (Priyadarsini et al. 2011).

Inhibition of Tumour Invasion and Angiogenesis

Matrix invasion and neovascularization play key roles in tumour growth, progression, and metastasis. During the process of invasion, matrix metalloproteinases

(MMPs) degrade the extracellular matrix (ECM) surrounding tumor tissues facilitating their migration into the blood vessel lumen and lymphatics for further dissemination (Decock et al. 2011). The MMPs are tightly regulated by tissue inhibitors of matrix metalloproteinases (TIMPs) and reversion induced cysteine rich protein with Kazal motifs (RECK) (Clark et al. 2007; Bourboulia and Stetler-Stevenson 2010). ECM processing by MMPs also triggers neovascularization through the production of several proangiogenic factors such as vascular endothelial growth factor (VEGF), hypoxia-inducible factor 1α (HIF-1α) epidermal growth factor (EGF), transforming growth factor-α (TGF-α), and platelet-derived growth factor (PDGF) (Deryugina and Quigley 2010). Quercetin was shown to inhibit MMPs, urokinase plasminogen activator (uPA), uPA receptor (uPAR), HIF-1α, and VEGF in various tumours (Lee and Lee 2008; Camargo et al. 2011; Senthilkumar et al. 2011). Quercetin was also found to inhibit AP-1 and prolyl isomerase Pin1, the key transcription factors for VEGF gene transcription (Oha et al. 2010). Quercetin also synergises with other dietary agents to inhibit epithelial-mesenchymal transition (EMT) by inhibiting the expression of vimentin, slug and snail (Tang et al. 2010). A study from our laboratory on the chemopreventive and chemotherapeutic potential of quercetin in the DMBA-induced HBP carcinogenesis model has revealed that quercetin inhibits tumour invasion and angiogenesis by modulating the expression of MMP-2, MMP-9, TIMP-2, RECK, PlGF, VEGF, VEGFR1 and HIF-1α (Priyadarsini et al. 2011).

Anti-inflammatory and Antioxidant Effects

Overexpression of the proinflammatory mediators- cyclooxygenase (COX) and lipooxygenase (LOX) results in overexpression of the antiapoptotic Bcl-2 family proteins, activation of antiapoptotic PI3K/Akt antiapoptotic pathways, and induction of matrix metalloproteinases and angiogenic factors (Kundu and Surh 2005). Quercetin was demonstrated to inhibit the production of inducible nitric oxide synthase (iNOS) and COX-2 in tumours (Choi et al. 2006; Warren et al. 2009). Quercetin packaged as nanoparticles was proven to be successful in "nanochemoprevention" and "nano-chemotherapy" by suppressing proinflammatory pathways (Nair et al. 2010). Quercetin also safeguards against oxidative stress induced damage to cellular macromolecules by quenching free radicals and reactive oxygen species (ROS) or by boosting the antioxidant defense mechanisms through upregulation of the antioxidant enzymes superoxide dismutase (SOD), catalase (CAT), reduced glutathione (GSH), glutathione peroxidase (GPx) and glutathione-S-transferase (GST) (De et al. 2000; Kamaraj et al. 2007; Vasquez-Garzon et al. 2009). The antioxidant potential of quercetin is chiefly attributed to the presence of two antioxidant pharmacophores within its structural moiety- the catechol group in ring B, and the hydroxyl groups at the third position of ring A and C that render optimal configuration for free radical scavenging (Heijnen et al. 2001).

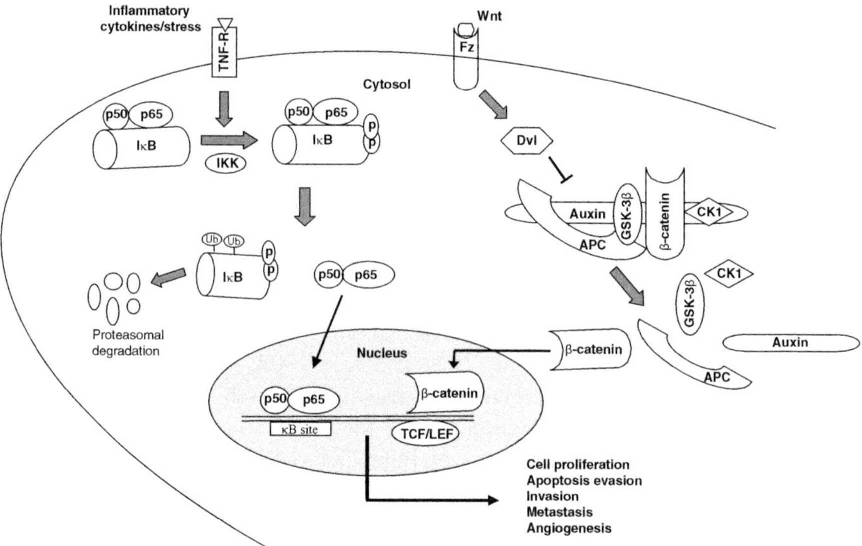

Fig. 1.3 Activation of the oncogenic signaling pathways-NFκB and Wnt within the cell. NF-κB exists in the cytoplasm as heterodimers complexed to IκB. Activation of TNF receptor by ligand binding results in the phoshorylation of IκB by IKK. This leads to polyubiquitination and proteasomal degradation of IκB, and translocation of NFκB heterodimer to the nucleus, and transactivation of various target genes. Wnt/ β-catenin signalling is activated by the binding of Wnt ligands to the frizzled receptor through Dvl recruitment. This results in the inhibition of APC/Axin/GSK3β multiprotein complex and accumulation of free cytoplasmic β-catenin, which eventually translocates to the nucleus and activates various downstream target genes by forming a transcriptional complex with LEF/TCF promoter element in DNA. APC-Adenamatous polyposis coli; Dvl- Dishevelled; Fz- Frizzled receptor; GSK3β- Glycogen synthase kinase-3β; IκB- Inhibitor of NF-κB; Ikk- IκB kinase; LEF- Lymphoid enhancer factor; TCF- β-Catenin/T-cell transcription factor

Modulation of Oncogenic Signaling Circuits

A wide range of oncogenic signaling pathways play an important role in initiating the carcinogenic event (Fig. 1.3). Quercetin has been identified to target various signaling circuits to inhibit tumour initiation and progression.

Nuclear Factor Kappa B (NF-κB)

Constitutive activation of NFκB, a redox sensitive transcription factor of the Rel family has been documented in various malignant neoplasms. In the resting state, NF-κB is found sequestered in the cytoplasm as a heterodimer of p65 and p50 subunits complexed with the inhibitory kappaB alpha (IκBα) protein. Phosphorylation with subsequent proteasomal degradation of IκB by ROS, radiation, and carcinogens is accompanied by nuclear translocation of NFκB that binds to the κB elements and transactivates target genes (Chaturvedi et al. 2011). NFκB is known to regulate the transcription of over 400 genes involved in the control of cell proliferation, cell cycle, apoptosis, invasion, metastasis, and angiogenesis (Sung et al. 2008). Quercetin was shown to inhibit the activation of NFκB by downregulating the expression and kinase activity of IKKβ, thereby impeding the phosphorylation and degradation of IκB (Hamalainen et al. 2007; Ying et al. 2008). Our own study has revealed that quercetin induces cell cycle arrest in HeLa cells by modulating the expression of the NF-κB family members -p50, p65, IκB, p-IκB-α, IKKβ as well as ubiquitin ligase (Vidya Priyadarsini et al. 2010).

Wnt/β-Catenin

NF-κB signaling is recognized to augment its oncogenic potential in various tumours by co-ordinately activating the canonical Wnt/β-catenin signaling pathway that regulates a wide variety of cellular processes including cell survival, proliferation, apoptosis, and differentiation (Khan et al. 2011; Moreau et al. 2011). β-Catenin, a multifunctional protein functions as key player of the canonical Wnt signaling pathway. Activation of the Wnt pathway through the binding of Wnt ligand to frizzled receptor inhibits the activity of GSK-3β multiprotein complex leading to the accumulation of free cytosolic β-catenin. Free β-catenin in the cytoplasmic pool, eventually translocates into the nucleus and initiates transcription of several oncogenes such as cyclin D1, c-Myc, c-Jun, uPA, MMPs and VEGF through binding to the TCF/LEF promoter (Akiyama 2000; Teiten et al. 2011). Quercetin has been reported to interfere with Wnt signaling through the modulation of beta-catenin expression, transcriptional activity and of the subsequent expression of Wnt target genes (Teiten et al. 2011). Quercetin was shown to inhibit the expression of nuclear beta-catenin, and the activity of LEF-1/TCF responsive reporter (Shan et al. 2009; Tang et al. 2010). Furthermore, quercetin is documented to suppress azoxymethane-induced colonic preneoplastic lesions in male C57BL/KsJ-db/db mice and F344 rats by inhibiting the formation of beta-catenin-accumulated crypts (BCACs) (Miyamoto et al. 2010). A multiple gene expression analysis conducted by van Erk et al. (2005) on the effect of quercetin in Caco-2 cells also revealed that quercetin significantly influences various genes involved in β-catenin/TCF signaling.

Epigenetic Remodelling

Chemical modifications in the DNA and histones that are not encoded by the DNA sequences referred to as 'epigenetic dysregulation' are known to make a profound impact on gene expression. DNA methylation catalyzed by DNA methyltransferase (DNMT) and histone acetylation and deacetylation catalyzed by histone acetyltransferases (HATs) and histone deacetylases (HDACs) respectively play a central role in the initiation and maintenance of cancer. While histone acetylation results in transcriptionally active chromatin, histone deacetylation and DNA hypermethylation results in transcriptional silencing (Ferguson et al. 2011). Quercetin was shown to promote histone H3 acetylation in human leukemic HL-60 cells by coordinately inducing the activation of HAT and inactivation of HDAC (Lee et al. 2011). Quercetin was also reported to inhibit HDAC and DNMT expression in DMBA-induced HBP carcinomas (Priyadarsini et al. 2011).

Targeting Cancer Stem Cells

Cancer stem cells (CSCs) that display the ability for proliferation and self-renewal by expressing anti-apoptotic and drug resistant proteins have attracted increasing attention in recent years. Eradication of CSCs is believed to be a promising strategy to prevent the initiation and progression of solid malignancies. Quercetin was found to synergize with EGCG to inhibit prostate cancer stem cell characteristics as well as invasion, migration, and epithelial-mesenchymal transition and induce apoptosis (Tang et al. 2010).

Modulation of Multidrug Resistance

Multidrug resistance as a result of the overexpression of P-glycoprotein (P-gp), a plasma membrane ATP-binding cassette (ABC) transporter is a major barrier for cancer chemotherapy. Quercetin was demonstrated to intensify the action of several cytostatic drugs by suppressing the multidrug resistance (MDR) phenomenon by attenuating the expression and function of P-gp, inhibiting the energy dependent drug interactions of P-gp with transporter enriched membranes, and sensitizing cells to reverse MDR activity (Shen et al. 2008; Borska et al. 2010).

DNA Microarray and Proteomic Analyses

Whole genome DNA microarray analysis of the effect of quercetin on gene expression in CO115 colon-adenocarcinoma cell line revealed differential expression of 5,060–7,000 genes, most of which were associated with cell-cycle control, apoptosis, and xenobiotic metabolism (van Erk et al. 2005). Transcriptome and proteome profiling of the colon mucosa of quercetin fed F344 rats indicated that quercetin significantly downregulated mitogen-activated protein kinase (MAPK) and heat shock proteins, and enhanced the expression of the phase I and II enzymes-Fmo5, Ephx1, Ephx2, and Gpx2, and the cell cycle involved proteins- Tp53, Pten, Msh2 and Mutyh (Dihal et al. 2008). A multiple gene expression analysis in quercetin treated Caco-2 cells showed that quercetin upregulates the expression of several tumor suppressor genes while simultaneously downregulating the expression of genes involved in cell cycle and cell proliferation, β-catenin/TCF signalling and MAPK signal transduction (Murtaza et al. 2006).

Clinical Trials

The promising anti-cancer effects of quercetin seen *in vitro, in vivo*, and in epidemiological studies have prompted phase I human clinical trials with quercetin. A phase I dose-escalation clinical trial conducted by Ferry et al. (1996) revealed that intravenous administration of quercetin at a bolus dose of 1,400 mg/m^2 to patients who were non-amenable to standard therapies resulted in inhibition of lymphocyte tyrosine kinase activity. Furthermore, in a hepatoma patient, quercetin administration was found to cause a significant decrease in the levels of serum alpha-fetoprotein. In an ovarian cancer patient refractory to cisplatin, quercetin administration resulted in a decline in CA 125 levels from 295 to 55 units/mL.

Synergism

Quercetin is shown to synergistically interact with other phytochemicals to enhance the anticancer effects. Chan et al. (2000) showed that micromolar concentrations of quercetin and resveratrol synergistically suppressed iNOS expression and nitric oxide production in RAW264.6 cells. Elattar and Virji (1999) showed that a combination of quercetin and resveratrol had greater inhibitory effects on the growth and DNA synthesis in squamous carcinoma cells. Low concentrations of quercetin and ellagic acid are demonstrated to synergistically influence cell proliferation and apoptosis in MOLT-4 human leukemia cells (Mertens-Talcott and Percival 2005). Co-administration of quercetin, epigallocatechin gallate and genistein to CWR22Rv1 CaP cells was shown to suppress proliferation of CWR22Rv1 cells by influencing the expression of androgen receptor, p53 and NQO1 (Hsieh and Wu 2009). In addition quercetin also synergises with anticancer therapeutic drugs such as tamoxifen potentiating its antineoplastic effects (Ma et al. 2004).

Adverse Effects

Despite its ability to block cell proliferation and survival, quercetin was found to interfere with cell cycle progression thereby diminishing the efficacy of microtubule-targeting drugs to arrest cells at G2/M (Samuel et al. 2010). Although quercetin displays chemopreventive potential, it induces expression of c-fos a cellular event that plays a key role in tumor promotion, unless it is stabilized by ascorbic acid (Olson et al. 2010). The oxidation products of quercetin in particular the thiol-reactive quinones formed during free radical scavenging are shown to induce cellular toxicity and cellular dysfunction by arylating protein thiols (Boots et al. 2011). Quercetin is also reported to induce mutations in *Salmonella typhimurium* TA102 and *Escherichia coli* WP-2 uvrA tester strains, and induce chromosomal aberrations and single strand breaks in hamster ovary and mouse lymphoma cells (Makena et al. 2009). An IARC monograph on the evaluation of carcinogenic risk of chemicals to humans showed that quercetin produced cytogenetic damage in both human and rodent cells (IARC 1983). Higher concentrations of quercetin are also reported to cause kidney toxicity and sperm abnormalities (Rastogi and Levin 1987; Dunnick and Hailey 1992; Verschoyle et al. 2007).

Conclusion and Future Perspectives

Extensive research over several decades has revealed that dietary quercetin exerts multi-functional effects such as carcinogen detoxification, antioxidant ability, anti-proliferation, apoptosis induction, inhibition of matrix invasion and angiogenesis, modulation of oncogenic signalling circuits, and epigenetic remodelling to inhibit tumour initiation and progression. In particular, the ability of quercetin to target multiple cellular checkpoints and signal transduction pathways that are aberrant in cancer holds promise for novel anti-cancer modalities as multi-targeted cancer prevention and therapy has assumed significance in recent years. However, the evidences from epidemiological studies and phase I human clinical trials need to be extensively investigated to initiate the translation of quercetin from the bench to the bedside.

Acknowledgement Financial support from the Indian Council of Medical Research, New Delhi, India in the form of a Senior Research Fellowship to Ms. R. Vidya Priyadarsini is gratefully acknowledged.

References

Akagi K, Hirose M, Hoshiya T, Mizoguchi Y et al (1995) Modulatory effects of ellagic acid, vanillin and quercetin in a rat medium term multi-organ carcinogenesis model. Cancer Lett 94(1):113–121

Akiyama T (2000) Wnt/β-catenin signaling. Cytokine Growth Factor Rev 11(4):273–282

Amin AR, Kucuk O, Khuri FR, Shin DM (2009) Perspectives for cancer prevention with natural compounds. J Clin Oncol 27(16):2712–2725

Androutsopoulos VP, Papakyriakou A, Vourloumis D, Spandidos DA (2011) Comparative CYP1A1 and CYP1B1 substrate and inhibitor profile of dietary flavonoids. Bioorg Med Chem 19(9):2842–2849

Ashida H, Fukuda I, Yamashita T, Kanazawa K et al (2000) Flavones and flavonols at dietary levels inhibit a transformation of aryl hydrocarbon receptor induced by dioxin. FEBS Lett 476(3):213–217

Boly R, Gras T, Lamkami T, Guissou P et al (2011) Quercetin inhibits a large panel of kinases implicated in cancer cell biology. Int J Oncol 38(3):833–842

Boots AW, Haenen GR, Bast A (2008) Health effects of quercetin: from antioxidant to nutraceutical. Eur J Pharmacol 585(2–3):325–337

Boots AW, Li H, Schins RP, Duffin R et al (2011) The quercetin paradox. Toxicol Appl Pharmacol 222(1):89–96

Borska S, Sopel M, Chmielewska M, Zabel M et al (2010) Quercetin as a potential modulator of P-glycoprotein expression and function in cells of human pancreatic carcinoma line resistant to daunorubicin. Molecules 15(2):857–870

Bourboulia D, Stetler-Stevenson WG (2010) Matrix metalloproteinases (MMPs) and tissue inhibitors of metalloproteinases (TIMPs): positive and negative regulators in tumor cell adhesion. Semin Cancer Biol 20(3):161–168

Bulzomi P, Galluzzo P, Bolli A, Leone S et al (2011) The pro-apoptotic effect of quercetin in cancer cell lines requires ERβ-dependent signals. J Cell Physiol. doi:10.1002/jcp. 22917

Camargo CA, da Silva ME, da Silva RA, Justo GZ et al (2011) Inhibition of tumor growth by quercetin with increase of survival and prevention of cachexia in Walker 256 tumor-bearing rats. Biochem Biophys Res Commun 406(4):638–642

Chan MM, Mattiacci JA, Hwang HS, Shah A et al (2000) Synergy between ethanol and grape polyphenols, quercetin, and resveratrol, in the inhibition of the inducible nitric oxide synthase pathway. Biochem Pharmacol 60(10):1539–1548

Chaturvedi MM, Sung B, Yadav VR, Kannappan R et al (2011) NF-κB addiction and its role in cancer: 'one size does not fit all'. Oncogene 30(14):1615–1630

Chen W, Wang X, Zhuang J, Zhang L et al (2007) Induction of death receptor 5 and suppression of survivin contribute to sensitization of TRAIL-induced cytotoxicity by quercetin in non-small cell lung cancer cells. Carcinogenesis 28(10):2114–2121

Choi SY, Park JH, Kim JS, Kim MK et al (2006) Effects of quercetin and beta-carotene supplementation on azoxymethane-induced colon carcinogenesis and inflammatory responses in rats fed with high-fat diet rich in omega-6 fatty acids. Biofactors 27(1–4):137–146

Choi EJ, Bae SM, Ahn WS (2008) Antiproliferative effects of quercetin through cell cycle arrest and apoptosis in human breast cancer MDA-MB-453 cells. Arch Pharm Res 31(10):1281–1285

Clark JC, Thomas DM, Choong PF, Dass CR (2007) RECK-a newly discovered inhibitor of metastasis with prognostic significance in multiple forms of cancer. Cancer Metastasis Rev 26(3–4):675–683

Clere N, Faure S, Martinez MC, Andriantsitohaina R (2011) Anticancer properties of flavonoids: roles in various stages of carcinogenesis. Cardiovasc Hematol Agents Med Chem 9(2):62–77

Cui Y, Morgenstern H, Greenland S, Tashkin DP et al (2008) Dietary flavonoid intake and lung cancer-a population-based case-control study. Cancer 112(10):2241–2248

Danial NN (2007) BCL-2 family proteins: critical checkpoints of apoptotic cell death. Clin Cancer Res 13(24):7254–7263

de Vries JH, Janssen PL, Hollman PC, van Staveren WA et al (1997) Consumption of quercetin and kaempferol in free-living subjects eating a variety of diets. Cancer Lett 114(1–2):141–144

De S, Chakraborty J, Chakraborty RN, Das S (2000) Chemopreventive activity of quercetin during carcinogenesis in cervix uteri in mice. Phytother Res 14(5):347–351

Decock J, Thirkettle S, Wagstaff L, Edwards DR (2011) Matrix metalloproteinases: protective roles in cancer. J Cell Mol Med 15(6):1254–1265

Deryugina EI, Quigley JP (2010) Pleiotropic roles of matrix metalloproteinases in tumor angiogenesis: contrasting, overlapping and compensatory functions. Biochim Biophys Acta 1803(1):103–120

Dihal AA, Woutersen RA, van Ommen B, Rietjens IM et al (2006) Stierum RH. Modulatory effects of quercetin on proliferation and differentiation of the human colorectal cell line Caco-2. Cancer Lett 238(2):248–259

Dihal AA, van der Woude H, Hendriksen PJ, Charif H et al (2008) Transcriptome and proteome profiling of colon mucosa from quercetin fed F344 rats point to tumor preventive mechanisms, increased mitochondrial fatty acid degradation and decreased glycolysis. Proteomics 8(1): 45–61

Dunnick JK, Hailey JR (1992) Toxicity and carcinogenicity studies of quercetin, a natural component of foods. Fundam Appl Toxicol 19(3):423–431

Ekström AM, Serafini M, Nyrén O, Wolk A et al (2011) Dietary quercetin intake and risk of gastric cancer: results from a population-based study in Sweden. Ann Oncol 22(2):438–443

Elattar TM, Virji AS (1999) The effect of red wine and its components on growth and proliferation of human oral squamous carcinoma cells. Anticancer Res 19(6B):5407–5414

Ferguson LR, Tatham AL, Lin Z, Denny WA (2011) Epigenetic regulation of gene expression as an anticancer drug target. Curr Cancer Drug Targets 11(2):199–212

Ferrandina G, Almadori G, Maggiano N, Lanza P et al (1998) Growth-inhibitory effect of tamoxifen and quercetin and presence of type II estrogen binding sites in human laryngeal cancer cell lines and primary laryngeal tumors. Int J Cancer 77(5):747–754

Ferry DR, Smith A, Malkhandi J, Fyfe DW et al (1996) Phase I clinical trial of the flavonoid quercetin: pharmacokinetics and evidence for in vivo tyrosine kinase inhibition. Clin Cancer Res 2(4):659–668

Fukuda I, Ashida H (2008) Suppressive effects of flavonoids on activation of the aryl hydrocarbon receptor induced by dioxins: Functional Foods and Health. In: Shibamoto T, Shahidi F, Kanazawa K, Ho CT (eds) ACS Symposium series. American Chemical Society, Washington DC, pp 368–374

Fukuda I, Mukai R, Kawase M, Yoshida K et al (2007) Interaction between the aryl hydrocarbon receptor and its antagonists, flavonoids. Biochem Biophys Res Commun 359(3):822–827

Garcia-Closas R, Gonzalez CA, Agudo A, Riboli E (1999) Intake of specific carotenoids and flavonoids and the risk of gastric cancer in Spain. Cancer Causes Control 10(1):71–75

Gates MA, Vitonis AF, Tworoger SS, Rosner B et al (2009) Flavonoid intake and ovarian cancer risk in a population-based case-control study. Int J Cancer 124(8):1918–1925

Gupta SC, Kim JH, Prasad S, Aggarwal BB (2010) Regulation of survival, proliferation, invasion, angiogenesis, and metastasis of tumor cells through modulation of inflammatory pathways by nutraceuticals. Cancer Metastasis Rev 29(3):405–434

Hamalainen M, Nieminen R, Vuorela P, Heinonen M et al (2007) Anti-inflammatory effects of flavonoids: genistein, kaempferol, quercetin, and daidzein inhibit STAT-1 and NF-kappaB activations, whereas flavone, isorhamnetin, naringenin, and pelargonidin inhibit only NF-kappaB activation along with their inhibitory effect on iNOS expression and NO production in activated macrophages. Mediators Inflamm 2007:45673

Hanahan D, Weinberg RA (2011) Hallmarks of cancer: the next generation. Cell 144(5):646–674

Heijnen CG, Haenen GR, van Acker FA, van der Vijgh WJ et al (2001) Flavonoids as peroxynitrite scavengers: the role of the hydroxyl groups. Toxicol In Vitro 15(1):3–6

Howells LM, Britton RG, Mazzoletti M, Greaves P et al (2010) Preclinical colorectal cancer chemopreventive efficacy and p53-modulating activity of 3′,4′,5′-trimethoxyflavonol, a quercetin analogue. Cancer Prev Res (Phila) 3(8):929–939

Hsieh TC, Wu JM (2009) Targeting CWR22Rv1 prostate cancer cell proliferation and gene expression by combinations of the phytochemicals EGCG, genistein and quercetin. Anticancer Res 29(10):4025–4032

Hung H (2007) Dietary quercetin inhibits proliferation of lung carcinoma cells. Forum Nutr 60:146–157

IARC (1983) IARC Monographs on the evaluation of carcinogenic risk of chemicals to humans, vol 31, Some food additives, feed additives and naturally occurring substances. IARC Press, Lyon, pp 213–229

Jemal A, Bray F, Center MM, Ferlay J et al (2011) Global cancer statistics. CA Cancer J Clin 61(2):134

Kamaraj S, Vinodhkumar R, Anandakumar P, Jagan S et al (2007) The effects of quercetin on antioxidant status and tumor markers in the lung and serum of mice treated with benzo(a)pyrene. Biol Pharm Bull 30(12):2268–2273

Khan MS, Halagowder D, Devaraj SN (2011) Methylated chrysin induces co-ordinated attenuation of the canonical Wnt and NF-kB signaling pathway and upregulates apoptotic gene expression in the early hepatocarcinogenesis rat model. Chem Biol Interact 193(1):12–21

Kundu JK, Surh YJ (2005) Breaking the relay in deregulated cellular signal transduction as a rationale for chemoprevention with anti-inflammatory phytochemicals. Mutat Res 591 (1–2):123–146

Kyle JA, Sharp L, Little J, Duthie GG et al (2010) Dietary flavonoid intake and colorectal cancer: a case-control study. Br J Nutr 103(3):429–436

Lam TK, Rotunno M, Lubin JH, Wacholder S et al (2010) Dietary quercetin, quercetin-gene interaction, metabolic gene expression in lung tissue and lung cancer risk. Carcinogenesis 31(4):634–642

Lee DH, Lee YJ (2008) Quercetin suppresses hypoxia-induced accumulation of hypoxia-inducible factor-1alpha (HIF-1alpha) through inhibiting protein synthesis. J Cell Biochem 105(2): 546–553

Lee YK, Hwang JT, Kwon DY, Surh YJ et al (2010) Induction of apoptosis by quercetin is mediated through AMPKalpha1/ASK1/p38pathway. Cancer Lett 292(2):228–236

Lee WJ, Chen YR, Tseng TH (2011) Quercetin induces FasL-related apoptosis, in part, through promotion of histone H3 acetylation in human leukemia HL-60 cells. Oncol Rep 25(2):583–591

Llambi F, Green DR (2011) Apoptosis and oncogenesis: give and take in the BCL-2 family. Curr Opin Genet Dev 21(1):12–20

Luo H, Jiang BH, King SM, Chen YC (2008) Inhibition of cell growth and VEGF expression in ovarian cancer cells by flavonoids. Nutr Cancer 60(6):800–809

Ma ZS, Huynh TH, Ng CP, Do PT et al (2004) Reduction of CWR22 prostate tumor xenograft growth by combined tamoxifen-quercetin treatment is associated with inhibition of angiogenesis and cellular proliferation. Int J Oncol 24(5):1297–1304

Makena PS, Pierce SC, Chung KT, Sinclair SE (2009) Comparative mutagenic effects of structurally similar flavonoids quercetin and taxifolin on tester strains Salmonella typhimurium TA102 and Escherichia coli WP-2 uvrA. Environ Mol Mutagen 50(6):451–459

Malumbres M (2007) Cyclins and related kinases in cancer cells. J BUON 12:S45–S52

Mertens-Talcott SU, Percival SS (2005) Ellagic acid and quercetin interact synergistically with resveratrol in the induction of apoptosis and cause transient cell cycle arrest in human leukaemia cells. Cancer Lett 218(2):141–151

Miyamoto S, Yasui Y, Ohigashi H, Tanaka T et al (2010) Dietary flavonoids suppress azoxymethane-induced colonic preneoplastic lesions in male C57BL/KsJ-db/db mice. Chem Biol Interact 183(2):276–283

Moreau M, Mourah S, Dosquet C (2011) β-Catenin and NF-κB cooperate to regulate the uPA/uPAR system in cancer cells. Int J Cancer 128(6):1280–1292

Murakami A, Ashida H, Terao J (2008) Multitargeted cancer prevention by quercetin. Cancer Lett 269(2):315–325

Murtaza I, Marra G, Schlapbach R, Patrignani A et al (2006) A preliminary investigation demonstrating the effect of quercetin on the expression of genes related to cell-cycle arrest, apoptosis and xenobiotic metabolism in human CO115 colon-adenocarcinoma cells using DNA microarray. Biotechnol Appl Biochem 45(Pt 1):29–36

Nair HB, Sung B, Yadav VR, Kannappan R et al (2010) Delivery of antiinflammatory nutraceuticals by nanoparticles for the prevention and treatment of cancer. Biochem Pharmacol 80(12):1833–1843

Nishiumi S, Miyamoto S, Kawabata K, Ohnishi K et al (2011) Dietary flavonoids as cancer-preventive and therapeutic biofactors. Front Biosci 3:1332–1362

Nothlings U, Murphy SP, Wilkens LR, Henderson BE et al (2007) Flavonols and pancreatic cancer risk: the multiethnic cohort study. Am J Epidemiol 166(8):924–931

Nothlings U, Murphy SP, Wilkens LR, Boeing H et al (2008) A food pattern that is predictive of flavonol intake and risk of pancreatic cancer. Am J Clin Nutr 88(6):1653–1662

Oha SJ, Kim O, Lee JS, Kim JA et al (2010) Inhibition of angiogenesis by quercetin in tamoxifen-resistant breast cancer cells. Food Chem Toxicol 48(11):3227–3234

Oi N, Hashimoto T, Kanazawa K (2008) Metabolic conversion of dietary quercetin from its conjugate to active aglycone following the induction of hepatocarcinogenesis in fisher 344 rats. J Agric Food Chem 56(2):577–583

Oliveira PA, Colaco A, Chaves R, Guedes-Pinto H et al (2007) Chemical carcinogenesis. An Acad Bras Cienc 79(4):593–616

Olson ER, Melton T, Dickinson SE, Dong Z et al (2010) Quercetin potentiates UVB-Induced c-Fos expression: implications for its use as a chemopreventive agent. Cancer Prev Res (Phila) 3(7):876–884

Pawlikowska-Pawlega B, Jakubowicz-Gil J, Rzymowska J, Gawron A (2001) The effect of quercetin on apoptosis and necrosis induction in human colon adenocarcinoma cell line LS180. Folia Histochem Cytobiol 39(2):217–218

Pereira MA, Grubbs CJ, Barnes LH, Li H et al (1996) Effects of the phytochemicals, curcumin and quercetin, upon azoxymethane-induced colon cancer and 7,12-dimethylbenz[a]anthracene-induced mammary cancer in rats. Carcinogenesis 17(6):1305–1311

Priyadarsini RV, Vinothini G, Murugan RS, Manikandan P et al (2011) The flavonoid quercetin modulates the hallmark capabilities of hamster buccal pouch tumors. Nutr Cancer 63(2): 218–226

Rastogi PB, Levin RE (1987) Induction of sperm abnormalities in mice by quercetin. Environ Mutagen 9(1):79–86

Ren W, Qiao Z, Wang H, Zhu L et al (2003) Flavonoids: promising anticancer agents. Med Res Rev 23(4):519–534

Rodriguez-Antona C, Gomez A, Karlgren M, Sim SC et al (2010) Molecular genetics and epigenetics of the cytochrome P450 gene family and its relevance for cancer risk and treatment. Hum Genet 127(1):1–17

Samanta SK, Bhattacharya K, Mandal C, Pal BC (2010) Identification and quantification of the active component quercetin 3-*O*-rutinoside from Barringtonia racemosa, targets mitochondrial apoptotic pathway in acute lymphoblastic leukemia. J Asian Nat Prod Res 12(8):639–648

Samuel T, Fadlalla K, Turner T, Yehualaeshet TE (2010) The flavonoid quercetin transiently inhibits the activity of taxol and nocodazole through interference with the cell cycle. Nutr Cancer 62(8):1025–1035

Senthilkumar K, Arunkumar R, Elumalai P, Sharmila G et al (2011) Quercetin inhibits invasion, migration and signalling molecules involved in cell survival and proliferation of prostate cancer cell line (PC-3). Cell Biochem Funct 29(2):87–95

Seo HS, Ju JH, Jang K, Shin I (2011) Induction of apoptotic cell death by phytoestrogens by up-regulating the levels of phospho-p53 and p21 in normal and malignant estrogen receptor α-negative breast cells. Nutr Res 31(2):139–146

Seufi AM, Ibrahim SS, Elmaghraby TK, Hafez EE (2009) Preventive effect of the flavonoid, quercetin, on hepatic cancer in rats via oxidant/antioxidant activity: molecular and histological evidences. J Exp Clin Cancer Res 28:80

Shan BE, Wang MX, Li RQ (2009) Quercetin inhibit human SW480 colon cancer growth in association with inhibition of cyclin D(1) and survivin expression through Wnt/beta-catenin signaling pathway. Cancer Invest 27(6):604–612

Shen J, Zhang W, Wu J, Zhu Y (2008) The synergistic reversal effect of multidrug resistance by quercetin and hyperthermia in doxorubicin-resistant human myelogenous leukemia cells. Int J Hyperthermia 24(2):151–159

Siegelin MD, Reuss DE, Habel A, Rami A et al (2009) Quercetin promotes degradation of survivin and thereby enhances death-receptor-mediated apoptosis in glioma cells. Neuro Oncol 11(2):122–131

Sporn MB, Dunlop NM, Newton DL, Smith JM (1976) Prevention of chemical carcinogenesis by vitamin A and its synthetic analogs (retinoids). Fed Proc 35(6):1332–1338

Sung B, Pandey MK, Ahn KS, Yi T et al (2008) Anacardic acid (6-nonadecyl salicylic acid), an inhibitor of histone acetyltransferase, suppresses expression of nuclear factor-kappaB-regulated gene products involved in cell survival, proliferation, invasion, and inflammation through inhibition of the inhibitory subunit of nuclear factor-kappaBalpha kinase, leading to potentiation of apoptosis. Blood 111(10):4880–4891

Tan XL, Spivack SD (2009) Dietary chemoprevention strategies for induction of phase II xenobiotic-metabolizing enzymes in lung carcinogenesis: a review. Lung Cancer 65(2): 129–137

Tang SN, Singh C, Nall D, Meeker D et al (2010) The dietary bioflavonoid quercetin synergizes with epigallocathechin gallate (EGCG) to inhibit prostate cancer stem cell characteristics, invasion, migration and epithelial-mesenchymal transition. J Mol Signal 5:14

Tanigawa S, Fujii M, Hou DX (2007) Action of Nrf2 and Keap1 in ARE-mediated NQO1 expression by quercetin. Free Radic Biol Med 42(11):1690–1703

Teiten MH, Gaascht F, Dicato M, Diederich M (2011) Targeting the Wingless signaling pathway with natural compounds as chemopreventive or chemotherapeutic agents. Curr Pharm Biotechnol

van Erk MJ, Roepman P, van der Lende TR, Stierum RH et al (2005) Integrated assessment by multiple gene expression analysis of quercetin bioactivity on anticancer-related mechanisms in colon cancer cells in vitro. Eur J Nutr 44(3):143–156

Vasquez-Garzon VR, Arellanes-Robledo J, Garcia-Roman R, Aparicio-Rautista DI et al (2009) Inhibition of reactive oxygen species and pre-neoplastic lesions by quercetin through an antioxidant defense mechanism. Free Radic Res 43(2):128–137

Verschoyle RD, Steward WP, Gescher AJ (2007) Putative cancer chemopreventive agents of dietary origin-how safe are they? Nutr Cancer 59(2):152–162

Vidya Priyadarsini R, Senthil Murugan R, Maitreyi S, Ramalingam K et al (2010) The flavonoid quercetin induces cell cycle arrest and mitochondria-mediated apoptosis in human cervical cancer (HeLa) cells through p53 induction and NF-κB inhibition. Eur J Pharmacol 649(1–3):84–91

Wang L, Lee IM, Zhang SM, Blumberg JB et al (2009) Dietary intake of selected flavonols, flavones, and flavonoid-rich foods and risk of cancer in middle-aged and older women. Am J Clin Nutr 89(3):905–912

Warren CA, Paulhill KJ, Davidson LA, Lupton JR et al (2009) Quercetin may suppress rat aberrant crypt foci formation by suppressing inflammatory mediators that influence proliferation and apoptosis. J Nutr 139(4):792

Yang JH, Hsia TC, Kuo HM, Chao PDL et al (2006) Inhibition of lung cancer cell growth by quercetin glucuronides via G2/M arrest and induction of apoptosis. Drug Metab Dispos 34(2):296–304

Ying B, Yang T, Song X, Hu X et al (2008) Quercetin inhibits IL-1 beta-induced ICAM-1 expression in pulmonary epithelial cell line A549 through the MAPK pathways. Mol Biol Rep 36(7):1825–1832

Chapter 2
Micronutrients and Cancer: Add Spice to Your Life

Sahdeo Prasad, Subash C. Gupta, and Bharat B. Aggarwal

Contents

Abstract Numerous lines of evidence from preclinical and clinical studies over the past several years have indicated that lifestyle factors play a major role in the pathogenesis of human cancers. High consumption of fruits and vegetables in diet are associated with reduced risk of cancer. The micronutrients present in diet are known to play an important role in both prevention and treatment of human cancers. How micronutrients exert anti-cancer activities is not completely understood. However, micronutrients have been shown to modulate multiple cell-signaling pathways closely linked to inflammation that plays a major role in tumor development. Among the dietary agents, spices have been consumed for centuries and are important ingredient of food. Spice constituents, such as curcumin, eugenol,

S. Prasad • S.C. Gupta • B.B. Aggarwal (✉)
Cytokine Research Laboratory, Department of Experimental Therapeutics, The University of Texas MD Anderson Cancer Center, 1515 Holcombe Blvd, Unit 1950, Houston, TX 77030, USA
e-mail: SPrasad@mdanderson.org; scgupta@mdanderson.org; aggarwal@mdanderson.org

S. Shankar and R.K. Srivastava (eds.), *Nutrition, Diet and Cancer*,
DOI 10.1007/978-94-007-2923-0_2,

cardamonin, capsaicin, anethol, zerumbone, diosgenin, piperine, and cinnamic acid, have been shown to affect all facets of tumor development, including cellular transformation and tumor cell survival, proliferation, invasion, angiogenesis, and metastasis. Due to high efficacy but limited toxicity noted in early-phase clinical studies, makes these agents an ideal candidate for large-scale, randomized clinical trials. How spice nutraceuticals affect tumor development and what are their different cancer targets are discussed in this chapter.

Introduction

An abundance of epidemiological evidence has shown that lifestyle plays a major role in the aetiology of human cancers. Approximately 90% of all cancers are caused by an adverse lifestyle, and as much as 30–40% of all cancers have been linked to diet. Consumption of a high-fat diet with low physical activity causes overweight and obesity, which is now recognized as a major cause of cancer in Western countries (Klurfeld and Kritchevsky 1986). Relatively low intake of fruit and vegetables is also a risk factor for many of the most important cancers (Block et al. 1992); in contrast, several epidemiological studies have revealed that greater consumption of fruits and vegetables is associated with a lower risk of cancer (Ames and Wakimoto 2002). How fruits and vegetables reduce cancer risk is not completely known. However, it has been hypothesized that this association is due to the presence of naturally occurring micronutrients or trace compounds that act as inhibitors of carcinogenesis. Micronutrients are essential and nonessential dietary components that are consumed in minute quantities and bring about a physiological effect. Polyphenols, which are found in different plants, phytoestrogens present in soy, and other phytochemicals are some examples of micronutrients.

Over the last few decades natural foods have been investigated as important sources of micronutrients and for their possible role against cancer. An early cohort study of cigarette smokers in Norway showed that men who consumed higher rather than lower amounts of vitamin A had substantially reduced risks of lung cancer (Kvale and Johansen 1982). This was a most interesting finding because cancer has already been identified in large majority of smokers. The lower risk of cancer in eastern countries than in western countries could be attributable to the higher production and consumption of fruits, vegetables and spices in the eastern countries (whereas in western countries the consumption of fruits, vegetables and spices is generally static or declining). Fruits and vegetables contain a huge range of other biologically active constituents that have been shown to exert anticarcinogenic effects in vitro and in animal models (He et al. 1997).

Among the natural compounds spices have their own particular importance. Some common spices are shown in Fig. 2.1. In general spices are consumed in the form of dried seed, fruit, root, bark, or vegetative substance. Spices are commonly used in nutritionally insignificant quantities as a food additive for flavor or color or as a preservative. Many spices are used for other purposes, such as medicine,

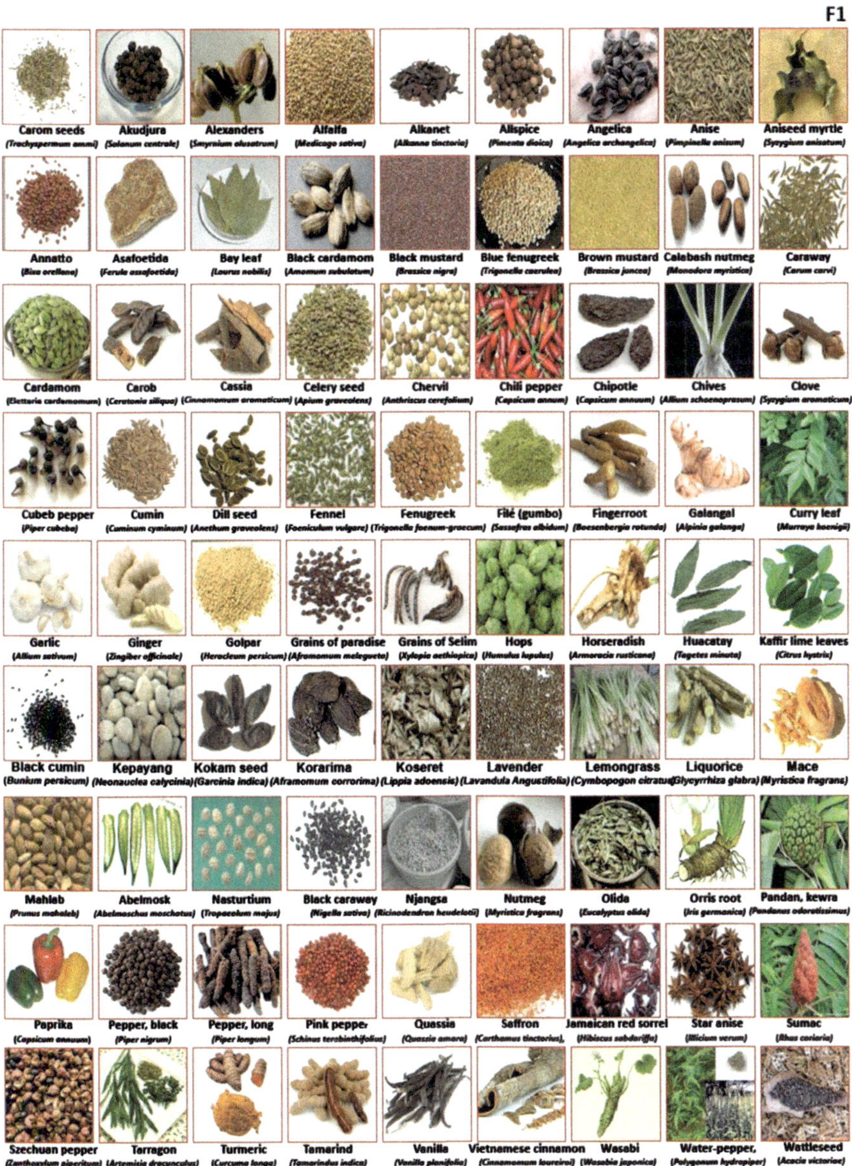

Fig. 2.1 Commonly used spices

religious rituals, cosmetics, perfumery, or for eating as vegetables. In this chapter we discuss the traditional uses and importance of spices in human well-being and in the prevention and treatment of cancer in experimental models. We also discuss the molecular mechanisms of spices and spice-derived nutraceuticals against cancer in experimental models.

History of Spices

The word "spice" originated from the Old French word "espice" which in turn derived from the Latin root "spec". This word refers to appearance, sort, or kind. The human use of spices in food dates back around 50,000 BC either purposely or accidentally. In Assyrian mythology the Gods drank sesame wine the night before they created the earth. The first concrete evidence of spices was the art work and writings of early civilizations. For example, hieroglyphs in the Great Pyramid at Giza showed workers eating garlic and onions for strength. And as archeologists discovered in the Egyptian tombs, as early as 3000 BC Egyptians were using various spices for flavoring food, in cosmetics, and for embalming their dead. These people believed that spices had strong connections or affiliations with different gods and offered a better chance of celestial help in travels into the afterlife. Around 400 BC the Greek physician Hippocrates described more than 400 medicines made with spices and herbs. During Roman times, spices were available only to the upper class, who valued them as highly as gold.

Spices were so desirable yet expensive that the Portuguese and Spanish searched for a cheaper way to obtain spices from the East, which led to the great Age of exploration and the discovery of the New World. The Portuguese explorer Vasco De Gama sailed around Africa's Cape of Good Hope to reach Calcutta, India, and discovered a sea route to the source of these spices. Along with pepper, cinnamon and ginger, he returned with jewels and trading deals with Indian princes. For similar reasons Christopher Columbus went westwards from Europe in 1492 to find a sea route to the lands of spices, but he found the Americas instead. And in 1519, Ferdinand Magellan from Spain sailed around the world. Although he died in the Philippines, his ship returned with pepper and other spices that made the trip financially successful. The Dutch, who in the beginning of the sixteenth century gained control of shipping and trading in northern Europe, had by the end of that century themselves entered the spice trade, overtaking Portuguese control. The Dutch made many expeditions to the East Indies and set up deals with local rulers. During the 1500s the English looked north for their own route to the spices in the east. Although a northern route was not found, in 1600 Elizabeth I chartered the British East India Company and began to take control in India.

North America also took an interest in the spice market. Boston-born Elihu Yale, a former clerk of the British East India Company in Madras, India, began his own spice business in 1672. In 1797 Captain Jonathan Carnes sailed into Salem, Massachusetts, from Indonesia with pepper, and he started trading directly with Asian natives rather than going through European countries. As a result, Salem became the center of spice trade in North America. As their influence grew, Americans contributed largely to the spice world. In 1883, chili powder was developed by Texan settlers for Mexican dishes; in 1889 a research facility in Watsonville, California, developed techniques for dehydrating onions and garlic; and in 1906 the first U.S. book of standards for spice purity was published by Eugene Durkee.

Production and Consumption of Spices

More than 80 varieties of spice are grown throughout the world. Asia still grows most of the spices that once ruled the trade, including cinnamon, pepper, nutmeg, cloves, ginger and others. India alone grows over 50 different varieties and has its own flavor and medicinal values. According to the United Nations' Food and Agriculture Organization (2003–2004), India produces 1,600,000 tonnes (86% of the world production) of spices. (China comes in at 99,000 tonnes (5%)). No other country in the world produces as many kinds of spices as India where the climate of the country is suitable for almost all spices. Because of these, India is known as the "the home of spices." Although India exports spices to more than 150 countries, its share of the world trade is only 45–50% by volume (25% in value) because the country exports only 8–10% of its production. Within India the consumption pattern varies with region, income, and other sample characteristics, but the estimated average per capita consumption of spices is 9.54 g (Uma Pradeep et al. 1993).

European countries grow mainly basil, bay leaves, celery leaves, chives, coriander, dill tips, thyme and water cress. The total European production of spices amounted to 124,000 tonnes in 2007; consumption was even higher and has increased from 265,000 tonnes in 2003–321,000 tonnes in 2007 (FAOSTAT 2008). The European market is also the one of largest market for spices and herbs in the world. In Europe, Germany is the leading consuming country, which accounts almost one fifth of total Europeon spice consumption, followed by the United Kingdom, Romania and Hungary. Mostly they consume pepper, paprika and allspice.

More and more spices, herbs, and aromatic seeds are being planted in the Western Hemisphere. Brazil is a major supplier of pepper, Grenada nutmeg, and Jamaica ginger and allspice. Nicaragua, El Salvador, and the United States grow sesame seed. California produces many herbs, and Canada grows several aromatic seeds. The consumption of spices in America has increased by 50% in the past decade. The demand for spices is growing due to increased consumer interest, availability of flavors and ingredients, and demand for ethnic foods. According to the new market research report on spices and seasonings, the United States represents the largest market for spices and seasonings worldwide.

Importance of Spices

Although spices enhance the flavor and aroma of any dish, they are also well known for their medicinal value. Different types of spices are important in health. Spices stimulate salivation and promote digestion. Ginger heats the stomach and improves digestion, nutmeg is beneficial for the spleen, and cinnamon, one of the most popular flavors in cooking, is considered particularly good for digestion and sore throats. Spices have been also used as preservatives. Spices can be mixed with salt to preserve meats, and they are also used for pickling. Aromatic spices, such as cloves and cardamon, have been used to conceal the foul breath of onion and garlic eaters. Hot, pungent spices are used more liberally in winter diets or to treat "cold" diseases accompanied by excess phlegm.

According to Ayurveda, spices help to maintain the balance of the three doshas, kapha, pitta, and vata. For example, turmeric promotes good digestion, increases vata and pitta if too much is consumed, and relieves kapha. Sesame increases pitta and kapha but decreases vata. In addition to relieving hemorrhoids and reducing vomiting, saffron increases vata and kapha and relieves pitta. In Traditional Chinese Medicine (TCM), spices are recommended not only for flavoring dishes but also for their nutritional benefits. According to the TCM star anise helps relieve cold stagnation. Ginger is used for nausea, indigestion, diarrhea and upset stomachs, and its warming effects boost the immune system and treat respiratory problems because the spice stimulates circulation of the blood and removes toxins from the body. Another warming herb, cinnamon, increases circulation and thus enhances cognitive thinking and increases metabolism.

Traditional Uses of Spices

Spices have historically been used to change the physical appearance of food and other products. For example, pepper sprinkled over dishes made them conspicuous, and turmeric changed the food color. Spices were also used to dye fabric, change the texture of food (such as coarse salt or sugar on snacks and desserts), and preserve meat and other foods that would otherwise spoil. Some spices are used because they are aromatic. Cinnamon is not only a popular flavor but is also widely used as a scent in candles, air fresheners and hand lotion. Lavender, known for its calming effects, is used in incense sticks, bath oils and tea.

Spices have long been used in home remedies as well. Garlic has been used for preserving memory and for a healthy heart. Turmeric is used against the common cold and influenza; it also enhances immune functions, improves digestion, and reduces the risk of heart attack. Turmeric is used in lotion to keep the face shiny and prevent pimples. Ginger has several medical properties: it helps prevent motion sickness, especially seasickness, and can be used to reduce the nausea and vomiting brought on by pregnancy. The medicinal uses of spice are many (Table 2.1). The use of herbal remedies among patients with cancer is prevalent throughout the world. In the United States alone, 68% of long-term survivors with lymphoma have used herbal medicines (Habermann et al. 2009). In European countries, 26.5% of patients with hematological cancers had used some form of herbal medicine, including spices, after a diagnosis of cancer (Molassiotis et al. 2005). In the past few decade scientists have paid more attention to the beneficial effects of spices on human health and discovered that spices contain antioxidants and anti-inflammatory agents helpful against several chronic diseases.

Table 2.1 Active components and traditional uses of spices

Spice (botanical name)	Active components	Traditional uses
1. Carom seeds (*Trachyspermum ammi*)	Thymol	Expectorant, anti-flatulent
2. Akudjura (*Solanum centrale*)		Restorative, phytoestrogenic, antimicrobial, anti-arthritic
3. Alexanders (*Smyrnium olusatrum*)	ND	
4. Alfalfa (*Medicago sativa*)	β-Carotene, octacosanol	Relieves osteoarthritis, rheumatoid arthritis, diabetes, upset stomach, kidney problems
5. Alkanet (*Alkanna tinctoria*)	Alkannin, Shikonin	Antimicrobial, wound healing
6. Allspice (*Pimenta dioica*)	Eugenol	Antiemetic, purgative
7. Angelica (*Angelica archangelica*)	Linalool, Coumarins, Borneol, Bergapten	Carminative, diaphoretic, sedative, emmenagogue, stomachic and tonic
8. Anise (*Pimpinella anisum*)	Anethol	Relieves asthma, bronchitis, cough, digestive disorders
9. Aniseed myrtle (*Syzygium anisatum*)	ND	Antiseptic, antiviral, antifungal; relieves colds, flu, chest congestion, digestive disorders
10. Annatto (*Bixa orellana*)	Bixim	Relieves asthma, colic, nausea, vomiting, blood pressure
11. Asafoetida (*Ferula assafoetida*)	Ferulic acid, Umbelliferone	Anti-helminthic, anti-tussive
12. Bay leaf (*Laurus nobilis*)	Costunolide	Embrocation, anti-rheumatic, antibacterial, anti-inflammatory
13. Black cardamom (*Amomum subulatum*)	Diphenyl-2-picrylhydrazyl	Antiseptic, antispasmodic, diuretic, carminative, digestive, expectorant, stimulant, stomachic and tonic
14. Black mustard (*Brassica nigra*)	Allyl isothiocyanate	Emetic, diuretic, nociceptive, anti-inflammatory, antibacterial
15. Blue fenugreek (*Trigonella caerulea*)	Diosgenin	Antidiabetic, anti-cholesterolemia
16. Brown mustard (*Brassica juncea*)	Allyl isothiocyanate, Sulforaphane	Stimulant, diuretic, purgative, rheumatism, relieves arthritis, chest congestion, aching back, sore muscles
17. Calabash nutmeg (*Monodora myristica*)	Cymene, α-phellandrene	Wound healing, relieves headache
18. Caraway (*Carum carvi*)	Carvacrol, Limonene	Diuretic, anti-spasmodic, galactogogue
19. Cardamom (*Elettaria cardamomum*)	Cineole	Antimicrobial, antispasmodic, antioxidant, anti-inflammotory, anti-depressant, relieves respiratory and digestive disorders

(continued)

Table 2.1 (continued)

Spice (botanical name)	Active components	Traditional uses
20. Carob (*Ceratonia siliqua*)	Tannins	Antioxidant, mucoprotective, anti-diarrhoeal, antibacterial
21. Cassia (*Cinnamomum aromaticum*)	Cinnamaldehyde	Treatment of atherosclerosis, eyesight, constipation, anemia, bronchitis, dysentery, fever, hemorrhoids, constipation, jaundice, dermatitis, weight loss, wounds
22. Celery seed (*Apium graveolens*)	Apigenin, Thalide	Diuretic, stimulant, sedative, anti-inflammatory
23. Chili pepper (*Capsicum spp.*)	Capsaicin	Relieves pain, lowers cholesterol
24. Chipotle (*Capsicum annuum*)	Capsanthin, Capsorubin, capsaicin	Relives cold, cough, nasal congestion, anti-oxidant, weight loss
25. Chives (*Allium schoenoprasum*)	Allicin	Relives stomach upset, bad breath, lower blood pressure, diuretic, antibacterial
26. Clove (*Syzygium aromaticum*)	Eugenol	Relives headache, nausea, toothache, hypertension, sore gums, chest pain, coughs, diarrhoea, arthritis, digestive and blisters problems
27. Cubeb pepper (*Piper cubeba*)	Kubebat acid, Kubebin, Piperine	Antioxidant, relieves flatulence and indigestion
28. Cumin (*Cuminum cyminum*)	Cuminaldehyde, Safranal, Apigenin, Luteolin, Caffeic acid, Ferulic acid, Chlorogenic acid	Anti-microbial, vermifuge diuretic
29. Curry leaf (*Murraya koenigii*)	Carbazole alkaloids	Diabetes, emaciation, skin disease, worm infection, neurosis, stimulate digestion
30. Dill seed (*Anethum graveolens*)	Carvone, Limonene, Myristicin, Anethole, Phellandrene, Eugenol	Relieves digestive disorders, cold, flu, cough, pain
31. Fennel (*Foeniculum vulgare*)	Anethole	Break kidney stones, nausea, aid digestion, prevent gout, hepatoprotective, treat jaundice
32. Fenugreek (*Trigonella foenum-graecum*)	Sotolon, Trigonelline, Doisgenin	Treat sore throats, bronchitis, improve digestion
33. Filé powder, gumbo filé (*Sassafras albidum*)	Safrole	Analgesic, antiseptic, treat scurvy, skin sores, toothache, kidney problems, rheumatism, menstrual disorders, swelling, sexually transmitted diseases, hypertension, bronchitis, dysentery
34. Fingerroot, krachai (*Boesenbergia rotunda*)	ND	Digestive, flatulence, anti-diarrheal, anti-dysentery

35. Galangal, greater (*Alpinia galanga*)	Kaempferid, Galangin, Alpinin, Galangol	Anti-nausea, digestion aid
36. Garlic (*Allium sativum*)	Diallyl sulfide, Allicin	Antimicrobial, antiarthitic, remove blood clot, lower cholesterol
37. Ginger (*Zingiber officinale*)	Gingerol, Shogaols	Aid digestion, stomach upset, treat diarrhea, nausea, arthritis
38. Golpar (*Heracleum persicum*)	Pimpinellin, Bergapten, Isobergapten	Relieve flatulence, stomach ache, improve appetite
39. Grains of paradise (*Aframomum melegueta*)	Paradol, Shogaal, Gingerol	Aphrodisiac, purgative, treat measles and leprosy
40. Grains of Selim (*Xylopia aethiopica*)	γ-Cadinene	Relieves stomachache, bronchitis, biliousness, dysentery, headache and neuralgia
41. Hops (*Humulus lupulus*)	α-Humulene	Relieves restlessness anxiety, digestive disorder, menstrual cycle
42. Horseradish (*Armoracia rusticana*)	Kaempferol, Quercetin, Catechin	Treat arthritis, rheumatism, vascular disorders, antidote, antiseptic
43. Huacatay (*Tagetes minuta*)	Ocimenone, Ocimene, Dihydrotagetone	Antiviral, relieve flatulence stomachache, improve appetite
44. Kaffir lime leaves (*Citrus hystrix*)	Hesperidin	Antimicrobial, antioxidant, improve digestion, promote gum health
45. Black cumin (*Bunium persicum*)	Thymoquinone, Nigellone, nigilline	Antiasthamatic, antioxidant, anti-inflammatory
46. Kepayang (*Neonauclea calycinia*)	Damnacanthal, morindone	Antimicrobial, antioxidant, anti-inflammatory
47. Kokam (*Garcinia indica*)	Garcinol	Digestive tonic, antihelminthic, cardiotonic anti-paralytic
48. Korarima (*Aframomum corrorima*)	Cineole, Nerolidol	Tonic, carminative, purgative
49. Koseret (*Lippia adoensis*)	Estragole, Carvacrol, Limonene	Antimicrobial
50. Lavender (*Lavandula Angustifolia*)	Linalyl acetate, Linalool, Cineol, Lavandulol, Terpineol, Limonene	Treats abscesses, abdominal cramps, anxiety, arthritis, bronchitis, burns, acne, dandruff, debility, depression, neuralgia, psoriasis, rheumatism
51. Lemongrass (*Cymbopogon citratus*)	Citral, Myrcene, Linalol, Farnesol	Antidepressant, anxiolytic, anticonvulsant, hypnotic,
52. Licorice, liquorice (*Glycyrrhiza glabra*)	Glycyrrhizin	Treat peptic ulcers, cough, asthma, eczema, canker sores,
53. Mace (*Myristica fragrans*)	Myristicin	Anti-diarrheal, stomachic, stimulant

(continued)

Table 2.1 (continued)

Spice (botanical name)	Active components	Traditional uses
54. Mahlab (*Prunus mahaleb*)	Herniarin, Vomifoliol	Cosmetic, anti-diarrhoeal
55. Marjoram (*Origanum majorana*)	Ursolic acid	Relieves hay fever, sinus, congestion, indigestion, asthma, stomach pain, headache, dizziness, colds, coughs, nervous disorders
56. Abelmosk (*Abelmoschus moschatus*)	Myricetin	Relieves digestive disorder and aching joints, insecticide, aphrodisiac
57. Nasturtium (*Tropaeolum majus*)	Benzylisothiocyanate, Isoquercitrin, Kaempferol	Insect repellant, heal pimples, bladder, kidney ailments, sore throats, coughs, colds, bronchitis
58. Nigella, black caraway (*Nigella sativa*)	Nigellone, Thymoquinone	Relieves respiratory, stomach, liver, and kidney problems, analgesic, anti-inflammatory, antiallergic, antioxidants
59. Njangsa (*Ricinodendron heudelotii*)	ND	Stimulant, facilitate digestion
60. Nutmeg (*Myristica fragrans*)	Trimyristin, Myristicin	Sedative, stimulant, relaxant, anti-inflammatory, antiseptic, bactericide
61. Olida (*Eucalyptus olida*)	Euclyptol	Relieves colds, flu, chest, congestion, sore throat, bronchitis, pneumonia
62. Orris root (*Iris germanica*)	Iridals	Relieves sore throat, colds, and dropsy, diuretic
63. Pandan (*Pandanus odoratissimus*)	Pyrroline	Relieves headache, pain, fever, treat leprosy, smallpox, wounds, and skin problem
64. Paprika (*Capsicum annuum*)	Capsaicin	Relieves colds, fever, headache, colic, gas, indigestion, fever and general pain, antidiabetic
65. Pepper black (*Piper nigrum*)	Piperine	Relieves respiratory disorders, cough, cold, constipation, digestion, anemia, impotency, muscular strains, dental care, pyorrhea, diarrhea, heart disease
66. Pepper, long (*Piper longum*)	Piperine	Expels mucus, digestive, anti- inflammatory, aphrodisiac, sedative, relieves cough, bronchitis and asthma
67. Pink pepper (*Schinus terebinthifolius*)	Schinol, Quercetin, Kaempferol	Diuretic, treats depression, tooth aches, menstrual disorders and rheumatism, insecticidal

68. Quassia (*Quassia amara*)	Quassin, Cinnamic aldehyde	Stimulates appetite, treats dysentery, antimalarial, insectcide
69. Saffron (*Crocus sativus*)	Zeaxanthin, lycopene	Treats depression, asthma, insomnia and baldness, antispasmodic, aphrodisiac, appetizer, emmenagogue, expectorant, sedative, diuretic
70. Jamaican red sorrel (*Hibiscus sabdariffa*)	Anthocyanidins	Diuretic, cholerectic, febrifugal, antispasmodic, antihelminthic, antibacterial, lowers hypertension, blood pressure
71. Star anise (*Illicium verum*)	Shikimic acid, Anethole	Stomachic, stimulant, diuretic, anti-influenza, anti-spasmodic, antimicrobial, anti-rheumatism
72. Sumac (*Rhus coriaria*)	Gallic acid	Diuretic, reducing fever, stomach upsets, refrigerant, emmenagogue, diaphoretic, cephalic
73. Szechuan pepper (*Zanthoxylum piperitum*)	Sanshool	Toothache remedy, heals wounds, stimulant, blood purifier and digestive
74. Tarragon (*Artemisia dracunculus*)	Artemisinin	Treats toothaches, digestive aid, sedative, antidote, anticardiac
75. Turmeric (*Curcuma longa*)	Curcumin	Treats epilepsy, bleeding disorders, skin disease, reduces fever, diarrhea, urinary disorders, insanity, poisoning, cough, analgesic, antibacterial, anti-inflammatory, anti-tumor, anti-allergic, antioxidant, antiseptic, antispasmodic, appetizer, astringent, cardiovascular, carminative, cholagogue, digestive, diuretic, stimulant, and vulnerary
76. Tamarind (*Tamarindus indica*)	Pinitol, Furan	Cathartic, astringent, febrifuge, antiseptic, refrigerant, laxative, blood purifier, sore throat
77. Vanilla (*Vanilla planifolia*)	Vanillin	Aphrodisiac, febrifuge, reduces fever
78. Vietnamese cinnamon (*Cinnamomum loureirii*)	ND	Anti-arthritic, anti-diabetic, anti-bacterial, regulates menstrual cycle
79. Wasabi (*Wasabia japonica*)	Isothiocyanate	Reduces blood clots, anti-bacterial, anti-fungal
80. Water-pepper (*Polygonum hydropiper*)	Polygodial, Indirubin, Tetrahydroxystilbene	Stimulant, diuretic, emmenagogue, antiseptic, diaphoretic, and vesicant
81. Wattleseed (*Acacia victoriae*)	Avicin, Saponins	Insecticide, treats flu, cough, colds, skin ailments

ND not determined

Spices Against Cancer

Extensive research over the past several years has indicated that spices contain nutritional agents called nutraceuticals (Fig. 2.2). Nutraceuticals have shown promise in modulating different stages of tumorigenesis, including tumor cell survival,

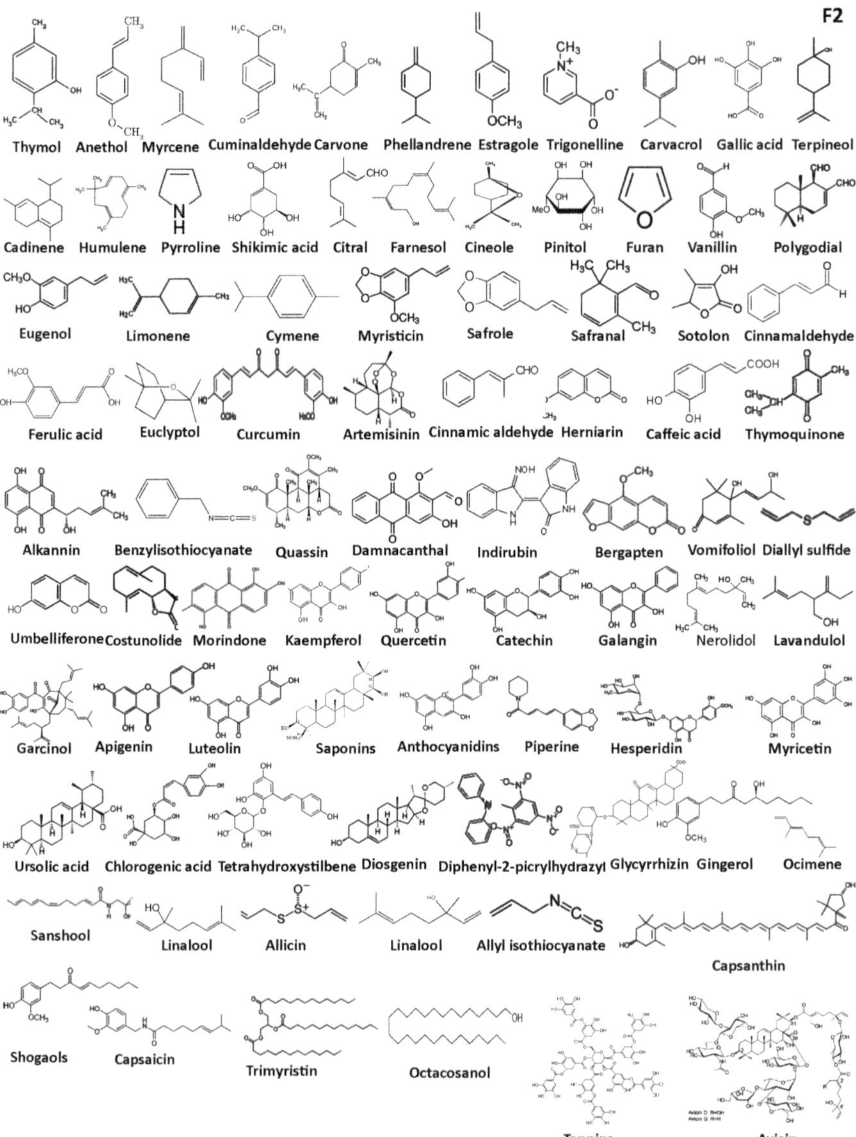

Fig. 2.2 Chemical structures of nutraceuticals derived from different spices

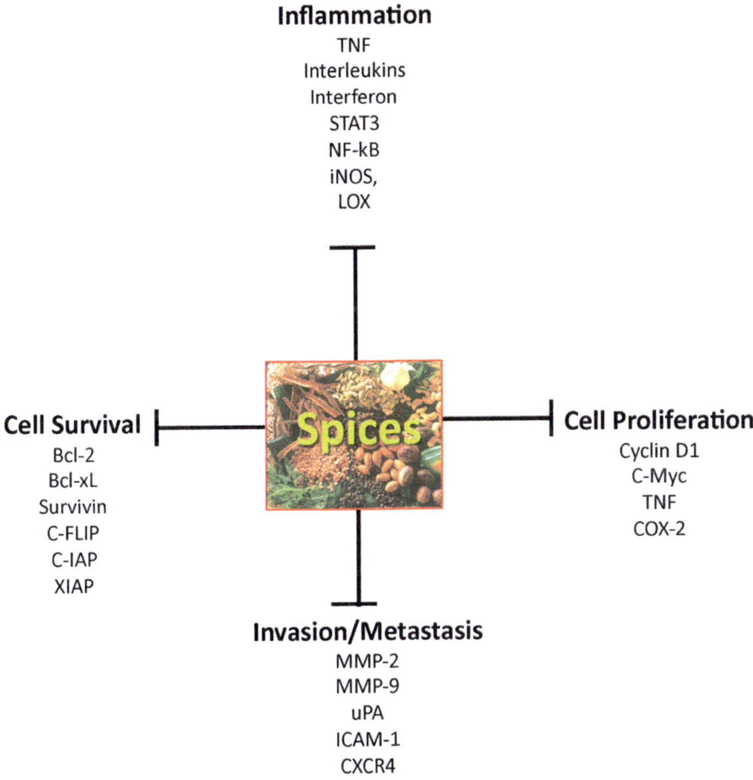

Fig. 2.3 Molecular targets of spices and spice derived nutraceuticals

proliferation, invasion and angiogenesis (Fig. 2.3). In this section, we discuss how spice-derived nutraceuticals modulate tumorigenesis. Because chronic inflammation is one of the major mediators of tumor progression, we will also discuss how nutraceuticals can affect inflammation. Because we cannot discuss all of the vast number of spice-derived anticancer nutraceuticals, we will focus on some of the most promising ones.

Role of Spices in Inflammation

Mounting evidence over the past two decades has indicated that at the molecular level cancer is caused by a dysregulated inflammatory response (Aggarwal and Gehlot 2009). One of the most important links between inflammation and cancer is the pro-inflammatory transcription factor nuclear factor-κB (NF-κB). NF-κB is a ubiquitous and evolutionary conserved transcription factor that regulates the expression of genes involved in the transformation, survival, proliferation, invasion, angiogenesis and metastasis of tumor cells. Therefore, inhibiting NF-kB activation can be used as a therapeutic strategy for preventing tumor development.

Our laboratory as well as others has shown that spice-derived nutraceuticals can exert anticancer activity by suppressing the NF-κB signaling pathway. Curcumin, which is derived from the ancient Indian medicine turmeric, has been widely studied. In one study, pretreatment of human colonic epithelial cells with curcumin resulted in an inhibition in tumor necrosis factor-α (TNF-α)–induced cyclooxygenase-2 (COX-2) gene transcription and NF-κB activation (Plummer et al. 1999). Curcumin has also been reported to suppress the TNF-α–induced nuclear translocation and DNA binding of NF-κB in a human myeloid leukemia cell line through the suppression of IκBα phosphorylation and subsequent degradation (Singh and Aggarwal 1995). Recently, we showed that curcumin has the potential to sensitize human colorectal cancer cells to the chemotherapeutic agent capecitabine by inhibiting NF-κB activation (Kunnumakkara et al. 2009).

Capsaicin obtained from pepper has also shown chemopreventive and chemoprotective effects (Aggarwal and Shishodia 2004; Surh and Lee 1995). Topical application of capsaicin has been associated with inhibition of phorbol 12-myristate 13-acetate (PMA)-induced mouse-skin tumor formation and NF-κB activation (Han et al. 2001). The inhibitory effect of capsaicin on NF-κB activation was attributed to blockage of IκBα degradation and NF-κB translocation into the nucleus. Caffeic acid phenethyl ester (CAPE), another spice-derived nutraceutical, has been shown to suppress NF-κB activation by suppressing the binding of the p50–p65 complex directly to DNA (Natarajan et al. 1996). Taken together, these studies suggest that nutraceuticals may block one or more steps in the NF-κB signaling pathway, such as IKK activity, IκBα phosphorylation, p65 nuclear translocation, and p65 DNA binding.

Other factors, such as TNF, interleukin (IL)-6, IL-8, IL-1β, and the proinflammatory transcription factor signal transducer and activator of transcription 3 (STAT3), have also been shown to link inflammation with cancer. Some nutraceuticals modulate the production of these factors (Table 2.2). Curcumin inhibits inflammatory cytokines such as IL-1 IL-6, IL-18, TNF-α, and lymphotoxin-β, and it inhibits inducible and constitutive STAT3 activation (Bharti et al. 2003). In PMA-activated HMC-1 cells, the neutraceutical apigenin was shown to inhibit the expression of the inflammatory cytokines TNF-α, IL-8, IL-6, COX-2, and granulocyte-macrophage colony-stimulating factor by decreasing the intracellular Ca(2+) level and inhibiting NF-κB activation; these results indicated that apigenin may be able to regulate inflammatory reactions (Kang et al. 2011). The nutraceuticals kaempferol and quercetin have been reported to inhibit lipopolysaccharide-induced IL-8 promoter activation in RAW 264.7 cells; in addition, the expression of TNF-α induced by burn injuries was decreased by kaempferol in mice (Park et al. 2010). Many other spice-derived compounds have been reported to effectively suppress inflammation and inflammatory cytokines (Table 2.2).

Table 2.2 Molecular targets of spice-derived nutraceuticals linked to tumorigenesis

Molecular target	Nutraceuticals
Inflammation	
NF-κB	Anethole, caffeic acid, capsaicin, carnosol, caryophyllene, cinnamaldehyde, curcumin, eugenol, 6-gingerol, galangin, humulene, pinitol, quercetin, sulforaphane, ursolic acid, thymol, vanillin, thymoquinone
TNF	Ajoene, allicin, apigenin, curcumin, eugenol, galangin, gingerol, humulene, kaempferol, piperine, pinitol, zingerone, thymol, vanillin
IL-6	Diallyl sulfide, phytic acid, piperine, pinitol, curcumin, capsaicin, thymoquinone, eugenol, 6-gingerol, ursolic acid, myricetin, vanillin
IL-8	Allicin, phytic acid, capsaicin, curcumin, pinitol, ursolic acid, myricetin, humulene
IL-1β	Allicin, apigenin, eugenol, gingerol, humulene, kaempferol, phytic acid, piperine, galangin, pinitol, capsaicin, curcumin, ursolic acid, myricetin, thymoquinone, vanillin
STAT3	Capsaicin, galangin, curcumin, myricetin, ursolic acid, thymoquinone
Lipoxygenase	Galangin, capsaicin, curcumin, eugenol, garcinol, ursolic acid, myricetin, thymoquinone, anethole, piperine
iNOS	Curcumin, eugenol, garcinol, α-humulene, ursolic acid, thymoquinone, lutein, vanillin, gingerol
Interferon-γ	Curcumin, α-humulene, piperine, vanillin
Cell survival	
Bax	Cinnamaldehyde, curcumin, diallyl sulfide, limonene, lutein, galangin, capsaicin, eugenol, garcinol, ursolic acid, myricetin, thymoquinone, 6-gingerol
Bcl-2	Garcinol, allyl isothiocyanate, capsaicin, carnosol, curcumin, diallyl sulfide, 6-gingerol, limonene, lutein, *S*-allylcysteine, sulforaphane, ursolic acid, galangin, pinitol, eugenol, myricetin, lutein, thymoquinone, piperine
Bcl-xL	Allyl isothiocyanate, capsaicin, sulforaphane, curcumin
Caspases	Allicin, cinnamaldehyde, diallyl sulfide, kaempferol, limonene, myristicin, paradol, shogaol, sulforaphane, ursolic acid, galangin, pinitol, capsaicin, curcumin, eugenol, garcinol, humulene, myricetin, thymoquinone, anethole, piperine, 6-gingerol
p53	Diallyl sulfide, limonene, lutein, shogaol, curcumin, eugenol, thymoquinone, 6 gingerol
Survivin	Capsaicin, curcumin, garcinol, ursolic acid, thymoquinone, 6-gingerol
Cell proliferation	
Cyclin D1	Apigenin, capsaicin, curcumin, lutein, sulforaphane, ursolic acid, pinitol, eugenol, thymoquinone, garcinol, myricetin, 6-gingerol
c-Myc	Apigenin, perillyl alcohol, curcumin, 6-gingerol, capsaicin, cinnamaldehyde
COX-2	Eugenol, curcumin, galangin, quercetin, myricetin, ursolic acid, 6-gingerol, sulforaphane, humulene, thymoquinone, eugenol, diallyl sulfide, capsaicin, shogaol, piperine

(continued)

Table 2.2 (continued)

Molecular target	Nutraceuticals
Invasion/Angiogenesis	
MMP-2	Allyl isothiocyanate, curcumin, diallyl disulfide, myricetin, quercetin
MMP-9	Allyl isothiocyanate, caffeic acid, carnosol, curcumin, diallyl disulfide, quercetin, ursolic acid, vanillin, pinitol, capsaicin, myricetin, thymoquinone, piperine
ICAM-1	Allicin, apigenin, crocetin, kaempferol, curcumin
CXCR4	Curcumin, ursolic acid, capsaicin
VEGF	Alliin, caffeic acid, capsaicin, curcumin, diallyl disulfide, diallyl sulfide, 6-gingerol, phytic acid, sulforaphane, galangin, pinitol, eugenol, ursolic acid, myricetin, thymoquinone

NF-κB nuclear factor-κB, *TNF* tumor necrosis factor, *IL* interleukin, *STAT3* signal transducer and activator of transcription 3, *iNOS* inducible nitric oxide synthase, *COX-2* cyclooxygenase-2, *MMP* matrix metalloproteinase, *ICAM* intracellular adhesion molecule, *CXCR-4* C-X-C chemokine receptor type 4, *VEGF* vascular endothelial growth factor

Role of Spices in Tumor Cell Survival

Under normal physiological conditions, the human body maintains homeostasis by eliminating unwanted, damaged, aged, and misplaced cells. Homeostasis is carried out in a genetically programmed manner by a process referred to as apoptosis (i.e., programmed cell death) (Song and Steller 1999; Steller 1995). Cancer cells are able to evade apoptosis and grow in a rapid and uncontrolled manner. A complex set of proteins, including caspases, proapoptotic and antiapoptotic B-cell lymphoma (Bcl)-2 family proteins, cytochrome-c, and apoptotic protease activating factor-1, execute apoptosis by either an intrinsic or an extrinsic pathway. The intrinsic pathway is mitochondria dependent, whereas the extrinsic pathway is triggered by death receptors (DRs). Some antiapoptotic proteins, such as Bcl-2 and Bcl-xL (Wang et al. 2003) and survivin (Ambrosini et al. 1997), are overexpressed in a wide variety of cancers. Therefore, the selective down-regulation of antiapoptotic proteins and up-regulation of proapoptotic proteins in cancer cells offers promise as a therapeutic intervention. A number of spice-derived nutraceuticals have shown promise against tumor cell survival by inducing apoptosis through a variety of mechanisms.

Some of the most common ways that nutraceuticals inhibit the survival of tumor cells are to activate caspases, induce proapoptotic proteins, and down-regulate antiapoptotic proteins. For example, curcumin has been reported to be a potent inducer of apoptosis in cancer cells. This spice induces the up-regulation of proapoptotic proteins Bax, Bcl-2–interacting mediator of cell death (Bim), Bak, p53-upregulated modulator of apoptosis (Puma), and PMA-induced protein 1 (Noxa) and the down-regulation of the antiapoptotic proteins Bcl-2 and Bcl-xL (Shankar and Srivastava 2007). Some nutraceuticals induce apoptosis through the up-regulation of DRs. For example, capsaicin and garcinol have been shown to sensitize cancer cells to TNF-related apoptosis-inducing ligand–mediated apoptosis via the up-regulation of DR5 and the down-regulation of anti-apoptotic proteins (Kim et al. 2010; Prasad et al. 2010).

Some nutraceuticals have the potential to inhibit the survival of tumor cells by modulating the STAT3 pathway. For example, capsaicin was reported to induce apoptosis in multiple myeloid cells by down-regulating STAT3-regulated expression of Bcl-2, Bcl-xL, and survivin (Bhutani et al. 2007). Some nutraceuticals inhibit NF-κB activation, thereby inhibiting NF-κB–regulated antiapoptotic proteins. For example, sulforaphane inhibited the survival of orthotopically implanted PC-3 tumors through the up-regulation of DR4, DR5, Bax, and Bak and the inhibition of NF-κB, phosphoinositide 3-kinase (PI3K)/AKT, and MAPK/ERK kinase (MEK) activation pathways (Shankar et al. 2008). Some other common spice-derived nutraceuticals that could inhibit tumor cell survival are listed in Table 2.2.

Role of Spices in Tumor Cell Proliferation

In normal cells, a delicate balance between growth and antigrowth signals regulates proliferation. Cancer cells, however, acquire the ability to generate their own growth signals and become insensitive to antigrowth signals (Hanahan and Weinberg 2000). Regulators of cell cycle such as cyclin-dependent kinases and CDK inhibitors are involved in the proliferation of cancer cells. In addition, the tumor suppressor proteins p53 and its downstream target p21, and activation of protooncogenes control cancer cell proliferation and growth (Soda et al. 1999). It has been also reported that COX-2 level are increased in both premalignant and malignant tissues (Soslow et al. 2000; Subbaramaiah and Dannenberg 2003) indicating its proliferative activity of cancer cells.

A number of inhibitors based on cell cycle regulators, including nutraceuticals, are being developed to prevent cancer. Nutraceuticals have this potential by targeting and halting one or more steps in the cell cycle. Most nutraceuticals prevent the transition of cancer cells from the G1 phase to the S phase. Some of these agents act through p53 and some through retinoblastoma (Rb). Curcumin is one of the most widely studied nutraceutical that has the potential to inhibit tumor proliferation. In gastric cancer cells, curcumin was shown to suppress the transition of cells from the G1 phase to the S phase, which was accompanied by a decrease in cyclin-D1 and p21-activated kinase-1 activity (Cai et al. 2009). NF-κB has been shown to bind to the promoter of genes involved in cellular proliferation. A few nutraceuticals, including curcumin, target one or more steps in NF-κB activation to regulate tumor cell proliferation. In an orthotopic murine model of ovarian cancer, curcumin was shown to inhibit tumor growth that correlated with inhibition of NF-κB and the STAT3 activation pathway (Lin et al. 2007). In another study, curcumin exhibited antiproliferative activity in association with decreased expression of cyclin-D1 and CDK-4 in the breast cancer cell lines MDA-MB-231 and BT-483 (Liu et al. 2009).

Quercetin was shown to induce cell cycle arrest at the G1 phase by elevating p53, p21, and p27 levels in a human hepatoma cell line in vitro (Mu et al. 2007). Sulforaphane suppressed the proliferation of epithelial ovarian cancer cells through G1 cell cycle arrest, pRb and free E2F-1 reduction, and Rb augmentation (Bryant et al. 2010). The antiproliferative activity of capsaicin correlated with the decreased expression of E2F-responsive proliferative genes such as cyclin-E, thymidylate synthase, cdc25A, and cdc6 in small cell lung cancer (Brown et al. 2010). In a benzo[a]pyrene-induced lung carcinogenesis mice model, an aqueous infusion of the spice clove inhibited tumor cell proliferation and induced apoptosis (Banerjee et al. 2006). The clove infusion up-regulated the expression of p53 and Bax and down-regulated the expression of Bcl-2 in the precancerous stages as well as the expression of the growth-promoting proteins COX-2, cMyc and Hras, indicating its potent antiproliferative activity. Crocetin, a carotenoid compound derived from saffron, exhibited antiproliferative activity in MIA-PaCa-2 pancreatic cancer cells, which was evident by the suppression of the cell proliferative Cdc-2, Cdc-25C, cyclin-B1, and epidermal growth factor receptor marker proteins (Dhar et al. 2009). The crocetin was also shown to cause regression in tumor growth by inhibiting the proliferation pancreatic cancer cells injected in mice; furthermore, it suppressed proliferating cell nuclear antigen and epidermal growth factor receptor expression in the tumor cells compared with control cells. Several other spices and spice-derived nutraceuticals have shown antiproliferative properties as well (Table 2.2).

Role of Spices in Tumor Cell Metastasis and Angiogenesis

Metastasis is the spread of tumor cells from their primary location in the body to other sites. Tumor cells penetrate into lymphatic and blood vessels, circulate through the bloodstream, and then invade and grow in normal tissues. The most common sites of cancer metastasis are the lungs, bones, and liver. The growth and proliferation of cancer cells require nutrients and oxygen, which can be provided by the development of new blood vessels (i.e., angiogenesis). Tumor metastasis and angiogenesis are regulated by the production of several stimulators, including matrix metalloproteinases (MMPs) and intracellular adhesion molecules (ICAMs). Pro-angiogenic factors also include IL-8, TNF, fibroblast growth factor-2, and platelet-derived growth factor. However, one of the most important factors in angiogenesis is vascular endothelial growth factor (VEGF), which is a potent stimulator of angiogenesis in vitro (McMahon 2000). These studies illustrate the importance of targeting these markers to block their production and release in tumor cell lines, possibly leading to stasis or tumor growth regression.

Agents that could suppress these biomarker-associated signaling pathways are urgently needed. Several chemotherapeutics drugs inhibit these biomarkers, but they have serious side effects and are enormously expensive. For example bevacizumab, a monoclonal antibody directed against VEGF for patients with metastatic colorectal cancer, has side effects such as complications in wound healing and even fatal pulmonary hemorrhage (www.avastin.com), and the treatment costs around $4,400 a month. In contrast, some natural compounds, including spices and spice-derived products, have been shown to inhibit invasion, metastasis and angiogenesis in both in vitro and in vivo models.

Curcumin has been shown to be highly potent in suppressing metastasis and angiogenesis. It suppressed MMP-9, ICAM-1 and VEGF expression in both in vitro and in vivo models (Kunnumakkara et al. 2008). In an MNNG-treated rat model, administration of eugenol induced apoptosis and inhibited invasion and angiogenesis, as evidenced by changes in the activities of MMPs and the expression of MMP-2, MMP-9, VEGF, VEGF receptor 1, Tissue Inhibitor of Metalloproteinases (TIMP)-2 and RECK (Manikandan et al. 2010). In contrast, kaempferol mildly inhibited cell viability but significantly reduced VEGF gene expression at the mRNA and protein levels in ovarian cancer cell lines. Hypoxia-inducible factor-1α, a regulator of VEGF, was down-regulated by kaempferol treatment in ovarian cancer cell lines (Luo et al. 2009). Apigenin prevented the activation of the downstream target gene VEGF and angiogenesis in hypoxic solid tumors (Mirzoeva et al. 2008). In ovarian tumor cells, apigenin inhibited VEGF and hypoxia-inducible factor-1 via the PI3K/AKT/p70S6K1 and HDM2/p53 pathways (Fang et al. 2005).

Capsaicin inhibited the VEGF-induced proliferation, chemotactic motility, and capillary-like tube formation of primary cultured human endothelial cells. Capsaicin has been also shown to suppress tumor-induced angiogenesis in a chick chorioallantoic membrane assay (Min et al. 2004). 6-Gingerol also blocked VEGF-induced capillary-like tube formation by endothelial cells, and it strongly inhibited the sprouting of endothelial cells in rat aorta and the formation of new blood vessel in mouse cornea in response to VEGF. In addition, it suppressed lung metastasis of intravenously injected B16F10 melanoma cells in mice (Kim et al. 2005). 6-Gingerol also inhibited the migration and motility of MDA-MB-231 cells through the suppression of MMP-2 or MMP-9 activity (Lee et al. 2008). Sulforaphane inhibited VEGF expression in human prostate cancer PC-3 cells (Xu et al. 2005). Diallyl sulfide reduced the serum level of VEGF in B16F-10 melanoma-bearing C57BL/6 mice (Thejass and Kuttan 2007). Allicin inhibited ICAM-1 expression induced by TNFα in human umbilical vein endothelial cells (Mo et al. 2003). Piperine suppressed MMP-9 production in B16F-10 melanoma cells (Pradeep and Kuttan 2004). Besides these, several other spice derived compounds are shown to have antiangiogenic and metastatic activities (Table 2.2).

Anticancer Effects of Spices in Combination

Because single agents may not always be sufficient to provide preventive or therapeutic efficacy, the concept of combining multiple agents or consuming "whole foods" has become an increasingly attractive area of investigation. A number of studies have shown that combining the active compounds of more than one spice or with other phytochemicals has been more effective than individual agents. The combination of *S*-allylcysteine, an organosulphur constituent of garlic, and lycopene, a tomato carotenoid, suppressed *N*-methyl-*N*′-nitro-*N*-nitroso-guanidine–induced gastric carcinogenesis in Wistar rats (Velmurugan et al. 2005), and the combination of garlic, turmeric and tomato suppressed 7, 12-dimethylbenz[a]anthracene–induced mutagenesis and oxidative stress in male Swiss mice (Chandra Mohan et al. 2004). In an in vitro study, piplartine, a component of spice piper species, or curcumin alone showed no or moderate cytotoxicity at given doses, but their combination resulted in significant cytotoxicity in rat histiocytoma cells (BC-8), mouse embryonal carcinoma cells (PCC4), mouse macrophages (P388D1 and J774), and human neuroblastoma cells (IMR32) (Jyothi et al. 2009). Thus, the combination of spice-derived phytochemicals is relevant for the enhancement of the anticancer effect.

Chemotherapeutic agents are routinely used to treat cancer patients, but the disease develops resistance to these drugs over time. Natural products, including spices, could be used with chemotherapeutic agents to provide additive or synergistic effects. Curcumin has been shown to potentiate the effect of the standard chemotherapeutic agent capecitabine against the growth and metastasis of colorectal cancer. This spice was shown to suppress inflammatory (NF-κB), cell proliferative (ki-67, cyclin-D1), cell survival (survivin, bcl-2, c-IAP) and metastatic (ICAM1, VEGF) markers both in vitro and in a nude mouse model (Kunnumakkara et al. 2009). Curcumin also enhanced the effect of gemcitabine, another standard chemotherapeutic drug, in suppressing pancreatic tumors (Kunnumakkara et al. 2007) and the drugs thalidomide and bortezomib against human multiple myeloma in a nude mice model (Sung et al. 2009).

Other neutraceuticals have shown promise as well. Eugenol, which is consumed by humans in the form of spices, combined with the endogenous estrogenic metabolite 2-methoxyestradiol inhibited the growth of prostate cancer cells more strongly and induced apoptosis at lower concentrations than either agent alone did (Ghosh et al. 2009). At its sublethal dose, eugenol synergistically enhanced the effect of gemcitabine in inducing the cyoitoxicity of cervical cancer cells, and eugenol and gemcitabine together synergistically down-regulated the expression levels of Bcl-2, COX-2 and IL-β (Hussain et al. 2011). The neutraceuticals capsaicin and lovastatin were synergistic in inducing the cytotoxicity of hepatocarcinoma Hep-G2 cells (Popovich et al. 2010). In another study, the treatment of human myeloid leukemia HL-60 cells with capsaicin alone resulted in a small increase in the number of differentiated cells but treatment with both capsaicin and 12-*O*-tetradecanoylphorbol-13-acetate (TPA) synergistically increased differentiation (Zheng et al. 2005); these results suggested that capsaicin may improve the therapeutic efficacy of TPA and help overcome resistance to TPA in some patients with myeloid leukemia.

In conclusion, several spices are known to enhance the affect of chemotherapeutic drugs or other cytotoxic agents.

Clinical Trials with Spices

Throughout the world spices and their active components are being tested for their potential in treating patients with cancer. Curcumin is one of the widely used nutraceuticals that being tested in clinical trials. For example, in a study with urinary bladder cancer, uterine cervical intraepithelial neoplasm, or oral leukoplakia patients, curcumin prevented further development of disease and was nontoxic (Cheng et al. 2001). In another study, curcumin (480 mg) in combination with quercetin (20 mg) was given orally three times a day to patients with familial adenomatous polyposis. After 6 months, all five patients had fewer and smaller (60.4%) polyps than at baseline (Cruz-Correa et al. 2006). Kuttan and colleagues assessed the use of turmeric as a topical treatment for 62 patients with oral cancer or leukoplakia and reported that 10% of the patients had smaller lesions (Kuttan et al. 1987). In a study of pancreatic cancer, oral treatment with up to 8 g of curcumin daily was well tolerated by the 25 enrolled patients (Dhillon et al. 2008). This treatment showed clinical biological activity in two patients: one had stable disease, and the other had brief, but marked, tumor regression (73%) accompanied by significant increases in serum cytokine levels (IL-6, IL-8, IL-10, and IL-1 receptor antagonists). In addition, the curcumin down-regulated the expression of NF-κB, COX-2, and phosphorylated STAT3 in peripheral blood mononuclear cells from all 25 patients (Dhillon et al. 2008).

Other phytochemicals from spices, such as isoflavons, have been assessed for their effects against cancer. A study of 124 premenopausal breast cancer patients found a threefold greater risk of estrogen receptor (ER)-negative tumors relative to ER-positive tumors with low intake of the isoflavons genistein and daidzein; however, low intake of the flavonoid kaempferol was associated with a decreased risk of ER-negative tumors (Touillaud et al. 2005). In another study, the isoflavon apigenin decreased the elevated levels of biomarkers (including phosphorylated Akt1, PDK-1, PTEN, and CK2) associated with cancer in the blood cells of patients with chronic lymphocytic leukemia (Shehata et al. 2010). Finally, sustained long-term treatment with apigenin was associated with a lower recurrence rate of colon neoplasia in patients with resected colon cancer: of 36 patients who had undergone surgical resection, the 14 who were treated with flavonoids (20 mg apigenin and 20 mg epigallocathechin-gallat daily) had no cancer recurrence, whereas 20% of the 22 untreated patients had cancer recurrence and 27% developed adenomas (Hoensch et al. 2008). Taken together, these study results indicate that flavonoids present in spices are effective in treating cancer patients.

Capsaicin is being tested as a pain reliever. In a study of 99 patients with postsurgical neuropathic pain, the subjects received 8 weeks of a 0.075% capsaicin cream followed by 8 weeks of an identical appearing placebo cream, or vice versa. During the first 8 weeks the capsaicin arm was associated with substantially more skin burning, skin redness, and coughing than the placebo was; however, during the second 8 weeks the capsaicin arm experienced substantially more pain relief (average pain reduction, 53% versus 17%) (Ellison et al. 1997). In another study, 21 patients with post-mastectomy pain syndrome were treated with capsaicin cream (0.025%) applied topically (3 daily applications for 2 months); out of 19 evaluable patients, 2 (10.5%) reported complete disappearance of all symptoms and 11 (57.9%) reported less pain (Dini et al. 1993). Several other spices, such as ginger (Levine et al. 2008) and garlic (Tanaka et al. 2006), are being used in clinical trials.

Safety, Efficacy, and Contraindications of Spices

The use of spices for flavoring food and in household remedies has long been known to be safe. Modern experimental studies have also shown that most of spices lack toxicity. The U.S. Food and Drug Administration has declared some spices and their active components as "generally regarded as safe," and in the United States most spices and their components are currently being used in cereals, chips, cheese, butter, and other products (see www.kalsec.com). However, some spices do have a low level of toxicity under certain conditions, such as at high doses or when used chronically (Deshpande et al. 1998; Shah et al. 1991).

Conclusion

Spices have been used for centuries for many purposes in a wide variety of cultures. Initially spices were used as flavoring agents, colorants, and preservatives. More recently spices have been explored as antibacterial, antiviral, anti-inflammatory, antitumor, antioxidant, antiseptic, cardioprotective, hepatoprotective, nephroprotective, radioprotective, and digestive agents. Because of their inherent medical qualities, spices have been tested for use against several chronic diseases, including cancer. To date the majority of spices and their active components have been tested in vitro, in animal models, or under preclinical conditions; only a few spices or their active components have been tested in clinical trials. More clinical trials and other studies with spices are needed to elucidate and understand their efficacy in the treatment and prevention of human cancer.

Acknowledgement We thank Lizzie Hess, Department of Scientific Publications for carefully editing the manuscript. Dr. Aggarwal is the Ransom Horne, Jr., Professor of Cancer Research. This work was supported by a core grant (CA-16672), and a program project grant from National Institutes of Health (NIH CA-124787-01A2), and a grant from the Center for Targeted Therapy of MD Anderson Cancer Center.

References

Aggarwal BB, Gehlot P (2009) Inflammation and cancer: how friendly is the relationship for cancer patients? Curr Opin Pharmacol 9(4):351–369

Aggarwal BB, Shishodia S (2004) Suppression of the nuclear factor-kappaB activation pathway by spice-derived phytochemicals: reasoning for seasoning. Ann NY Acad Sci 1030:434–441

Ambrosini G, Adida C, Altieri DC (1997) A novel anti-apoptosis gene, survivin, expressed in cancer and lymphoma. Nat Med 3(8):917–921

Ames BN, Wakimoto P (2002) Are vitamin and mineral deficiencies a major cancer risk? Nat Rev Cancer 2(9):694–704

Banerjee S, Panda CK, Das S (2006) Clove (Syzygium aromaticum L.), a potential chemopreventive agent for lung cancer. Carcinogenesis 27(8):1645–1654

Bharti AC, Donato N, Aggarwal BB (2003) Curcumin (diferuloylmethane) inhibits constitutive and IL-6-inducible STAT3 phosphorylation in human multiple myeloma cells. J Immunol 171(7):3863–3871

Bhutani M, Pathak AK, Nair AS, Kunnumakkara AB, Guha S, Sethi G, Aggarwal BB (2007) Capsaicin is a novel blocker of constitutive and interleukin-6-inducible STAT3 activation. Clin Cancer Res 13(10):3024–3032

Block G, Patterson B, Subar A (1992) Fruit, vegetables, and cancer prevention: a review of the epidemiological evidence. Nutr Cancer 18(1):1–29

Brown KC, Witte TR, Hardman WE, Luo H, Chen YC, Carpenter AB, Lau JK, Dasgupta P (2010) Capsaicin displays anti-proliferative activity against human small cell lung cancer in cell culture and nude mice models via the E2F pathway. PLoS One 5(4):e10243

Bryant CS, Kumar S, Chamala S, Shah J, Pal J, Haider M, Seward S, Qazi AM, Morris R, Semaan A, Shammas MA, Steffes C, Potti RB, Prasad M, Weaver DW, Batchu RB (2010) Sulforaphane induces cell cycle arrest by protecting RB-E2F-1 complex in epithelial ovarian cancer cells. Mol Cancer 9:47

Cai XZ, Wang J, Li XD, Wang GL, Liu FN, Cheng MS, Li F (2009) Curcumin suppresses proliferation and invasion in human gastric cancer cells by downregulation of PAK1 activity and cyclin D1 expression. Cancer Biol Ther 8(14):1360–1368

Chandra Mohan KV, Abraham SK, Nagini S (2004) Protective effects of a mixture of dietary agents against 7,12-dimethylbenz[a]anthracene-induced genotoxicity and oxidative stress in mice. J Med Food 7(1):55–60

Cheng AL, Hsu CH, Lin JK, Hsu MM, Ho YF, Shen TS, Ko JY, Lin JT, Lin BR, Ming-Shiang W, Yu HS, Jee SH, Chen GS, Chen TM, Chen CA, Lai MK, Pu YS, Pan MH, Wang YJ, Tsai CC, Hsieh CY (2001) Phase I clinical trial of curcumin, a chemopreventive agent, in patients with high-risk or pre-malignant lesions. Anticancer Res 21(4B):2895–2900

Cruz-Correa M, Shoskes DA, Sanchez P, Zhao R, Hylind LM, Wexner SD, Giardiello FM (2006) Combination treatment with curcumin and quercetin of adenomas in familial adenomatous polyposis. Clin Gastroenterol Hepatol 4(8):1035–1038

Deshpande SS, Lalitha VS, Ingle AD, Raste AS, Gadre SG, Maru GB (1998) Subchronic oral toxicity of turmeric and ethanolic turmeric extract in female mice and rats. Toxicol Lett 95(3):183–193

Dhar A, Mehta S, Dhar G, Dhar K, Banerjee S, Van Veldhuizen P, Campbell DR, Banerjee SK (2009) Crocetin inhibits pancreatic cancer cell proliferation and tumor progression in a xenograft mouse model. Mol Cancer Ther 8(2):315–323

Dhillon N, Aggarwal BB, Newman RA, Wolff RA, Kunnumakkara AB, Abbruzzese JL, Ng CS, Badmaev V, Kurzrock R (2008) Phase II trial of curcumin in patients with advanced pancreatic cancer. Clin Cancer Res 14(14):4491–4499

Dini D, Bertelli G, Gozza A, Forno GG (1993) Treatment of the post-mastectomy pain syndrome with topical capsaicin. Pain 54(2):223–226

Ellison N, Loprinzi CL, Kugler J, Hatfield AK, Miser A, Sloan JA, Wender DB, Rowland KM, Molina R, Cascino TL, Vukov AM, Dhaliwal HS, Ghosh C (1997) Phase III placebo-controlled trial of capsaicin cream in the management of surgical neuropathic pain in cancer patients. J Clin Oncol 15(8):2974–2980

Fang J, Xia C, Cao Z, Zheng JZ, Reed E, Jiang BH (2005) Apigenin inhibits VEGF and HIF-1 expression via PI3K/AKT/p70S6K1 and HDM2/p53 pathways. FASEB J 19(3):342–353

Ghosh R, Ganapathy M, Alworth WL, Chan DC, Kumar AP (2009) Combination of 2-methoxyestradiol (2-ME2) and eugenol for apoptosis induction synergistically in androgen independent prostate cancer cells. J Steroid Biochem Mol Biol 113(1–2):25–35

Habermann TM, Thompson CA, LaPlant BR, Bauer BA, Janney CA, Clark MM, Rummans TA, Maurer MJ, Sloan JA, Geyer SM, Cerhan JR (2009) Complementary and alternative medicine use among long-term lymphoma survivors: a pilot study. Am J Hematol 84(12):795–798

Han SS, Keum YS, Seo HJ, Chun KS, Lee SS, Surh YJ (2001) Capsaicin suppresses phorbol ester-induced activation of NF-kappaB/Rel and AP-1 transcription factors in mouse epidermis. Cancer Lett 164(2):119–126

Hanahan D, Weinberg RA (2000) The hallmarks of cancer. Cell 100(1):57–70

He L, Mo H, Hadisusilo S, Qureshi AA, Elson CE (1997) Isoprenoids suppress the growth of murine B16 melanomas in vitro and in vivo. J Nutr 127(5):668–674

Hoensch H, Groh B, Edler L, Kirch W (2008) Prospective cohort comparison of flavonoid treatment in patients with resected colorectal cancer to prevent recurrence. World J Gastroenterol 14(14):2187–2193

Hussain A, Priyani A, Sadrieh L, Brahmbhatt K, Ahmed M, Sharma C (2011) Concurrent sulforaphane and eugenol induces differential effects on human cervical cancer cells. Integr Cancer Ther

Jyothi D, Vanathi P, Mangala Gowri P, Rama Subba Rao V, Madhusudana Rao J, Sreedhar AS (2009) Diferuloylmethane augments the cytotoxic effects of piplartine isolated from Piper chaba. Toxicol In Vitro 23(6):1085–1091

Kang OH, Lee JH, Kwon DY (2011) Apigenin inhibits release of inflammatory mediators by blocking the NF-kappaB activation pathways in the HMC-1 cells. Immunopharmacol Immunotoxicol 33(3):473–479

Kim EC, Min JK, Kim TY, Lee SJ, Yang HO, Han S, Kim YM, Kwon YG (2005) [6]-Gingerol, a pungent ingredient of ginger, inhibits angiogenesis in vitro and in vivo. Biochem Biophys Res Commun 335(2):300–308

Kim JY, Kim EH, Kim SU, Kwon TK, Choi KS (2010) Capsaicin sensitizes malignant glioma cells to TRAIL-mediated apoptosis via DR5 upregulation and survivin downregulation. Carcinogenesis 31(3):367–375

Klurfeld DM, Kritchevsky D (1986) The Western diet: an examination of its relationship with chronic disease. J Am Coll Nutr 5(5):477–485

Kunnumakkara AB, Guha S, Krishnan S, Diagaradjane P, Gelovani J, Aggarwal BB (2007) Curcumin potentiates antitumor activity of gemcitabine in an orthotopic model of pancreatic cancer through suppression of proliferation, angiogenesis, and inhibition of nuclear factor-kappaB-regulated gene products. Cancer Res 67(8):3853–3861

Kunnumakkara AB, Anand P, Aggarwal BB (2008) Curcumin inhibits proliferation, invasion, angiogenesis and metastasis of different cancers through interaction with multiple cell signaling proteins. Cancer Lett 269(2):199–225

Kunnumakkara AB, Diagaradjane P, Anand P, Harikumar KB, Deorukhkar A, Gelovani J, Guha S, Krishnan S, Aggarwal BB (2009) Curcumin sensitizes human colorectal cancer to capecitabine by modulation of cyclin D1, COX-2, MMP-9, VEGF and CXCR4 expression in an orthotopic mouse model. Int J Cancer 125(9):2187–2197

Kuttan R, Sudheeran PC, Josph CD (1987) Turmeric and curcumin as topical agents in cancer therapy. Tumori 73(1):29–31

Kvale G, Johansen A (1982) [Lung cancer in Norway. A review based on the Cancer Registry of Norway]. Tidsskr Nor Laegeforen 102(8):480–484

Lee SH, Cekanova M, Baek SJ (2008) Multiple mechanisms are involved in 6-gingerol-induced cell growth arrest and apoptosis in human colorectal cancer cells. Mol Carcinog 47(3):197–208

Levine ME, Gillis MG, Koch SY, Voss AC, Stern RM, Koch KL (2008) Protein and ginger for the treatment of chemotherapy-induced delayed nausea. J Altern Complement Med 14(5):545–551

Lin YG, Kunnumakkara AB, Nair A, Merritt WM, Han LY, Armaiz-Pena GN, Kamat AA, Spannuth WA, Gershenson DM, Lutgendorf SK, Aggarwal BB, Sood AK (2007) Curcumin inhibits tumor growth and angiogenesis in ovarian carcinoma by targeting the nuclear factor-kappaB pathway. Clin Cancer Res 13(11):3423–3430

Liu Q, Loo WT, Sze SC, Tong Y (2009) Curcumin inhibits cell proliferation of MDA-MB-231 and BT-483 breast cancer cells mediated by down-regulation of NFkappaB, cyclinD and MMP-1 transcription. Phytomedicine 16(10):916–922

Luo H, Rankin GO, Liu L, Daddysman MK, Jiang BH, Chen YC (2009) Kaempferol inhibits angiogenesis and VEGF expression through both HIF dependent and independent pathways in human ovarian cancer cells. Nutr Cancer 61(4):554–563

Manikandan P, Murugan RS, Priyadarsini RV, Vinothini G, Nagini S (2010) Eugenol induces apoptosis and inhibits invasion and angiogenesis in a rat model of gastric carcinogenesis induced by MNNG. Life Sci 86(25–26):936–941

McMahon G (2000) VEGF receptor signaling in tumor angiogenesis. Oncologist 5(Suppl 1):3–10

Min JK, Han KY, Kim EC, Kim YM, Lee SW, Kim OH, Kim KW, Gho YS, Kwon YG (2004) Capsaicin inhibits in vitro and in vivo angiogenesis. Cancer Res 64(2):644–651

Mirzoeva S, Kim ND, Chiu K, Franzen CA, Bergan RC, Pelling JC (2008) Inhibition of HIF-1 alpha and VEGF expression by the chemopreventive bioflavonoid apigenin is accompanied by Akt inhibition in human prostate carcinoma PC3-M cells. Mol Carcinog 47(9):686–700

Mo SJ, Son EW, Rhee DK, Pyo S (2003) Modulation of TNF-alpha-induced ICAM-1 expression, NO and H2O2 production by alginate, allicin and ascorbic acid in human endothelial cells. Arch Pharm Res 26(3):244–251

Molassiotis A, Margulies A, Fernandez-Ortega P, Pud D, Panteli V, Bruyns I, Scott JA, Gudmundsdottir G, Browall M, Madsen E, Ozden G, Magri M, Selvekerova S, Platin N, Kearney N, Patiraki E (2005) Complementary and alternative medicine use in patients with haematological malignancies in Europe. Complement Ther Clin Pract 11(2):105–110

Mu C, Jia P, Yan Z, Liu X, Li X, Liu H (2007) Quercetin induces cell cycle G1 arrest through elevating Cdk inhibitors p21 and p27 in human hepatoma cell line (HepG2). Methods Find Exp Clin Pharmacol 29(3):179–183

Natarajan K, Singh S, Burke TR Jr, Grunberger D, Aggarwal BB (1996) Caffeic acid phenethyl ester is a potent and specific inhibitor of activation of nuclear transcription factor NF-kappa B. Proc Natl Acad Sci U S A 93(17):9090–9095

Park BK, Lee S, Seo JN, Rhee JW, Park JB, Kim YS, Choi IG, Kim YE, Lee Y, Kwon HJ (2010) Protection of burn-induced skin injuries by the flavonoid kaempferol. BMB Rep 43(1):46–51

Plummer SM, Holloway KA, Manson MM, Munks RJ, Kaptein A, Farrow S, Howells L (1999) Inhibition of cyclo-oxygenase 2 expression in colon cells by the chemopreventive agent curcumin involves inhibition of NF-kappaB activation via the NIK/IKK signalling complex. Oncogene 18(44):6013–6020

Popovich DG, Tiaras F, Yeo CR, Zhang W (2010) Lovastatin interacts with natural products to influence cultured hepatocarcinoma cell (hep-g2) growth. J Am Coll Nutr 29(3):204–210

Pradeep CR, Kuttan G (2004) Piperine is a potent inhibitor of nuclear factor-kappaB (NF-kappaB), c-Fos, CREB, ATF-2 and proinflammatory cytokine gene expression in B16F-10 melanoma cells. Int Immunopharmacol 4(14):1795–1803

Prasad S, Ravindran J, Sung B, Pandey MK, Aggarwal BB (2010) Garcinol potentiates TRAIL-induced apoptosis through modulation of death receptors and antiapoptotic proteins. Mol Cancer Ther 9(4):856–868

Shah AH, Qureshi S, Ageel AM (1991) Toxicity studies in mice of ethanol extracts of Foeniculum vulgare fruit and Ruta chalepensis aerial parts. J Ethnopharmacol 34(2–3):167–172

Shankar S, Srivastava RK (2007) Involvement of Bcl 2 family members, phosphatidylinositol 3′-kinase/AKT and mitochondrial p53 in curcumin (diferulolylmethane)-induced apoptosis in prostate cancer. Int J Oncol 30(4):905–918

Shankar S, Ganapathy S, Srivastava RK (2008) Sulforaphane enhances the therapeutic potential of TRAIL in prostate cancer orthotopic model through regulation of apoptosis, metastasis, and angiogenesis. Clin Cancer Res 14(21):6855–6866

Shehata M, Schnabl S, Demirtas D, Hilgarth M, Hubmann R, Ponath E, Badrnya S, Lehner C, Hoelbl A, Duechler M, Gaiger A, Zielinski C, Schwarzmeier JD, Jaeger U (2010) Reconstitution of PTEN activity by CK2 inhibitors and interference with the PI3-K/Akt cascade counteract the antiapoptotic effect of human stromal cells in chronic lymphocytic leukemia. Blood 116(14):2513–2521

Singh S, Aggarwal BB (1995) Activation of transcription factor NF-kappa B is suppressed by curcumin (diferuloylmethane) [corrected]. J Biol Chem 270(42):24995–25000

Soda G, Antonaci A, Bosco D, Nardoni S, Melis M (1999) Expression of bcl-2, c-erbB-2, p53, and p21 (waf1-cip1) protein in thyroid carcinomas. J Exp Clin Cancer Res 18(3):363–367

Song Z, Steller H (1999) Death by design: mechanism and control of apoptosis. Trends Cell Biol 9(12):M49–M52

Soslow RA, Dannenberg AJ, Rush D, Woerner BM, Khan KN, Masferrer J, Koki AT (2000) COX-2 is expressed in human pulmonary, colonic, and mammary tumors. Cancer 89(12):2637–2645

Steller H (1995) Mechanisms and genes of cellular suicide. Science 267(5203):1445–1449

Subbaramaiah K, Dannenberg AJ (2003) Cyclooxygenase 2: a molecular target for cancer prevention and treatment. Trends Pharmacol Sci 24(2):96–102

Sung B, Kunnumakkara AB, Sethi G, Anand P, Guha S, Aggarwal BB (2009) Curcumin circumvents chemoresistance in vitro and potentiates the effect of thalidomide and bortezomib against human multiple myeloma in nude mice model. Mol Cancer Ther 8(4):959–970

Surh YJ, Lee SS (1995) Capsaicin, a double-edged sword: toxicity, metabolism, and chemopreventive potential. Life Sci 56(22):1845–1855

Tanaka S, Haruma K, Yoshihara M, Kajiyama G, Kira K, Amagase H, Chayama K (2006) Aged garlic extract has potential suppressive effect on colorectal adenomas in humans. J Nutr 136(3 Suppl):821S–826S

Thejass P, Kuttan G (2007) Antiangiogenic activity of diallyl sulfide (DAS). Int Immunopharmacol 7(3):295–305

Touillaud MS, Pillow PC, Jakovljevic J, Bondy ML, Singletary SE, Li D, Chang S (2005) Effect of dietary intake of phytoestrogens on estrogen receptor status in premenopausal women with breast cancer. Nutr Cancer 51(2):162–169

Uma Pradeep K, Geervani P, Eggum BO (1993) Common Indian spices: nutrient composition, consumption and contribution to dietary value. Plant Foods Hum Nutr 44(2):137–148

Velmurugan B, Mani A, Nagini S (2005) Combination of S-allylcysteine and lycopene induces apoptosis by modulating Bcl-2, Bax, Bim and caspases during experimental gastric carcinogenesis. Eur J Cancer Prev 14(4):387–393

Wang S, Yang D, Lippman ME (2003) Targeting Bcl-2 and Bcl-XL with nonpeptidic small-molecule antagonists. Semin Oncol 30(5 Suppl 16):133–142

Xu C, Shen G, Chen C, Gelinas C, Kong AN (2005) Suppression of NF-kappaB and NF-kappaB-regulated gene expression by sulforaphane and PEITC through IkappaBalpha, IKK pathway in human prostate cancer PC-3 cells. Oncogene 24(28):4486–4495

Zheng X, Ryan A, Patel N, Klemons S, Hansson A, Shih WJ, Lin Y, Huberman E, Chang RL, Conney AH (2005) Synergistic stimulatory effect of 12-O-tetradecanoylphorbol-13-acetate and capsaicin on macrophage differentiation in HL-60 and HL-525 human myeloid leukemia cells. Int J Oncol 26(2):441–448

Chapter 3
Chemoprevention of Prostate Cancer with Cruciferous Vegetables: Role of Epigenetics

Laura M. Beaver, David E. Williams, Roderick H. Dashwood, and Emily Ho

Contents

L.M. Beaver • D.E. Williams • R.H. Dashwood • E. Ho (✉)
Linus Pauling Institute, Oregon State University, Corvallis, OR 97331-6512, USA

L.M. Beaver • E. Ho
Department of Nutrition and Exercise Sciences, Oregon State University, 117 Milam Hall, Corvallis, OR 97331, USA
e-mail: beaver@onid.orst.edu; Emily.Ho@oregonstate.edu

D.E. Williams • R.H. Dashwood
Department of Environmental and Molecular Toxicology, Oregon State University, Corvallis, OR, USA
e-mail: david.williams@oregonstate.edu; rod.dashwood@oregonstate.edu

S. Shankar and R.K. Srivastava (eds.), *Nutrition, Diet and Cancer*,
DOI 10.1007/978-94-007-2923-0_3,

Abstract Globally, prostate cancer is the second most frequently diagnosed cancer in men although the incidence of cancer varies greatly throughout the world. Nutrition and diet are important modifiable risk factors for prostate cancer development. Epidemiological studies have shown an inverse association between cruciferous vegetable intake and the risk of developing prostate cancer. Here we focus specifically on the molecular mechanisms by which phytochemicals in cruciferous vegetables, sulforaphane (SFN), indole-3-carbinol (I3C) and its derivative 3,3′-diindolylmethane (DIM), may prevent the initiation of prostate cancer and slow tumorigenesis. We have particularly emphasized a possible role for epigenetics in this process as many dietary factors can modulate epigenetic alterations and alter susceptibility to disease. We have identified known and possible epigenetic mechanisms by which these phytochemicals can alter detoxification pathways, sex hormone signaling, and genes that regulate cell cycle, apoptosis, inflammation, angiogenesis and metastasis. The ability of SFN, I3C or DIM to target aberrant epigenetic patterns, in addition to their effects on detoxification/carcinogen metabolism, may make them effective chemoprevention agents at multiple stages of the prostate carcinogenesis pathway. The identification of dietary epigenetic modulators and their use either alone or in combination, may increase efficacy of anti-cancer therapies and prevention strategies, without serious side effects.

Introduction

Globally, prostate cancer is the second most frequently diagnosed cancer in men (International Agency for Research on Cancer 2010). North American countries have some of the highest incidences of prostate cancer whereas Asian countries tend to have the lowest incidence (International Agency for Research on Cancer 2010). Other than skin cancer, prostate cancer is the most prevalent cancer in American men and the second leading cause of cancer-related death (Jemal et al. 2011; American Cancer Society 2011). In the United States 1 in 6 men will develop prostate cancer during their lifetime and in 2011 approximately 240,890 new cases of prostate cancer were diagnosed (Howlader et al. 2011; American Cancer Society 2011). These numbers illustrate the great burden of this disease both in the US and throughout the world. Nutrition and diet appear to be important modifiable risk factors for prostate cancer development. For example, the risk of developing prostate cancer increases with obesity (Hsing et al. 2007) and increased consumption of red meats (John et al. 2011). In contrast, increased consumption of fruits and vegetables has been associated with a decreased risk for prostate cancer (Ambrosini et al. 2008; Kolonel et al. 2000). Given the potential of fruits and vegetables to prevent prostate cancer or delay the onset of cancer, identification of specific dietary components that alter disease outcomes has become a great public health and research interest. Examination of the literature reveals that many compounds found in the diet may reduce prostate cancer incidence. This includes, but is not limited to, organosulfur compounds found in garlic, lycopene found in the tomato, tea catechins, soy isoflavones, and the microminerals zinc and selenium (Colli and Amling 2009; Ho and Song 2009; Venkateswaran and Klotz 2010).

In particular, epidemiological and experimental based studies support a possible role for cruciferous vegetables in the prevention of prostate cancer (Higdon et al. 2007). The family of cruciferous vegetables (*Brassicaceae*) includes vegetables such as broccoli, cauliflower, cabbage, collard greens, Brussels sprouts, watercress, bok choy and kale (Higdon et al. 2007). These vegetables are widely regarded as healthy because they are a good source of a variety of nutrients and phytochemicals with cancer chemopreventative properties including fiber, folate, carotenoids, chlorophyll and glucosinolates. Glucosinolates are sulfur-containing compounds that give cruciferous vegetables their characteristic pungent aroma and spicy or bitter taste (Higdon et al. 2007). Glucosinolates are also the source of the anti-carcinogenic phytochemicals sulforaphane (SFN) and indole-3-carbinol (I3C) (Steinbrecher et al. 2009). The mean daily intake of cruciferous vegetables in Chinese and Japanese diets is 40 g and 55 g per day, compared to the 12 g/day consumed by the average person in the United States (International Agency For Research On Cancer 2010). Epidemiological studies have shown an inverse association between cruciferous vegetable intake and cancer risk in many tissues including the prostate (Table 3.1). Interestingly, a recent analysis of the EPIC-Heidelberg cohort study showed that the risk of prostate cancer decreased significantly when specifically comparing glucosinolate intake (Steinbrecher et al. 2009).

Prostate cancer is the uncontrolled growth of abnormal cells originating from the prostate, a small gland in the male reproductive system. The "hallmarks" of this disease includes the capacity of the abnormal cells to resist cell death, evade growth suppression, and induce proliferative signals, genomic instability, tumor-promoting inflammation, angiogenesis, invasion and metastasis to distant organs (Hanahan and Weinberg 2011). These hallmarks are driven by dysregulation of expression of genes that control these cellular phenotypes. Historically, mutations in DNA and genetic abnormalities have been cited as the cause for this dysregulation but epigenetic mechanisms that alter gene expression are also fundamental in cancer development (Boumber and Issa 2011). Epigenetics is defined as heritable changes in gene expression that are not caused by changes in DNA sequence (Feinberg 2007). Modification of histones, methylation of DNA, and interfering micro RNAs (miRNA) are all epigenetic mechanisms that play an important role in prostate cancer development (Abbas and Gupta 2008; Dobosy et al. 2007). Importantly, dietary factors and specific nutrients can modulate epigenetic alterations and alter susceptibility to disease. In this chapter we will focus on the mechanisms by which the dietary compounds derived from cruciferous vegetables, specifically SFN and I3C, may act to prevent prostate cancer. Furthermore, we will examine if these phytochemicals can act through epigenetic mechanisms in order to reduce cancer development.

Table 3.1 Cruciferous vegetables and prostate cancer risk in humans

Reference	Year	Study population	Food source	Finding for prostate cancer
Steinbrecher et al. (2009)	2009	11,405 men in the EPIC-Heidelberg cohort study	Glucosinolates	Reduced risk
Ambrosini et al. (2008)	2008	11,798 individuals in Australia	23 Fruit and vegetables	Reduced risk with increased consumption of broccoli
Joseph et al. (2004)	2004	456 men with prostate cancer and 537 controls	– Cruciferous vegetables – Broccoli	– Reduced risk – Reduced risk
Key et al. (2004)	2004	130,544 men in 7 countries in Europe (EPIC)	– Fruit and vegetables – Cruciferous vegetables	– No significant association – No significant association
Giovannucci et al. (2003)	2003	47,365 men in the Health Professionals Follow-Up Study	Cruciferous vegetables	– Trend, reduced risk of organ confined prostate cancer – Trend of reduced risk was stronger in men < 65 years
Kolonel et al. (2000)	2000	1619 men with prostate cancer and 1618 controls in USA and Canada	Fruits, vegetables, soy and legumes	– Reduced risk of prostate cancer with increased consumption of cruciferous vegetables
Cohen et al. (2000)	2000	628 men with prostate cancer and 602 controls in USA	– Fruits and vegetables – Cruciferous vegetables	– No significant association – Reduced risk of prostate cancer
Jain et al. (1999)	1999	617 men with prostate cancer and 636 population controls in Canada	Cruciferous vegetables	Reduced risk
Schuurman et al. (1998)	1998	610 men in Netherlands Cohort Study	21 Vegetables and 8 fruits	– Did not reduce the risk – Consumption of kale had a trend towards reduced risk
Le Marchand et al. (1991)	1991	452 men with prostate cancer, 899 controls, Hawaii	Cruciferous vegetables	– No significant association
Hsing et al. (1990)	1990	17,633 white men in Lutheran Brotherhood study	35 Food items	– No association between consumption of fruit and vegetables and prostate cancer
Graham et al. (1983)	1983	260 men with prostate cancer and controls in USA	Cruciferous vegetables	Trend towards reduced risk

Sulforaphane (SFN)

Cruciferous vegetables contain high concentrations of glucosinolates, which are hydrolyzed to isothiocyanates (ITCs) by myrosinase, an enzyme endogenous in the plant and present in colonic microflora (Shapiro et al. 1998). Within the plant, glucosinolate content can vary greatly between and within members of the Cruciferae family depending on cultivation environment and genotype (Kushad et al. 1999) and there are over 120 glucosinolates in the various varieties of cruciferous vegetables, each yielding different aglycone metabolic products including isothiocyanates (Mithen 2001). The general structure of glucosinolate consists of a β-D-thioglucose group, a sulfonated oxime group, and a variable side chain. Many of the anticancer effects observed from cruciferous vegetables have been attributed to the ITCs rather than their parent glucosinolates. SFN is a well studied ITC derived from the glucosinolate glucoraphanin (Fig. 3.1a), which is

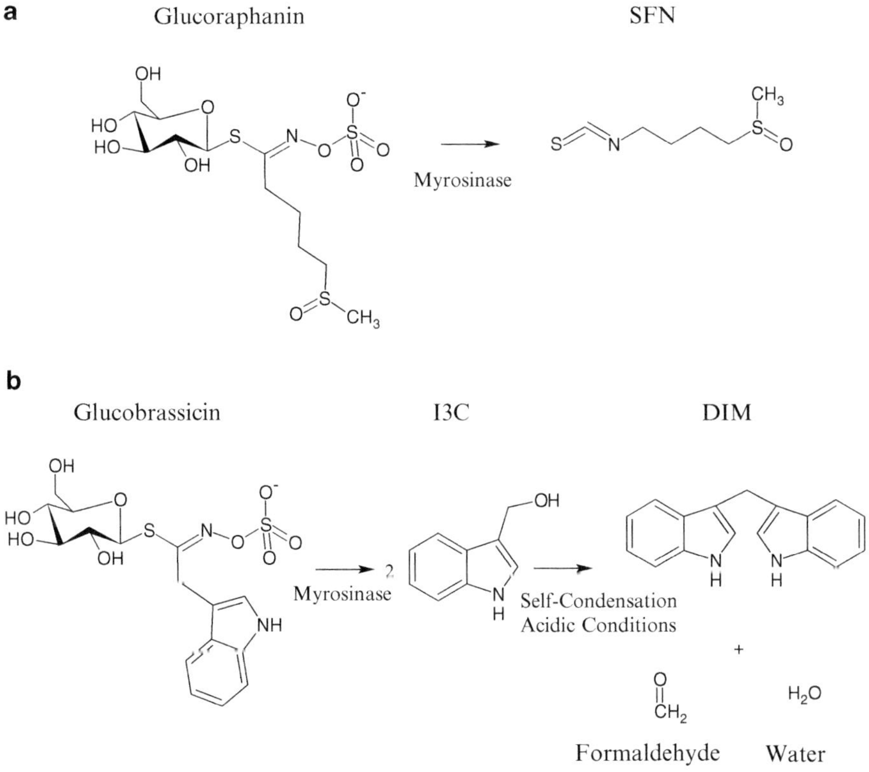

Fig. 3.1 Chemical structures of several phytochemicals from cruciferous vegetables. (**a**) SFN is produced through the hydrolysis of glucoraphanin by the enzyme myrosinase. (**b**) I3C is produced by the breakdown of glucobrassicin by the myrosinase enzyme. Under acidic conditions I3C undergoes self-condensation and the primary product is DIM. Water and formaldehyde are also produced in this reaction

abundant in broccoli and broccoli sprouts. After absorption, SFN is predominantly metabolized via the mercapturic acid pathway. In these reactions, the electrophilic central carbon of the –N=C=S group in SFN reacts with the sulfhydryl group of GSH to form a dithiocarbamate GSH conjugate. The enzymes that catalyze GSH conjugation to SFN are the family of glutathione-*S*-transferase (GST) enzymes. The final steps in SFN metabolism is formation of SFN-cysteine (SFN-Cys) followed by SFN-*N*-acetylcysteine (SFN-NAC) (Kassahun et al. 1997; Rajendran et al. 2011b).

Pharmacokinetic studies in both rats and humans also support that SFN can be distributed in the body and reach μM concentrations in the blood. In rats, following a 50 μmol gavage of SFN, detectable SFN was evident after 1 h and peaked at 20 μM at 4 h, with a half life of approximately 2.2 h (Hu et al. 2004). In another study, mice supplemented with 300 or 600 ppm SFN, accumulated SFN and SFN-GSH plasma concentrations of 124–254 nM and 579–770 nM, respectively. Also SFN and SFN-GSH concentrations in the small intestine were between 3 and 13 nmol/g of tissue and 14–32 nmol/g of tissue, respectively, which is equivalent to roughly 3–30 μM of total SFN. Notably, the accumulation of SFN in colonic tissue corresponded with decreased adenoma formation in these animals (Hu et al. 2006). In mouse gavage studies, administration of 5 μmol SFN caused increases in SFN content in tissues including brain, liver, kidney, small intestine (SI) mucosa, colonic mucosa, lung and prostate at 2 and 6 h. Concentrations were highest in the SI, prostate, kidney and lung, and lowest in the brain. In the prostate, the total sum of all SFN metabolites was 0.066 nmol/mg tissue 2 h following a dose of 5 μmol SFN by gavage (Clarke et al. 2011). Interestingly, free SFN is not the major compound present in tissues of mice given SFN, but rather the glutathione, cysteinyl, and *N*-acetylcysteine conjugates of SFN are the most abundant. In, human subjects given a single dose of 200 μmol broccoli sprouts preparation (largely SFN with lesser amounts of other ITCs), ITC plasma concentrations peaked between 0.943 and 2.27 μM 1 h after feeding, with a half life of 1.77 ± 0.13 h (Ye et al. 2002). In humans, SFN and its metabolites were excreted with first-order kinetics (Shapiro et al. 1998; Ye et al. 2002) and most data indicate that SFN and its metabolites are cleared from the body within 72 h of dosing (Cramer and Jeffery 2011). To date bioavailability of SFN to the prostate in humans is unknown. However, in human mammary tissue, an oral dose 1 h prior to breast surgery of broccoli sprout preparation containing 200 μmol SFN showed that mean epithelial-/stromal-enriched breast tissue dithiocarbamate concentrations were 1.45 ± 1.12 and 2.00 ± 1.95 pmol/mg tissue for the right and left breast, respectively (Cornblatt et al. 2007). From these data it can be extrapolated that maintenance of SFN concentrations in the body can be achieved by consuming recommended servings of cruciferous vegetables once a day. Collectively, the published data indicate that SFN can be absorbed, reach μM concentrations in the blood, accumulate in tissues, and be maintained to achieve the anticancer effects.

Sulforaphane and Prostate Cancer: Preclinical and Clinical Studies

In preclinical rodent models, there is significant data supporting the chemopreventive effects of SFN at several stages of carcinogenesis. Administration of SFN by gavage or in the diet reduces the growth of prostate cancer xenografts in immune-deficient mice (Myzak et al. 2007; Singh et al. 2004). Oral gavage of 6 μmol SFN three times weekly also reduced prostate tumor growth and pulmonary metastasis in the Transgenic Adenocarcinoma of Mouse Prostate (TRAMP) mouse model of prostate cancer (Singh et al. 2009). Dietary SFN, given in the form of broccoli sprouts (240 mg/day), also slows prostate tumor growth in TRAMP mice (Keum et al. 2009). To date very few human clinical trials have evaluated the effects of SFN on prostate bioavailability and/or cancer outcome, however, several pilot and phase 1 human SFN trials have been conducted utilizing different sources of SFN (Egner et al. 2011). In one randomized study a placebo-controlled, double-blind, phase 1 clinical trial of healthy volunteers was undertaken and used glucoraphanin or isothiocyanate as the SFN source (Shapiro et al. 2006). The phase 1 trial consisted of three study groups; 25 μmol of glucosinolate, 100 μmol of glucosinolate, or 25 μmol ITC for 7 days and examined parameters of safety, tolerance, and pharmacokinetics. Importantly, there were no significant toxicities associated with taking the extracts at the doses employed. In women given an oral dose of broccoli sprout preparation, the transcript levels of detoxification genes NAD(P)H:quinone oxidoreductase (NQO1) and heme oxygenase-1 (HO-1) targets of NRF2, were measured in both breasts of all subjects (Cornblatt et al. 2007). This data provides a proof of principle that these measures can be detected in a clinical trial (Cornblatt et al. 2007). Interventions with broccoli rich diets for 6 or 12 months did not induce NRF2-regulated genes in gastric mucosa or prostate tissue (Gasper et al. 2007; Traka et al. 2008). However, the 6 month broccoli-rich diets did result in changes in insulin and epidermal growth factor (EGF) signaling in the prostate tissue of men diagnosed with high grade Prostatic Intraepithelial Neoplasia (PIN) (Traka et al. 2008). It has been hypothesized that enhanced AKT phosphorylation are also targets of SFN, especially in the absence of PTEN (Traka et al. 2010). These clinical trials provide the important link to human relevance for SFN as a promising cancer prevention agent.

Molecular Targets of SFN

SFN acts through diverse cellular mechanisms at various stages of prostate cancer development including initiation, promotion and metastasis. At the initiation stage, early research has focused on Phase II enzyme induction by SFN, as well as the inhibition of Phase I enzymes (Clarke et al. 2008). These enzymes are involved in the metabolism and activation of carcinogens (Clarke et al. 2008). The mechanisms contributing to this "blocking activity" of SFN, has focused on Nrf2 signaling and antioxidant response element (ARE)-driven gene expression (Clarke et al. 2008). For example, the chemoprotective effects of SFN have been attributed to its ability to up-regulate (HO-1) and the Phase II detoxification systems such as NQO1 epoxide hydrolase, and gamma-glutamylcysteine synthetase (rate-limiting enzyme in glutathione synthesis). This occurs through activation via ARE sites in the 5′-flanking region of the corresponding genes. Upregulation of Phase II metabolism is likely a critical mechanism leading to cancer prevention by SFN in the "initiation" phase, helping to more rapidly eliminate genotoxins from the body.

Recent studies also suggest that SFN offers protection against tumor development during the "post-initiation" phase and mechanisms for "suppression" effects of SFN are of particular interest. Multiple mechanisms have been postulated for the effects of SFN post-initiation including activation of mitogen-activated protein kinases (MAPK), suppression of AKT phosphorylation, inhibition of nuclear factor κ-B (NF-κB) and AP1, modulation of androgen receptor (AR) and the induction of reactive oxygen species (ROS) (reviewed in Clarke et al. 2008). In vivo, regression of prostate tumors in TRAMP mice correlates with an induction of Nrf2 and upregulation of pro-apoptotic markers cleaved caspase-3, cleaved PARP and Bax (Keum et al. 2009). It has also been proposed that SFN administration inhibits prostate cancer progression and metastasis by increasing cytotoxicity of natural killer cells (Singh et al. 2009).

In particular, SFN affects pathways involved in cell cycle arrest and the induction of apoptosis. *In vitro* experiments with SFN indicate a pronounced role for cell cycle arrest in its anticancer properties. Cell cycle progression is controlled by cyclin-dependent kinases (CDKs) and their activities are further regulated by cyclins and CDK inhibitors. The expression of these proteins, in conjunction with cell cycle checkpoint regulators like Chk kinases and Cdc phosphatases, determines if the cell arrests or moves through various points of the cell cycle. In LnCap prostate cancer cells, a dramatic increase in G_2/M phase arrest occurred in a concentration- and time-dependent manner concomitant with induction of cyclin B1, Chk2 kinase, and down-regulation of Cdk1 and Cdc25C protein levels (Herman-Antosiewicz et al. 2007). In addition, 10 μM SFN treatment in DU145 prostate cancer cells reduced cell viability and induced G_2/M cell cycle arrest (Cho et al. 2005). Although G_2/M arrest is the predominant stage of cell cycle arrest induced by SFN (Gamet-Payrastre 2006; Parnaud et al. 2004), arrest at other phases of the cell cycle occurs in both prostate cells. A G_1/S block in LnCap and DU145 prostate cells has also been reported at concentrations at or below 10 μM (Chiao et al. 2002; Wang et al. 2004). The tumor suppressor and cell cycle inhibitor protein p21 appears to play an important role in SFN-induced cell cycle arrest. An induction of p21 is consistently observed regardless of cell type and p53 status (Clarke et al. 2011; Herman-Antosiewicz et al. 2007; Myzak et al. 2006b; Nian et al. 2009; Shen et al. 2006). In mice, dietary SFN supplementation also induced the expression of genes involved in cell cycle arrest and apoptosis, specifically in the prostate where genetics was used to create a PTEN-null tissue, but this was not observed in wild-type tissues (Traka et al. 2010).

Kallifatidis et al., recently found that SFN also sensitizes pancreatic and prostate cancer cells to chemotherapeutics such as cisplatin, gecitabine, doxorubicin and 5-fluorouracil (Kallifatidis et al. 2011).

Role of Epigenetics in the Action of SFN

DNA is associated with histone proteins in the nucleus of cells. Histone proteins interact with each other and the DNA in order to form a structure termed the nucleosome (Fig. 3.2a). When DNA tightly interacts with histones through their protein tails, a closed DNA structure is formed which is transcriptionally inert (Fig. 3.2a and reviewed in Perry et al. 2010). This is usually accompanied by a high level of methylation of the DNA at cytosine residues which is regulated by DNA methyltransferases (DNMTs). This closed chromatin structure is also generally associated with the hypoacetylation of histone tails. This is achieved through the deacetylation of histones by histone deacetylases (HDACs) (Fig. 3.2a). Acetylation of histones by histone acetyltransferases (HATs) and removal of DNA methylation causes the DNA structure to become more accessible to transcription factors, which bind DNA and activate gene transcription (Fig. 3.2b). In cancer cells, the balance between HAT and HDAC activities is disrupted and higher levels of HDAC proteins are commonly observed causing the epigenetic silencing of tumor suppressor genes (reviewed in Perry et al. 2010). Cancer cells are also characterized by global hypomethylation of DNA and site specific hypermethylation of specific genes involved in cancer progression (reviewed in Perry et al. 2010).

HDAC inhibition is emerging as a promising field in cancer chemoprevention and therapy. Increased HDAC activity and expression can result in repression of transcription that results in a de-regulation of differentiation, cell cycle and apoptotic mechanisms. Moreover, tumor suppressor genes, such as *p21*, appear to be targets of HDACs and are "turned off", or transcriptionally silenced, by deacetylation. HDAC1, a class I HDAC, is over-expressed and localized in the nucleus in hormone-refractory prostate cancer (Halkidou et al. 2004). It has also been shown that Sirt1, the predominant class III NAD^+ dependent HDAC, is over-expressed in both human and mouse prostate cancers (Huffman et al. 2007). In human patient samples, global decreases in histone acetylation corresponded with increased grade of cancer and risk of prostate cancer recurrence (Seligson et al. 2005). Taken together these findings support the hypothesis that overactive HDAC activity and hypoacetylation may contribute to prostate cancer progression. Several clinical trials are currently ongoing aimed at establishing the chemotherapeutic efficacy of HDAC inhibitors, based on evidence that cancer cells undergo cell cycle arrest, differentiation and apoptosis *in vitro*, and that tumor volume and/or tumor number may be reduced in animal models. Strikingly, the effects of HDAC inhibition occur preferentially in cancer cells and not normal cells (Johnstone 2002).

According to several reports, SFN may act as a dietary epigenetic modulator in cancer cells with the strongest evidence as an HDAC inhibitor and modulator

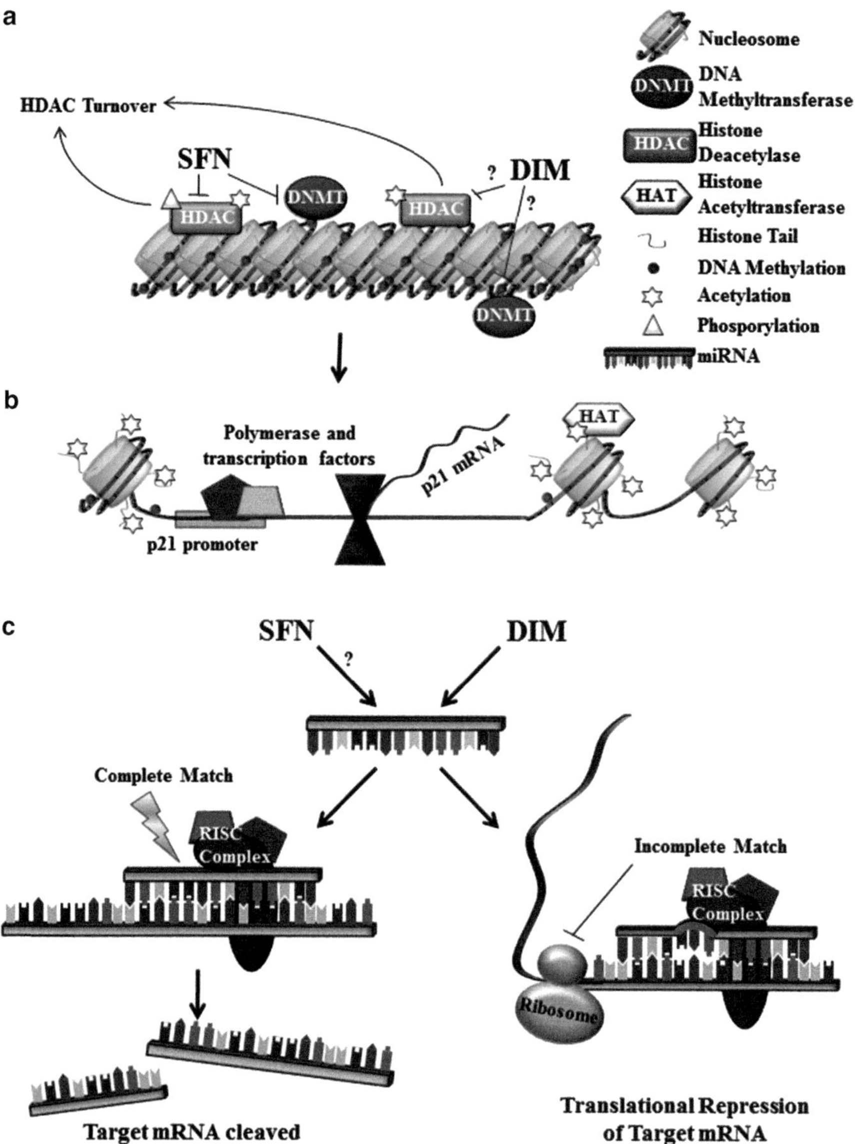

Fig. 3.2 Epigenetic Mechanisms that SFN and I3C/DIM May Effect Gene Expression. (**a**) A closed chromatin structure is generally associated with hypoacetylation achieved by histone deacetylases (HDACs) and a high level of DNA methylation which is regulated by DNA methyltransferases (DNMTs). SFN inhibits HDACs (Clarke et al. 2011) and DNMTs (Hsu et al. 2011). SFN and DIM treatments lead to turnover of HDAC proteins (Li et al. 2010a; Rajendran et al. 2011a) (**b**) SFN facilitates an open chromatin structure and expression of tumor suppressor genes. The open chromatin structure is associated with increased acetylation of histone tails by histone acetyltransferases (HATs). (**c**) miRNAs disrupt the translation of mRNA through an interact with the target mRNA and the RISC protein complex. DIM has been shown to change expression of miRNAs in prostate cancer cells (Li et al. 2009)

of DNA methylation. Biochemical assays found that SFN metabolites did indeed inhibit HDAC activity *in vitro*, the greatest inhibition involving SFN-NAC and SFN-Cys. Molecular modeling in the active site of an HDAC enzyme provided evidence that SFN-Cys is acting as a competitive inhibitor (Myzak et al. 2004). In addition to competitive inhibition, recent research has shown that SFN causes a decrease in specific HDAC protein expression. Treatment of transformed prostate cells with 15 μM SFN causes a selective decrease in both Class I (HDAC3) and Class II HDAC (HDAC6) proteins (Clarke et al. 2011). The loss of Class II HDACs has important implications in modulating the acetylation of non-histone proteins such as tubulin and HSP90, which have roles in controlling apoptosis/autophagy pathways and androgen receptor stability, respectively. The loss of HDAC3 protein may be related to alteration in HDAC protein turnover and disruption of the HDAC3/SMRT co-repressor complex (Rajendran et al. 2011a). Interestingly, similar to pharmacological HDAC inhibitors, we have found that 15 μM SFN causes potent HDAC inhibition and G2/M arrest in LnCaP and PC3 cancer cells, but has no effect on normal prostate epithelial cells (Clarke et al. 2011). These data support the hypothesis that HDAC inhibition may be an important mechanism of chemoprevention for SFN and the cytotoxic effects are specific to cancer, not normal cells.

SFN-mediated epigenetic alterations may not only be limited to HDAC regulation. Recent studies suggest that SFN may play an important role in methyl CpG-binding proteins' recruitment of HDAC family members (Traka et al. 2005). In breast cancer cells, SFN suppresses DNA methylation in the promoter of the telomerase reverse transcriptase gene (*hTERT*), leading to transcriptional repression of a gene that is upregulated in most cancers (Meeran et al. 2010). Studies in our own lab have also demonstrated significant decreases in DNA methyltransferase expression in LnCaP cells that is coupled with hypomethylation of the cyclinD2 promoter following SFN treatment (unpublished data). The effects of SFN on miRNA targets are currently unclear (Fig. 3.2c). Many of the molecular targets discussed for SFN can also be linked to alteration of epigenetics and will be discussed in the following section.

Pre-initiation Mechanisms and SFN: Role of Epigenetics

Detoxification Mechanism

Kelch-like ECH-associated protein 1 (Keap1) is a cysteine rich protein which, in its dimeric form, interacts with Nrf2 sequestering it the cytosol, thereby inhibiting its transcriptional activity. Several models have been suggested to explain how Keap1 regulates Nrf2. In the most widely accepted model, two cysteine residues, C273 and C288, are important for the dissociation of Keap1 from Nrf2. The traditional dogma is that SFN is able to react with the thiol groups of Keap1 and form thionacyl adducts promoting Nrf2 dissociation from Keap1 and subsequent activation of

ARE-driven gene expression. The disruption of Keap1 and the induction nrf2/ARE-related genes has for many years been the "classic" chemoprevention mechanism associated with SFN. However, several SFN intervention studies in rodents and humans have shown no increase in the expression of Nrf2-regulated genes with SFN treatments. Treatment with 1 μmol SFN/g diet for up to 8 weeks in PTEN-null and wild-type mice did not induce Nrf2-regulated genes in the prostate (Traka et al. 2010). In human volunteers, acute administration of a standard broccoli meal or a 12 month intervention of a broccoli-rich diet did not induce Nrf2-related gene expression in gastric mucosa (Gasper et al. 2007) or prostate (Traka et al. 2008), respectively.

Regardless, Nrf2 itself is epigenetically regulated and there exist several possible interrelationships between Nrf2 activation and epigenetic regulation. Yu and colleagues demonstrated that Nrf2 expression was suppressed in prostate tumors derived from TRAMP mice (Yu et al. 2010). Moreover, the silencing of Nrf2 was attributed to both promoter hypermethylation and histone modifications. The addition of pharmacological DNMT inhibitors and/or HDAC inhibitors restored the expression and activity of Nrf2 (Yu et al. 2010). Thus, the addition of dietary DNMT or HDAC inhibitors, such as sulforaphane, may have effects on Nrf2 activation at the epigenetic level in addition to its effects on Keap1. Although Nrf2 activation may be controlled, in part, by epigenetic mechanisms, it does not appear that the epigenetic effects of SFN depend on Nrf2. HT-29 colon cancer cells, which lack endogenous Nrf2 protein, and Nrf2$^{-/-}$ mouse embryonic fibroblasts, both exhibited an HDAC inhibitory response to SFN treatment (unpublished results). These results indicated the possibility of a separate SFN chemoprevention pathway distinct from the classic Nrf2 pathway.

In contrast to the intense study of covalent modifications that drive the dissociation of Keap1 and activation of Nrf2, the covalent modifications that control the activity of Nrf2 after it has been released from Keap1 are not as well understood. There exists increasing evidence in the literature that post-translation modifications to Nrf2 following dissociation also play a role in its transcriptional activity. More recently, Kawai etal. demonstrated that direct acetylation of Nrf2 in the nucleus via acetyltransferases such as CBP facilitates its binding to the ARE and subsequent transcriptional activation. In contrast, deacetylation, likely by Sirt1 disrupts ARE binding, decreases transcriptional activity and results in nuclear export of Nrf2 (Kawai et al. 2011; Mercado et al. 2011). In addition to direct epigenetic modification of Nrf2, downstream factors of Nrf2 also appear to be modulated by epigenetics. Hypermethylation of the π family of glutathione-S-transferase (GSTp1), a Nrf2-inducible gene, is one of the most frequent epigenetic modifications in prostate cancer (DeMarzo et al. 2003; Dobosy et al. 2007; Gonzalgo et al. 2003; Harden et al. 2003; Jeronimo et al. 2004; Li et al. 2005a) and has been investigated as an alternative to Prostate Specific Antigen (PSA) as an early detection biomarker. In fact, many of the commonly silenced genes include tumor suppressor genes and genes involved in carcinogen detoxification, hormonal responses and cell cycle control (Baylin et al. 2001; Baylin and Ohm 2006; Herman and Baylin 2003; Li et al. 2005a). Since DNA hypermethylation-based silencing may couple with and depend on histone deacetylation, dietary HDAC and/or DNMT inhibitors could have a profound effect on the expression of these silenced detoxification genes. For example, phenethyl isothiocyanate (PEITC), another ITC found in cruciferous vegetables such as watercress, was able to reverse hypermethylation of *GSTP1* promoter elements in androgen-dependent and androgen-independent prostate cancer cells. Concurrent with demethylation effects, PEITC (2–5 μM) was able to inhibit HDAC activity and increase acetylated histones. The effectiveness of PEITC on promoter demethylation and HDAC inhibition was greater than the chemical DNMT and HDAC inhibitors, 5-aza and TSA (Wang et al. 2007). Currently the effects of SFN on Nrf2 acetylation or methylation of GSTP1 and subsequent re-expression are unknown.

Post-initiation Mechanisms and SFN: Role of Epigenetics

Apoptosis and Cell Cycle Arrest

Over-expression of Class I HDACs have been reported in prostate cancer tumors (Nakagawa et al. 2007; Weichert et al. 2008). Moreover, inhibition of Class I HDACs has direct effects that result in cell cycle arrest and apoptosis (Li et al. 2005a; Weichert et al. 2008). The best documented epigenetic target of SFN is the inhibition of HDACs in cancer cells and the subsequent upregulation of p21 and Bax expression. More specifically, in BPH1, PC3, and LnCap prostate cancer cells, SFN inhibited HDAC activity and expression of some HDACs with a concomitant increase in global histone acetylation (Clarke et al. 2011; Myzak et al. 2006b). This was also shown to increase acetylated histone interactions with the *p21* and *Bax* promoter, and induction of p21 and Bax mRNA and protein levels (Clarke et al. 2011; Myzak et al. 2006b). This HDAC inhibition coincided with the induction of G_2/M phase cell cycle arrest and apoptosis as indicated by multi-caspase activation (Myzak et al. 2006b). Furthermore, in prostate cancer xenograft studies, dietary SFN supplementation resulted in significant HDAC inhibition and slower tumor growth (Dashwood and Ho 2007). Taken together, these studies provide compelling evidence that the changes in class I HDAC proteins and histone acetylation may be responsible for the changes in cell fate.

These data on SFN inhibiting HDACs and inducing p21 and Bax expression in prostate cancer are supported by literature on SFN and colon cancer. *In vivo*, mice were given a single oral gavage dose of 10 μM SFN or SFN-NAC and HDAC inhibition was observed with a concomitant increase in acetylated histones and induction of p21 in the colonic mucosa. In dietary studies, *Apc*^{min} mice were fed 6 μmol SFN/day for 10 weeks. In these experiments a significant decrease in intestinal polyps and an increase in global acetylated histones H3 and H4 were observed, with specific increases at the *Bax* and *p21* promoters (Myzak et al. 2006a). Another report showed that siRNA knockdown of HDAC3 in SW480 colon cancer cells increased acetylated H4-K12 at the *p21* promoter, induced p21 expression and potentiated butyrate induced cell cycle arrest and growth inhibition (Spurling et al. 2008). From these prostate and colon cancer studies it can be concluded that HDAC inhibition represents a novel chemoprevention mechanism by which SFN might promote cell cycle arrest and apoptosis.

Another epigenetic mechanism by which SFN may affect cell cycle involves the G1 to S phase transition which is controlled by D-type cyclins (D1, D2, and D3) (Zhang 1999). Dysregulation of cyclin Ds disrupts cell cycle control and promotes neoplastic transformation. *Cyclin D2/ CCND2* has been identified in several cancers as a proto-oncogene. In prostate cancer, increased *cyclin D2* promoter methylation corresponds to a decrease in *cyclin D2* mRNA expression, and correlates with higher Gleason scores and pathologic features of tumor aggressiveness (Henrique et al. 2006). Recent results indicate that SFN may act as a DNA methyltransferase (DNMT) inhibitor resulting in de-methylation of the *cyclin D2* promoter and de-repression of *cyclin D2* expression, suggesting a novel mechanism behind SFN's growth inhibitory effects on prostate cancer cells (Hsu et al. 2011).

When discussing SFN and apoptosis, it is also important to note that SFN also modulates Class II HDACs, such as HDAC6 (Clarke et al. 2011). Over-expression of HDAC6 rescues PC3 cells from SFN-induced decreases in cell viability suggesting that HDAC6 plays a critical role in mediating its cytotoxicity (Clarke et al. 2011). The inhibition of HDAC6 could play a key role in the stabilization of microtubule networks, disruption of tubulin polymerization and ultimately contribute to the mitotic cell cycle arrest observed with SFN treatment (Azarenko et al. 2008; Jackson and Singletary 2004). The link between tubulin acetylation and selectively toxicity towards cancer cells has been reported after treatment with the HDAC6 specific inhibitor tubacin. Treatment with tubacin induced a dose and time dependent increase in α-tubulin acetylation and ultimately cytotoxicity in several multiple myeloma cell lines and bone marrow plasma cells, but had no effect in normal peripheral blood mononuclear cells (Hideshima et al. 2005). Autophagy is another cellular response that is partially mediated by HDAC6 because it functions to deliver polyubiquitinated proteins to aggresomes for degradation by binding both the polyubiquitinated proteins and the microtubule motor dynein (Rodriguez-Gonzalez et al. 2008). SFN treatment in PC3 and LNCaP prostate cells results in an induction of autophagy and partial inhibition of cytochrome C release and apoptosis (Herman-Antosiewicz et al. 2006). The decrease in HDAC6 protein we observed in BPH1, LnCap and PC3 cells may divert the cell away from survival (autophagy) and towards cell death (apoptosis) by decreasing the formation of autophagic aggresomes.

Nuclear Factor Kappa-B (NF-κB) Inhibition

NF-κB is a heterodimeric transcription factor that consists of a p50 and p65 subunit and, when active, promotes inflammatory gene expression, cell proliferation and cell survival. Constitutive activation of NF-κB is common in various human malignancies, including prostate cancer, and leads to up-regulation of genes encoding adhesion molecules, inflammatory cytokines, growth factors, and anti-apoptotic genes (Baldwin 2001; Rayet and Gelinas 1999). NF-κB plays an important role in regulating apoptosis, inflammation, angiogenesis and metastasis. Thus, inhibition of NF-κB activation has been postulated as a key target at multiple stages of cancer development.

Several labs have shown down-regulation of NF-κB activity with SFN administration in prostate cancer cells. This was observed in PC3 cells treated with 20 μM SFN in which reduced nuclear localization of p65-NF-κB occurred after 1 h (Choi et al. 2007). Additionally, in PC3 cells inhibition of NF-κB activity coincided with expression of downstream targets, VEGF, cyclin D1, and Bcl-X_L. Decreased nuclear translocation and activation of p65-NF-κB was attributed to the inhibition of I kappa B kinase (IKK), thereby attenuating phosphorylation and degradation of the NF-κB inhibitor, IκBα (Xu et al. 2005). The inhibitor of apoptosis (IAP) family is one of the downstream factors up-regulated by NF-κB activation. In LnCap and PC3 cells, the modulation of IAP levels was proportional to the level of NF-κB activity (Choi et al. 2007). Collectively, these results indicate that SFN can affect proliferation signals and apoptotic signals via modulation of NF-κB activity. Inhibition of HDAC has also been closely linked with inhibition of NF-κB. Treatment with benzylisothiocyanate (BITC), which is structurally similar to sulforaphane isothiocyanate, inhibits activity and expression of HDAC1 and HDAC3 and inhibited NF-κB selectively in pancreatic cancer cells. Overexpression of HDAC1 or HDAC3 rescued the effects of BITC, suggesting that inhibition of HDAC1/HDAC3 may be related to NF-κB inactivation by BITC (Batra et al. 2010). It is plausible that SFN- mediated NF-κB inhibition may also be related to HDAC inhibition or direct acetylation of NF-κB.

Androgen-Receptor (AR)

AR is a ligand-activated transcription factor belonging to the steroid receptor superfamily. It is a critical transcription factor in the development the male reproductive organ function and in prostate cancer progression. Moreover, AR is believed to be a major player in the transition from hormone-sensitive to androgen-independent prostate cancer (Hotte and Saad 2010). Hormone ablation therapy is often a first-line treatment for early-stage prostate cancer and novel strategies to effectively target and block AR signaling are being actively sought for the treatment of prostate cancer. Kim and Singh demonstrated that SFN causes transcription repression of AR and inhibition of AR nuclear translocation in LnCaP and C4-2 prostate cancer cells showing for the first time a link between SFN and AR signaling (Kim and Singh 2009). Gibbs et al., found that HDAC6 over-expression in LnCap cells abrogated the effects of SFN on HSP90 acetylation and inhibited its association with AR (Gibbs et al. 2009). Thus, this study provided further evidence that inhibition of HDAC6 was a specific target of sulforaphane and HDAC inhibition had profound effects for AR signaling.

Indole-3-Carbinol (I3C) and 3,3′-Diindolylmethane (DIM)

I3C is produced by the breakdown of the glucosinolate glucobrassicin during the consumption of cruciferous vegetables (Fig. 3.1b) (Aggarwal and Ichikawa 2005). Broccoli, Brussels sprouts, cabbage, and cauliflower are food sources that contain glucobrassicin. When these foods are chopped, chewed or consumed glucobrassicin comes into contact with the enzyme myrosinase and I3C is formed (Fig. 3.1b and reviewed in Higdon et al. 2007). In the acidic environment of the stomach I3C undergoes extensive and rapid self condensation and produces many oligomeric products (Aggarwal and Ichikawa 2005; Sarkar and Li 2004). A major condensation product is DIM, which is formed from 2 molecules of I3C (Fig. 3.1b) (Sarkar and Li 2004). In prostate cancer cells the current literature suggests that DIM, which is a prominent condensation product, is the active agent responsible for the observed changes in cancer cell physiology (Bradlow and Zeligs 2010). This remains controversial as I3C has been shown to have some distinct effects from DIM as shown by the ability of I3C, but not DIM, to reduce carcinogen induced mammary tumors in an animal model (Lubet et al. 2011). DIM appears to enter the cell passively, with 10% of DIM in treated cells remaining in the cytosol and 30–40% located in the nucleus (Staub et al. 2006).

Importantly, studies on prostate cancer animal models support the anti-carcinogenic effects of I3C/DIM. The experimental details by which I3C or DIM was introduced and the method of cancer induction differed in each study but they all concluded I3C/DIM inhibited prostate carcinogenesis and decreased proliferation and increased apoptosis were commonly observed (Cho et al. 2011; Fares et al. 2010; Nachshon-Kedmi et al. 2004a; Souli et al. 2008). A study of C57BL/6 mice inoculated with prostate cancer cells demonstrated that I3C, injected intraperitonially at a dose of 20 mg/kg body weight, decreased tumor volume by 78% and altered angiogenesis by decreasing microvessel density (Souli et al. 2008). A TRAMP mouse model study showed that mice fed DIM, 10 or 20 mg/kg body weight by gavage, had inhibited growth of prostate cancer cells and altered expression of genes that regulate cell cycle including CDK2, CDK4, p27 and Bax (Cho et al. 2011). It has also been shown that the phytochemical did not affect animal weight or liver and kidney functions (Fares et al. 2010; Nachshon-Kedmi et al. 2004a; Souli et al. 2008). Furthermore, one study supports the use of DIM as both a therapeutic and preventative phytochemical for prostate cancer formation (Souli et al. 2008). Epidemiology studies of humans also provide modest support that the intake of high levels of cruciferous vegetables, the dietary source of I3C/DIM, can reduce prostate cancer risk (Table 3.1 and reviewed in Kristal and Lampe 2002). Furthermore, a clinical study in humans shows that a single dose of the bioavailable DIM is well tolerated up to 200 mg and DIM was detectable in the blood of treated individuals (Reed et al. 2008).

Pharmacokinetic studies in animals have established that, following oral administration, I3C or DIM are effectively absorbed and distributed to the bloodstream and tissues (previously reviewed by Howells et al. (2007)). Briefly, after oral administration of 250 mg/kg of I3C in mice I3C was observed in plasma at levels up to 28 μM and 20–170 μM in tissues with the highest concentrations found in the kidney and liver, followed by the lung and heart, and low levels in the brain (Anderton et al. 2004b). When pure DIM (250 mg/kg) or an equivalent amount of a bioavailable formulation (833 mg/kg) were dosed by gavage, 24 μM DIM was found in plasma and 32–200 μM concentrations in tissues with the highest concentrations found in the liver, followed by the kidney, lung, heart, and the brain respectively (Anderton et al. 2004a). Fifty percent higher concentrations were detected in the tissues with the bioavailable DIM as compared to pure DIM (Anderton et al. 2004a). While these are important studies it is worth noting that the dose given to a 70 kg person would equal 17,500 mg in a day which is well above the levels which are currently tested in humans. A bioavailable formulation of DIM has been shown to be well tolerated in prostate cancer patients and a Phase II study has been recommended at a 225 mg dose given orally twice daily (Heath et al. 2010). At this time we are not aware of a publication evaluating the amount of neither I3C nor DIM in prostate tissue following treatment.

Molecular Targets of I3C and DIM

Alteration of Carcinogen Metabolism

Acid condensation products of I3C can influence the metabolism of xenobiotic compounds through an interaction with the aryl hydrocarbon receptor. More specifically, binding of I3C condensation products to the aryl hydrocarbon receptor in the cytoplasm results in its movement to the nucleus where it interacts with the nuclear receptor called aryl hydrocarbon receptor nuclear translocator (Arnt) (reviewed in Higdon et al. 2007). This complex then interacts with DNA sequences containing a xenobiotic response element and causes the upregulation of a number of Phase I and Phase II enzymes. This phenomenon of increased Phase I and Phase II enzymes was also reported in prostate cancer cells analyzed by microarrays after treatment with 60 μM I3C or 40 μM DIM (Li et al. 2003). Interestingly, these treatments induced the upregulation of CYP1A1 as early as 6 h after treatment and persisted up to 48 h post treatment (Li et al. 2003). Upregulation of these enzymes by I3C/DIM illustrates that treatment can cause cells to have an increased capacity for detoxification of exogenous compounds including carcinogens (Li et al. 2003; Takahashi et al. 1995). While this is generally considered an important mechanism by which I3C/DIM may prevent cancer formation, we should note that some studies suggest that it is not completely straight forward. This is in part due to a report that demonstrated that DIM can directly inhibit the activity of some P450 enzymes including CYP1A1, CYP1A2 and CYP2B1 (Stresser et al. 1995).

Alteration of Sex Hormone Metabolism and Signaling

The levels and types of sex hormones play a critical role in the development and progression of prostate cancer. Hormone ablation therapies are common in patients diagnosed with prostate cancer and the sensitivity of the tumor to this treatment is dependent on sex hormone status. Examination of the literature on the relationship between I3C/DIM and hormones shows that these phytochemicals have an effect on both testosterone and estrogen but the details vary depending on the chemical, dose and experimental system. DIM and other I3C condensation products have been shown to influence the form and amount of testosterone and estrogen derivative compounds in mammals (Wortelboer et al. 1992 and reviewed in Higdon et al. 2007). Historically, many studies have emphasized that DIM can alter both estrogen metabolism through CYP1A1 expression and estrogen receptor signaling but the majority of this literature has been focused on breast cancer studies (reviewed in Weng et al. 2008). I3C/DIM has been shown to influence the metabolism of testosterone, its ability to bind to its receptor, and the AR signaling pathway. Specifically, DIM treatment caused the upregulation of Phase II enzymes and coordinately increased 7 α-hydroxylation of testosterone and decreased 16α- and 2α-testosterone hydroxylation (Wortelboer et al. 1992). A screening study also identified I3C as showing antiandrogenic activity only, whereas DIM had both an estrogenic mode of action with an antiandrogenic activity (Bovee et al. 2008). This was measured by a fluorescent reporter system coupled to the human androgen receptor or estrogen receptor in yeast which identified these phytochemicals as agonistic compounds (Bovee et al. 2008). It is of interest to note that I3C has been shown to inhibit ligand-inducible AR activity (Fan et al. 2006). Additionally, a study on DIM and ring-substituted DIM analogs identified the capacity of these compounds to inhibit testosterone-stimulated growth of androgen sensitive prostate cancer cells and suggests that DIM analogs have the potential to be a new therapy for treating hormone-sensitive prostate cancers (Abdelbaqi et al. 2011).

At the receptor level Hsu et al. showed that I3C inhibited the expression of AR protein and mRNA levels within 12 h of treatment while DIM had no affect on AR expression (Hsu et al. 2005). However, two additional studies in prostate cancer cells have shown opposing data, where DIM induced a down-regulation in the levels of AR (Chinnakannu et al. 2009; Garikapaty et al. 2006b). Interestingly I3C also inhibited ligand-inducible AR activity in conjunction with induction the tumor suppressor genes BRCA1 and BRCA2 (Fan et al. 2006). Downstream of AR, both I3C and DIM inhibited androgen and estrogen-mediated pathways in prostate cancer cells including the classic output gene of the androgen pathway PSA (Hsu et al. 2005; Wang et al. 2011).

Inhibit Growth

Perhaps one of the best documented mechanisms by which I3C/DIM inhibits prostate cancer development is through the inhibition of cell growth. This is seen in animal models were I3C/DIM treated animals had a reduction in tumor volume and a decline in the rate of proliferation of cancer cells (Garikapaty et al. 2005; Nachshon-Kedmi et al. 2004a; Souli et al. 2008). Many different types of cultured human prostate cancer cells, ranging in androgen-dependence and presence of a functional p53 signaling cascade, have shown growth inhibition following I3C/DIM treatment (Chinnakannu et al. 2009; Chinni et al. 2001; Li et al. 2005b; Vivar et al. 2009). Considerable effort has been made to define the underlying molecular changes that drive the growth inhibitory effect of I3C/DIM. A microarray study identified that I3C and DIM down-regulated the expression of genes that are critically involved in the regulation of signal transduction, cell cycle and cell growth (Li et al. 2003). This is supported by additional studies that showed that I3C/DIM induces a down regulation of a signaling cascade which plays a key role in cancer growth, namely the epidermal growth factor receptor (EGFR), phosphoinositide 3-kinase (PI3K), and Akt pathway (Chinni and Sarkar 2002; Li et al. 2005b). This is also accompanied by the activation of a G1 cell cycle arrest due to the up-regulation of genes regulating this checkpoint (Chinnakannu et al. 2009; Chinni et al. 2001; Vivar et al. 2009). More specifically, I3C/DIM can cause the upregulation of the CDK inhibitors p21(WAF1) and p27(Kip1) along with down-regulation of AR, CDK2, CDK4, and CDK6 and changes in the phosphorylation status of Rb (Chinnakannu et al. 2009; Chinni et al. 2001; Vivar et al. 2009). This *in vitro* work was confirmed in the TRAMP model of prostate cancer where DIM was used as an intervention (Cho et al. 2011). DIM reduced the number of proliferating cells in the prostate and reduced the expression of cyclin A, CDK2, CDK4 (Cho et al. 2011). Taken together, research shows that one mechanism by which DIM inhibits prostate carcinogenesis is through the inhibition of cell cycle progression.

Promote Apoptosis

I3C/DIM treatment of prostate cancer in animal models and cells consistently results in the induction of apoptosis (Cho et al. 2011; Garikapaty et al. 2006a, b; Nachshon-Kedmi et al. 2004a). At the molecular level, consumption of DIM also resulted in the reduction of Bcl-xL expression and increased Bax expression in prostate cancer tumors (Cho et al. 2011). To further determine the specific pathways that lead to DIM-induced apoptosis researchers examined cell death in a wide range of human prostate cancer cells. I3C/DIM consistently altered the expression of the Bcl 2 family of proteins (which regulate apoptosis) including the up-regulation of Bax and down-regulation of Bcl-2 Bcl-x(L), and BAD (Chinni et al. 2001; Chinni and Sarkar 2002). I3C and DIM treatment also increased the level of activated p53 and inactivated NF-κB signaling which was associated with cell death (Chinnakannu et al. 2009; Hsu et al. 2006; Nachshon-Kedmi et al. 2003). DIM also induced apoptosis in prostate cancer cells lacking p53, through the mitochondrial pathway (Nachshon-Kedmi et al. 2004b). DIM induced the release of cytochrome c from the mitochondria, activation of caspases 9, 3 and 6, and lead to PARP cleavage and apoptosis in PC-3 prostate cancer cells (Nachshon-Kedmi et al. 2004b). I3C has also been shown to sensitize prostate cancer cells to TRAIL induced death through the induction of the death receptors DR4 and DR5 (Jeon et al. 2003).

Disrupt Inflammation, Angiogenesis, and Metastasis

NF-κB plays an important role in regulating the transcription of genes that drive the inflammatory response, angiogenesis and metastasis. A sustained and hyperactive level of NF-κB has been observed in prostate cancer cells and animal models and is associated with chronic inflammation (Gasparian et al. 2002; Hsu et al. 2011). DIM causes a down regulation of NF-κB signaling in cultured prostate cancer cells but not in normal prostate cells as observed by increased IκBα levels, decreased nuclear NF-κB and decreased binding of NF-κB to DNA, resulting in altered expression of NF-κB target genes (Chinnakannu et al. 2009; Li et al. 2005b). It is possible that the down regulation of NF-κB by DIM could be a driving mechanism for the reduce inflammation and angiogenesis observed in animal models through inhibition of cytokines and Hypoxia Inducible Factor (HIF) levels respectively (Souli et al. 2008). Furthermore, the DIM induced decline in NF-κB could play a role in the lower level of prostate metastases that was observed in a rat model of prostate cancer treated with I3C (Garikapaty et al. 2005).

I3C/DIM and Epigenetic Regulation

There is strong evidence that I3C/DIM alters the expression of tumor suppressors and oncogenes but the potential of this phytochemical to exert these affects through epigenetic means has not been investigated extensively in prostate cancer. However, DIM has been shown to alter epigenetic markers, namely HDACs and miRNAs in other cancer sites. More specifically, colon cancer cells treated with 0–60 μM DIM had decreased levels of HDAC1, HDAC2, HDAC3 and HDAC8 along with a decline in the expression of survivin and Cyclin B1 (Bhatnagar et al. 2009; Li et al. 2010a). DIM also produced a decline in the expression of class I HDACs in mice bearing colon cancer xenografts (Li et al. 2010a). The change in HDAC expression was associated with increases in Bax, p21 and p27 expression (classic HDAC target genes) and increased cell cycle arrest and apoptosis of the cancer xenografts (Bhatnagar et al. 2009; Li et al. 2010a). Class II HDACs were not affected by DIM treatment (Li et al. 2010a) and the selective degradation of class I HDACs was shown to be mediated by the proteasome (Li et al. 2010a).

DIM can also alter aggressiveness of pancreatic cancer through epigenetic changes, specifically via miRNA expression. miRNAs have been traditionally shown to disrupt the translation of mRNA through an interaction with the target mRNA and the RISC protein complex (Fig. 3.2c) (Parasramka et al. 2011). If the miRNA has complete complementation with the target mRNA then this results in cleavage of the mRNA. If there is only partial complementation of the target mRNA then the target mRNA is transcriptionally repressed at the ribosome (Fig. 3.2c). Expression of miR-146a is low in pancreatic cancer cells compared with normal pancreatic epithelial cells (Li et al. 2010b). Treatment of pancreatic cancer cells with DIM increased miR-146a expression (Li et al. 2010b). This caused the down regulation of EGFR, MTA-2, IRAK-1, and NF-κB, resulting in an inhibition of cell invasion (Li et al. 2010b). Furthermore, miRNA microarrays revealed that DIM treatments caused alterations in the expression of 28 different miRNAs in pancreatic cancer cells (Li et al. 2009). Upregulation of miRNAs from the miR-200 and let-7 families were of particular interest as they resulted in the down-regulation of the proteins ZEB1, slug, and vimentin and the reversal of a phenotype associated with cancer cell invasion and metastasis (Li et al. 2009). While these studies provide direct evidence that DIM can alter epigenetic mechanisms they do not address the question in the context of prostate cancer. In the following sections we will highlight where epigenetic mechanisms could be at work to reduce prostate cancer tumorigenesis.

Pre-initiation Mechanisms and I3C/DIN: Possible Role of Epigenetics

At this time there is very few studies exploring an interconnection between I3C/DIM induced changes in epigenetics and the classic Phase I and II target genes. The most promising epigenetic mechanism by which DIM may affect xenobiotic metabolism is through Ahr and P450 genes. HDAC inhibitors have been shown to regulate the promoter region of Ahr in cultured murine cells (Garrison et al. 2000) and cause a significant increase in the activity of CYP enzymes in breast cancer cells (Hooven et al. 2005). Thus, it is possible that DIM, as a dietary HDAC inhibitor, may also modulate the activity of Ahr- regulated gene expression and CYP expression. In addition, both Ahr and several CYP enzymes are regulated by DNA methylation. In particular Cyp1B1 and Cyp7B1 methylation has been implicated in prostate cancer causing overexpression of these genes in cancer tissues (Olsson et al. 2007; Tokizane et al. 2005). Since the condensation of I3C to DIM creates a formaldehyde group (Fig. 3.1b), it is possible the I3C may contribute to the methylation pool through this byproduct and alter DNA methylation patterns. Alternatively I3C or DIM may modulate DNA methyltransferase expression/activity similar to SFN. It will be of interest to determine if the observed changes in the expression of CYP genes following I3C/DIM treatment occur through epigenetic mechanisms.

There is also very little literature exploring an interconnection between epigenetics, I3C/DIM, and sex hormone levels. However, it has been previously shown that AR expression levels are decreased by HDAC inhibitors in androgen sensitive prostate cancer cells (Trtkova et al. 2010). If DIM inhibits HDACs in prostate cancer cells, then it is possible that AR expression may be repressed in this same mechanism. We have preliminary evidence supporting this possibility, as DIM treatment causes a decrease in HDAC activity and HDAC6 protein in PC-3 prostate cancer cells (Beaver, unpublished data). HDAC6 can also effect hormone signaling as it modulates the acetylation levels of HSP90 and effects the interaction of between HSP90 and AR (Ai et al. 2009). Knockdown of HDAC6 in prostate cancer cells results in impaired nuclear localization of AR, inhibition of PSA expression and cell growth (Ai et al. 2009). Further research is needed to examine if DIM acts through epigenetic mechanisms to change hormone levels and signaling.

Post-initiation Mechanisms and I3C/DIN: Possible Role of Epigenetics

Growth Inhibition

The most likely mechanism by which DIM could influence epigenetics and inhibit cell growth would be through targeting genes that mediate cell cycle. As previously mentioned, DIM-induced inhibition of class I HDACs was associated with a cell cycle arrest in colon cancer cells (Li et al. 2010a). This was triggered by the down regulation of the cell cycle regulatory genes p21, p27, cyclin B1, cyclin D1, and CDK4 (Li et al. 2010a). Inhibition of HDAC activity by other phytochemicals is associated with increased histone acetylation, the binding of transcription factors to the p21 promoter, and elevated p21 protein levels (Clarke et al. 2011; Nian et al. 2009). Given the decreased levels of HDAC proteins in DIM treated colon cancer cells and the increased expression of p21 found following DIM treatment, it is easy to hypothesize that DIM is acting through this epigenetic mechanism to upregulate p21 in prostate cancer cells (Fig. 3.2). An HDAC independent mechanism by which DIM may influence cell cycle arrest may also be through the up-regulation of the miR-200 family of miRNA (Li et al. 2009). Increased expression of the miR-200a/141 cluster has been shown to cause increased p27/Kip1 and decreased CDK6 expression resulting in the arrest of cell growth at the G1/S checkpoint (Uhlmann et al. 2010).

Promote Apoptosis

Another likely epigenetic mechanism by which I3C/DIM could promote apoptosis is through inhibition of HDAC activity. At this time there are no published studies showing an interconnection between DIM target miRNAs and the known apoptosis pathways affected by DIM treatment. In contrast, pharmacological HDAC inhibitors are potent inducers of cell death, especially in rapidly dividing cancer cells. For example, the HDAC inhibitors trichostatin A and sodium butyrate triggered apoptosis in ovarian and human glioma cancer cells through the increased expression of Bad (Sawa et al. 2001; Strait et al. 2005). Trichostatin A also decreased expression of anti-apoptotic Bcl-2 and Bcl-XL proteins and activated apoptosis through caspase-3, caspase-8 and PARP cleavage and cytochrome c release from the mitochondria (Kim et al. 2006). Since DIM selectively inhibits class I HDACs in colon cancer cells, it would be interesting to test the hypothesis that DIM can inhibit HDAC activity in prostate cancer cells and act to promote apoptosis through the epigenetic regulation of the Bcl-2 family of proteins.

Disrupt Inflammation, Angiogenesis, and Metastasis

If DIM causes a decline in HDAC levels and activity in prostate cancer in a similar manner to what was observed in colon cancer cells then DIM may inhibit inflammation, angiogenesis, and metastasis through an epigenetic mechanism. For example, pharmacological HDAC inhibitors have anti-inflammatory properties *in vitro* and *in vivo* and can reduce EGFR expression (Chou et al. 2011; Glauben et al. 2009). These results are similar to those previously described with DIM treatment in animal studies. The reduction in EGFR, which plays an important role in tumor growth and metastasis, by HDAC inhibitors was achieved through the dissociation of SP1, HDAC3 and CBP from the EGFR promoter (Chou et al. 2011).

Another possible epigenetic mechanism involves HDACs. HDAC1 localizes to kappa B binding sites, as shown by ChIP, and affects cancer related outcomes including inflammation and angiogenesis (Aurora et al. 2010; Elsharkawy et al. 2010). HDAC1 also regulates cancer cell motility and invasion through the regulation of the adhesion molecule E-cadherin (Kim et al. 2011). HDAC1 was shown to be downregulated in colon cancer cells by DIM (Bhatnagar et al. 2009; Li et al. 2010a). Thus, if DIM causes a similar decline in HDAC1 in prostate cancer this could alter the NF-κB signaling pathway and E-cadherin resulting in changes in inflammation, angiogenesis and metastasis (Elsharkawy et al. 2010).

Alternatively, DIM may also modulate NF-κB activity via miRNAs. Treatment of pancreatic cancer cells with DIM increased miR-146a, caused a downregulation of EGFR and NF-κB and resulted in an inhibition of pancreatic cancer cell invasion (Li et al. 2010b). Furthermore, miR-146a has been implicated as a negative feedback regulator of NF-κB and knockout of miR-146a has been shown to increased transcription of NF-κB –regulated genes (Zhao et al. 2011). This interconnection between DIM, miR-146a and NF-κB is a possible mechanism by which DIM could affect prostate cancer progression. Additionally, miRNA's from the miR-200 family, which are upregulated by DIM, have been shown to affect EGFR levels and tumor cell adhesion, migration, invasion and metastasis in other cancer cell types (Adam et al. 2009; Mongroo and Rustgi 2010). Whether DIM can regulate these pathways in prostate cancer remains to be determined and is an interesting future research area.

Conclusions

There are clear indicators that a man's diet can affect his risk for developing prostate cancer. In this chapter we have focused specifically on the molecular mechanisms by which phytochemicals in cruciferous vegetables may prevent the initiation of prostate cancer and slow tumorigenesis. We have particularly emphasized a possible role for epigenetics in this process. We have outlined some of the known and possible mechanisms by which SFN and I3C/DIM specifically alter epigenetic mechanisms which may function to prevent or slow prostate cancer progression. To date there is still a great deal more research needed to fully evaluate the means by which these phytochemicals act to regulate epigenetic mechanisms.

It is clear that the consumption of cruciferous vegetables is likely to have multiple benefits for human health. Compounds containing SFN and DIM have been shown to be safe in preliminary studies of healthy volunteers (Cornblatt et al. 2007; Cramer and Jeffery 2011; Reed et al. 2008). Further study of these phytochemicals are needed to inform if these supplements are as effective as eating the whole food. Also, further study is needed to establish how much of these chemicals should be taken, at what interval, and what are the long term effects of supplement use. These are important studies, particular in the case of I3C and DIM where some animal studies suggest that high dose supplementation of these compounds could promote growth of established colon, thyroid, pancreas and liver cancers (reviewed in Dashwood 1998; Stoner et al. 2002).

Targeting the epigenome is an evolving strategy for cancer chemoprevention and both SFN and DIM have shown promise in cancer clinical trials. The ability of SFN, I3C or DIM to target aberrant epigenetic patterns, in addition to effects on detoxification/carcinogen metabolism, may make it an effective chemoprevention agent at multiple stages of the carcinogenesis pathway. The identification of dietary epigenetic modulators and their use either alone or in combination, may increase efficacy of anti-cancer therapies/prevention strategies, without serious side effects. Much more additional work needs to be done to define molecular mechanisms and human bioavailability for these compounds. Together, these types of studies provide the important link to human relevance for the use of cruciferous vegetable phytochemicals as promising anticancer agents and provide a strong scientific foundation for future trials to identify effective dietary intervention strategies that will significantly reduce the burden of prostate cancer.

Acknowledgements Research conducted in the authors' laboratory is supported by NIH grants CA90890, CA65525, CA122906, CA122959, CA80176, and by NIEHS Center grant P30 ES00210.

References

Abbas A, Gupta S (2008) The role of histone deacetylases in prostate cancer. Epigenetics 3: 300–309

Abdelbaqi K, Lack N, Guns ET, Kotha L, Safe S, Sanderson JT (2011) Antiandrogenic and growth inhibitory effects of ring-substituted analogs of 3,3′-diindolylmethane (ring-DIMs) in hormone-responsive LNCaP human prostate cancer cells. Prostate 71:1401–1412

Adam L, Zhong M, Choi W, Qi W, Nicoloso M, Arora A, Calin G, Wang H, Siefker-Radtke A, McConkey D, Bar-Eli M, Dinney C (2009) miR-200 expression regulates epithelial-to-mesenchymal transition in bladder cancer cells and reverses resistance to epidermal growth factor receptor therapy. Clin Cancer Res 15:5060–5072

Aggarwal BB, Ichikawa H (2005) Molecular targets and anticancer potential of indole-3-carbinol and its derivatives. Cell Cycle 4:1201–1215

Ai J, Wang Y, Dar JA, Liu J, Liu L, Nelson JB, Wang Z (2009) HDAC6 regulates androgen receptor hypersensitivity and nuclear localization via modulating Hsp90 acetylation in castration-resistant prostate cancer. Mol Endocrinol 23:1963–1972

Ambrosini GL, de Klerk NH, Fritschi L, Mackerras D, Musk B (2008) Fruit, vegetable, vitamin A intakes, and prostate cancer risk. Prostate Cancer Prostatic Dis 1:61–66

American Cancer Society (2011) Cancer facts & figures 2011. http://www.cancer.org/Research/CancerFactsFigures/CancerFactsFigures/cancer-facts-figures-2011

Anderton MJ, Manson MM, Verschoyle R, Gescher A, Steward WP, Williams ML, Mager DE (2004a) Physiological modeling of formulated and crystalline 3,3’-diindolylmethane pharmacokinetics following oral administration in mice. Drug Metab Dispos 32:632–638

Anderton MJ, Manson MM, Verschoyle RD, Gescher A, Lamb JH, Farmer PB, Steward WP, Williams ML (2004b) Pharmacokinetics and tissue disposition of indole-3-carbinol and its acid condensation products after oral administration to mice. Clin Cancer Res 10:5233–5241

Aurora AB, Biyashev D, Mirochnik Y, Zaichuk TA, Sanchez-Martinez C, Renault MA, Losordo D, Volpert OV (2010) NF-kappaB balances vascular regression and angiogenesis via chromatin remodeling and NFAT displacement. Blood 116:475–484

Azarenko O, Okouneva T, Singletary KW, Jordan MA, Wilson L (2008) Suppression of microtubule dynamic instability and turnover in MCF7 breast cancer cells by sulforaphane. Carcinogenesis 29:2360–2368

Baldwin AS (2001) Control of oncogenesis and cancer therapy resistance by the transcription factor NF-kappa-B. J Clin Invest 107:241–246

Batra S, Sahu RP, Kandala PK, Srivastava SK (2010) Benzyl isothiocyanate-mediated inhibition of histone deacetylase leads to NF-kappaB turnoff in human pancreatic carcinoma cells. Mol Cancer Ther 9:1596–1608

Baylin SB, Ohm JE (2006) Epigenetic gene silencing in cancer - a mechanism for early oncogenic pathway addiction? Nat Rev Cancer 6:107–116

Baylin SB, Esteller M, Rountree MR, Bachman KE, Schuebel K, Herman JG (2001) Aberrant patterns of DNA methylation, chromatin formation and gene expression in cancer. Hum Mol Genet 10:687–692

Bhatnagar N, Li X, Chen Y, Zhou X, Garrett SH, Guo B (2009) 3,3’-diindolylmethane enhances the efficacy of butyrate in colon cancer prevention through down-regulation of survivin. Cancer Prev Res 2:581–589

Boumber Y, Issa JP (2011) Epigenetics in cancer: what’s the future? Oncology (Williston Park) 25:220–226, 228

Bovee TF, Schoonen WG, Hamers AR, Bento MJ, Peijnenburg AA (2008) Screening of synthetic and plant-derived compounds for (anti)estrogenic and (anti)androgenic activities. Anal Bioanal Chem 390:1111–1119

Bradlow HL, Zeligs MA (2010) Diindolylmethane (DIM) spontaneously forms from indole-3-carbinol (I3C) during cell culture experiments. In Vivo 24:387–391

Chiao JW, Chung FL, Kancherla R, Ahmed T, Mittelman A, Conaway CC (2002) Sulforaphane and its metabolite mediate growth arrest and apoptosis in human prostate cancer cells. Int J Oncol 20:631–636

Chinnakannu K, Chen D, Li Y, Wang Z, Dou QP, Reddy GP, Sarkar FH (2009) Cell cycle-dependent effects of 3,3'-diindolylmethane on proliferation and apoptosis of prostate cancer cells. J Cell Physiol 219:94–99

Chinni SR, Sarkar FH (2002) Akt inactivation is a key event in indole-3-carbinol-induced apoptosis in PC-3 cells. Clin Cancer Res 8:1228–1236

Chinni SR, Li Y, Upadhyay S, Koppolu PK, Sarkar FH (2001) Indole-3-carbinol (I3C) induced cell growth inhibition, G1 cell cycle arrest and apoptosis in prostate cancer cells. Oncogene 20:2927–2936

Cho SD, Li G, Hu H, Jiang C, Kang KS, Lee YS, Kim SH, Lu J (2005) Involvement of c-Jun N-terminal kinase in G2/M arrest and caspase-mediated apoptosis induced by sulforaphane in DU145 prostate cancer cells. Nutr Cancer 52:213–224

Cho HJ, Park SY, Kim EJ, Kim JK, Park JH (2011) 3,3'-Diindolylmethane inhibits prostate cancer development in the transgenic adenocarcinoma mouse prostate model. Mol Carcinog 50: 100–112

Choi S, Lew KL, Xiao H, Herman-Antosiewicz A, Xiao D, Brown CK, Singh SV (2007) D, L-Sulforaphane-induced cell death in human prostate cancer cells is regulated by inhibitor of apoptosis family proteins and Apaf-1. Carcinogenesis 28:151–162

Chou CW, Wu MS, Huang WC, Chen CC (2011) HDAC inhibition decreases the expression of EGFR in colorectal cancer cells. PLoS One 6:e18087

Clarke JD, Dashwood RH, Ho E (2008) Multi-targeted prevention of cancer by sulforaphane. Cancer Lett 269:291–304

Clarke JD, Hsu A, Yu Z, Dashwood RH, Ho E (2011) Differential effects of sulforaphane on histone deacetylases, cell cycle arrest and apoptosis in normal prostate cells versus hyperplastic and cancerous prostate cells. Mol Nutr Food Res 55:999–1009

Cohen JH, Kristal AR, Stanford JL (2000) Fruit and vegetable intakes and prostate cancer risk. J Natl Cancer Inst 92:61–68

Colli JL, Amling CL (2009) Chemoprevention of prostate cancer: what can be recommended to patients? Curr Urol Rep 10:165–171

Cornblatt BS, Ye L, Dinkova-Kostova AT, Erb M, Fahey JW, Singh NK, Chen MSA, Stierer T, Garrett-Mayer E, Argani P, Davidson NE, Talalay P, Kensler TW, Visvanathan K (2007) Preclinical and clinical evaluation of sulforaphane for chemoprevention in the breast. Carcinogenesis 28:1485–1490

Cramer JM, Jeffery EH (2011) Sulforaphane absorption and excretion following ingestion of a semi-purified broccoli powder rich in glucoraphanin and broccoli sprouts in healthy men. Nutr Cancer 63:196–201

Dashwood RH (1998) Indole-3-carbinol: anticarcinogen or tumor promoter in brassica vegetables? Chem Biol Interact 110:1–5

Dashwood RH, Ho E (2007) Dietary histone deacetylase inhibitors: from cells to mice to man. Semin Cancer Biol 17:363–369

DeMarzo AM, Nelson WG, Isaacs WB, Epstein JI (2003) Pathological and molecular aspects of prostate cancer. Lancet 361:955–964

Dobosy JR, Roberts JLW, Fu VX, Jarrard DF (2007) The expanding role of epigenetics in the development, diagnosis and treatment of prostate cancer and benign prostatic hyperplasia. J Urol 177:822–831

Egner PA, Chen JG, Wang JB, Wu Y, Sun Y, Lu JH, Zhu J, Zhang YH, Chen YS, Friesen MD, Jacobson LP, Munoz A, Ng D, Qian GS, Zhu YR, Chen TY, Botting NP, Zhang Q, Fahey JW, Talalay P, Groopman JD, Kensler TW (2011) Bioavailability of sulforaphane from two broccoli sprout beverages: results of a short-term, cross-over clinical trial in Qidong, China. Cancer Prev Res 4:384–395

Elsharkawy AM, Oakley F, Lin F, Packham G, Mann DA, Mann J (2010) The NF-kappaB p50:p50: HDAC-1 repressor complex orchestrates transcriptional inhibition of multiple pro-inflammatory genes. J Hepatol 53:519–527

Fan S, Meng Q, Auborn K, Carter T, Rosen EM (2006) BRCA1 and BRCA2 as molecular targets for phytochemicals indole-3-carbinol and genistein in breast and prostate cancer cells. Br J Cancer 94:407–426

Fares F, Azzam N, Appel B, Fares B, Stein A (2010) The potential efficacy of 3,3'-diindolylmethane in prevention of prostate cancer development. Eur J Cancer Prev 19:199–203

Feinberg AP (2007) Phenotypic plasticity and the epigenetics of human disease. Nature 447: 433–440

Gamet-Payrastre L (2006) Signaling pathways and intracellular targets of sulforaphane mediating cell cycle arrest and apoptosis. Curr Cancer Drug Targets 6:135–145

Garikapaty VP, Ashok BT, Chen YG, Mittelman A, Iatropoulos M, Tiwari RK (2005) Anti-carcinogenic and anti-metastatic properties of indole-3-carbinol in prostate cancer. Oncol Rep 13:89–93

Garikapaty VP, Ashok BT, Tadi K, Mittelman A, Tiwari RK (2006a) 3,3'-Diindolylmethane down-regulates pro-survival pathway in hormone independent prostate cancer. Biochem Biophys Res Commun 340:718–725

Garikapaty VP, Ashok BT, Tadi K, Mittelman A, Tiwari RK (2006b) Synthetic dimer of indole-3-carbinol: second generation diet derived anti-cancer agent in hormone sensitive prostate cancer. Prostate 66:453–462

Garrison PM, Rogers JM, Brackney WR, Denison MS (2000) Effects of histone deacetylase inhibitors on the Ah receptor gene promoter. Arch Biochem Biophys 374:161–171

Gasparian AV, Yao YJ, Kowalczyk D, Lyakh LA, Karseladze A, Slaga TJ, Budunova IV (2002) The role of IKK in constitutive activation of NF-kappaB transcription factor in prostate carcinoma cells. J Cell Sci 115:141–151

Gasper AV, Traka M, Bacon JR, Smith JA, Taylor MA, Hawkey CJ, Barrett DA, Mithen RF (2007) Consuming broccoli does not induce genes associated with xenobiotic metabolism and cell cycle control in human gastric mucosa. J Nutr 137:1718–1724

Gibbs A, Schwartzman J, Deng V, Alumkal J (2009) Sulforaphane destabilizes the androgen receptor in prostate cancer cells by inactivating histone deacetylase 6. Proc Natl Acad Sci U S A 106:16663–16668

Giovannucci E, Rimm EB, Liu Y, Stampfer MJ, Willett WC (2003) A prospective study of cruciferous vegetables and prostate cancer. Cancer Epidemiol Biomarkers Prev 12:1403–1409

Glauben R, Sonnenberg E, Zeitz M, Siegmund B (2009) HDAC inhibitors in models of inflammation-related tumorigenesis. Cancer Lett 280:154–159

Gonzalgo ML, Pavlovich CP, Lee SM, Nelson WG (2003) Prostate cancer detection by GSTP1 methylation analysis of postbiopsy urine specimens. Clin Cancer Res 9:2673–2677

Graham S, Haughey B, Marshall J, Priore R, Byers T, Rzepka T, Mettlin C, Pontes JE (1983) Diet in the epidemiology of carcinoma of the prostate gland. J Natl Cancer Inst 70:687–692

Halkidou K, Gaughan L, Cook S, Leung HY, Neal DE, Robson CN (2004) Upregulation and nuclear recruitment of HDAC1 in hormone refractory prostate cancer. Prostate 59:177–189

Hanahan D, Weinberg RA (2011) Hallmarks of cancer: the next generation. Cell 144:646–674

Harden SV, Guo Z, Epstein JI, Sidransky D (2003) Quantitative GSTP1 methylation clearly distinguishes benign prostatic tissue and limited prostate adenocarcinoma. J Urol 169: 1138–1142

Heath EI, Heilbrun LK, Li J, Vaishampayan U, Harper F, Pemberton P, Sarkar FH (2010) A phase I dose-escalation study of oral BR-DIM (BioResponse 3,3'- Diindolylmethane) in castrate-resistant, non-metastatic prostate cancer. Am J Transl Res 2:402–411

Henrique R, Costa VL, Cerveira N, Carvalho AL, Hoque MO, Ribeiro FR, Oliveira J, Teixeira MR, Sidransky D, Jeronimo C (2006) Hypermethylation of Cyclin D2 is associated with loss of mRNA expression and tumor development in prostate cancer. J Mol Med 84:911–918

Herman JG, Baylin SB (2003) Gene silencing in cancer in association with promoter hypermethylation. N Engl J Med 349:2042–2054

Herman-Antosiewicz A, Johnson DE, Singh SV (2006) Sulforaphane causes autophagy to inhibit release of cytochrome c and apoptosis in human prostate cancer cells. Cancer Res 66: 5828–5835

Herman-Antosiewicz A, Xiao H, Lew KL, Singh SV (2007) Induction of p21 protein protects against sulforaphane-induced mitotic arrest in LNCaP human prostate cancer cell line. Mol Cancer Ther 6:1673–1681

Hideshima T, Bradner JE, Wong J, Chauhan D, Richardson P, Schreiber SL, Anderson KC (2005) Small-molecule inhibition of proteasome and aggresome function induces synergistic antitumor activity in multiple myeloma. Proc Natl Acad Sci U S A 102:8567–8572

Higdon JV, Delage B, Williams DE, Dashwood RH (2007) Cruciferous vegetables and human cancer risk: epidemiologic evidence and mechanistic basis. Pharmacol Res 55:224–236

Ho E, Song Y (2009) Zinc and prostatic cancer. Curr Opin Clin Nutr Metab Care 12:640–645

Hooven LA, Mahadevan B, Keshava C, Johns C, Pereira C, Desai D, Amin S, Weston A, Baird WM (2005) Effects of suberoylanilide hydroxamic acid and trichostatin A on induction of cytochrome P450 enzymes and benzo[a]pyrene DNA adduct formation in human cells. Bioorg Med Chem Lett 15:1283–1287

Hotte SJ, Saad F (2010) Current management of castrate-resistant prostate cancer. Curr Oncol 17(Suppl 2):S72–S79

Howells LM, Moiseeva EP, Neal CP, Foreman BE, Andreadi CK, Sun YY, Hudson EA, Manson MM (2007) Predicting the physiological relevance of in vitro cancer preventive activities of phytochemicals. Acta Pharmacol Sin 28:1274–1304

Howlader N, Noone AM, Krapcho M, Neyman N, Aminou R, Waldron W, Altekruse SF, Kosary CL, Ruhl J, Tatalovich Z, Cho H, Mariotto A, Eisner MP, Lewis DR, Chen HS, Feuer EJ, Cronin KA, Edwards BK (2011) SEER cancer statistics review, 1975–2008. National Cancer Institute, Bethesda

Hsing AW, McLaughlin JK, Schuman LM, Bjelke E, Gridley G, Wacholder S, Chien HT, Blot WJ (1990) Diet, tobacco use, and fatal prostate cancer: results from the Lutheran Brotherhood Cohort Study. Cancer Res 50:6836–6840

Hsing AW, Sakoda LC, Chua SC (2007) Obesity, metabolic syndrome, and prostate cancer. Am J Clin Nutr 86:843S–857S

Hsu JC, Zhang J, Dev A, Wing A, Bjeldanes LF, Firestone GL (2005) Indole-3-carbinol inhibition of androgen receptor expression and downregulation of androgen responsiveness in human prostate cancer cells. Carcinogenesis 26:1896–1904

Hsu JC, Dev A, Wing A, Brew CT, Bjeldanes LF, Firestone GL (2006) Indole-3-carbinol mediated cell cycle arrest of LNCaP human prostate cancer cells requires the induced production of activated p53 tumor suppressor protein. Biochem Pharmacol 72:1714–1723

Hsu A, Bruno RS, Lohr CV, Taylor AW, Dashwood RH, Bray TM, Ho E (2011) Dietary soy and tea mitigate chronic inflammation and prostate cancer via NFkappaB pathway in the Noble rat model. J Nutr Biochem 22:502–510

Hu R, Hebbar V, Kim BR, Chen C, Winnik B, Buckley B, Soteropoulos P, Tolias P, Hart RP, Kong AN (2004) In vivo pharmacokinetics and regulation of gene expression profiles by isothiocyanate sulforaphane in the rat. J Pharmacol Exp Ther 310:263–271

Hu R, Khor TO, Shen G, Jeong WS, Hebbar V, Chen C, Xu C, Reddy B, Chada K, Kong AN (2006) Cancer chemoprevention of intestinal polyposis in ApcMin/+ mice by sulforaphane, a natural product derived from cruciferous vegetable. Carcinogenesis 27:2038–2046

Huffman DM, Grizzle WE, Bamman MM, Kim JS, Eltoum IA, Elgavish A, Nagy TR (2007) SIRT1 is significantly elevated in mouse and human prostate cancer. Cancer Res 67:6612–6618

International Agency for Research on Cancer (2010) GLOBOCAN 2008, Cancer fact sheet: prostate cancer. http://globocan.iarc.fr/factsheets/cancers/prostate.asp

Jackson SJ, Singletary KW (2004) Sulforaphane: a naturally occurring mammary carcinoma mitotic inhibitor, which disrupts tubulin polymerization. Carcinogenesis 25:219–227

Jain MG, Hislop GT, Howe GR, Ghadirian P (1999) Plant foods, antioxidants, and prostate cancer risk: findings from case-control studies in Canada. Nutr Cancer 34:173–184

Jemal A, Bray F, Center MM, Ferlay J, Ward E, Forman D (2011) Global cancer statistics. CA Cancer J Clin 61:69–90

Jeon KI, Rih JK, Kim HJ, Lee YJ, Cho CH, Goldberg ID, Rosen EM, Bae I (2003) Pretreatment of indole-3-carbinol augments TRAIL-induced apoptosis in a prostate cancer cell line, LNCaP. FEBS Lett 544:246–251

Jeronimo C, Henrique R, Hoque MO, Mambo E, Ribeiro FR, Varzim G, Oliveira J, Teixeira MR, Lopes C, Sidransky D (2004) A quantitative promoter methylation profile of prostate cancer. Clin Cancer Res 10:8472–8478

John EM, Stern MC, Sinha R, Koo J (2011) Meat consumption, cooking practices, meat mutagens, and risk of prostate cancer. Nutr Cancer 63:525–537

Johnstone RW (2002) Histone-deacetylase inhibitors: novel drugs for the treatment of cancer. Nat Rev Drug Discov 1:287–299

Joseph MA, Moysich KB, Freudenheim JL, Shields PG, Bowman ED, Zhang Y, Marshall JR, Ambrosone CB (2004) Cruciferous vegetables, genetic polymorphisms in Glutathione S-Transferases M1 and T1, and prostate cancer risk. Nutr Cancer 50:206–213

Kallifatidis G, Labsch S, Rausch V, Mattern J, Gladkich J, Moldenhauer G, Buchler MW, Salnikov AV, Herr I (2011) Sulforaphane increases drug-mediated cytotoxicity toward cancer stem-like cells of pancreas and prostate. Mol Ther 19:188–195

Kassahun K, Davis M, Hu P, Martin B, Baillie T (1997) Biotransformation of the naturally occurring isothiocyanate sulforaphane in the rat: identification of Phase I metabolites and glutathione conjugates. Chem Res Toxicol 10:1228–1233

Kawai Y, Garduno L, Theodore M, Yang J, Arinze IJ (2011) Acetylation-deacetylation of the transcription factor Nrf2 (nuclear factor erythroid 2-related factor 2) regulates its transcriptional activity and nucleocytoplasmic localization. J Biol Chem 286:7629–7640

Keum YS, Khor TO, Lin W, Shen G, Kwon KH, Barve A, Li W, Kong AN (2009) Pharmacokinetics and pharmacodynamics of broccoli sprouts on the suppression of prostate cancer in transgenic adenocarcinoma of mouse prostate (TRAMP) mice: implication of induction of Nrf2, HO-1 and apoptosis and the suppression of Akt-dependent kinase pathway. Pharm Res 26:2324–2331

Key TJ, Allen N, Appleby P, Overvad K, Tjonneland A, Miller A, Boeing H, Karalis D, Psaltopoulou T, Berrino F, Palli D, Panico S, Tumino R, Vineis P, Bueno-De-Mesquita HB, Kiemeney L, Peeters PH, Martinez C, Dorronsoro M, Gonzalez CA, Chirlaque MD, Quiros JR, Ardanaz E, Berglund G, Egevad L, Hallmans G, Stattin P, Bingham S, Day N, Gann P, Kaaks R, Ferrari P, Riboli E (2004) Fruits and vegetables and prostate cancer: no association among 1104 cases in a prospective study of 130544 men in the European Prospective Investigation into Cancer and Nutrition (EPIC). Int J Cancer 109:119–124

Kim SH, Singh SV (2009) D, L-Sulforaphane causes transcriptional repression of androgen receptor in human prostate cancer cells. Mol Cancer Ther 8:1946–1954

Kim HR, Kim EJ, Yang SH, Jeong ET, Park C, Lee JH, Youn MJ, So HS, Park R (2006) Trichostatin A induces apoptosis in lung cancer cells via simultaneous activation of the death receptor-mediated and mitochondrial pathway? Exp Mol Med 38:616–624

Kim NH, Kim SN, Kim YK (2011) Involvement of HDAC1 in E-cadherin expression in prostate cancer cells; its implication for cell motility and invasion. Biochem Biophys Res Commun 404:915–921

Kolonel LN, Hankin JH, Whittemore AS, Wu AH, Gallagher RP, Wilkens LR, John EM, Howe GR, Dreon DM, West DW, Paffenbarger RS (2000) Vegetables, fruits, legumes and prostate cancer: a multiethnic case-control study. Cancer Epidemiol Biomarkers Prev 9:795–804

Kristal AR, Lampe JW (2002) Brassica vegetables and prostate cancer risk: a review of the epidemiological evidence. Nutr Cancer 42:1–9

Kushad MM, Brown AF, Kurilich AC, Juvik JA, Klein BP, Wallig MA, Jeffrey EH (1999) Variation of glucosinolates in vegetable crops of *Brassica oleracea*. J Agric Food Chem 47:1541–1548

Le Marchand L, Hankin JH, Kolonel LN, Wilkens LR (1991) Vegetable and fruit consumption in relation to prostate cancer risk in Hawaii: a reevaluation of the effect of dietary beta-carotene. Am J Epidemiol 133:215–219

Li Y, Li X, Sarkar FH (2003) Gene expression profiles of I3C- and DIM-treated PC3 human prostate cancer cells determined by cDNA microarray analysis. J Nutr 133:1011–1019

Li LC, Carroll PR, Dahiya R (2005a) Epigenetic changes in prostate cancer: implication for diagnosis and treatment. J Natl Cancer Inst 97:103–115

Li Y, Chinni SR, Sarkar FH (2005b) Selective growth regulatory and pro-apoptotic effects of DIM is mediated by AKT and NF-kappaB pathways in prostate cancer cells. Front Biosci 10: 236–243

Li Y, VandenBoom TG, Kong D, Wang Z, Ali S, Philip PA, Sarkar FH (2009) Up-regulation of miR-200 and let-7 by natural agents leads to the reversal of epithelial-to-mesenchymal transition in gemcitabine-resistant pancreatic cancer cells. Cancer Res 69:6704–6712

Li Y, Li X, Guo B (2010a) Chemopreventive agent 3,3'-diindolylmethane selectively induces proteasomal degradation of class I histone deacetylases. Cancer Res 70:646–654

Li Y, Vandenboom TG, Wang Z, Kong D, Ali S, Philip PA, Sarkar FH (2010b) miR-146a suppresses invasion of pancreatic cancer cells. Cancer Res 70:1486–1495

Lubet RA, Heckman BM, De Flora SL, Steele VE, Crowell JA, Juliana MM, Grubbs CJ (2011) Effects of 5,6-benzoflavone, indole-3-carbinol (I3C) and diindolylmethane (DIM) on chemically-induced mammary carcinogenesis: is DIM a substitute for I3C? Oncol Rep 26: 731–736

Meeran SM, Patel SN, Tollefsbol TO (2010) Sulforaphane causes epigenetic repression of hTERT expression in human breast cancer cell lines. PLoS One 5:e11457

Mercado N, Thimmulappa R, Thomas CM, Fenwick PS, Chana KK, Donnelly LE, Biswal S, Ito K, Barnes PJ (2011) Decreased histone deacetylase 2 impairs Nrf2 activation by oxidative stress. Biochem Biophys Res Commun 406:292–298

Mithen R (2001) Glucosinolates – biochemistry, genetics and biological activity. Plant Growth Regul 34:91–103

Mongroo PS, Rustgi AK (2010) The role of the miR-200 family in epithelial-mesenchymal transition. Cancer Biol Ther 10:219–222

Myzak MC, Karplus PA, Chung FL, Dashwood RH (2004) A novel mechanism of chemoprotection by sulforaphane: inhibition of histone deacetylase. Cancer Res 64:5767–5774

Myzak MC, Dashwood WM, Orner GA, Ho E, Dashwood RH (2006a) Sulforaphane inhibits histone deacetylase in vivo and suppresses tumorigenesis in Apc-minus mice. FASEB J 20: 506–508

Myzak MC, Hardin K, Wang R, Dashwood RH, Ho E (2006b) Sulforaphane inhibits histone deacetylase activity in BPH-1, LnCaP and PC-3 prostate epithelial cells. Carcinogenesis 27:811–819

Myzak MC, Tong P, Dashwood WM, Dashwood RH, Ho E (2007) Sulforaphane retards the growth of human PC-3 xenografts and inhibits HDAC activity in human subjects. Exp Biol Med 232:227–234

Nachshon-Kedmi M, Yannai S, Haj A, Fares FA (2003) Indole-3-carbinol and 3,3'-diindolylmethane induce apoptosis in human prostate cancer cells. Food Chem Toxicol 41:745–752

Nachshon-Kedmi M, Fares FA, Yannai S (2004a) Therapeutic activity of 3,3'-diindolylmethane on prostate cancer in an in vivo model. Prostate 61:153–160

Nachshon-Kedmi M, Yannai S, Fares FA (2004b) Induction of apoptosis in human prostate cancer cell line, PC3, by 3,3'-diindolylmethane through the mitochondrial pathway. Br J Cancer 91:1358–1363

Nakagawa M, Oda Y, Eguchi T, Aishima S, Yao T, Hosoi F, Basaki Y, Ono M, Kuwano M, Tanaka M, Tsuneyoshi M (2007) Expression profile of class I histone deacetylases in human cancer tissues. Oncol Rep 18:769–774

Nian H, Delage B, Ho E, Dashwood RH (2009) Modulation of histone deacetylase activity by dietary isothiocyanates and allyl sulfides: studies with sulforaphane and garlic organosulfur compounds. Environ Mol Mutagen 50:213–221

Olsson M, Gustafsson O, Skogastierna C, Tolf A, Rietz BD, Morfin R, Rane A, Ekstrom L (2007) Regulation and expression of human CYP7B1 in prostate: overexpression of CYP7B1 during progression of prostatic adenocarcinoma. Prostate 67:1439–1446

Parasramka MA, Ho E, Williams DE, Dashwood RH (2011) MicroRNAs, diet, and cancer: New mechanistic insights on the epigenetic actions of phytochemicals. Mol Carcinog 51:213–230

Parnaud G, Li P, Cassar G, Rouimi P, Tulliez J, Combaret L, Gamet-Payrastre L (2004) Mechanism of sulforaphane-induced cell cycle arrest and apoptosis in human colon cancer cells. Nutr Cancer 48:198–206

Perry AS, Watson RW, Lawler M, Hollywood D (2010) The epigenome as a therapeutic target in prostate cancer. Nat Rev Urol 7:668–680

Rajendran P, Delage B, Dashwood WM, Yu TW, Wuth B, Williams DE, Ho E, Dashwood RH (2011a) Histone deacetylase turnover and recovery in sulforaphane-treated colon cancer cells: competing actions of 14-3-3 and Pin1 in HDAC3/SMRT corepressor complex dissociation/reassembly. Mol Cancer 10:68

Rajendran P, Williams DE, Ho E, Dashwood RH (2011b) Metabolism as a key to histone deacetylase inhibition. Crit Rev Biochem Mol Biol 46:181–199

Rayet B, Gelinas C (1999) Aberrant rel/nfkb genes and activity in human cancer. Oncogene 18:6938–6947

Reed GA, Sunega JM, Sullivan DK, Gray JC, Mayo MS, Crowell JA, Hurwitz A (2008) Single-dose pharmacokinetics and tolerability of absorption-enhanced 3,3'-diindolylmethane in healthy subjects. Cancer Epidemiol Biomarkers Prev 17:2619–2624

Rodriguez-Gonzalez A, Lin T, Ikeda AK, Simms-Waldrip T, Fu C, Sakamoto KM (2008) Role of the aggresome pathway in cancer: targeting histone deacetylase 6-dependent protein degradation. Cancer Res 68:2557–2560

Sarkar FH, Li Y (2004) Indole-3-carbinol and prostate cancer. J Nutr 134:3493S–3498S

Sawa H, Murakami H, Ohshima Y, Sugino T, Nakajyo T, Kisanuki T, Tamura Y, Satone A, Ide W, Hashimoto I, Kamada H (2001) Histone deacetylase inhibitors such as sodium butyrate and trichostatin A induce apoptosis through an increase of the bcl-2-related protein Bad. Brain Tumor Pathol 18:109–114

Schuurman AG, Goldbohm RA, Dorant E, van den Brandt PA (1998) Vegetable and fruit consumption and prostate cancer risk: a cohort study in The Netherlands. Cancer Epidemiol Biomarkers Prev 7:673–680

Seligson DB, Horvath S, Shi T, Yu H, Tze S, Grunstein M, Kurdistani SK (2005) Global histone modification patterns predict risk of prostate cancer recurrence. Nature 435:1262–1266

Shapiro TA, Fahey JW, Wade KL, Stephenson KK, Talalay P (1998) Human metabolism and excretion of cancer chemoprotective glucosinolates and isothiocyanates of cruciferous vegetables. Cancer Epidemiol Biomarkers Prev 7:1091–1100

Shapiro TA, Fahey JW, Dinkova-Kostova AT, Holtzclaw WD, Stephenson KK, Wade KL, Ye L, Talalay P (2006) Safety, tolerance, and metabolism of broccoli sprout glucosinolates and isothiocyanates: a clinical phase I study. Nutr Cancer 55:53–62

Shen G, Xu C, Chen C, Hebbar V, Kong AN (2006) p53-independent G1 cell cycle arrest of human colon carcinoma cells HT-29 by sulforaphane is associated with induction of p21CIP1 and inhibition of expression of cyclin D1. Cancer Chemother Pharmacol 57:317–327

Singh AV, Xiao D, Lew KL, Dhir R, Singh SV (2004) Sulforaphane induces caspase-mediated apoptosis in cultured PC-3 human prostate cancer cells and retards growth of PC-3 xenografts in vivo. Carcinogenesis 25:83–90

Singh SV, Warin R, Xiao D, Powolny AA, Stan SD, Arlotti JA, Zeng Y, Hahm ER, Marynowski SW, Bommareddy A, Desai D, Amin S, Parise RA, Beumer JH, Chambers WH (2009) Sulforaphane inhibits prostate carcinogenesis and pulmonary metastasis in TRAMP mice in association with increased cytotoxicity of natural killer cells. Cancer Res 69:2117–2125

Souli E, Machluf M, Morgenstern A, Sabo E, Yannai S (2008) Indole-3-carbinol (I3C) exhibits inhibitory and preventive effects on prostate tumors in mice. Food Chem Toxicol 46:863–870

Spurling CC, Godman CA, Noonan EJ, Rasmussen TP, Rosenberg DW, Giardina C (2008) HDAC3 overexpression and colon cancer cell proliferation and differentiation. Mol Carcinog 47: 137–147

Staub RE, Onisko B, Bjeldanes LF (2006) Fate of 3,3'-diindolylmethane in cultured MCF-7 human breast cancer cells. Chem Res Toxicol 19:436–442

Steinbrecher A, Nimptsch K, Husing A, Rohrmann S, Linseisen J (2009) Dietary glucosinolate intake and risk of prostate cancer in the EPIC-Heidelberg cohort study. Int J Cancer 125: 2179–2186

Stoner G, Casto B, Ralston S, Roebuck B, Pereira C, Bailey G (2002) Development of a multi-organ rat model for evaluating chemopreventive agents: efficacy of indole-3-carbinol. Carcinogenesis 23:265–272

Strait KA, Warnick CT, Ford CD, Dabbas B, Hammond EH, Ilstrup SJ (2005) Histone deacetylase inhibitors induce G2-checkpoint arrest and apoptosis in cisplatinum-resistant ovarian cancer cells associated with overexpression of the Bcl-2-related protein Bad. Mol Cancer Ther 4: 603–611

Stresser DM, Bjeldanes LF, Bailey GS, Williams DE (1995) The anticarcinogen 3,3'-diindolylmethane is an inhibitor of cytochrome P-450. J Biochem Toxicol 10:191–201

Takahashi N, Dashwood RH, Bjeldanes LF, Williams DE, Bailey GS (1995) Mechanisms of indole-3-carbinol (I3C) anticarcinogenesis: inhibition of aflatoxin B1-DNA adduction and mutagenesis by I3C acid condensation products. Food Chem Toxicol 33:851–857

Tokizane T, Shiina H, Igawa M, Enokida H, Urakami S, Kawakami T, Ogishima T, Okino ST, Li LC, Tanaka Y, Nonomura N, Okuyama A, Dahiya R (2005) Cytochrome P450 1B1 is overexpressed and regulated by hypomethylation in prostate cancer. Clin Cancer Res 11: 5793–5801

Traka M, Gasper AV, Smith JA, Hawkey CJ, Bao Y, Mithen RF (2005) Transcriptome analysis of human colon Caco-2 cells exposed to sulforaphane. J Nutr 135:1865–1872

Traka M, Gasper AV, Melchini A, Bacon JR, Needs PW, Frost V, Chantry A, Jones AM, Ortori CA, Barrett DA, Ball RY, Mills RD, Mithen RF (2008) Broccoli consumption interacts with GSTM1 to perturb oncogenic signalling pathways in the prostate. PLoS One 3:e2568

Traka MH, Spinks CA, Doleman JF, Melchini A, Ball RY, Mills RD, Mithen RF (2010) The dietary isothiocyanate sulforaphane modulates gene expression and alternative gene splicing in a PTEN null preclinical murine model of prostate cancer. Mol Cancer 9:189

Trtkova K, Paskova L, Matijescukova N, Strnad M, Kolar Z (2010) Binding of AR to SMRT/N-CoR complex and its co-operation with PSA promoter in prostate cancer cells treated with natural histone deacetylase inhibitor NaB. Neoplasma 57:406–414

Uhlmann S, Zhang JD, Schwager A, Mannsperger H, Riazalhosseini Y, Burmester S, Ward A, Korf U, Wiemann S, Sahin O (2010) miR-200bc/429 cluster targets PLCgamma1 and differentially regulates proliferation and EGF-driven invasion than miR-200a/141 in breast cancer. Oncogene 29:4297–4306

Venkateswaran V, Klotz LH (2010) Diet and prostate cancer: mechanisms of action and implications for chemoprevention. Nat Rev Urol 7:442–453

Vivar OI, Lin CL, Firestone GL, Bjeldanes LF (2009) 3,3'-Diindolylmethane induces a G(1) arrest in human prostate cancer cells irrespective of androgen receptor and p53 status. Biochem Pharmacol 78:469–476

Wang L, Liu D, Ahmed T, Chung FL, Conaway C, Chiao JW (2004) Targeting cell cycle machinery as a molecular mechanism of sulforaphane in prostate cancer prevention. Int J Oncol 24: 187–192

Wang LG, Beklemisheva A, Liu XM, Ferrari AC, Feng J, Chiao JW (2007) Dual action on promoter demethylation and chromatin by an isothiocyanate restored GSTP1 silenced in prostate cancer. Mol Carcinog 46:24–31

Wang TT, Schoene NW, Milner JA, Kim YS (2012) Broccoli-derived phytochemicals indole-3-carbinol and 3,3′-diindolylmethane exerts concentration-dependent pleiotropic effects on prostate cancer cells: Comparison with other cancer preventive phytochemicals. Mol Carcinog 51:244–256

Weichert W, Roske A, Gekeler V, Beckers T, Stephan C, Jung K, Fritzsche FR, Niesporek S, Denkert C, Dietel M, Kristiansen G (2008) Histone deacetylases 1, 2 and 3 are highly expressed in prostate cancer and HDAC2 expression is associated with shorter PSA relapse time after radical prostatectomy. Br J Cancer 98:604–610

Weng JR, Tsai CH, Kulp SK, Chen CS (2008) Indole-3-carbinol as a chemopreventive and anti-cancer agent. Cancer Lett 262:153–163

Wortelboer HM, de Kruif CA, van Iersel AA, Falke HE, Noordhoek J, Blaauboer BJ (1992) Acid reaction products of indole-3-carbinol and their effects on cytochrome P450 and phase II enzymes in rat and monkey hepatocytes. Biochem Pharmacol 43:1439–1447

Xu C, Shen G, Chen C, Gelinas C, Kong AN (2005) Suppression of NF-kappa-B and NF-kappa-B-regulated gene expression by sulforaphane and PEITC through IkappaBalpha, IKK pathway in human prostate cancer PC-3 cells. Oncogene 24:4486–4495

Ye L, Dinkova-Kostova AT, Wade KL, Zhang Y, Shapiro TA, Talalay P (2002) Quantitative determination of dithiocarbamates in human plasma, serum, erythrocytes and urine: pharmacokinetics of broccoli sprout isothiocyanates in humans. Clin Chim Acta 316:43–53

Yu S, Khor TO, Cheung KL, Li W, Wu TY, Huang Y, Foster BA, Kan YW, Kong AN (2010) Nrf2 expression is regulated by epigenetic mechanisms in prostate cancer of TRAMP mice. PLoS One 5:e8579

Zhang P (1999) The cell cycle and development: redundant roles of cell cycle regulators. Curr Opin Cell Biol 11:655–662

Zhao JL, Rao DS, Boldin MP, Taganov KD, O'Connell RM, Baltimore D (2011) NF-{kappa}B dysregulation in microRNA-146a-deficient mice drives the development of myeloid malignancies. Proc Natl Acad Sci U S A 108:9184–9189

Chapter 4
Molecular Insight and Preclinical Perspective of Thymoquinone as Chemopreventive Agent and Therapeutic Adjunct in Cancer

Sanjeev Banerjee, Mansi Parasramka, Fazlul H. Sarkar, and Ramzi M. Mohammad

Contents

S. Banerjee (✉) • M. Parasramka • F.H. Sarkar • R.M. Mohammad
Department of Pathology and Internal Medicine, School of Medicine, Barbara Ann Karmanos Cancer Institute, Wayne State University, Room-715 HWCRC Bldg., 4100 John R Street, Detroit, MI, 48201, USA
e-mail: sbanerjee@wayne.edu; aw9624@wayne.edu; fsarkar@med.wayne.edu; mohammar@karmanos.org

S. Shankar and R.K. Srivastava (eds.), *Nutrition, Diet and Cancer*, DOI 10.1007/978-94-007-2923-0_4, © Springer Science+Business Media B.V. 2012

Abstract Thymoquinone (TQ) is the predominant bioactive constituent present in black seed oil (*Nigella sativa*) and tested for its anecdotal efficacy against several diseases including their potent anticancer and adjunctive therapeutic potential. We present information from literature highlighting molecular insight for anti-tumor functions of TQ largely due to its pleiotropic mechanism of action and ability to prevent tumor growth in preclinical models. Thymoquinone has anti-inflammatory effects and inhibits tumor cell proliferation through modulation of apoptosis signaling, inhibition of angiogenesis, metastasis and exert cytostatic as well as cytotoxic effect on several cancer cell lines. Collectively the results, thus far, points to efficacy of this compound in enhancing therapeutic benefit against tumors that are resistant to therapy. TQ targets cellular niches considered as molecular determinants for chemo resistant phenotype and responsible for their survival and progression. Novel analogs of TQ directed towards better efficacy and sensitizing potential than parent TQ have been reported. Further in-depth studies are warranted including investigation on its bioavailability and pharmacokinetics. From clinical perspective, information on maximum tolerated dose (MTD) and dosing schedule in human subjects are lacking in literature. Nevertheless, existing preclinical knowledge strongly support advancement of TQ to phase-I clinical trial for intervention strategies that prevent or slows down the disease process and contribute to reduced incidence of cancer.

Introduction

Cancer subsists as major global threat to public health and projected to reach over 11 million cases by 2030. According to SEER Cancer Statistics Review, of the 1,529,560 men and women diagnosed with cancer in 2010, 569,490 succumbed to this disease despite advancements in therapy. Thus, from a global perspective, there is strong rationale to focus on cancer prevention activities. Corollary to this conception, numerous studies examined the role of non-nutritive dietary agents with pleiotropic effects in high risk individuals as subject of intervention study. Some of these agents have attracted considerable attention because of their ability to modulate myriad of deregulated signaling pathways that lead to abnormal cellular proliferation associated with ontogeny of cancer. The outcome has therefore been conceptualized as a rational approach to prevent development of cancer in high risk patients. This led our attention to evaluate the beneficial therapeutic effects of bioactive compounds present in *Nigella sativa*, also known as Black Caraway seed /Black seed /Black cumin which is endorsed in the Bible as ‘Curative Black Cumin’, and described as ‘Melanthion’ of Hippocrates and Dioscorides and as Gith of Pliny. Other subjective description includes a common Islamic belief that black seed is a remedy for all ailments except death.

Nigella sativa is an annual dicotyledonous herb belonging to *Ranunculaceae* family and its seeds have been used in folklore and traditional medicine as

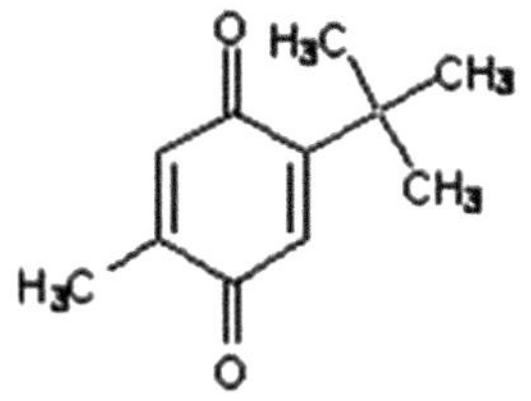

Fig. 4.1 Molecular structure of thymoquinone (TQ): 2-Isopropyl-5-methyl-1,4-benzoquinone (Other relevant information includes: Molecular formula – $C_{10}H_{12}O_2$, Molecular weight – 164.20, CAS # 490-91-5)

a supplement to maintain and promote health and treat various diseases. It is native to the Mediterranean region and southwestern Asian countries including India, Pakistan and Afghanistan. Thymoquinone (TQ) is the bioactive compound derived from black seed [Nigella sativa] oil. The compound exists in tautomeric forms including the enol form, the keto form and its mixtures. The keto form is the major fraction (90%) as deduced by thin layer chromatography (TLC) and high performance liquid chromatography (HPLC) analyses and responsible for the pharmacological properties of TQ (Alkharfy et al. 2011). Over the last few years, TQ have been the subject of extensive research elucidating the multifaceted role of this bioactive phytochemical compound harboring therapeutic/ chemopreventive potential. In folklore medicine, the seed is considered as a remedy for diverse ailments including bronchial asthma, dysentery, headache, gastrointestinal problems, eczema, hypertension and obesity. Accumulating evidences reveal therapeutic value of TQ due to its pleiotropic actions, many of which are closely related to the underlying patho-physiological cause of diseases. This article focuses on understanding and extends current knowledge about TQ as a therapeutic and chemopreventive agent with potential for intervention efficacy in high-risk individuals in context of oncologic diseases. A systematic review reveals growing evidence for TQ being associated with anti-cancer properties in several cell line models including breast, pancreas, colon, ovary, prostate, larynx, lung, myeloblastic leukemia and osteosarcoma (Rooney and Ryan 2005; Shoieb et al. 2003; Gali-Muhtasib et al. 2004a; Roepke et al. 2007; Wilson-Simpson et al. 2007; El-Mahdy et al. 2005). Mechanistically, from current data researchers have inferred and postulated that TQ reportedly induces apoptosis in tumor cells by suppressing NF-κB, Akt activation and extracellular signal-regulated kinase signaling pathways along with inhibition of tumor angiogenesis (Chehl et al. 2009; Yi et al. 2008; Banerjee et al. 2009; Sethi et al. 2008). The chemical structure of thymoquinone and an overview of its pleiotropic effect has been summarized in Figs. 4.1 and 4.2, and presented in the following sections below. This review lead credence to our belief that TQ could be a putative adjunct to conventional chemotherapeutics, impending issues related to comprehensive pharmaco-kinetic and pharmaco-dynamic related studies and side effects to assess risk benefits of TQ.

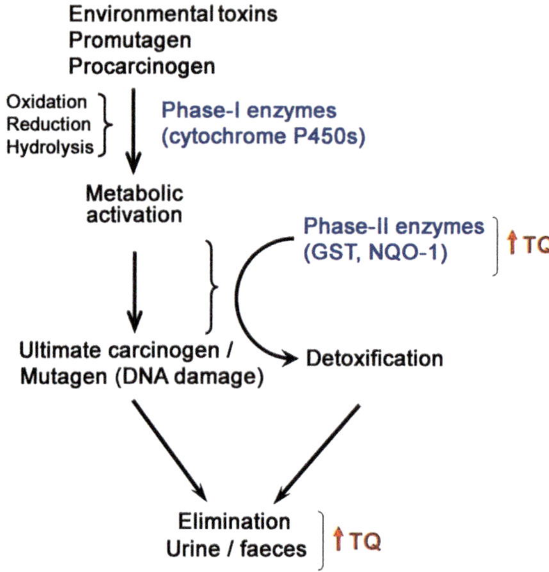

Fig. 4.2 Schematic representation of phase I and II reactions and its modulation by TQ

TQ and Phase-I and II Carcinogen and Xenobiotic Detoxification

Ever since Dr. Lee Wattenberg ascribed that non-nutrient dietary chemicals can inhibit chemical carcinogenesis, modulation of Phase-I and II components have remained a key perspective in rational application of chemoprevention strategies. The cytochrome P450s superfamily of heme-containing monooxygenases (CYP) catalyzes the oxidative metabolism of exogenous and endogenous compounds, mostly resulting in increased hydrophilicity and elimination (Morse and Stoner 1993; Wattenberg 1985). The capacity of dietary factors to prevent cancer has been shown by their ability to inhibit metabolic activation by the P450 system or through the induction of chemical detoxification and antioxidant defense (Fig. 4.3). Of relevance to chemoprevention, TQ act as phase-II enzyme inducer; phase-II enzyme inducers are more attractive than CYP because the duration of their prospective effects will be lasting longer. TQ has been documented to downregulate CYP3A1 in liver and kidney tissues in renal ischaemia – reperfusion model (Awad et al. 2011). It is interesting to speculate that carcinogens and xenobiotics whose biotransformation is dependent on CYP3A may result in inhibiting the appearance of their metabolites.

The glutathione S-transferase (GST) family of phase II detoxification enzymes catalyzes the reaction of glutathione with electrophiles and has been a target of interest for chemoprevention of cancer (Hayes and Pulford 1995). Of interest, TQ

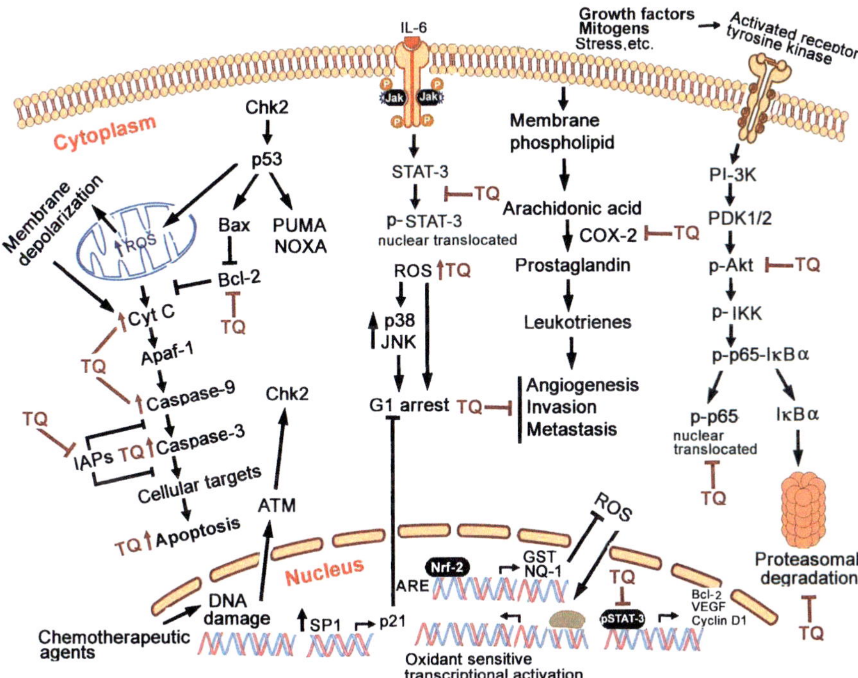

Fig. 4.3 A schematic summary of the molecular targets and cell signaling pathways altered by TQ. TQ is able to stimulate ROS production in mitochondria and downregulates Bcl-2 and IAP protein expression causing activation of the caspase cascade leading to apoptosis. Multiple growth factor receptors are activated at the cell surface during cancer. TQ promotes transcriptional activation of a battery of detoxification and antioxidant proteins. The P13K- Akt, NF-κB and STAT-3 pathways are of significance and targets of TQ. By dephosphorylating these molecules, TQ modulates downstream signaling pathways impinging on proliferation, angiogenesis and apoptosis. NF-κB pathway is inactive as a result of the binding of p50 and p65 to I-κBα. When I-κBα is phosphorylated by IKKs and degraded, p50 and p65 are set free and are translocated into the nucleus to activate a specific set of genes. This pathway has been shown to be inhibited both in vitro and in vivo. TQ inhibits COX-2 enzyme and reduces PGE2 levels

has been found effective in increasing the activities of glutathione transferase along with quinone reductase (*NQ-1*) in mouse liver and in fibrosarcoma animal model (Nagi and Almakki 2009; Badary and Gamal El-Din 2001). This suggests TQ as a promising prophylactic agent against chemical carcinogenesis and toxicity. Insight into molecular interaction between TQ and Nrf-2 that regulates the basal and inducible expression of phase-II genes (e.g., *GST and NQ-1*) by binding to the Antioxidant Response Element (ARE) in their promoters; have not been explored despite our knowledge regarding the pivotal role of Nrf-2 transcription factor in the regulation of antioxidant signaling for many chemopreventive agents.

Pro- and Anti-oxidant Activities of TQ

Natural products have been envisaged as potential resource for principles with ability to modulate the intracellular redox-sensitive mechanism in context of cancer prevention and therapy. Significant scientific evidence has shown that during aerobic metabolism, reactive oxygen species (ROS) are being constantly generated and a dynamic balance exists between the amount of free radicals produced in the body and antioxidant enzymes, such as SOD, catalase, glutathione peroxidase, and to a lesser extent GST. These enzymes detoxify biologically reactive oxidative intermediates protecting the body against deleterious effects.

TQ exacerbates as a 'pro-oxidant' and undergoes redox cycling by cellular oxido-reductases generating reactive oxygen species (ROS) radicals that subsequently provokes cell death by mitochondrial membrane disruption (Nohl et al. 1998; Gali-Muhtasib et al. 2008a; Koka et al. 2010; El-Najjar et al. 2010). In tumor cells, TQ-induced-ROS has been shown to complement growth inhibition through pathways including depletion of glutathione (GSH) levels, activation of Jun kinase (JNK) and caspases, and over-expression of GADD45a (Giovannini et al. 2004; Bower et al. 2006; Higuchi 2004; Finkel and Holbrook 2000). In p53-deficient cancer cells, TQ induces apoptosis through generation of intracellular ROS through transcriptional activation of cell cycle check point regulator, *p*73 gene, considered as structural and functional homolog of *p*53 with similar functions (Alhosin et al. 2010). Thus, from therapeutic angle TQ stimulates production of ROS, inhibits Akt phosphorylation and depletes GSH. Overall, these have been proposed as mechanism of inhibition of the growth of prostate cancer, colon and primary effusion lymphoma (PEL) cell lines (Koka et al. 2010; El-Najjar et al. 2010; Hussain et al. 2011). A 3-fold increase in ROS levels have been observed with TQ treatment in prostate cancer cells independent of androgen receptor status and inhibiting growth of these cells (Koka et al. 2010).

Paradoxically, the effect of TQ in improving oxidative damage and tissue inflammation have also been cited in several reports, indicating that different tissues may respond differently to TQ. The protective effects of TQ in sepsis, and by extension in preventive oncology can be attributed at least partially, to its ability to function as an antioxidant that defend different vital biological components from the harmful effects of ROS (Alkharfy et al. 2011; Badary et al. 2003). Furthermore, the broad spectrum antioxidant potential of TQ has been linked with its potential to stop the radical reaction chain through upregulation of antioxidant enzymes and glutathione under different experimental conditions (Mansour et al. 2002; Hamdy and Taha 2009). TQ rich fraction has been cited to improve plasma antioxidant capacity and expression of antioxidant genes in hypercholesterolemic rats (Ismail et al. 2009). It has been proposed that TQ exerts antioxidant activity through the inhibition of NF-κB which is a key transcription factor for the production of many inflammatory cytokines (Sayed and Morcos 2007; Moine et al. 2000). Like TQ, a number of flavonoids, for instance, apigenin and chrysin have also been documented to have both pro-and antioxidant effects on cells (Miyoshi et al. 2007; Kachadourian et al. 2007).

Under normal circumstances, lipid soluble antioxidants α-tocopherol and β-carotene play complementary roles in protecting lipids from lipid peroxidation. Lower antioxidant enzyme activity is also responsible for the increased lipid peroxidation, which leads to loss of membrane fluidity, membrane integrity, and finally loss of cell functions leading to leakage of free radicals to circulation. Thus far, studies cited in the literature suggest that TQ protects the kidney against ifosfamide, mercuric chloride, cisplatin and doxorubicin- induced damage by preventing renal GSH depletion and anti-lipid peroxidation product accumulation thereby improving renal functioning (Badary et al. 1997; Badary 1999; Fouda et al. 2008). TQ supplementation in diet of Sprague-Dawley rats inhibited malonaldehyde content in liver suggestive of reduction in the lipid peroxide formation (Al-Johar et al. 2008). The protective effects of TQ in phaeochromocytoma PC12 cells against serum/glucose deprivation-induced cytotoxicity has been reported occurring via antioxidant mechanisms mediated by inhibition of the intracellular ROS production (Mousavi et al. 2010).

Anti-inflammatory Activity of TQ

The critical role of inappropriate inflammation and cancer is well recognized since approximately 20% of all human cancer in adults result from chronic inflammatory state or have inflammatory etiology (Balkwill and Coussens 2004). Several lines of evidence indicate pro-inflammatory mediators such as cyclooxygenase-2 (COX-2), prostaglandins (PGs), inducible nitric oxide synthase (iNOS), nitric oxide (NO) and proinflammatory cytokine (such as TNF-α and interleukin-1) augment tumor growth by multiple mechanisms such as by stimulating angiogenesis, metastasis and inhibiting apoptosis through the activation of different oncogenes (Buchanan and DuBois 2006; Wang and DuBois 2008). The first evidence that TQ is useful in inflammatory conditions was reported by Hajhashemi et al.,using carrageenan-induced paw oedema in rats and croton oil-induced ear oedema in mice as model of acute inflammation (Hajhashemi et al. 2004). Subsequent studies revealed TQ alleviates *in vivo* production of PGs and Th2 cytokine driven immune response in mouse model of allergic airway inflammation (El Mezayen et al. 2006). Attenuation of inflammation by TQ has been cited presumably to occur via induction of glutathione (El-Gouhary et al. 2005). Subsequently, TQ has been reported previously to be a potent inhibitor of eicosanoid generation, namely thromboxane B_2 and leukotrienes B_4 in peritoneal leukocytes stimulated with calcium ionophore A23187 by inhibiting COX-2 and 5-lipooxygenase (5-LOX), respectively (Houghton et al. 1995). Additionally, TQ has been found to be a potent inhibitor of leukotrienes formation in human and rat blood cells through its effect on 5-lipooxgenase and Leucotriene-C4-synthase (LT4synthase) activity (Mansour and Tornhamre 2004; El-Dakhakhny et al. 2002). However, no studies describing the potential of TQ in inhibiting leukotrienes have yet been recorded in cancer models.

TQ supplementation have shown to produce significantly less nitrite/nitrate in animal model of acetaminophen-induced oxidative stress, and nitric oxide (NO) in lipopolysaccharide (LPS)-stimulated rat peritoneal macrophages indicating the potential of TQ to inhibit NO production (El-Mahmoudy et al. 2002; Nagi et al. 2010).Consistent with these observation TQ has also been shown to suppress the expression of iNOS which may be useful in not only in ameliorating inflammatory conditions but also contributing to anti-carcinogenic effects since NO has been implicated in the regulation of tumorigenecity and metastasis (Wink et al. 1998; Xie and Fidler 1998). This prediction about TQ chemoprotection in tumor models had been confirmed by Chehl et al. in pancreatic ductal adenocarcinoma cells (Chehl et al. 2009). Available information reveals inhibition of different proinflammatory cytokines and chemokines (monocyte chemoattractant protein-1, TNF-α, interleukin-1β) and COX-2 by TQ, and the effect was more dramatic than a specific HDAC inhibitor-Trichostatin A (Chehl et al. 2009). A related study revealed that TQ blocks GATA transcription factor expression and promoter binding that inhibits LPS-induced pro-inflammatory cytokine (IL-5 and IL-13) production (El Gazzar 2007).

Mounting evidence indicates that prostaglandin E_2 (PGE_2), the proinflammatory product of elevated COX-2 activity plays a direct role in malignant progression of most solid tumors including pancreatic cancer. In line, a study from author's laboratory demonstrated that TQ suppresses PGE_2 synthesis and inhibits COX-2 expression in PaCa cell line (Banerjee et al. 2009). The therapeutic benefit of NSAIDs derives from inhibition of COX-2 at the site of inflammation. Taken together, the foregoing studies collectively support the notion that TQ could be useful in intervening the inflammatory cascade probably with substantial safety advantage over existing NSAIDs, which may lead to the inhibition of cancer progression, and thus improving patient's morbidity and mortality.

Signaling Molecules and Molecular Targets of TQ

TQ and Redox Sensitive Transcription Factor NF-κB

NF-κB is considered to be a survival factor that activates the expression of various anti-apoptotic genes and the production and secretion of cytokines, which in turn serves as stimulus for NF-κB activation and induction of chemoresistance. Compelling evidence have also emerged from several research groups that led to the widely held belief that most cancer preventive agents are NF-κB inhibitors. As reported by us and others, NF-κB is a molecular target of TQ in cancer (Chehl et al. 2009; Banerjee et al. 2009; Sethi et al. 2008). Furthermore, Sethi et al. reported the suppression of TNF-α induced NF-κB activation by TQ in a dose- and time-dependent manner, and TQ also inhibited NF-κB activation induced by various carcinogens and inflammatory stimuli (Sethi et al. 2008). Of interest,

NF-κB activation correlated with sequential inhibition of the activation of IκBα kinase, IκBα phosphorylation, IκBα degradation, p65 phosphorylation, p65 nuclear translocation, and the NF-κB dependent reporter gene expression (Sethi et al. 2008). TQ specifically suppressed the direct binding of nuclear p65 and recombinant p65 to the DNA, and this binding was reversed by DTT (Sethi et al. 2008). We reported that TQ is effective in down regulating constitutively nuclear activated, as well as chemotherapeutic agents- gemcitabine and oxaliplatin, induced NF-κB activation in HPAC (mutant *k-ras* and p53 status) and BxPc-3 (wild type *k-ras*; mutant p53 status) pancreatic cancer cell lines (Banerjee et al. 2009). Corollary to our findings, Chehl also pointed abrogation of constitutive and TNF induced NF-κB in another pancreatic cancer cell line- HS766 (Chehl et al. 2009). Prior to these extensive reports, Mohamed et al. (2005) and Sayed and Morcos (2007) reported the inhibitory effects of TQ on activation of NF-κB in experimental autoimmune encephalomyelitis and human proximal tubular epithelial cells (pTECs) stimulated with advanced glycation end products (AGEs). A significant reduction of AGE-induced NF-κB-activation and IL-6 expression was observed which points to the potential anti-oxidatant qualities of TQ (Sayed and Morcos 2007). In the stimulated non-tumorigenic cell line model (rat mast cells, RBL-2H3) TQ had no effect on the expression of AP-1 protein subunits, c-Jun, c-Fos, and phospho-c-Jun but markedly reduced the transcription of GATA-1 and −2 genes (El Gazzar 2007). GATA transcription factors are involved in the transcription of IL-5 and IL-13. Collectively, the above results strongly suggest that further in-depth research on the role of TQ in modulation of the redox sensitive transcription factors is warranted.

TQ and Signal Transducer and Activator of Transcription (STAT)

Constitutive activation of the signal transducer and activator of transcription 3 (STAT3) pathways is frequently encountered in various human tumors through phosphorylation of STAT3- an immediate early step in STAT3 nuclear translocation, and its DNA binding. In multiple myeloma cells, TQ inhibits both constitutive and IL-6-inducible STAT3 phosphorylation and nuclear translocation along with inhibition of c-Src and JAK2 activation (Li et al. 2010). As a fall out of TQ induced suppression of STAT3 activation, the expression of various STAT3-regulated anti-apoptotic genes products, such as cyclin D1, Bcl-2, Bcl-xL, survivin, Mcl-1, and STAT-3 regulated vascular endothelial growth factor affecting angiogenesis have also been described (Li et al. 2010) Upregulation of STAT-1 has been shown to play a role in MUC-4 induction (Andrianifahanana et al. 2007). Furthermore, TQ intervenes with phosphorylation at Ser727 of STAT-1 in highly aggressive pancreatic cancer cell line- Colo 357/FG (Torres et al. 2010). These supporting evidence raises potential for further testing of TQ and evaluation for application in the prevention and treatment of MM and other cancers as well.

TQ and Regulation of the Akt Pathway

The phosphatidylinositol 3-kinase (PI3K)/Akt axis is frequently activated in cancer because most human cancers display reduced expression of the Akt inhibitor PTEN (the tumor suppressor phosphatase and tensin homologue deleted on chromosome 10). Activated Akt is a protein kinase that phosphorylates unwarranted downstream substrates involved in the regulation of cell survival, cell cycle progression, and cellular growth considered as attractive target for therapeutic intervention. TQ has been found to inhibit cancer cell growth and induce apoptosis through the inhibition of Akt signaling in breast, prostate and in primary effusion lymphoma cells (Yi et al. 2008; Hussain et al. 2011; Arafa el et al. 2011). Moreover, in doxorubicin-resistant breast cancer with constitutively active Akt, the ability of TQ to induce apoptosis implies the importance of the inhibition of phosphorylated Akt signaling as a clinically significant strategy (Arafa el et al. 2011). In addition, several downstream targets of Akt such as Forkhead family of transcription factor (FOXO1), GSK-3β and proapoptotic protein Bad have been shown to undergo dephosphorylation by TQ treatment allowing cells to undergo apoptosis (Hussain et al. 2011). In spot of clinical drug development, TQ mediates the inhibition of angiogenic features of human umbilical vein endothelial cells *in vitro*, which correlated with inactivation of Akt and suppression of extracellular signal regulate kinase signaling pathway compromising angiogenesis in vivo and in vitro (Yi et al. 2008).

TQ and MAPK Signaling

There are three major subfamilies of MAPK in mammalian cells: the extracellular signal regulated kinases (ERKs), c-Jun N-terminal kinases (JNK) and p38 kinases. El Naggar et al., reported in human colon cancer cells the generation of ROS lead to activation of the MAPK [phospho-JNK and phospho- ERK1/2, but not phospho-p38] pathway causing TQ induced apoptosis (El-Najjar et al. 2010). Although the results are quite opposite to the common role played by JNK and ERK in apoptosis, it has been hypothesized that these signaling mechanism bypass the stress injury caused by ROS generation, allowing cells to undergo apoptosis (El-Najjar et al. 2010). Contradictory to this report, TQ suppresses VEGF-induced ERK activation in human umbilical vein endothelial cells (HUVEC) causing inhibition of HUVEC migration, invasion and tube formation (Yi et al. 2008). Also in model of human rheumatoid arthritis fibroblast like synoviocytes (FLS), TQ have been found to block LPS induced phospho-p38 and phospho- ERK1/2 MAPK (Vaillancourt et al. 2011).

Antiproliferative Activity of TQ

Pivotal to chemoprevention strategy and therapeutic modalities including chemotherapy and radiotherapy, impeding proliferation of tumor cells and by extension tumor growth is a crucial factor. Thus far, TQ has been shown to inhibit cell proliferation in cultured cells derived from human breast and ovarian adenocarcinoma (Shoieb et al. 2003), myeloblastic leukemia cells, HL-60 (El-Mahdy et al. 2005), squamous carcinoma (SCC VII; Ivankovic et al. 2006), fibrosarcoma (FSaR; Ivankovic et al. 2006), laryngeal neoplastic cells-Hep-2 (Womack et al. 2006), prostate and pancreatic cancer (PC) cell lines (Yi et al. 2008; Banerjee et al. 2009; Kaseb et al. 2007; Tan et al. 2006). Interestingly, human pancreatic ductal epithelial cells (HPDE cells), non-cancerous (BPH-1) prostate epithelial cells, normal human intestinal cells (FGs74Int), kidney cells, lung fibroblast (IMR-90) and normal human osteoblasts are relatively resistant to inhibitory effect of TQ as reported by several investigators (Roepke et al. 2007; Banerjee et al. 2009; El-Najjar et al. 2010; Kaseb et al. 2007; Gurung et al. 2010). With respect to p53 mutational status, Roepe et al. (2007) evaluated the anti-proliferative and pro-apoptotic effect of TQ in two human osteosarcoma cells lines- p53-null (MG63) cells and p53-mutant (MNNG/HOS) cells- and concluded that, despite differential involvement of the mitochondrial pathway in apoptosis induction in these two cell lines, TQ functioned in p53-independent manner in inducing apoptosis in these cell lines. This highlights the potential importance of TQ in the clinical setting for the treatment of this cancer because loss of p53 function is frequently observed in osteosarcoma patients. In addition to the study reported by Kaseb et al. (2007) suggesting that TQ is a chemopreventive agent for prostate cancer, Richard et al. (2006) reported the effectiveness of TQ in retarding the growth of androgen dependent human prostate cancer cell line LNCaP.

The beneficial effect of TQ as a neuroprotective agent in inhibiting viability of human neuroblastoma cell line- SH-SY5Y in conjunction with L-dopa has been explored and reported by Martin et al. (2006). We, along with others, reported the anti-cell viability of TQ in PC cell lines with differences in molecular signatures related to k-*ras* oncogene status and concluded that TQ inhibits cell proliferation independent of the k-*ras* mutation status (Banerjee et al. 2009; Tan et al. 2006). According to Womack et al., a single dose of 5 μM of TQ caused a 50% reduction in laryngeal carcinoma- Hep-2 cell numbers after 24 h, and a 4-fold decline in cell number after 48 h. These results clearly attest the ability of TQ in a sub-therapeutic dose to alter cellular viability (Womack et al. 2006). As a spin-off to the anti-proliferative effect of TQ, McDermott et al. evaluated the potential of TQ against an important industrial solvent and ambient air pollutant-n-hexane induced toxicity and proliferation in Jurkat T-cells. They found that TQ not only inhibited cell proliferation but also significantly reduced n-hexane-induced LDH leakage to the control levels (McDermott et al. 2008). Additionally, Gali-Muhtasib et al. reported suppression of C26 mouse colorectal carcinoma growth in three-dimensional spheroids with significantly increasing signs of apoptosis and a 50% decreased C26 cell invasion by TQ (Gali-Muhtasib et al. 2008b).

Cell Cycle Regulation by TQ

Evidence so far indicates the effectiveness of TQ in arresting tumor cells at different stages of their progression. The progression of the cell cycle through the four phases G1, S, G2 and M is regulated by cyclin dependent kinases (CDK) molecules and cyclins, which drives the cell from one phase to the next. Despite limited studies reported for cell cycle regulating protein modification by TQ, it reportedly induces G1 cell cycle arrest in osteosarcoma cells (COS31), as well as in human colon cancer cells (HCT-116) which correlates with reduced expression of CDK inhibitor p16 and down regulation of cyclin D1 (Shoieb et al. 2003; Gali-Muhtasib et al. 2004a). In HCT-116 cells, Gali-Muhtasib et al. conducted an extensive study and reported that G1-arrest was associated with up-regulation of $p21^{WAF}$ which suggest the principal transcriptional target of TQ is p53 in the context of the G1 checkpoint arrest (Gali-Muhtasib et al. 2004a). It has been hypothesized that the resulting up-regulation of $p21^{WAF1}$ blocks cdk2 activity and possibly cdk4 and cdk6 activities leading to G1 arrest. In androgen dependent LNCaP prostate cancer cells, TQ treatment caused a dramatic increase in $p21^{WAF1/Cip1}$, $p27^{Kip1}$, and block the progression of synchronized LNCaP cells from G1 to S phase, along with reduction in androgen receptor (AR) and E2F-1 transcription factor along with E2F-1-regulated proteins necessary for cell cycle progression (Kaseb et al. 2007). Immunoblot performed on C4-2B derived tumors from nude mice that were treated with TQ, revealed dramatic decrease in AR, E2F-1, and cyclin A (Kaseb et al. 2007); these results suggest that TQ might be an effective agent in treating hormone-sensitive and hormone-refractory prostate cancers with a reasonable degree of selectivity, and possibly other cancers as well. Of interest, is the novel finding that TQ also causes up-regulation of p53 expression. Since virtually all human tumors harbor either deregulated pRB or p53 pathway, or sometimes both, the unique effects of TQ on p53 protein clearly warrant further studies in determining the precise molecular targets of TQ (Yamasaki 2003). In spindle cell carcinoma, TQ induced growth inhibition by inducing G2/M cell-cycle arrest which was associated with an increase in p53 expression and down-regulation of cyclin B1 protein. In Jurkat cells, TQ inhibits the growth by promoting cell cycle arrest at the G0/G1 phase (Alhosin et al. 2010). Clearly, more in-depth studies are highly desirable to investigate the effects of TQ on other proteins that are involved in cell cycle arrest to unravel the mechanism(s) by which TQ may function as an inhibitor of cell cycle progression and as antitumor agent. In pancreatic cancer cells (HPAC) TQ pre-treatment followed by gemcitabine led to increased cell population at the G0-G1 phase, whereas oxaliplatin treatment augments S phase arrest while the proportion of G2-M phase cells decreased (Banerjee et al. 2009). These studies indicate that TQ pretreatment potentiates the arrest of cells in the progression of the cell cycle.

TQ and Apoptosis

Tumor cells tend to elude apoptosis by deregulating genes that perpetuate programmed cell death (apoptosis). Several studies to date, mostly limited to *in vitro* cell experiments, document TQ mediated apoptosis by regulating multiple targets in the apoptotic machinery. Although evidence for reduced cell viability has been observed in response to TQ treatment in breast, colon, bone, leukemia, larynx, prostate and PC cells, the classical hallmark of apoptosis such as chromatin condensation, translocation of phosphatidyl serine across plasma membrane and DNA fragmentation have been documented in TQ treated cells. Furthermore, TQ has been shown by us and others to activate the mitochondrial/intrinsic pathway which involves release of cytochrome c from the mitochondria into the cytosol, which in turn binds to the apoptosis protease activation factor-1 (Apaf-1) and leads to the activation of the initiator caspase-9. Activation of caspase-9 has been described following exposure of human myeloblastic leukemia HL-60 cells (El-Mahdy et al. 2005) and PC cells to TQ (Banerjee et al. 2009). Thus, one mechanism of apoptosis induction by TQ involves interference with mitochondrial integrity. There has been no studies reported implicating TQ with the activation of the death receptor/extrinsic pathway of apoptosis in cancer cells. Another molecular entity closely linked to apoptosis is the pro-apoptotic Bcl-2 family of proteins which includes Bax and Bak which are activated by TQ pretreatment (Banerjee et al. 2009; Yamasaki 2003). In several cell lines prolonged incubation with TQ showed induction of apoptosis by up-regulation of pro-apoptotic Bax protein along with down-regulation of anti-apoptotic Bcl-2 proteins, resulting in an enhanced Bax/Bcl-2 ratio. In a recent study reported by Gali-Muhtasib et al., checkpoint kinase 1 homolog-CHEK1, a serine/ threonine kinase, has been pointed out as one of the targets of TQ, leading to apoptosis in p53+/+ colon cancer cells (Gali-Muhtasib et al. 2008a). Upon comparing the effect of TQ on p53+/+ as well as p53−/− HCT116 colon cancer cells, p53+/+ cells were found to be more sensitive to TQ in terms of DNA damage and apoptosis-induction; it was noted that CHEK1 was 9 folds up-regulated in p53-null HCT116 cells. The results are in agreement with *in vivo* experimental findings demonstrating that tumors lacking p53 had higher levels of CHEK1 which was associated with poorer apoptosis, advance tumor stages and worse prognosis. In related context, Alhosin et al. studied the effect of TQ on p53 deficient lymphoblastic leukemia Jurkat cells and found TQ treatment produced intracellular ROS promoting a DNA damage-related cell cycle arrest and triggered apoptosis through p73-dependent mitochondrial and cell cycle signalling pathway. This was followed by down-regulation of UHRF1 which prevented epigenetic code replication and hindered the cancer signature to be inherited in daughter cancer cells (Alhosin et al. 2010). This highlights pivotal potency of TQ to stimulate cells lacking functional p53 to undergo apoptosis through p73 component of signaling cascade when p73 is expressed.

In a recent published study by Torres et al., the expression of Mucin-4 (Muc-4) was investigated in pancreatic cancer cells and found that TQ downregulates

Muc-4 expression through the proteasomal pathway and induces apoptosis by the activation of c-Jun NH2-terminal kinase and p38 mitogen-activated protein kinase pathways (Torres et al. 2010). In agreement with previous studies, the decrease in MUC4 expression correlated with an increase in apoptosis, decreased motility, and decreased migration of pancreatic cancer cells. Accordingly, MUC4 transient silencing showed that c-Jun NH2-terminal kinase and p38 mitogen-activated protein kinase pathways become activated in pancreatic cancer cells, indicating that the activation of these pathways by TQ is directly related to the MUC4 downregulation induced by the drug (Torres et al. 2010).

Anti-invasive and Anti-metastatic Effect of TQ

Cancer metastasis represents primary source of clinical morbidity and mortality in large majority of solid tumors. This is attributable, at least, in part to invasion of tumor cells through tumor associated stroma, and entry of tumor cells into the systemic circulation (intravasation), survival in circulation, extravasation to distant organs, and finally growth of cancer cells resulting in secondary tumors. In multiple assay systems, TQ has been shown to interfere with invasive potential of cancer cells. In metastatic pancreatic tumor cells (Colo357/FG), TQ treatment correlates with decrease in the phosphorylation of focal adhesion kinase (FAK), which indicates that the drug has potential in reducing tumor metastasis. FAK controls cell migration and anchorage – dependent differentiation, and is over-expressed in invasive and metastatic tumors. Complimenting with alterations in FAK expression, the motility of two metastatic pancreatic tumor cells lines (Colo 357/FG and CD18/HPAF) were found reduced after treatment with TQ when subjected to evaluation by wound healing (qualitative measure) and in Transwell assays (quantitative measure) (Torres et al. 2010). TQ also inhibits invasion of C26 colon cancer cells across Matrigel-coated filters without compromising on cell viability (Gali-Muhtasib et al. 2008b). Furthermore, endothelial cell migration is an important step of angiogenesis; TQ has been found to inhibit HUVEC migration, invasion and its tube forming capability in concentration dependent manner by decreasing Akt/ERK activation (Yi et al. 2008). In breast cancer cells (MDA MB231) TQ was effective in inhibiting the metastatic process *in vitro* through reduction in cell migration and invasion (Woo et al. 2011). Other molecules of relevance to metastasis are the proteolytic enzymes- MMP-2 and MMP-9; these are known to promote and enhance the metastatic phenotype of cancer cells and inhibited by TQ (Sethi et al. 2008).

TQ Inhibits Angiogenesis and Endothelial Cell Functions

Of relevance to tumor growth; angiogenesis is a prerequisite for supplying oxygen and nutrients to sustain growth beyond a critical size and metastasis. Using the human umbilical vein endothelial cells (HUVECs) and aortic ring assay as a model of angiogenesis, it is inferred that TQ have no direct effect on vascular endothelial growth factor receptor- 2 activation which plays a major role in VEGF-dependent angiogenesis, but instead it modulates vessel outgrowth and various steps of angiogenesis (Yi et al. 2008). TQ inhibits proangiogenic factor (VEGF) induced ERK activation, and inhibits tube formation on matrigel and induces dose-dependent decrease in the proliferative activity of endothelial cells (Yi et al. 2008). These findings indicate that TQ interferes with all essential steps of neovascularization from proangiogenic signaling to endothelial cell migration, and tube formation.

Secondary Targets of TQ

The ubiquitin–proteasome pathway represents a non-lysosomal protein degradation system responsible for degrading both damaged and unfolded proteins dangerous for normal cell growth and critical regulatory proteins related to apoptosis, cell cycle regulation, gene expression and DNA repair. This complex has been cited as a target of TQ action (Cecarini et al. 2010). In TQ treated malignant glioma cells, 20S and 26S proteasome activity measurement reveals inhibition of the complex alongside accumulation of p53 and Bax- two proteasome substrates with pro-apoptotic activity confirming that TQ mediated proteasome inhibition as basis for induction of apoptosis. Furthermore, accumulating data reveal existence of a correlation between reduction of UHRF1 (Ubiquitin-like, containing PHD and RING Finger domains, 1) expression level and cell cycle arrest and apoptosis. This nuclear protein is over expressed in numerous cancer cell lines and tissues (Jenkins et al. 2005; Bronner et al. 2007). TQ induces activation of the cell cycle checkpoint regulator p73, which in turn represses UHFR1 expression (Alhosin et al. 2010). This attests UHFR1 as a target for executing TQ action in tumor cells.

It has been reported that TQ facilitate telomere attrition by inhibiting the activity of telomerase (Gurung et al. 2010). Other studies points to the regulation of low density lipoprotein receptor and 3-hydroxy-3-methyglutaryl coenzyme A reductase gene expression by TQ in HepG2 cells (Al-Naqeep et al. 2009). Narrowing down, one may conclude that TQ regulates genes involved in cholesterol metabolism by two mechanisms viz., the uptake of low density lipoprotein cholesterol via the upregulation of the LDLR gene and inhibition of cholesterol synthesis via the suppression of the HMGCR gene.

Peroxisome proliferators activated receptors (PPARγ) are ligand activated transcription factors with pleiotropic effects on cell fate and has been extensively evaluated as a target for anti-cancer therapy in preclinical models (Panigrahy et al. 2005). In line with speculation that PPARγ activity induces apoptosis, Woo et al. recently reported TQ as PPARγ agonist (Woo et al. 2011). Moreover, TQ down regulates PPARγ related genes, including Bcl-2, Bcl-xL and survivin at mRNA and protein expression level (Woo et al. 2011).

In Vivo Anti-tumor and Chemopreventive Activity of TQ

Complimenting aforementioned studies reporting multi-targeted cellular, molecular and biological effects of TQ, the anti-tumor efficacy of TQ appear promising in cancer chemoprevention strategy as well as, in preventing drug induced toxicity. As pointed previously, TQ displays some selectivity to cancer cells since normal cells are resistant to the apoptotic effect of TQ (Banerjee et al. 2009; Gali-Muhtasib et al. 2004b). We reviewed preclinical studies reported thus far on site specific anti-tumor effect of TQ. However randomized clinical trials are warranted to ascertain with confidence the use of TQ as a rational chemopreventive agent and as a therapeutic adjunct.

Oral Cancer

The chemopreventive efficacy of TQ based upon its membrane stabilizing effects on cell surface glycoconjugates and cytokeratin expression during DMBA induced hamster buccal pouch carcinogenesis have been reported (Rajkamal et al. 2010). TQ (30 mg/kg body weight) was administered orally 1 week before exposure to the carcinogen and continued every alternate days for 14 weeks; this schedule resulted in reduction of tumor formation and protected against development of abnormalities on cell surface glycoconjugates during genesis of buccal pouch carcinogenesis (Rajkamal et al. 2010). In a xenograft model of squamous cell cancer (SCCVII), the antitumor efficacy of TQ administered intraperitoneally was found to be encouraging with predilection for further improvement of its antitumor effect with increase in TQ dose (Ivankovic et al. 2006).

GI Cancers: Colon Cancer

The chemopreventive potential of TQ in 1, 2-dimethyl hydrazine (DMH) induced murine colon cancer model has been reported (Gali-Muhtasib et al. 2008b). TQ was injected intraperitoneally and the multiplicity, size and distribution of aberrant crypt foci (ACF) and tumors were determined at initiation, and post-initiation phase at weeks 10, 20 and 30. TQ significantly reduced the numbers and sizes of ACF by 86%, and tumor multiplicity at week 20 was reduced from 17.8 in the DMH group to 4.2 in mice injected with TQ. The antitumor effect persisted and tumors did not re-grow even when TQ was discontinued for 10 weeks. Immunostaining for cleaved caspase 3 in remnant tumors confirmed increased apoptosis in response to TQ. Another study reported reduction in the aberrant crypt foci by TQ treatment in colon cancer induced by azoxymethane (Al-Johar et al. 2008).

In preclinical xenograft model induced by HCT116 cells, TQ treatment (20 mg/kg, i.p., for 21 days) significantly delayed growth of tumor with augmented evidence of apoptosis in xenograft tumors. This supports the potential use of TQ as a therapeutic agent in human colorectal cancer (Gali-Muhtasib et al. 2008b).

Forestomach Cancer

The chemopreventive efficacy of TQ against benzo(a)pyrene induced forestomach carcinogenesis and chromosomal aberrations (CAs) in bone marrow cells of mice has been reported (Badary et al. 1999). TQ administration during peri- and post-initiation stage, significantly reduced the frequency of CAs and damaged cells compared to the highly clastogenic activity of B(a)P alone. In addition, tumor incidence and multiplicity was also seen inhibited as much as 70% and 67%, respectively following TQ treatment.

Hepatic Cancer

The effect of TQ during the 'initiation' phase of hepatocarcinogenesis induced by diethylnitrosamine (DENA) in rats have been reported (Sayed-Ahmed et al. 2010). TQ supplementation reversed the biochemical changes elicited by DENA treatment by reducing oxidative stress and reversing the activity and mRNA expression of antioxidant enzymes (glutathione peroxidase, catalase, and glutathione S-transferase) and histopathological changes induced by DENA to the control values (Sayed-Ahmed et al. 2010).

Breast Cancer

Connelly et al. investigated the effect of TQ treatment on palpable tumors generated by orthotopic injection of a transgenic cell line- PyVT cells (Connelly et al. 2011). TQ treatment resulted in the reduction of tumor volume and tumor weight compared to vehicle-treated control. Based on the findings the authors propose that epithelial NF-κB is an active contributor to tumor progression and that inhibition of NF-κB by TQ have a significant therapeutic impact even at later stages of mammary tumor progression.

Fibrosarcoma

In a murine model of fibrosarcoma induced by 20-methylcholanthrene (MCA), the growth inhibitory and anti-tumor effects of TQ was investigated (Badary and Gamal

El-Din 2001). The results confirm TQ effectiveness not only in inhibiting tumor incidence and tumor burden significantly (34% compared to 100% in control tumor bearing mice), it also delayed the onset of the tumors attesting chemopreventive potential of TQ against fibrosarcoma development. Additionally, in a xenograft model induced by mouse fibrosarcoma cells, TQ exhibited significant anticancer effects (Ivankovic et al. 2006).

Prostate Cancer

Kaseb et al. reported in a xenograft prostate tumor model that TQ inhibits the growth of C4-2B derived tumors in nude mice (50% reduction relative to untreated control) associated with decrease in androgen receptor, transcription factor E2F-1 and cyclin A in tumor tissue (Kaseb et al. 2007). The findings clearly suggest that TQ may prove as an efficient agent in treating hormone-sensitive, as well as hormone-refractory prostate cancers with reasonable degree of selectivity. TQ has also been shown in another study of human prostate cancer (PC3 cells) xenograft to inhibit the tumor growth and blocked angiogenesis with almost no toxic side effects (Yi et al. 2008).

TQ and Chemo- and Radio-Sensitization of Cancer

From clinical perspective, to overcome conventional drug resistance and to enhance therapeutic efficacy, additional treatments such as chemotherapy and radiotherapy along with TQ may shift the treatment paradigm of cancer therapy. In this direction of development preclinical studies reported till date reveal the potential of TQ in improving the therapeutic effect of anti-cancer drugs and protect non-tumor tissues against chemotherapy induced damages. For example, TQ ameliorated nephrotoxicity and cardiotoxicity by cisplatin, ifosfamide and doxorubicin (Badary et al. 1997, 2000; al-Shabanah et al. 1998). Additionally, TQ have shown to reduce the destructive effect of methotrexate on testicular tissue (Gokce et al. 2011). Furthermore, TQ have also shown to lower the cyclophosphomide induced toxicity by upregulation of antioxidant mechanisms (Alenzi et al. 2010). The superoxide scavenging and anti-lipid peroxidation ability of TQ have been documented to confer a protective advantage against doxorubicin induced cardio toxicity in preclinical setup (Nagi and Mansour 2000). No Phase-I pilot study has so far been reported evaluating its promising anti-cancer effect in human subjects. Of interest, Gali-Muhtasib et al. (2004b) noted that TQ induces increase in p16 protein levels within 2 h of treatment; this observation is of interest, since as mentioned by Gali-Muhtasib et al. (2006) and Hochhauser (1997), modulation of p16 protein expression increases tumor sensitivity to chemotherapeutic drugs.

Barron et al., evaluated a combined dose of TQ and selenium on proliferation of osteoblasts cells (MG 63) and reported reduced cell proliferation, along with increased cell damage and reduce levels of alkaline phosphatase and glutathione signifying that the combined use of TQ and selenium (Se) may be an efficient treatment option against human osteosarcoma (Barron et al. 2008). We reported chemo-sensitizing effect of TQ against conventional chemo-therapeutic agents both *in vitro* and as well as *in vivo* in an orthotopic model of pancreatic cancer (PaCa). *In vitro* studies revealed that pre-exposure with TQ followed by gemcitabine or oxaliplatin resulted in 60–80% loss of viable tumor cells compared to 15–25% when gemcitabine or oxaliplatin was used as monotherapy. TQ synergized killing of PaCa cells by down-regulating NF-κB, Bcl-2 family and NF-κB dependent anti-apoptotic protein members – XIAP's and survivin. We and others have previously shown that NF-κB gets activated upon exposure to conventional chemo-therapeutic agents (Banerjee et al. 2005, 2007). Interestingly, TQ treatment results in down-regulation of activated NF-κB *in vitro*, resulting in chemo-sensitization effect. Similar findings were recapitulated in orthotopic model of pancreatic cancer (Banerjee et al. 2009). Using *in vitro* model system the efficacy and selectivity of doxorubicin was improved by adjuvant treatment with TQ in multidrug resistant MCF-7/TOPO breast carcinoma cells (Effenberger-Neidnicht and Schobert 2011). Similar findings have been reported for doxorubicin in HL-60 leukemia cells, 518A2 melanoma, KB-V1 cervix and HT-29 colon cancer cells and their multidrug resistant variants (Effenberger-Neidnicht and Schobert 2011). In human myeloid KBM-5 cells, pretreatment of cells with TQ significantly enhanced the cytotoxic effects of TNF, paclitaxel and doxorubicin (Sethi et al. 2008). The effect of TQ in increasing the efficacy of 5-Fluorouracil in breast cancer cells (MCF-7) by approximately 2.5 times has also been recently reported (Woo et al. 2011). It is presumed the potential of TQ as superoxide radical scavenger and inhibitor of lipid peroxidation is responsible for many of the observed effects of TQ. Furthermore, subtoxic doses of TQ have been shown to sensitize human primary effusion lymphoma (PEL) cells to TRAIL induced apoptosis via up-regulation of DR5 (Hussain et al. 2011).

In context of translational drug development in lung cancer Jafri et al. contemplated TQ and CDDP as an active therapeutic combination in both- non-small cell lung cancer (NSCLC) and small cell lung cancer (SCLC) cell lines (Jafri et al. 2010).The combination regimen showed synergism that was further complimented by validation of their hypothesis in a mouse xenograft model. The authors also demonstrated that combination of TQ and CDDP significantly reduces tumor volume and tumor weight in dose responsive manner [up to 79% relative to untreated control]. Furthermore, the prognostic value of TQ in chemosensitizing multiple myeloma (MM) cells has been reported (Li et al. 2010). The authors report TQ significantly improves the apoptotic effects of thalidomide and bortezomib in MM cells driven via modulation of STAT-3 signaling pathway. In doxorubicin-resistant human breast cancer cells, Arafa et al. found TQ up-regulates PTEN expression and induces apoptosis (Arafa el et al. 2011). Their provocative finding provides insight into a novel molecular basis for TQ action, since most human cancers display reduced expression of the Akt inhibitor – PTEN.

Badary et al. predicted possible augmentation of the anti- tumor activity of cisplatin by TQ in Ehrlich ascites carcinoma (EAC) bearing mice, and reported that TQ potentiates the anti-tumor activity of cisplatin (Badary et al. 1997). Another related study by Badary et al. in mice bearing Ehrlich ascites carcinoma (EAC) xenograft, documented that TQ (10 mg/kg per day) in drinking water significantly enhances the anti-tumor effect of Ifosfamide (Badary 1999). These observations assert that TQ may improve the therapeutic efficacy of Ifosfamide and cisplatin and in addition reverses Ifosfamide and cisplatin- induced nephrotoxicity by preventing renal glutathione depletion and lipid peroxide generation thereby improving anti-tumor efficacy of the agents.

In addition to chemotherapy, radiotherapy is another conventional modality commonly used for treatment of solid tumors. Nevertheless, de novo as well as acquired radioresistance of local recurrent tumor, or advanced and metastatic tumors reflect limitations of radiotherapy. The potential of TQ in radiosensitization of human breast carcinoma cells have been reported (Velho-Pereira et al. 2011). Human breast adenocarcinoma cells MCF7 (wild type p53) and ductal carcinoma cells T47D (mutant p53) when subjected to a single dose of radiation (2.5 Gy) along with TQ exert supra-additive cytotoxic effects with enhanced apoptosis and cell cycle modulation as underlying basis of TQ mediated radiosensitization.

TQ Analogs

Attempts have been made to synthesize novel analogs of TQ exhibiting superior efficacy against tumors. Conjugates of TQ with various monoterpenes, sesquiterpenes, and the cytotoxic triterpene betulinic acid have been synthesized and evaluated for better anti-cancer activity (Effenberger et al. 2010). These derivatives were tested for growth inhibition of human cancer cell lines- HL-60 (leukemia), 518A2 (melanoma), multidrug-resistant KB-V1/Vbl (cervix carcinoma), and MCF-7/Topo (breast adenocarcinoma) cells, and non-malignant foreskin fibroblasts. Some of the analogs exhibited far more efficacious than the parent drug, while being considerably less toxic to non-malignant human fibroblasts. From mechanistic viewpoint the effects of these analogs on the mitochondrial membrane potential and cellular levels of reactive oxygen species (ROS) was evaluated as basis for their cellular mechanism of action (Effenberger et al. 2010). Our laboratory recently reported and evaluated the effect of TQ analogs against a spectrum of PaCa cell lines (Banerjee et al. 2010). Out of 27 analogs synthesized, 3 compounds exhibited activity that was greater than TQ at equimolar concentration (10 μM). Further, the select compounds were evaluated for sensitivity to cytotoxic chemotherapeutic agents in pancreatic cancer cells and were found superior to parent TQ with reference to viability and apoptosis induction (Banerjee et al. 2010). Other attempts in this direction include a study by Ravindran et al. reporting TQ encapsulated in biodegradable nanoparticulate formulation (based on poly (lactide-co-glycolide) (PLGA) and the stabilizer polyethylene glycol (PEG)-5000) augmenting anti-proliferative, anti-inflammatory and chemosensitization potential (Ravindran et al. 2010). One analog (TQ-NP) was more potent than TQ in suppressing proliferation of colon cancer, breast cancer, prostate cancer, and multiple myeloma cells and exposed to be more potent than TQ in sensitizing leukemic cells to TNF and paclitaxel-induced apoptosis (Ravindran et al. 2010).

Conclusion

In conclusion, this article provides a global overview suggesting that TQ could have potential benefit for chemoprevention and also as an adjunct to conventional therapeutics for the treatment of human malignancies in the future. Furthermore, the therapeutic potential of TQ should not be undermined despite extreme heterogeneity of cancer cells and lack of any study accounting their bioavailability which needs to be pursued. The foregoing narrative are "proof-of-principle" that must be tested in controlled clinical trials especially because diet derived molecules such as TQ have pleiotropic molecular mechanism with different molecular targets including its action on cell cycle, cell apoptotic processes, angiogenesis, invasion, and metastasis. Moreover, with emerging technologies including the use of genetically modified mouse models of human diseases and computational analysis, further molecular insights into basic, translational and clinical research will aid in the advancement of our knowledge to prove or disprove whether TQ could fulfill its promise as a chemopreventive and/or therapeutic agent against human cancers. However, the data available in the literature to-date provide strong support in favor of the use of TQ as a cancer preventive and therapeutic agent for human malignancies, and suggest the need for definitive clinical trial results. Meanwhile, efforts should continue focusing on laboratory research to gain further in-depth understanding on its molecular mechanism of action as well as devise strategy to devise potent analogs with minimum to low side effects with the ultimate goal of translating the benefits of this nature endowed compound for therapeutic uses for diseases afflicting mankind.

References

Alenzi FQ, El-Bolkiny Yel S, Salem ML (2010) Protective effects of Nigella sativa oil and thymoquinone against toxicity induced by the anticancer drug cyclophosphamide. Br J Biomed Sci 67(1):20–28

Alhosin M et al (2010) Induction of apoptosis by thymoquinone in lymphoblastic leukemia Jurkat cells is mediated by a p73-dependent pathway which targets the epigenetic integrator UHRF1. Biochem Pharmacol 79(9):1251–1260

Al-Johar D et al (2008) Role of Nigella sativa and a number of its antioxidant constituents towards azoxymethane-induced genotoxic effects and colon cancer in rats. Phytother Res 22(10):1311–1323

Alkharfy KM et al (2011) The protective effect of thymoquinone against sepsis syndrome morbidity and mortality in mice. Int Immunopharmacol 11(2):250–254

Al-Naqeep G, Ismail M, Allaudin Z (2009) Regulation of low-density lipoprotein receptor and 3-hydroxy-3-methylglutaryl coenzyme a reductase gene expression by thymoquinone-rich fraction and thymoquinone in HepG2 cells. J Nutrigenet Nutrigenomics 2(4–5):163–172

al-Shabanah OA et al (1998) Thymoquinone protects against doxorubicin-induced cardiotoxicity without compromising its antitumor activity. J Exp Clin Cancer Res 17(2):193–198

Andrianifahanana M et al (2007) IFN-gamma-induced expression of MUC4 in pancreatic cancer cells is mediated by STAT-1 upregulation: a novel mechanism for IFN-gamma response. Oncogene 26(51):7251–7261

Arafa E-SA et al (2011) Thymoquinone up-regulates PTEN expression and induces apoptosis in doxorubicin-resistant human breast cancer cells. Mutat Res 706(1–2):28–35

Awad AS, Kamel R, Sherief MA (2011) Effect of thymoquinone on hepatorenal dysfunction and alteration of CYP3A1 and spermidine/spermine N-1-acetyl-transferase gene expression induced by renal ischaemia-reperfusion in rats. J Pharm Pharmacol 63(8):1037–1042

Badary OA (1999) Thymoquinone attenuates ifosfamide-induced Fanconi syndrome in rats and enhances its antitumor activity in mice. J Ethnopharmacol 67(2):135–142

Badary OA, Gamal El-Din AM (2001) Inhibitory effects of thymoquinone against 20-methylcholanthrene-induced fibrosarcoma tumorigenesis. Cancer Detect Prev 25(4):362–368

Badary OA et al (1997) Thymoquinone ameliorates the nephrotoxicity induced by cisplatin in rodents and potentiates its antitumor activity. Can J Physiol Pharmacol 75(12):1356–1361

Badary OA et al (1999) Inhibition of benzo(a)pyrene-induced forestomach carcinogenesis in mice by thymoquinone. Eur J Cancer Prev 8(5):435–440

Badary OA et al (2000) The influence of thymoquinone on doxorubicin-induced hyperlipidemic nephropathy in rats. Toxicology 143(3):219–226

Badary OA et al (2003) Thymoquinone is a potent superoxide anion scavenger. Drug Chem Toxicol 26(2):87–98

Balkwill F, Coussens LM (2004) Cancer: an inflammatory link. Nature 431(7007):405–406

Banerjee S et al (2005) Molecular evidence for increased antitumor activity of gemcitabine by genistein in vitro and in vivo using an orthotopic model of pancreatic cancer. Cancer Res 65(19):9064–9072

Banerjee S et al (2007) In vitro and in vivo molecular evidence of genistein action in augmenting the efficacy of cisplatin in pancreatic cancer. Int J Cancer 120(4):906–917

Banerjee S et al (2009) Antitumor activity of gemcitabine and oxaliplatin is augmented by thymoquinone in pancreatic cancer. Cancer Res 69(13):5575–5583

Banerjee S et al (2010) Structure-activity studies on therapeutic potential of Thymoquinone analogs in pancreatic cancer. Pharm Res 27(6):1146–1158

Barron J, Benghuzzi H, Tucci M (2008) Effects of thymoquinone and selenium on the proliferation of MG 63 cells in tissue culture. Biomed Sci Instrum 44:434–440

Bower JJ et al (2006) As(III) transcriptionally activates the gadd45a gene via the formation of H2O2. Free Radic Biol Med 41(2):285–294

Bronner C et al (2007) The UHRF family: oncogenes that are drugable targets for cancer therapy in the near future? Pharmacol Ther 115(3):419–434

Buchanan FG, DuBois RN (2006) Connecting COX-2 and Wnt in cancer. Cancer Cell 9(1):6–8

Cecarini V et al (2010) Effects of thymoquinone on isolated and cellular proteasomes. FEBS J 277(9):2128–2141

Chehl N et al (2009) Anti-inflammatory effects of the Nigella sativa seed extract, thymoquinone, in pancreatic cancer cells. HPB (Oxford) 11(5):373–381

Connelly L et al (2011) Inhibition of NF-kappa B activity in mammary epithelium increases tumor latency and decreases tumor burden. Oncogene 30(12):1402–1412

Effenberger K, Breyer S, Schobert R (2010) Terpene conjugates of the Nigella sativa seed-oil constituent thymoquinone with enhanced efficacy in cancer cells. Chem Biodivers 7(1):129–139

Effenberger-Neidnicht K, Schobert R (2011) Combinatorial effects of thymoquinone on the anticancer activity of doxorubicin. Cancer Chemother Pharmacol 67(4):867–874

El-Dakhakhny M et al (2002) Nigella sativa oil, nigellone and derived thymoquinone inhibit synthesis of 5-lipoxygenase products in polymorphonuclear leukocytes from rats. J Ethnopharmacol 81(2):161–164

El Gazzar MA (2007) Thymoquinone suppressses in vitro production of IL-5 and IL-13 by mast cells in response to lipopolysaccharide stimulation. Inflamm Res 56(8):345–351

El-Gouhary I et al (2005) Comparison of the amelioration effects of two enzyme inducers on the inflammatory process of experimental allergic encephalitis (EAE) using immunohistochemical technique. Biomed Sci Instrum 41:376–381

El-Mahdy MA et al (2005) Thymoquinone induces apoptosis through activation of caspase-8 and mitochondrial events in p53-null myeloblastic leukemia HL-60 cells. Int J Cancer 117(3):409–417

El Mahmoudy A et al (2002) Thymoquinone suppresses expression of inducible nitric oxide synthase in rat macrophages. Int Immunopharmacol 2(11):1603–1611

El Mezayen R et al (2006) Effect of thymoquinone on cyclooxygenase expression and prostaglandin production in a mouse model of allergic airway inflammation. Immunol Lett 106(1):72–81

El Najjar N et al (2010) Reactive oxygen species mediate thymoquinone-induced apoptosis and activate ERK and JNK signaling. Apoptosis 15(2):183–195

Finkel T, Holbrook NJ (2000) Oxidants, oxidative stress and the biology of ageing. Nature 408(6809):239–247

Fouda AM et al (2008) Thymoquinone ameliorates renal oxidative damage and proliferative response induced by mercuric chloride in rats. Basic Clin Pharmacol Toxicol 103(2):109–118

Gali-Muhtasib H et al (2004a) Thymoquinone extracted from black seed triggers apoptotic cell death in human colorectal cancer cells via a p53-dependent mechanism. Int J Oncol 25(4):857–866

Gali-Muhtasib HU et al (2004b) Molecular pathway for thymoquinone-induced cell-cycle arrest and apoptosis in neoplastic keratinocytes. Anticancer Drugs 15(4):389–399

Gali-Muhtasib H, Roessner A, Schneider-Stock R (2006) Thymoquinone: a promising anti-cancer drug from natural sources. Int J Biochem Cell Biol 38(8):1249–1253

Gali-Muhtasib H et al (2008a) Thymoquinone triggers inactivation of the stress response pathway sensor CHEK1 and contributes to apoptosis in colorectal cancer cells. Cancer Res 68(14):5609–5618

Gali-Muhtasib H et al (2008b) Thymoquinone reduces mouse colon tumor cell invasion and inhibits tumor growth in murine colon cancer models. J Cell Mol Med 12(1):330–342

Giovannini C et al (2004) Checkpoint effectors CDKN1A and Gadd45 correlate with oxidative DNA damage in human prostate carcinoma. Anticancer Res 24(6):3955–3960

Gokce A et al (2011) Protective effect of thymoquinone against methotrexate-induced testicular injury. Hum Exp Toxicol 30(8):897–903

Gurung RL et al (2010) Thymoquinone induces telomere shortening, DNA damage and apoptosis in human glioblastoma cells. PLoS One 5(8):e12124

Hajhashemi V, Ghannadi A, Jafarabadi H (2004) Black cumin seed essential oil, as a potent analgesic and antiinflammatory drug. Phytother Res 18(3):195–199

Hamdy NM, Taha RA (2009) Effects of Nigella sativa oil and thymoquinone on oxidative stress and neuropathy in streptozotocin-induced diabetic rats. Pharmacology 84(3):127–134

Hayes JD, Pulford DJ (1995) The glutathione S-transferase supergene family: regulation of GST and the contribution of the isoenzymes to cancer chemoprotection and drug resistance. Crit Rev Biochem Mol Biol 30(6):445–600

Higuchi Y (2004) Glutathione depletion-induced chromosomal DNA fragmentation associated with apoptosis and necrosis. J Cell Mol Med 8(4):455–464

Hochhauser D (1997) Modulation of chemosensitivity through altered expression of cell cycle regulatory genes in cancer. Anticancer Drugs 8(10):903–910

Houghton PJ et al (1995) Fixed oil of Nigella sativa and derived thymoquinone inhibit eicosanoid generation in leukocytes and membrane lipid peroxidation. Planta Med 61(1):33–36

Hussain AR et al (2011) Thymoquinone suppresses growth and induces apoptosis via generation of reactive oxygen species in primary effusion lymphoma. Free Radic Biol Med 50(8):978–987

Ismail M, Al-Naqeep G, Chan KW (2009) Nigella sativa thymoquinone-rich fraction greatly improves plasma antioxidant capacity and expression of antioxidant genes in hypercholesterolemic rats. Free Radic Biol Med 48(5):664–672

Ivankovic S et al (2006) The antitumor activity of thymoquinone and thymohydroquinone in vitro and in vivo. Exp Oncol 28(3):220–224

Jafri SH et al (2010) Thymoquinone and cisplatin as a therapeutic combination in lung cancer: in vitro and in vivo. J Exp Clin Cancer Res 29:87

Jenkins Y et al (2005) Critical role of the ubiquitin ligase activity of UHRF1, a nuclear RING finger protein, in tumor cell growth. Mol Biol Cell 16(12):5621–5629

Kachadourian R, Leitner HM, Day BJ (2007) Selected flavonoids potentiate the toxicity of cisplatin in human lung adenocarcinoma cells: a role for glutathione depletion. Int J Oncol 31(1):161–168

Kaseb AO et al (2007) Androgen receptor and E2F-1 targeted thymoquinone therapy for hormone-refractory prostate cancer. Cancer Res 67(16):7782–7788

Koka PS et al (2010) Studies on molecular mechanisms of growth inhibitory effects of thymoquinone against prostate cancer cells: role of reactive oxygen species. Exp Biol Med (Maywood) 235(6):751–760

Li F, Rajendran P, Sethi G (2010) Thymoquinone inhibits proliferation, induces apoptosis and chemosensitizes human multiple myeloma cells through suppression of signal transducer and activator of transcription 3 activation pathway. Br J Pharmacol 161(3):541–554

Mansour M, Tornhamre S (2004) Inhibition of 5-lipoxygenase and leukotriene C4 synthase in human blood cells by thymoquinone. J Enzyme Inhib Med Chem 19(5):431–436

Mansour MA et al (2002) Effects of thymoquinone on antioxidant enzyme activities, lipid peroxidation and DT-diaphorase in different tissues of mice: a possible mechanism of action. Cell Biochem Funct 20(2):143–151

Martin TM, Benghuzzi H, Tucci M (2006) The effect of conventional and sustained delivery of thymoquinone and levodopa on SH-SY5Y human neuroblastoma cells. Biomed Sci Instrum 42:332–337

McDermott C, O'Donoghue MH, Heffron JJ (2008) n-Hexane toxicity in Jurkat T-cells is mediated by reactive oxygen species. Arch Toxicol 82(3):165–171

Miyoshi N et al (2007) Dietary flavonoid apigenin is a potential inducer of intracellular oxidative stress: the role in the interruptive apoptotic signal. Arch Biochem Biophys 466(2):274–282

Mohamed A et al (2005) Thymoquinone inhibits the activation of NF-kappaB in the brain and spinal cord of experimental autoimmune encephalomyelitis. Biomed Sci Instrum 41:388–393

Moine P et al (2000) NF-kappaB regulatory mechanisms in alveolar macrophages from patients with acute respiratory distress syndrome. Shock 13(2):85–91

Morse MA, Stoner GD (1993) Cancer chemoprevention: principles and prospects. Carcinogenesis 14(9):1737–1746

Mousavi SH et al (2010) Protective effect of Nigella sativa extract and thymoquinone on serum/glucose deprivation-induced PC12 cells death. Cell Mol Neurobiol 30(4):591–598

Nagi MN, Almakki HA (2009) Thymoquinone supplementation induces quinone reductase and glutathione transferase in mice liver: possible role in protection against chemical carcinogenesis and toxicity. Phytother Res 23(9):1295–1298

Nagi MN, Mansour MA (2000) Protective effect of thymoquinone against doxorubicin-induced cardiotoxicity in rats: a possible mechanism of protection. Pharmacol Res 41(3):283–289

Nagi MN et al (2010) Thymoquinone supplementation reverses acetaminophen-induced oxidative stress, nitric oxide production and energy decline in mice liver. Food Chem Toxicol 48(8–9):2361–2365

Nohl H, Gille L, Kozlov AV (1998) Prooxidant functions of coenzyme Q. Subcell Biochem 30:509–526

Panigrahy D et al (2005) PPARgamma as a therapeutic target for tumor angiogenesis and metastasis. Cancer Biol Ther 4(7):687–693

Rajkamal G et al (2010) Evaluation of chemopreventive effects of Thymoquinone on cell surface glycoconjugates and cytokeratin expression during DMBA induced hamster buccal pouch carcinogenesis. BMB Rep 43(10):664–669

Ravindran J et al (2010) Thymoquinone poly (lactide-co-glycolide) nanoparticles exhibit enhanced anti-proliferative, anti-inflammatory, and chemosensitization potential. Biochem Pharmacol 79(11):1640–1647

Richards LR et al (2006) The physiological effect of conventional treatment with epigallocatechin-3-gallate, thymoquinone, and tannic acid on the LNCaP cell line. Biomed Sci Instrum 42:357–362

Roepke M et al (2007) Lack of p53 augments thymoquinone-induced apoptosis and caspase activation in human osteosarcoma cells. Cancer Biol Ther 6(2):160–169

Rooney S, Ryan MF (2005) Effects of alpha-hederin and thymoquinone, constituents of Nigella sativa, on human cancer cell lines. Anticancer Res 25(3B):2199–2204

Sayed AA, Morcos M (2007) Thymoquinone decreases AGE-induced NF-kappaB activation in proximal tubular epithelial cells. Phytother Res 21(9):898–899

Sayed-Ahmed MM et al (2010) Thymoquinone attenuates diethylnitrosamine induction of hepatic carcinogenesis through antioxidant signaling. Oxid Med Cell Longev 3(4):254–261

Sethi G, Ahn KS, Aggarwal BB (2008) Targeting nuclear factor-kappa B activation pathway by thymoquinone: role in suppression of antiapoptotic gene products and enhancement of apoptosis. Mol Cancer Res 6(6):1059–1070

Shoieb AM et al (2003) In vitro inhibition of growth and induction of apoptosis in cancer cell lines by thymoquinone. Int J Oncol 22(1):107–113

Tan M et al (2006) Effects of (−)epigallocatechin gallate and thymoquinone on proliferation of a PANC-1 cell line in culture. Biomed Sci Instrum 42:363–371

Torres MP et al (2010) Effects of thymoquinone in the expression of mucin 4 in pancreatic cancer cells: implications for the development of novel cancer therapies. Mol Cancer Ther 9(5):1419–1431

Vaillancourt F et al (2011) Elucidation of molecular mechanisms underlying the protective effects of thymoquinone against rheumatoid arthritis. J Cell Biochem 112(1):107–117

Velho-Pereira R et al (2011) Radiosensitization in human breast carcinoma cells by thymoquinone: role of cell cycle and apoptosis. Cell Biol Int 35(10):1025–1029

Wang D, DuBois RN (2008) Pro-inflammatory prostaglandins and progression of colorectal cancer. Cancer Lett 267(2):197–203

Wattenberg LW (1985) Chemoprevention of cancer. Cancer Res 45(1):1–8

Wilson-Simpson F, Vance S, Benghuzzi H (2007) Physiological responses of ES-2 ovarian cell line following administration of epigallocatechin-3-gallate (EGCG), thymoquinone (TQ), and selenium (SE). Biomed Sci Instrum 43:378–383

Wink DA et al (1998) The multifaceted roles of nitric oxide in cancer. Carcinogenesis 19(5):711–721

Womack K et al (2006) Evaluation of bioflavonoids as potential chemotherapeutic agents. Biomed Sci Instrum 42:464–469

Woo CC et al (2011) Anticancer activity of thymoquinone in breast cancer cells: possible involvement of PPAR-gamma pathway. Biochem Pharmacol 82(5):463–475

Xie K, Fidler IJ (1998) Therapy of cancer metastasis by activation of the inducible nitric oxide synthase. Cancer Metastasis Rev 17(1):55–75

Yamasaki L (2003) Role of the RB tumor suppressor in cancer. Cancer Treat Res 115:209–239

Yi T et al (2008) Thymoquinone inhibits tumor angiogenesis and tumor growth through suppressing AKT and extracellular signal-regulated kinase signaling pathways. Mol Cancer Ther 7(7):1789–1796

Chapter 5
Dietary Biofactors in the Management of Cancer: Myth or Reality?

Vidushi S. Neergheen-Bhujun, K.S. Kang, O.I. Aruoma, and T. Bahorun

Contents

Abstract In 400 B.C. Hippocrates said, "Let thy food be thy medicine and thy medicine be thy food." Despite technological and cultural advances, the essence of these words has seen contemporary resurgence through renewed interest in food and

---

V.S. Neergheen-Bhujun (✉)
Department of Health Sciences, Faculty of Science and ANDI Centre of Excellence for Biomedical and Biomaterials Research, CBBR Building. MSIRI, University of Mauritius, Réduit, Republic of Mauritius
e-mail: v.neergheen@uom.ac.mu

K.S. Kang
Adult Stem Cell Research Center, Laboratory of Stem Cell and Tumor Biology, Department of Veterinary Public Health College of Veterinary Medicine, Seoul National University, Sillim-Dong, Seoul, 151-742 Korea
e-mail: kangpub@snu.ac.kr

O.I. Aruoma
School of Biomedical Sciences and School of Pharmacy, American University of Health Sciences, Signal Hill, USA
e-mail: oaruoma@auhs.edu

T. Bahorun
ANDI Centre of Excellence for Biomedical and Biomaterials Research, CBBR Building, MSIRI, University of Mauritius, Réduit, Republic of Mauritius
e-mail: tbahorun@uom.ac.mu

S. Shankar and R.K. Srivastava (eds.), *Nutrition, Diet and Cancer*,
DOI 10.1007/978-94-007-2923-0_5,

their ability to reduce the incidence of chronic diseases. Thus, the search for novel and effective cancer chemopreventive agents has led to the identification of various naturally occurring compounds from the diet. Over the last decade, there has been extensive preclinical and clinical research to validate the role of dietary factors in the management of cancer. Ideally, the biofactor is expected to restore normal growth control to preneoplastic or cancerous cells by targeting multiple biochemical and physiological pathways involved in tumor development, while minimizing toxicity in normal tissues. A number of the dietary biofactors has the capacity to interact with multiple molecular targets and appears to be relatively nontoxic, at least at the doses tested. Since cancer has a long latency period, the role of diet and diet-derived components has gained considerable attention. Nevertheless, a number of factors in particular low systemic availability of the parent compound due to insolubility and rapid metabolism limit the therapeutic value of these components. However, much work is in the pipeline to improve the bioavailability of these dietary biofactors via nanoparticle delivery system thereby increasing therapeutic application and pharmacologic properties in the different target tissues, and to better understand the mechanisms of action in order to predict their respective efficacy. This chapter aims at examining the current state of knowledge of the effects of dietary biofactors in the management of cancer.

Introduction

Burgeoningevidence from preclinical and clinical studies in the last decade has provided unprecedented clues that chemoprevention is a promising strategy for reducing cancer incidence both in well defined "high-risk" groups and also in the general population with "low-risk" of developing cancer. The term 'chemoprevention' was first coined by Michael B Sporn in 1976, referring to the prevention of cancer development by natural forms of vitamin A along with its synthetic analogs and since, a number of studies have indicated the potential role of several dietary biofactors in the management of cancer (Veronesi and Bonanni 2005). Chemoprevention entails the use of specific naturally occurring dietary and/or synthetic agents to thwart cancer development and progression and has gained significant recognition by the National Cancer Institute (NCI) prevention branch, American Society of Clinical Oncology (ASCO), American Cancer Society (ACS), American Association for Cancer Research (AACR) and some private foundations such as American Institute for Cancer Research (AICR) and Cancer Research and Prevention Foundation (CRPF).

However, the successful implementation of chemoprevention depends heavily on a mechanistic understanding of carcinogenesis at the molecular, cellular and tissue levels. Carcinogenesis is a multifactorial and multistage process consisting of three distinct phases: initiation, promotion and progression phases. In addition, the latter involves a series of genetic and epigenetic alterations that begin with genomic instability and terminate with the development of cancer (Dolinoy et al.

2007; Laconi et al. 2008). At the molecular level, carcinogenesis involves the activation of oncogenes, loss of function of tumor suppressor genes, modulation in genes related to growth regulation, cell cycle, apoptosis, metastases, angiogenesis, as well as aberrant promoter hypermethylation associated with inappropriate gene silencing. These successive genetic and molecular alterations are subsequently translated to the cellular and tissue levels, leading to a gradual transition, usually occurring over several years or even decades, from normal to increasing grades of dysplasia, and finally resulting in an invasive and metastatic phenotype. This long and complex process and the different interplays present opportunities for the development of clinical interventions both in preventing cancer initiation, progression and promotion.

Epidemiological studies have shown marked variations in cancer incidence and mortality across different geographic regions, a number of researchers have attributed these findings to the role of nutrition in cancer risk (Gregorio et al. 2004; Wu and Li 2007). Furthermore, despite the intense cancer surveillance, surgical prophylaxis (i.e., prophylactic mastectomy), and preventive therapy against cancer, there has been a constant rise in the cancer prevalence/mortality rate during the last decade and statistics indicate that man are largely plagued by lung, colon, rectum and prostate cancer whilst woman increasingly suffer from breast, colon rectum and stomach cancer. Over the past several years, cancer has been the leading cause of death worldwide, accounting for 7.9 million deaths (approximately 13%) in 2007 (WHO 2011). According to the WHO (2011), deaths from cancer worldwide are projected to continue rising, with an estimated death of 12 millions in 2030. Thus, recognition of the limitations of current diagnostic, surgical, and therapeutic approaches to cancer has resulted in a new focus on cancer chemoprevention. It has been reported that >30% of human cancers could be prevented by an alternative strategy of appropriate dietary modification.

Case-control and cohort studies have consistently shown that regular consumption of fruits, vegetables and spices is associated with reduced risk of developing cancer (Smith-Warner et al. 2003). It has been suggested that the health benefits of fruits and vegetables are attributed to the complex mixture of the additive and synergistic effects of phytochemicals present in whole foods, rather than to a single compound (Neergheen et al. 2010). In a meta-analysis of 16 case-control studies and 3 cohort studies, a 25% lower breast cancer risk was found for high versus low consumption of vegetables and a 6% lower risk for high versus low consumption of fruits (Gandini et al. 2000). A recent epidemiological study including 322 lung cancer patients showed that green leafy and vegetables consumption was linked to a lower risk of lung cancer (Dosil-Díaz et al. 2008). However, some cohort studies do not show the same protective effect (Kabat et al. 2010).

Epidemiological and experimental studies thus highlight the protective roles of dietary phytochemicals including sulforaphane, resveratrol, genistein, curcumin, epigallocatechin-3-gallate (EGCG), gingerol, diallyl sulfide, brassinin and caffeic acid phenyl ester as well as whole food extracts for the control and containment of carcinogenesis (Arai et al. 2000; Bettuzzi et al. 2006; Chan et al. 2009; Kale et al. 2008; Knekt et al. 1997; Kundu and Surh 2005; Surh 2003). Diet-derived phytochemicals play a prominent role in modern day pharmaceutical care and research has been directed towards the use of total plant extracts mainly because of the synergistic effects of the cocktail of plant metabolites and the multiple points of intervention in chemoprevention. The preventive mechanisms of tumor promotion by natural phytochemicals range from the inhibition of genotoxic effects, increased antioxidant and anti-inflammatory activity, inhibition of proteases and cell proliferation, protection of intercellular communications to modulation of apoptosis and signal transduction pathways due to their multiple cell-regulatory activities within cancer cells. (Chen and Kong 2005; De Flora and Ferguson 2005; Holmes-McNary and Baldwin 2000; Hwang et al. 2005; Shimizu et al. 2005; Yu and Kensler 2005; Aruoma et al. 2005; Soobrattee et al. 2006). However, well-controlled randomized clinical trials are warranted to ascertain the chemopreventive efficacy of these phytochemicals.

Recent progress in understanding the molecular changes that underlie cancer development offer the prospect of specifically targeting malfunctioning molecules and pathways to achieve more effective and rational cancer therapy. Despite the positive associations between dietary factors and the incidence of cancer, there are a number of issues that need to be addressed. For instance, genetic polymorphisms in the population which might influence such associations due to inherited differences in the capacity of individuals to metabolise and eliminate these products. Besides, the potential role of the dietary factors to attenuate the efficacy of anti-cancer drugs is of prime importance. Although each biofactor has the potential to affect etiology and development of cancer, it is important to strategically proceed for the design and selection of the biofactor in order to demonstrate clinical benefit with the minimum of adverse effects.

Curcumin, Cucurminoids and Turmeric

Curcumin, a well-known component of turmeric (*Curcuma longa*), has long been reported to prevent various diseases such as diabetes, obesity, and cancer and accumulating evidence indicates that curcumin may exert its pharmacological activities on a wide range of molecular targets (Miguel 2008; Hatcher et al. 2008). The analogues of curcumin including demethoxycurcumin and bisdemethoxycurcumin have been reported to possess similar biological activities to curcumin and therefore are interesting bioactive compounds. A study by Lee et al. (2009) reported the stimulation of AMP activated protein kinase (AMPK) by curcumin which resulted in the down-regulation of peroxisome proliferatoractivated receptor-γ (PPAR) in 3T3-L1 adipocytes and a decrease in cycloxygenase-2 (COX-2) in MCF-7 breast cancer cells. The activation of AMPK in curcumin treated breast cancer cells was observed with the concomitant growth inhibition and cell cycle arrest at the sub G1 phase possibly via the alteration of the VEGF survival gene or p53 and p21 apoptosis-related genes. In 12-*O*-tetrade tetradecanoylphorbol-13-acetate (TPA) challenged breast cancer cells, the curcumin treatment resulted in an activation of AMPK, with a significant decrease in the expressions of ERK1/2, p38, and COX-2, which could be responsible for the antiproliferatory effect of curcumin (Kunnumakkara et al. 2008). Demethoxycurcumin and bisdemethoxycurcumin showed an effect on the regulation of matrix metalloproteinases (MMPs) and urokinase plasminogen activator (uPA) components which play an important role in cancer cell invasion by cleavage of extracellular matrix (ECM) in HT1080 human fibrosarcoma and NIH3T3 fibroblasts. The data highlighted that demethoxycurcumin and bisdemethoxycurcumin suppressed MMP-2 activity in a dose-dependent manner and to a greater extent than curcumin while inhibition of collagenase and MMP-9 was comparable for the three components (Yodkeeree et al. 2009).

Pre-clinical studies in a variety of cancer cell lines and animal models have consistently shown that curcumin possesses anti-cancer activity (Aggarwal et al. 2003; Tian et al. 2008). In addition, in vitro studies using colon, gastric, hepatic, leukemia, ovarian, pancreatic, and prostate cancer cell lines have been performed showing that curcumin displays a potentiating effect with traditional pharmaceuticals such as 5-fluorouracil(5-FU), all-trans retinoic acid, cisplatin, celecoxib, and doxorubicin (Du et al. 2006; Lev-Ari et al. 2005a, b; Notarbartolo et al. 2005; Koo et al. 2004; Chan et al. 2003; Hour et al. 2002). Whilst the in vitro mechanisms of action ranged from induction of apoptosis via the activation of caspase 3, 8 and 9 (Reuter et al. 2008) to modulation of cell signaling pathways associated with induction of detoxifying enzymes and inhibition of metastasis and angiogenesis (Hua et al. 2010; Prasad et al. 2009; Kang et al. 2007) to activation of transcription factors (Suphim et al. 2010) to regulation of cell cycle proteins (Aggarwal et al. 2007) and inhibition of COX-2 enzymes, there is significant interest on the reduction of cancers in vivo. Despite being a highly pleiotropic molecule with an excellent safety profile, targeting multiple diseases and strong evidence on the molecular level, curcumin could not achieve its optimum therapeutic outcome in past clinical trials (Basnet and Skalko-Basnet 2011) primarily due to its low solubility and poor bioavailability. Nevertheless, with a wide array of information on the chemopreventive aspect of curcumin, its role in cancer chemoprevention cannot be discarded. The latter can be developed as a therapeutic drug through improvement in formulation properties or delivery systems in particular nanoparticulate delivery systems, enabling its enhanced absorption and cellular uptake. A recent investigation by Kanai et al. (2011) reported the efficacy of a newly developed nanoparticle curcumin with increased water solubility in healthy human volunteers. The latter safely increased the plasma curcumin levels in a dose-dependent manner thereby improving the bioavailability of curcumin.

Isothiocyanates and Cruciferous Vegetables

Isothiocyanates are low molecular weight organic compounds and sulfur-containing compounds, stored as glucosinolate precursors in plants and are responsible for the pungent aromas and spicy taste (Drewnowski and Gomez-Carneros 2000).

Isothiocyanates are abundant in cruciferous vegetables. Literature abounds in examples where consumption of cruciferous vegetables has been intrinsically linked to a reduction of cancers in particular that of the lung, colorectal, breast and prostate (Higdon et al. 2007). A small clinical trial showed that the consumption of 250 g/day of broccoli and 250 g/day of Brussels sprouts significantly increased the urinary excretion of a potential carcinogen found in well-done meat, namely 2-amino-1-methyl- 6-phenylimidazo[4,5-b]pyridine (Walters et al. 2004). Thus, the study concluded that high cruciferous vegetable intake might decrease colorectal cancer risk by enhancing the elimination of the potential carcinogen and related dietary heterocyclic amine carcinogens. Furthermore, a prospective study of Dutch adults showed that high intakes of cruciferous vegetables (averaging 58 g/day) were significantly associated with reduced risk of developing colon cancer in men and women than those with the lowest intakes (averaging 11 g/day) (Voorrips et al. 2000).

It is widely accepted that isothiocyanates are the bioactive constituents present in cruciferous vegetables. The mechanisms by which isothiocyanates exert their potential chemopreventive effects are likely to be multifactorial as indicated in cancer cell lines and in animals models (Cavell et al. 2011; Yuan et al. 2008). Many isothiocyanates, particularly sulforaphanes, have been discussed as potent inducers of phase II enzymes in cultured human cells. Under physiological conditions, these enzymes are expressed constitutively at relatively low levels and the expression levels can be enhanced in response to several classes of compounds including members of the group isothiocyanates. Although, these compounds can induce the phase I and II detoxifying enzymes, however major interest is focused on inducers of phase II detoxifying enzymes for the biotransformation and elimination of potential carcinogens. These natural chemopreventive compounds can serve as transcriptional activators for the expression of glutathione S-transferase, NAD(P)H:quinone oxidoreductase (NQO), heme oxygenase 1 (HO1),γ-glutamylcysteine synthetase (γGCS) and antioxidant enzymes via the antioxidant/electrophile response element (ARE/EpRE) (Yuan et al. 2008) (Fig. 5.1). However, limited data from clinical trials suggests that glucosinolate-rich foods can increase phase II enzyme activity in humans.

Other mechanisms by which isothiocyanates mediate their action is via modulation of cell signaling pathways and regulation of transcription factors. For instance, a sub-toxic dose of sulforaphane was shown to attenuate TNF-α-induced NF-κB activity, thereby sensitizing TNF-α-resistant leukemia cells to TNF-α-mediated apoptosis. The mechanism of action of the sulforaphane was via non-specific inhibition of NF-κB activation by suppressing IκBα phosphorylation and degradation stimulated with TNF-α, and down-regulation of the expression of NF-κB-regulated gene products involved in cellular proliferation (c-Myc, cyclin D1, and COX-2), metastasis (VEGF and MMP-9), and anti-apoptosis (IAP- 1, IAP-2, XIAP, Bcl-2, and Bcl-xL) (Cavell et al. 2011; Srivastava and Singh 2004). Thus sulforaphane can be potentially used in combination with TNFα as the latter may provide a good strategy for the treatment of a variety of human cancers that are

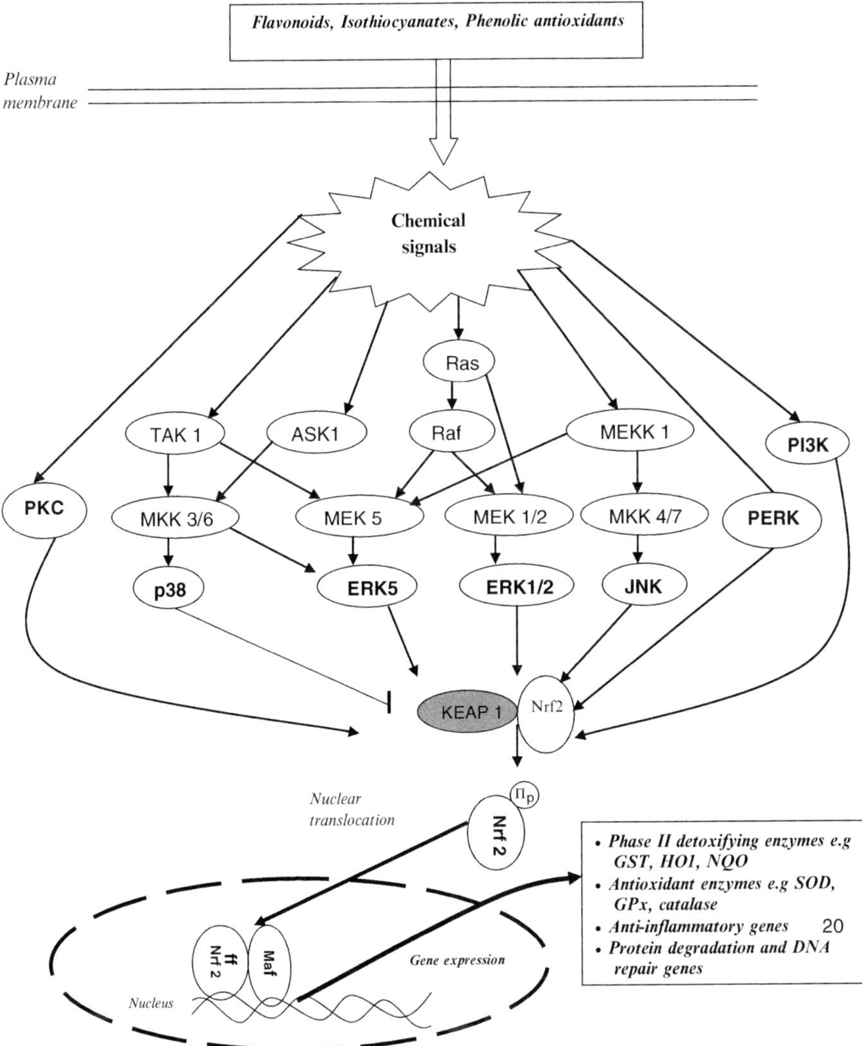

Fig. 5.1 Regulation of the Nrf2-mediated pathways by natural phytochemicals, providing multiple modes of resistance to chemical induced carcinogenesis. Nrf2 is thethered in the cytoplasm by the KEAP 1 actin binding protein. The function and localization of Nrf2 is regulated by multiple upstream kinases (JNK, ERK, PKC, PERK, PI3K). Activation by these signaling pathways elicit positive influences on Nrf2 and subsequent translocation to the nucleus and binding to ARE sequences in the promoter regions of many genes encoding cytoprotective enzymes (Adapted from Neergheen et al. 2010)

resistant to TNF-α treatment alone (Moon et al. 2009). Besides, sulforaphane has been found to reduce proliferation in MCF-7 cells and inhibited COX-2 expression in M13SV1 cells treated with TPA. These chemopreventive effects were associated with p38 mitogen-activated protein kinase suggesting its important role in cell survival/apoptosis regulation and stabilization of COX-2 (Jo et al. 2007).

Another interesting target of indole-3-carbaminol, a component of the isothiocyanate family, in breast cancer has been the ability to inhibit the transcription of estrogen-responsive genes thereby reducing the risk of developing estrogen-sensitive cancer (Ashok et al. 2001; Meng et al. 2000). Although, clinical studies are not very conclusive about the potential role of isothiocyanates in abrogating the incidence of cancer, a number of prospective cohort studies have given an indication about the link (Feskanich et al. 2000; Giovannucci et al. 2003).

Isoflavonoids and Soy-Products

Most members of the Leguminosae family contain significant quantities of isoflavones and due to the wide diversity of these molecules, the isoflavones have been reported to have diverse effects on human health (Cornwell et al. 2004).

For instance, genistein with phytoestrogenic activity is one of the isoflavones found principally in soy beans and has been particularly studied. In addition to the plethora of biological activities, genistein has been shown to inhibit growth of cancer cells through modulation of genes involved in homeostatic control of cell cycle and apoptosis (Aggarwal 2000). Genistein mediate its effect by inhibiting the activation of nuclear transcription factor, P13K/Akt and NF-κB signaling pathway, and regulate estrogen- and androgen-mediated signaling pathways in prostate carcinogenesis *in vitro* (Sarkar and Li 2002).

A study on male Sprague-Dawley rats showed that dietary genistein down-regulated expression of the androgen receptor and estrogen receptors -α and -β in the rat prostate at concentrations comparable to those found in humans on a soy diet. The study concluded that down-regulated sex steroid receptor expression may be responsible for the lower incidence of prostate cancer in populations on a diet containing high levels of phytoestrogens (Fritz et al. 2002). Dietary glycine soya, on the other hand, has been reported to enhance the therapeutic efficacy of tamoxifen against mammary tumors in rats with 7, 12-dimethylbenz[a] anthracene (DMBA)-induced mammary tumor The efficacy was resulted via a combination of tumor cell apoptosis and inhibition of tumor cell proliferation and suppression of the growth of glutathione-S-transferase (GST-P)-expressing preneoplastic liver lesions thereby minimizing tamoxifen's hepatocarcinogenesis promotion potential (Mishra et al. 2011).

A randomised, double-blind, placebo-controlled crossover study using a dietary supplement containing soy and isoflavones in 49 patients with a history of prostate cancer and rising prostate specific antigen (PSA) levels showed a delayed PSA progression (Schröder et al. 2005). In addition, Atteritano et al. (2008) showed that following 12 month administration of the phytoestrogen genistein in a randomized placebo-controlled study, the level of plasma cytogenetic biomarkers was significantly reduced in postmenopausal women. Thus the protective effect against genomic damage appeared to be a particularly promising tool in reducing the risk of cancer. Further clinical studies ascertaining the potential of genistein in the fight against cancer, a case-control study of diet and prostate cancer in Japan, indicated that the Japanese diet which is rich in soy-based products was associated with a reduced risk of prostate cancer in the general population (Sonoda et al. 2004). In addition, consumption of soy foods was observed to be associated with a significant decrease in prostate cancer risk in Scottish men (Heald et al. 2007). These clinical data indicated the benefits underlying the consumption of soy and its products and a better understanding of how these factors interact through further studies with a multi-ethnic perspective will facilitate appropriate public health strategies to include and/or maintain these protective factors in the diet.

Resveratrol and Grapes

Resveratrol, chemically known as a 3,5,4'-trihydroxy stilbene, is a naturally occurring polyphenolic antioxidant compound produced by a wide variety of plants. The cancer chemopreventive properties of resveratrol were first recognised when Jang et al. demonstrated that resveratrol possessed cancer chemopreventive activity against all the three major stages of carcinogenesis (Jang et al. 1997). Besides its ability to suppress the proliferation of a wide variety of tumor cells, including lymphoid and myeloid cancers; breast, colon, pancreas, stomach, prostate, head and neck, ovary, liver, lung and cervical cancers; melanoma and muscles, resveratrol has been found to prevent cancer in animal models (Athar et al. 2007).

The mechanism of actions underlying the G1 phase arrest in resveratrol treated HepG2 cells showed that a decrease in the proliferation cell nuclear antigen expression, a decrease in the expression of cyclin D1 as well as p38 MAP kinase, Akt and Pak1 suggesting that growth inhibitory activity of resveratrol is associated with the downregulation of cell proliferation and survival pathways (Parekh et al. 2011). Extensive data in human cell cultures indicate that resveratrol has the ability to modulate multiple pathways involved in cell growth, apoptosis, and inflammation. In addition, the anti-carcinogenic effects of resveratrol appear to be closely associated with its antioxidant activity, and it has been shown to inhibit cyclooxygenase, hydroperoxidase, protein kinase C, Bcl-2 phosphorylation, Akt, focal adhesion kinase, NFκB, matrix metalloprotease-9, and cell cycle regulators (Athar et al. 2007). Besides, grape extracts from 13 varieties demonstrated significant ability to induce mammalian phase II detoxification enzymes, quinone reductase, in Hepa1c1c7 murine hepatoma cells (Yang and Liu 2009).

In order to substantiate the *in vitro* data, accumulating experiments indicate the role of resveratrol in alleviating cancer in animal models. For instance, the topical application of a dose of 10 μmol resveratrol per animal, 30 min prior to each UVB exposure reduced skin hyperplasia by modulating cell cycle regulatory proteins (Reagan-Shaw et al. 2004). Soleas et al. (2002) also found a 60% reduction in papillomas following topical application of resveratrol, which could be related to its cytotoxic and free radical scavenging activities (Kapadia et al. 2002). Orally administered resveratrol was also shown to inhibit DMBA/croton oil-induced mouse skin papillomas, which correlated with prolonging the latent period of tumor occurrence and inhibiting croton oil-induced enhancement of epidermal ODC activities (Fu et al. 2004).

The in vivo efficacy of resveratrol in animal models of colorectal cancer, in particular dimethylhydrazine -induced AOM which share many histopathologic similarities with human tumors showed that an oral administration of 200 μg/kg/day in the drinking water, significantly decreased the number of AOM-induced aberrant crypt foci (ACF) associated with changes in Bax and p21 expression (Tessitore et al. 2000). In addition, doses of 2.5 and 10 mg/kg resveratrol were also found to significantly reduce the tumor volume (42%), tumor weight (44%) and metastatic potential (56%) in mice bearing highly metastatic Lewis lung carcinomas. The mechanism of reduction was through the inhibition of DNA synthesis and neovascularization and tube formation of HUVEC (Kimura and Okuda 2001).

Howells et al. (2011) recently showed that micronized resveratrol, was found to be well tolerated patients with colorectal cancer and hepatic metastases scheduled to undergo hepatectomy. Data from this phase 1 randomised double-blind pilot study indicated that cleaved caspase-3 was significantly increased in malignant hepatic tissue following resveratrol treatment, compared to tissue from the placebo-treated patients thereby highlighting the apoptotic-inducing effect in the cancerous cells. Although the supporting research in laboratory models is quite substantial, the evidence for benefits of resveratrol in humans remains too sparse to be conclusive (Smoliga et al. 2011) yet, the limited data that are available, combined with a growing list of animal studies, provide a strong justification for further clinical studies.

Catechins and Green Tea

The important role of green, black and oolong tea in the prevention of a number of chronic diseases has been advocated by multiple lines of evidence from epidemiologic and laboratory studies using animal and *in vitro* cell culture models, indicating that tea consumption is inversely associated with the risk of several types of human cancer and cardiovascular diseases (Adhami et al. 2003; Geleijnse et al. 1999; Kaur et al. 2007; Kundu et al. 2005; Park and Surh 2004). The health-promoting effects of regular tea consumption are mainly ascribed to its polyphenol content (35% of their dry weight in the leaves) with the major phenolics being the flavan-3-ols ((epi)catechins, (epi)gallocatechins and their gallate esters), the flavonols (mono-, di-, and tri-glycoside conjugates of myricetin, quercetin and kaempferol), the flavones and quinic acid esters of gallic, coumaric and caffeic acids. There are four major catechins in green tea, of which (−)-epigallocatechin gallate (EGCG) is dominant and constitutes more than 50% of total catechins (Hara 2006) and much of the health-promoting effects have been ascribed to the catechins.

Accumulating data from various cell line studies indicate that tea catechins possesses strong antiproliferative properties, for instance intraperitoneal injection of green tea (-)-EGCG inhibited the growth and rapidly reduced the size of human prostate tumours in nude mice formed by the human prostate cancer cell lines PC-3 and LNCaP 104R (Liao et al. 1995). A nutrient mixture containing ascorbic acid, lysine, proline, arginine and green tea extract significantly inhibited human bladder (T-24) and human ovarian (SK-OV-3) cancer cell proliferation whilst simultaneously inhibiting cell secretion of matrix mellaproteinase −2 and −9 thereby reducing the invasiveness of cancerous cells (Roomi et al. 2006). Even black tea, which has a reduced content of tea catechins, has been shown to reduce the proliferation of MCF-7 primary tumours and also to increase the apoptotic rate (Zhou et al. 2004) while (-)-EGCG slowed growth and induced death of ER-negative breast cancer cell lines including MDAMB 231, D3-1 and Hs 578T cell lines in a dose-dependent manner (Kavanagh et al. 2001) while promoting apoptosis in human bladder cancer cells (T24) (Qin et al. 2007).

The first clinical study to prove the effectiveness of green tea catechins was conducted in a randomized, double-blind, placebo-controlled study involving 60 subjects The data suggest 90% reduction in developing prostate cancer among the male volunteers after 1 year (Bettuzzi et al. 2006). Successively in a larger, randomized, double-blind, placebo-controlled trial with 262 subjects, the supplementation of standardised green tea extract resulted in a significant reduction in serum levels of prostate serum antigens, hepatocyte growth factor, and vascular endothelial growth factor in men with prostate cancer, with no elevation of liver enzymes (McLarty et al. 2009). A meta-analysis reported a significant association between green tea consumption and lung cancer risk. Furthermore, an increase in green tea consumption of two cups/day was associated with an 18% decreased risk of developing lung cancer (RR = 0.82, 95% CI = 0.71 − 0.96) (Tang et al. 2009). In the same vein, Butler and Wu (2011) reported inverse associations for green tea intake and risk of ovarian cancer (odds ratio [OR] = 0.66; 95% confidence interval [CI]: 0.54, 0.80), and for green tea and risk of endometrial cancer (OR = 0.78, 95% CI: 0.62, 0.98).

L-Ergothioneine and Mushrooms

L-Ergothioneine (EGT) is a dietary water-soluble sulfur-containing histidine derivative abundantly found in mushrooms. As opposed to other naturally occurring thiols (e.g., glutathione, N-acetylcysteine), EGT is present in aqueous solutions predominantly as a thione rather than a tautomeric thiol structure and as a consequence is a very stable antioxidant that is nonautoxidizable at physiologic pH. L-Ergothioneine is well-known for its antioxidant properties (Hartman 1990; Akanmu et al. 1991) and nowadays there are claims regarding its role in cancer chemoprevention (Obayashi et al. 2005).

A study conducted by Botta et al. (2008) indicated the ability of ergothioneine to reduce the genotoxic effect of visible light and UVA light on human keratinocytes and CHO cells. A maximal protective effect of 97.9% for ergothioneine at a concentration of 0.5 mM against visible light while 59.8% against UVA/visible light was observed. In addition, ergothioneine has been found to alleviate the potential side-effects of cisplatin an anti- drug tumour. Whilst the neurotoxic and cytotoxic effects of cisplatin have been widely reported, ergothioneine has been found to prevent cisplatin-induced decreased in PC12 cells proliferation and inhibition of the growth of axon and dendrite of primary cortical neuron cells. Furthermore, an *in vivo* study showed that ergothioneine enhanced cognition, possibly through the inhibition of oxidative stress and restoration of acetyl cholinesterase activity in neuronal cells in mice treated with cisplatin (Song et al. 2010).

Despite a wide interest in ergothioneine, there is limited preclinical and clinical data to validate its role in protecting against cancer. Nevertheless, there is a great deal of data on mushrooms which contain high proportion of ergothioneine in cancer. Yang et al. (2006) studied the ability of *Antrodia camphorate*, a mushroom used in traditional Chinese medicine, to induce apoptosis in cultured MCF-7 breast cancer cells. The latter exhibited an antiproliferative effect through the induction of apoptosis, associated with cytochrome c translocation, caspase 3 activation, PARP degradation, and dysregulation of Bcl-2 and Bax in MCF-7 cells; thus, suggesting the potency of *A. camphorata* in terms of its chemotherapeutic and cytostatic activity in human breast cancer cells. *A. camphorata* was also reported to exhibit significant apoptotic cell death against leukemia HL-60 cells (Hseu et al. 2004).

Among other species of mushrooms, the crude extracts of *Ganoderma lucidum* were found to exhibit anticancer activity in in-vitro systems against a variety of cancer cells like leukemia, lymphoma, breast, human bladder and prostate, liver, lung and myeloma cell lines (Lu et al. 2004; Aida et al. 2009). Mahajna et al. (2009) suggested several mechanisms of action of this species including the inhibition of proliferation, induction of apoptosis, induction of cell cycle arrest, inhibition of invasive behaviour and suppression of tumour angiogenesis in many experimental systems including prostate cancer. Other studies by Sarangi et al. (2006) and Shah et al. (2007) also reported the immunomodulatory and antitumor properties of proteoglycan derived from fruiting body and mycelia of *P. ostreatus*. Species of mushrooms including *Phellinus rimosus*, *Pleurotus florida*, *Pleurotus pulmonaris* and Inonotus obliquus have also been credited for their significant antimutagenic and anticarcinogenic activities (Park et al. 2006; Thekkuttuparambil and Kainoor 2007). The bioactive constituents from mushrooms could serve as novel source of anti-cancer agents with potential health benefits. However, clinical studies with appropriate endpoints and surrogate markers for the anticancer response would help to evaluate the potential role and application of mushroom-derived biofactors against cancer.

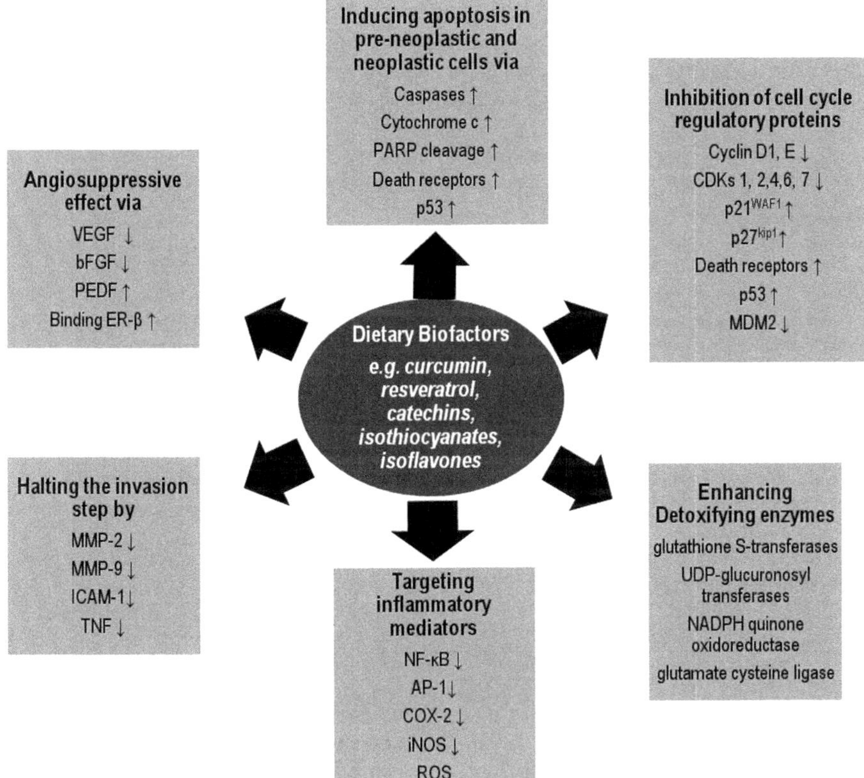

Fig. 5.2 Schematic representation of the possible cellular and molecular targets of dietary biofactors against cancer. *CDKs* cyclin-dependent kinases, *MDM2* murine double minute-2, *PARP* poly ADP ribose polymerase, *VEGF* vascular endothelial growth factor, *bFGF* basic fibroblast growth factor, *PEDF* pigment epithelium-derived factor, *ER-b* estrogen receptor β, *MMP* matrix metalloproteinase, *ICAM-1* intercellular adhesion molecule-1, *TNF* tumor necrosis factor, *NF-kB* nuclear factor kB, *COX-2* cyclooxygenase-2, *AP- 1* activator protein-1, *iNOS* inducible nitric oxide synthase, *ROS* reactive oxygen species

Conclusion

From this point of view, chemoprevention has been successfully achieved in numerous *in vitro* and as well as *in vivo* studies. The pleiotropic effects of the dietary biofactors in a network of multiple cell-regulatory activities support further investigations in improving the bioavailability and pharmacologic properties in the different target tissues, and in better understanding their mechanisms of action (Fig. 5.2). However intensive clinical studies with appropriate endpoints and surrogate markers for anticancer response are mandatory to justify any purported claim. Despite extensive interest and effort, and continuing promising results from basic research and clinical trials, the therapeutic application of these biofactors is limited by poor water solubility, fast metabolism and low bioavailability, therefore attempt to circumvent these pitfalls primarily by nanocarriers seems a promising strategy in making cancer chemoprevention a reality.

References

Adhami VM, Afaq F, Ahmad N (2003) Suppression of ultraviolet B exposure-mediated activation of NF-kappaB in normal human keratinocytes by resveratrol. Neoplasia 5(1):74–82

Aggarwal R (2000) Cell signaling and regulators of cell cycle as molecular targets for prostate cancer prevention by dietary agents. Biochem Pharmacol 60(8):1051–1059

Aggarwal BB, Kumar A, Bharti AC (2003) Anticancer potential of curcumin: preclinical and clinical studies. Anticancer Res 23(1):363–398

Aggarwal BB, Banerjee S, Bharadwaj U, Sung B et al (2007) Curcumin induces the degradation of cyclin E expression through ubiquitin-dependent pathway and up-regulatescyclin-dependent kinase inhibitors p21 and p27 in multiple human tumor cell lines. Biochem Pharmacol 73(8):1024–1032

Aida FMNA, Shuhaimi M, Yazid M, Maaruf AG (2009) Mushroom as a potential source of prebiotics: a review. Trends Food Sci Technol 20(11):567–575

Akanmu D, Cecchini R, Aruoma OI, Halliwell B (1991) The antioxidant action of ergothioneine. Arch Biochem Biophys 298(1):10–16

Arai Y, Watanabe S, Kimira M, Shimoi K et al (2000) Dietary intakes of flavonols, flavones and isoflavones by Japanese women and the inverse correlation between quercetin intake and plasma LDL cholesterol concentration. J Nutr 130(9):2243–2250

Aruoma OI, Bahorun T, Clement Y, Mersch-Sundermann V (2005) Inflammation, cellular and redox signalling mechanisms in cancer and degenerative diseases. Mutat Res 579(1):1–5

Ashok BT, Chen Y, Liu X, Bradlow HL et al (2001) Abrogation of estrogen-mediated cellular and biochemical effects by indole-3-carbinol. Nutr Cancer 41:180–187

Athar M, Back J, Tang X, Kim KH et al (2007) Resveratrol: a review of preclinical studies for human cancer prevention. Toxicol Appl Pharmacol 224(3):274–283

Atteritano M, Pernice F, Mazzaferro S, Mantuano S et al (2008) Effects of phytoestrogen genistein on cytogenetic biomarkers in postmenopausal women: 1 year randomized, placebo-controlled study. Eur J Pharmacol 589(1–3):22–26

Basnet P, Skalko-Basnet N (2011) Curcumin: an anti-inflammatory molecule from a curry spice on the path to cancer treatment. Molecules 16(6):4567–4598

Bettuzzi S, Brausi M, Rizzi F, Castagnetti G et al (2006) Chemoprevention of human prostate cancer by oral administration of green tea catechins in volunteers with high-grade prostate intraepithelial neoplasia: a preliminary report from a one-year proof-of-principle study. Cancer Res 66(2):1234–1240

Botta C, Di Giorgio C, Sabatier A, De Méo M (2008) Genotoxicity of visible light (400–800 nm) and photoprotection assessment of ectoin, L-ergothioneine and mannitol and four sunscreens. J Photochem Photobiol B Biol 91(1):24–34

Butler LM, Wu AH (2011) Green and black tea in relation to gynecologic cancers. Mol Nutr Food Res 55(6):931–934

Cavell BE, Alwi SSA, Donlevy A, Packham G (2011) Anti-angiogenic effects of dietary isothiocyanates: mechanisms of action and implications for human health. Biochem Pharmacol 81(2):327–336

Chan MM, Fong D, Soprano KJ, Holmes WF et al (2003) Inhibition of growth and sensitization to cisplatinmediated killing of ovarian cancer cells by polyphenolic chemopreventive agents. J Cell Physiol 194(1):63–70

Chan R, Lok K, Woo J (2009) Prostate cancer and vegetable consumption. Mol Nutr Food Res 53(2):201–216

Chen C, Kong ANT (2005) Dietary cancer-chemopreventive compounds: from signalling and gene expression to pharmacological effects. Trends Pharmacol Sci 26(6):318–326

Cornwell T, Cohick W, Raskin I (2004) Dietary phytoestrogens and health. Phytochemistry 65(8):995–1016

De Flora S, Ferguson LR (2005) Overview of mechanisms of cancer chemopreventive agents. Mutat Res 591(1–2):8–15

Dolinoy DC, Weidman JR, Jirtle RL (2007) Epigenetic gene regulation: linking early developmental environment to adult disease. Reprod Toxicol 23(3):297–307

Dosil-Díaz O, Ruano-Ravina A, Gestal-Otero J, Barros-Dios JM (2008) Consumption of fruit and vegetables and risk of lung cancer: a case-control study in Galicia. Spain Nutr 24(5):407–413

Drewnowski A, Gomez-Carneros C (2000) Bitter taste, phytonutrients, and the consumer: a review. Am J Clin Nutr 72:1424–1435

Du B, Jiang L, Xia Q, Zhong L (2006) Synergistic inhibitory effects of curcumin and 5-fluorouracil on the growth of the human colon cancer cell line HT-29. Chemotherapy 52(1):23–28

Feskanich D, Ziegler RG, Michaud DS, Giovannucci EL et al (2000) Prospective study of fruit and vegetable consumption and risk of lung cancer among men and women. J Natl Cancer Inst 92(22):1812–1823

Fritz WA, Wang J, Eltoum IE, Lamartiniere CA (2002) Dietary genistein down-regulates androgen and estrogen receptor expression in the rat prostate. Mol Cell Endocrinol 186(1):89–99

Fu ZD, Cao Y, Wang KF, Xu SF et al (2004) Chemopreventive effect of resveratrol to cancer. Ai zheng (Chin J Cancer) 23:869–873

Gandini S, Merzenich H, Robertson C, Boyle P (2000) Meta-analysis of studies on breast cancer risk and diet: the role of fruit and vegetable consumption and the intake of associated micronutrients. Eur J Cancer 36(5):636–646

Geleijnse JM, Laurer LJ, Hofman A, Pols HAP et al (1999) Tea flavonoids may protect against atherosclerosis: the Rotterdam Study. Arch Intern Med 159:2170–2174

Giovannucci E, Rimm EB, Liu Y, Stampfer MJ et al (2003) A prospective study of cruciferous vegetables and prostate cancer. Cancer Epidemiol Biomarkers Prev 12(12):1403–1409

Gregorio D, Kulldorff M, Sheehan TJ, Samociuk H (2004) Geographic distribution of prostate cancer incidence in the era of PSA testing, connecticut, 1984 to 1998. Urology 63(1):78–82

Hara Y (2006) Prophylactic functions of tea catechins. In: Jain NK, Siddiqi MA, Weisburger JH (eds) Protective effects of tea on human health. CABI, Oxfordshire, UK, pp 16–24

Hartman PE (1990) Ergothioneine as antioxidant. Methods Enzymol 186:310–318

Hatcher H, Planalp R, Cho J, Torti FM et al (2008) Curcumin: from ancient medicine to current clinical trials. Cell Mol Life Sci 65(11):1631–1652

Heald CL, Ritchie MR, Bolton-Smith C, Morton MS et al (2007) Phyto-oestrogens and risk of prostate cancer in Scottish men. Br J Nutr 98(2):388–396

Higdon JV, Delage B, Williams DE, Dashwood RH (2007) Cruciferous vegetables and human cancer risk: epidemiologic evidence and mechanistic basis. Pharmacol Res 55(3):224–236

Holmes-McNary M, Baldwin ASB Jr (2000) Chemopreventive properties of trans-resveratrol are associated with inhibition of activation of the IκB kinase. Cancer Res 60(13):3477–3483

Hour TC, Chen J, Huang CY, Guan JY et al (2002) Curcumin enhances cytotoxicity of chemotherapeutic agents in prostate cancer cells by inducing p21(WAF1/CIP1) and C/EBPbeta expressions and suppressing NF-kappaB activation. Prostate 51(3):211–218

Howells LM, Berry DP, Elliott PJ, Jacobson EW et al (2011) Phase I randomised double-blind pilot study of micronized resveratrol(SRT501) in patients with hepatic metastases – safety, pharmacokinetics and pharmacodynamics. Cancer Prev Res (Phila) 4(9):1419–1425

Hseu YC, Yang HL, Lai YC, Lin JG et al (2004) Induction of apoptosis by Antrodia camphorate in human premyelocytic leukemia HL-60 cells. Nutr Cancer 48:189–197

Hua WF, Fu YS, Liao YJ, Xia WJ et al (2010) Curcumin induces down-regulation of EZH2 expression through the MAPK pathway in MDA-MB-435 human breast cancer cells. Eur J Pharmacol 637(1–3):16–21

Hwang JT, Ha J, Park OJ (2005) Combination of 5-fluorouracil and genistein induces apoptosis synergistically in chemo resistant cancer cells through the modulation of AMPK and COX-2 signaling pathways. Biochem Biophys Res Commun 332(2):433–440

Jang M, Cai L, Udeani GO, Slowing K et al (1997) Cancer chemopreventive activity of resveratrol, a natural product derived from grapes. Science 275(5297):218–220

Jo EH, Kim SH, Ahn NS, Park JS et al (2007) Efficacy of sulforaphane is mediated by p38 MAP kinase and caspase-7 activations in ER-positive and COX-2-expressed human breast cancer cells. Eur J Cancer Prev 16(6):505–510

Kabat GC, Park Y, Hollenbeck AR, Schatzkin A et al (2010) Intake of fruits and vegetables, and risk of endometrial cancer in the NIH-AARP diet and health study. Cancer Epidemiol 34(5):568–573

Kale A, Gawande S, Kotwal S (2008) Cancer phytotherapeutics: role for flavonoids at the cellular level. Phytother Res 22(5):567–577

Kanai M, Imaizumi A, Otsuka Y, Sasaki H et al (2011) Dose-escalation and pharmacokinetic study of nanoparticle curcumin, a potential anticancer agent with improved bioavailability, in healthy human volunteers. Cancer Chemother Pharmacol 69(1):65–70

Kang ES, Woo IS, Kim HJ, Eun SY et al (2007) Up-regulation of aldose reductase expression mediated by phosphatidylinositol 3-kinase/Akt and Nrf2 is involved in the protective effect of curcumin against oxidative damage. Free Radic Biol Med 43(4):535–545

Kapadia GJ, Azuine MA, Tokuda H, Takasaki M et al (2002) Chemopreventive effect of resveratrol, sesamol, sesame oil and sunflower oil in the Epstein–Barr virus early antigen activation assay and the mouse skin two-stage carcinogenesis. Pharmacol Res 45(6):499–505

Kaur S, Greaves P, Cooke DN, Edwards R, Steward WP et al (2007) Breast cancer prevention by green tea catechins and black tea theaflavins in the C3 (1) SV40 T, t antigen transgenic mouse model is accompanied by increased apoptosis and a decrease in oxidative DNA adducts. J Agric Food Chem 55(9):3378–3385

Kavanagh KT, Hafer LT, Kim DW, Mann KK et al (2001) Green tea extracts decrease carcinogen-induced mammary tumour burden in rats and rate of breast cancer cell proliferation in culture. J Cell Biochem 82(3):387–398

Kimura Y, Okuda H (2001) Resveratrol isolated from Polygonum cuspidatum root prevents tumor growth and metastasis to lung and tumor-induced neovascularization in Lewis lung carcinoma-bearing mice. J Nutr 131:1844–1849

Knekt P, Jarvinen R, Seppanen R, Heliövaara M et al (1997) Dietary flavonoids and the risk of lung cancer and other malignant neoplasms. Am J Epidemiol 146(2):223–230

Koo JY, Kim HJ, Jung KO, Park KY (2004) Curcumin inhibits the growth of AGS human gastric carcinoma cells in vitro and shows synergism with 5-fluorouracil. J Med Food 7(2):117–121

Kundu JK, Surh YJ (2005) Breaking the relay in deregulated cellular signal transduction as a rationale for chemoprevention with anti-inflammatory phytochemicals. Mutat Res 591(1–2):123–146

Kundu T, Dey S, Roy M, Siddiqi M et al (2005) Induction of apoptosis in human leukemia cells by black tea and its polyphenol theaflavin. Cancer Lett 230(1):111–121

Kunnumakkara AB, Anand P, Aggarwal BB (2008) Curcumin inhibits proliferation, invasion, angiogenesis and metastasis of different cancers through interaction with multiple cell signaling proteins. Cancer Lett 269(2):199–225

Laconi E, Doratiotto S, Vineis P (2008) The microenvironments of multistage carcinogenesis. Semin Cancer Biol 18:322–329

Lee YK, Lee WS, Hwang JT, Kwon DY et al (2009) Curcumin exerts antidifferentiation effect through AMPK-PPAR- in 3T3-L1 adipocytes and antiproliferatory effect through AMPK-COX-2 in cancer cells. J Agric Food Chem 57(1):305–310

Lev-Ari S, Strier L, Kazanov D, Madar-Shapiro L et al (2005a) Celecoxib and curcumin synergistically inhibit the growth of colorectal cancer cells. Clin Cancer Res 11(18):6738–6744

Lev-Ari S, Zinger H, Kazanov D, Yona D et al (2005b) Curcumin synergistically potentiates the growth inhibitory and proapoptotic effects of celecoxib in pancreatic adenocarcinoma cells. Biomed Pharmacother 59(suppl 2):S276–S280

Liao S, Umekita Y, Guo J, Kokontis JM et al (1995) Growth inhibition and regression of human prostate and breast tumours in athymic mice by tea epigallocatechin gallate. Cancer Lett 96(2):239–243

Lu QY, Jin YS, Zhang Q, Zhang Z et al (2004) Ganoderma lucidum extracts inhibit growth and induce actin polymerization in bladder cancer cells in vitro. Cancer Lett 216(1):9–20

Mahajna J, Dotan N, Zaidman BZ, Petrova RD et al (2009) Pharmacological values of medicinal mushrooms for prostate cancer therapy: the case of Ganoderma lucidum. Nutr Cancer 61(1):16–26

McLarty J, Bigelow RL, Smith M, Elmajian D et al (2009) Tea polyphenols decrease serum levels of prostate-specific antigen, hepatocyte growth factor, and vascular endothelial growth factor in prostate cancer patients and inhibit production of hepatocyte growth factor and vascular endothelial growth factor in vitro. Cancer Prev Res (Phila) 2(7):673–682

Meng Q, Goldberg ID, Rosen EM, Fan S (2000) Inhibitory effects of indole-3- carbinol on invasion and migration in human breast cancer cells. Breast Cancer Res Treat 63:147–152

Miguel LL (2008) Anticancer and carcinogenic properties of curcumin: considerations for its clinical development as a cancer chemopreventive and chemotherapeutic agent. Mol Nutr Food Res 52(1):1–12

Mishra R, Bhadauria S, Murthy PK, Murthy PSR (2011) Glycine soya diet synergistically enhances the suppressive effect of tamoxifen and inhibits tamoxifen-promoted hepatocarcinogenesis in 7,12-dimethylbenz[a]anthracene-induced rat mammary tumor model. Food Chem Toxicol 49(2):434–440

Moon DO, Kim MO, Kang SH, Choi YH et al (2009) ulforaphane suppresses TNF-a-mediated activation of NF-jB and induces apoptosis through activation of reactive oxygen species-dependent caspase-3. Cancer Lett 274(1):132–142

Neergheen VS, Bahorun T, Taylor EW, Jen LS et al (2010) Targeting specific cell signaling transduction pathways by dietary and medicinal phytochemicals in cancer chemoprevention. Toxicology 278(2):229–241

Notarbartolo M, Poma P, Perri D, Dusonchet L et al (2005) *Antitumor effects of curcumin, alone or in combination with cisplatin or doxorubicin, on human hepatic cancer cells.* Analysis of their possible relationship to changes in NF-jB activation levels and in IAP gene expression. Cancer Lett 224(1):53–65

Obayashi K, Kurihara K, Okano Y, Masaki H et al (2005) Ergothioneine scavenges superoxide and singlet O and suppresses TNF-α and MMP-1 expression in UV-irradiated human dermal fibroblasts. J Cosmet Sci 56(1):17–27

Parekh P, Motiwale L, Naik N, Rao KVK (2011) Downregulation of cyclin D1 is associated with decreased levels of p38 MAP kinases, Akt/PKB and Pak1 during chemopreventive effects of resveratrol in liver cancer cells. Exp Toxicol Pathol 63(2):167–173

Park OJ, Surh YJ (2004) Chemopreventive potential of epigallocatechin gallate and genistein: evidence from epidemiological and laboratory studies. Toxicol Lett 150(1):43–56

Park JR, Park JS, Jo EH, Hwang JW et al (2006) Reversal of the TPA-induced inhibition of gap junctional intercellular communication by Chaga mushroom (Inonotus obliquus) extracts: effects on MAP kinases. Biofactors 27(1–4):147–155

Prasad CP, Rath G, Mathur S, Bhatnagar D et al (2009) Potent growth suppressive activity of curcumin in human breast cancer cells: modulation of Wnt/β-catenin signaling. Chem Biol Interact 181(2):263–271

Qin J, Xie LP, Zheng XY, Wang YB et al (2007) A component of green tea, (−)-epigallocatechin-3-gallate, promotes apoptosis in T24 human bladder cancer cells via modulation of the PI3K/Akt pathway and Bcl2 family proteins. Biochem Biophys Res Commun 354(4):852–857

Reagan-Shaw S, Afaq F, Aziz MH, Ahmad N (2004) Modulations of critical cell cycle regulatory events during chemoprevention of ultraviolet Bmediated responses by resveratrol in SKH-1 hairless mouse skin. Oncogene 23(30):5151–5160

Reuter S, Eifes S, Dicato M, Aggarwal BB et al (2008) Modulation of anti-apoptotic and survival pathways by curcumin as a strategy to induce apoptosis in cancer cells. Biochem Pharmacol 76(11):1340–1351

Roomi MW, Ivanov V, Kalinovsky T, NiedzwieckI A et al (2006) Inhibition of matrix metalloproteinase-2 secretion and invasion of human ovarian cancer cell line SK-OV-3 with lysine, proline, arginine, ascorbic acid and green tea extract. J Obstet Gynaecol Res 32(2):148–154

Sarangi I, Ghosh D, Bhutia SK, Mallick SK et al (2006) Anti-tumor and immunomodulating effects of Pleurotus ostreatus mycelia-derived proteoglycans. Int Immunopharmacol 6(8):1287–1297

Sarkar FH, Li Y (2002) Mechanisms of cancer chemoprevention by soy isoflavone genistein. Cancer Metastasis Rev 21(3–4):265–280

Schröder FH, Roobol MJ, Boevé ER, de Mutsert R et al (2005) Randomized, double-blind, placebo-controlled crossover study in men with prostate cancer and rising PSA: effectiveness of a dietary supplement. Eur Urol 48(6):922–931

Shah S, Ghosh D, Mallick SK, Sarangi I et al (2007) Immunomodulatory and anti-tumor activities of water-soluble proteoglycanisolated from the fruiting bodies edible mushroom Pleurotus ostreatus. Int J Med Mushrooms 9:123–138

Shimizu M, Deguchi A, Hara Y, Moriwaki H et al (2005) EGCG inhibits activation of the insulin-like growth factor-1 receptor in human colon cancer cells. Biochem Biophys Res Commun 334(3):947–953

Smith-Warner SA, Spiegelman D, Yaun SS, Albanes D et al (2003) Fruits, vegetables and lung cancer: a pooled analysis of cohort studies. Int J Cancer 107(6):1001–1011

Smoliga JM, Baur JA, Hausenblas HA (2011) Resveratrol and health – A comprehensive review of human clinical trials. Mol Nutr Food Res. doi:10.1002/mnfr.201100143

Soleas GJ, Grass L, Josephy PD, Goldberg DM et al (2002) A comparison of the anticarcinogenic properties of four red wine polyphenols. Clin Biochem 35(2):119–124

Song TY, Chen CL, Liao JW, Ou HS et al (2010) Ergothioneine protects against neuronal injury induced by cisplatin both in vitro and in vivo. Food Chem Toxicol 48(12):3492–3499

Sonoda T, Nagata Y, Mori M, Miyanaga N et al (2004) A case-control study of diet and prostate cancer in Japan: possible protective effect of traditional Japanese diet. Cancer Sci 95(3):238–242

Soobrattee MA, Bahorun T, Aruoma OI (2006) Chemopreventive actions of polyphenolic compounds in cancer. Biofactors 27(1):19–35

Srivastava SK, Singh SV (2004) Cell cycle arrest, apoptosis induction and inhibition of nuclear factor kappa B activation in anti-proliferative activity of benzyl isothiocyanate against human pancreatic cancer cells [J]. Carcinogenesis 25(9):1701–1709

Suphim B, Prawan A, Kukongviriyapan U, Kongpetch S et al (2010) Redox modulation and human bile duct cancer inhibition by curcumin. Food Chem Toxicol 48(8–9):2265–2272

Surh YJ (2003) Cancer chemoprevention with dietary phytochemicals. Nat Rev Cancer 3(10):768–780

Tang N, Wu Y, Vhou B, Wang B et al (2009) Green tea, black tea consumption and risk of lung cancer: a meta-analysis. Lung Cancer 65(3):274–283

Tessitore L, Davit A, Sarotto I, Caderni G (2000) Resveratrol depresses the growth of colorectal aberrant crypt foci by affecting bax and p21(CIP) expression. Carcinogenesis 21(8):1619–1622

Thekkuttuparambil AA, Kainoor KJ (2007) Indian medicinal mushrooms as a source of antioxidant and antitumor agents. J Clin Biochem Nutr 40(3):157–162

Tian B, Wang Z, Zhao Y, Wang D et al (2008) Effects of curcumin on bladder cancer cells and development of urothelial tumors in a rat bladder carcinogenesis model. Cancer Lett 264(2):299–308

Veronesi U, Bonanni B (2005) Chemoprevention: from research to clinical oncology. Eur J Cancer 41(13):1833–1841

Voorrips LE, Goldbohm RA, van Poppel G, Sturmans F et al (2000) Vegetable and fruit consumption and risks of colon and rectal cancer in a prospective cohort study: the Netherlands cohort study on diet and cancer. Am J Epidemiol 152(11):1081–1092

Walters DG, Young PJ, Agus C, Knize MG et al (2004) Cruciferous vegetable consumption alters the metabolism of the dietary carcinogen 2-amino-1-methyl-6-phenylimidazo[4,5-b]pyridine (PhIP) in humans. Carcinogenesis 25(9):1659–1669

WHO (2011) Cancer statistics http://www.who.int/cancer/en/

Wu K, Li K (2007) Association between esophageal cancer and drought in China by using geographic information system. Environ Int 33(5):603–608

Yang J, Liu RH (2009) Induction of phase II enzyme, quinone reductase, in murine hepatoma cells in vitro by grape extracts and selected phytochemicals. Food Chem 114(3):898–904

Yang H, Chen C, Chang W, Lu F et al (2006) Growth inhibition and induction of apoptosis in MCF-7 breast cancer cells by Antrodia camphorata. Cancer Lett 231(2):215–227

Yodkeeree S, Chaiwangyen W, Garbisa S, Limtrakul P (2009) Curcumin, demethoxycurcumin and bisdemethoxycurcumin differentially inhibit cancer cell invasion through the down-regulation of MMPs and uPA. J Nutr Biochem 20(2):87–95

Yu X, Kensler T (2005) Nrf 2 as a target for cancer chemoprevention. Mutat Res 591(1–2):93–102

Yuan P, Chen BA, Liu DL (2008) Anticancer mechanisms and researches of isothiocyanates. Chin J Nat Med 6(5):325–332

Zhou JR, Yu L, Mai Z, Blackburn GL (2004) Combined inhibition of estrogen-dependent human breast carcinoma by soy and tea bioactive components in mice. Int J Cancer 108(1):8–14

Chapter 6
Nutritional Compounds as Chemopreventive Agents by Proteasome Inhibition

Kristin Landis-Piwowar, Elizabeth Smerczak, Jian Zuo, and Q. Ping Dou

Contents

Abstract Nutritional phytochemicals, distributed throughout the plant kingdom, possess anticancer activities associated with their consumption. This chapter will focus on the cellular activities of phytochemicals, their potential molecular targets

K. Landis-Piwowar (✉) • E. Smerczak
Biomedical Diagnostic and Therapeutic Sciences, School of Health Sciences, Oakland University, 321 HHS, 2100N. Squirrel Rd, Rochester, MI 48309, USA
e-mail: landispi@oakland.edu

J. Zuo • Q.P. Dou (✉)
The Developmental Therapeutics Program, Barbara Ann Karmanos Cancer Institute, and Departments of Oncology, Pharmacology and Pathology, School of Medicine, Wayne State University, 540.1 HWCRC, 4100 John R Rd, Detroit, MI 48201, USA
e-mail: doup@karmanos.org

S. Shankar and R.K. Srivastava (eds.), *Nutrition, Diet and Cancer*,
DOI 10.1007/978-94-007-2923-0_6,

and biological effects on cancer cells with a focus on the proteasome inhibition. The proteasome is a large multicatalytic, proteinase complex located in the cytosol and the nucleus of eukaryotic cells. The ubiquitin-proteasome system is responsible for the degradation of most intracellular proteins and therefore plays an essential regulatory role in critical cellular processes including cell cycle progression, proliferation, differentiation, angiogenesis, and apoptosis. Normal cell function and homeostasis depends on proteasome activity, however, cancer cells are more sensitive to proteasome inhibitors than normal cells, indicating that the inhibition of the ubiquitin-proteasome system could be used as an approach for cancer therapy and understanding chemoprevention.

Introduction

Although the cancer mortality rate has decreased in recent years, cancer claims more lives than heart disease in individuals less than 85 years of age. Cancer is a public health burden worldwide, and in the year 2011 it is predicted that nearly 1.6 million new cases and 570,000 deaths will occur in the United States alone (Jemal et al. 2010). While novel therapeutic agents should be utilized to reduce cancer mortality rates, cancer control by application of chemopreventive agents should also be studied to reduce incidence of cancer cases.

Chemotherapy is often the most effective cancer treatment, yet patient toxicity and drug resistant tumors are common obstacles in achieving and maintaining a cancer-free status (Landis-Piwowar et al. 2006). While new chemotherapeutic strategies and anticancer agents are continuously developed, the status quo of chemotherapy is less than acceptable, especially in advanced disease (Bendell and Goldberg 2007; Carver et al. 2007). The evolution of chemotherapy that kills proliferating cells indiscriminately to molecularly targeted agents holds promise in cancer therapy. However, the molecular profile of specific tumors and a better understanding of drug mechanisms of action are necessary to provide predictive outcomes for the clinical efficacy of molecularly targeted agents.

Chemotherapy is a necessary tool for advanced cancers, but practical objectives in cancer therapy should include a decrease in the incidence of invasive cancer and the integration of pharmacological mediators that promote prevention rather than cure. This defines a growing field of oncology, termed chemoprevention, which focuses on the use of natural or synthetic products to inhibit carcinogenesis at all three stages, initiation, promotion, and progression (Russo 2007). Chemopreventive compounds from plant sources, known as phytochemicals, have been studied extensively in cell culture and animal models, and some are entering clinical trials (Landis-Piwowar et al. 2006).

The applications of non-toxic nutritional compounds for the treatment of various diseases including cancer have found great popularity in recent years. Likewise, the proteasome has become an increasingly important molecular target in cancer and drug resistance research. The proteasome inhibitor, bortezomib (co-developed by

Millenium Pharmaceuticals Inc., Cambridge, MA, USA and Johnson Pharmaceutical Research and Development, L.L.C., Raritan, NJ, USA) has received regular approval from the US Food and Drug Administration for the treatment of multiple myeloma and mantle cell lymphoma. However, treatment with bortezomib has predictable toxic side effects (Landis-Piwowar et al. 2006), indicating that there is still a need for less toxic proteasome inhibitors, e.g., from naturally occurring compounds. This chapter will focus on phytochemical chemopreventive/therapeutic agents and their interaction with the proteasome and other potential molecular targets.

The Proteasome

Because the ubiquitin (Ub)-proteasome pathway is the predominant means of proteolysis in eukaryotic cells, its functionality is critical for controlling the intracellular levels of a variety of proteins and maintaining normal cellular function. This pathway involves two successive steps: conjugation of multiple ubiquitin molecules to the protein substrate, and degradation of the tagged protein by the 26S proteasome (Fig. 6.1). Ubiquitin is a highly conserved 76-amino acid protein that is covalently ligated to a target protein by a multi-enzymatic system consisting of Ub-activating (E1), Ub-conjugating (E2), and the Ub-ligating (E3) enzymes, which act in a sequential manner. This is a three-stage process that starts with activation of ubiquitin by the E1 enzyme in an ATP- requiring reaction that generates a high-energy thiol ester intermediate, E1-S ~ ubiquitin. Activated ubiquitin is then transferred from E1 to one of several ubiquitin-conjugating enzymes, E2, *via* an additional high-energy thiol-ester intermediate, E2-S ~ ubiquitin. The activated ubiquitin can be then transferred directly from E2 to the E3-bound substrate, or via a third high-energy thiol ester inter- mediate, E3-S ~ ubiquitin, to a protein substrate (Ciechanover et al. 2000a) (Fig. 6.1).

Ubiquitinated proteins are recognized by the 26S proteasome, a large multi-subunit protease complex that is localized in the nucleus and cytosol and selectively degrades intracellular proteins. Only proteins containing polyubiquitin chains on sequential lysine residues are recognized and degraded by the 26S proteasome, and the ubiquitin is released and recycled (Fig. 6.1). The proteolytic core of this complex, the 20S proteasome, contains multiple peptidase activities and functions as the catalytic machine. This core is com- posed of 28 subunits arranged in four heptameric, tightly stacked rings (α7, β7, β7, α7) to form a cylindrical structure (Groll et al. 1999). The α-subunits make up the two outer and the β-subunits the two inner rings of the stack (Fig. 6.1). The entrance of substrate proteins to the active site of the complex is guarded by the α-subunits that allow access only to unfolded polypeptides. The proteolytic activities are confined to the β-subunits conferring the unique and distinguishing proteasome feature of multiple peptidase activities that include chymotrypsin-like (cleavage after hydrophobic side chains, mediated by the β5 subunit), peptidylglutamyl peptide hydrolyzing-like or

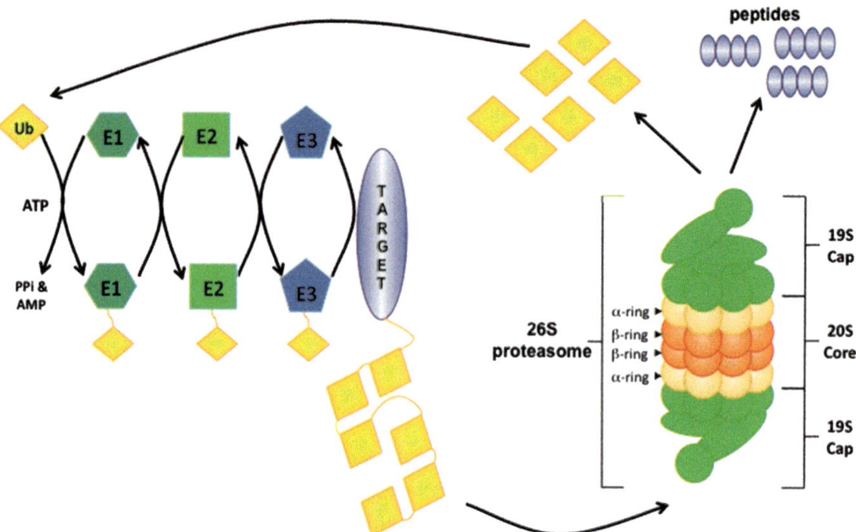

Fig. 6.1 The ubiquitin proteasome pathway. Ubiquitin (*Ub*) is covalently ligated to target proteins by a multi-enzymatic system consisting of Ub-activating (*E1*), Ub-conjugating (*E2*), and the Ub-ligating (*E3*) enzymes. E1 activates an Ub monomer at its C-terminal cysteine residue to a high-energy thiol ester bond that is then transferred to a reactive cysteine residue of the E2 enzyme. The final transfer of Ub to a reactive lysine residue of a target protein is brought about by the E3 enzyme. Ubiquitinated proteins are escorted to the 26S proteasome, through the 19S cap and to the catalytic 20S core for degradation into oligopeptides. The Ub is then released and recycled to begin the process anew

PGPH-like (cleavage after acidic side chains, mediated by the β1 subunit), and trypsin-like (cleavage after basic side chains, mediated by the β2 subunit) activities (Groll et al. 1999).

The ubiquitin-proteasome pathway is vital in the degradation of proteins involved in cell cycle progression, proliferation, and apoptosis and the vast majority of abnormal proteins that result from oxidative damage and mutations. The proteasome can therefore contribute to the pathological state of several human diseases including cancer, in which some regulatory proteins are either stabilized due to decreased degradation or lost due to accelerated degradation (Ciechanover 1998).

Almost all regulated proteolysis in eukaryotic cells occurs through the actions of the ubiquitin-proteasome pathway (Ciechanover et al. 2000b). Although it would seem disastrous to alter the activity of this crucial protein degradation system, proteasome inhibition has been well established as a rational strategy for multiple myeloma (Richardson et al. 2005), mantle cell lymphoma, non-Hodgkin lymphoma and some other solid tumors (Ruschak et al. 2011). Understanding the mechanism of action has led to integration into combination regimens using both proteasome inhibitors and standard chemotherapeutics.

Proteasome Targets and Cellular Consequences

The primary, immediate consequence of proteasome inhibition is a decrease of overall rates of protein breakdown in cells. Various proteins involved in carcinogenesis and cancer survival have been identified as targets of the proteasome, including cyclins A, B, D and E (Glotzer et al. 1991; Won and Reed 1996; Diehl et al. 1997; Chen et al. 2004), tumor suppressor protein p53 (Blagosklonny 2002), pro-apoptotic protein Bax (Li and Dou 2000), cyclin-dependent kinase inhibitor (CKI) p27 (Sun et al. 2001), and the NFkB inhibitor, IkB-a (Perkins 2000). A brief description of particular target proteins and their contributions to the pathology of cancer is described below.

The cell cycle is driven by the activation/induction of cyclin- dependent kinases (Cdks), while CKIs lead to growth arrest (Polyak et al. 1994; Sherr and Roberts 1999). Progression through the cell cycle requires tightly regulated proteolysis of both cyclins and CKIs and numerous data support the roles for the CKIs, p16, p21, and p27, as tumor suppressor proteins (Deng et al. 1995; Sherr and Roberts 1995). In fact, cell cycle arrest, due to an accumulation of the CKIs p21 and p27, occurs following treatment with proteasome inhibitors (Katayose et al. 1997) and their accumulation is furthermore linked to mechanisms of apoptosis (Sun et al. 2001).

In addition to CKIs, the ubiquitin/proteasome pathway also regulates degradation of cyclins. Cyclin D1 degradation is mediated by phosphorylation-triggered, ubiquitin-dependent proteolysis and its degradation allows the cell passage out of G_1 (Diehl et al. 1997). Similarly, Cyclin E protein must be degraded to allow the cell entry into S phase (Won and Reed 1996). Cyclin A must be degraded to allow the cell to pass through S into G_2 and Cyclin B is required for mitosis completion and return to G_1 phase (Glotzer et al. 1991). Accumulation of these proteins following proteasome inhibition leads to a halt in cell cycle progression.

The ratio of pro-apoptotic to anti-apoptotic proteins is also critically involved in cellular survival. Members of the pro- apoptotic Bcl-2 family of proteins, such as Bax, contribute to the release of cytochrome c while their anti-apoptotic counterparts, such as Bcl-2 and Bcl-X_L, promote cell survival (Green and Reed 1998). Bax degradation *via* the proteasome pathway is critical to maintain cancer cell survival and its accumulation is important for reducing the progression of some cancers (Li and Dou 2000). Several studies have demonstrated that proliferating cells are more sensitive to proteasome inhibition than non-proliferating cells (Drexler 1997; An et al. 1998; Orlowski et al. 1998; Drexler et al. 2000; Soligo et al. 2001) and proteasome inhibition leads to apoptosis induction (Landis-Piwowar et al. 2006, 2007). The greater sensitivity of proliferating cells to apoptosis following proteasome inhibition is most likely a consequence of the accumulation of the pro-apoptotic proteins and their effects on cellular activities.

Nutritional Compounds Inhibit Proteasome Activity

The cancer-preventive and anticancer effects of dietary polyphenols such as green tea polyphenols (GTPs) and flavonoids (Fig. 6.2) are widely supported by results from epidemiological, cell culture, and animal studies. A number of these plant polyphenols have been implicated as natural proteasome inhibitors and might be able to sensitize tumor cells to chemotherapeutic agents and radiation therapy by interfering in pathways that lead cancer cells to drug resistance (Garg et al. 2005).

Green Tea Polyphenols

Tea is the most widely consumed beverage in the world, second only to water, and epidemiological studies indicate that green tea consumption is associated with cancer preventive benefits. Biologically active components of green tea include polyphenolic catechins, (-)-epicatechin [(-)-EC], (-)-epicatechin-3-gallate [(-)-ECG], (-)-epigallocatechin [(-)-EGC], and (-)-epigallocatechin-3-gallate [(-)-EGCG] (Gupta et al. 2003). Several studies indicate that (-)-EGCG (Fig. 6.2) is the

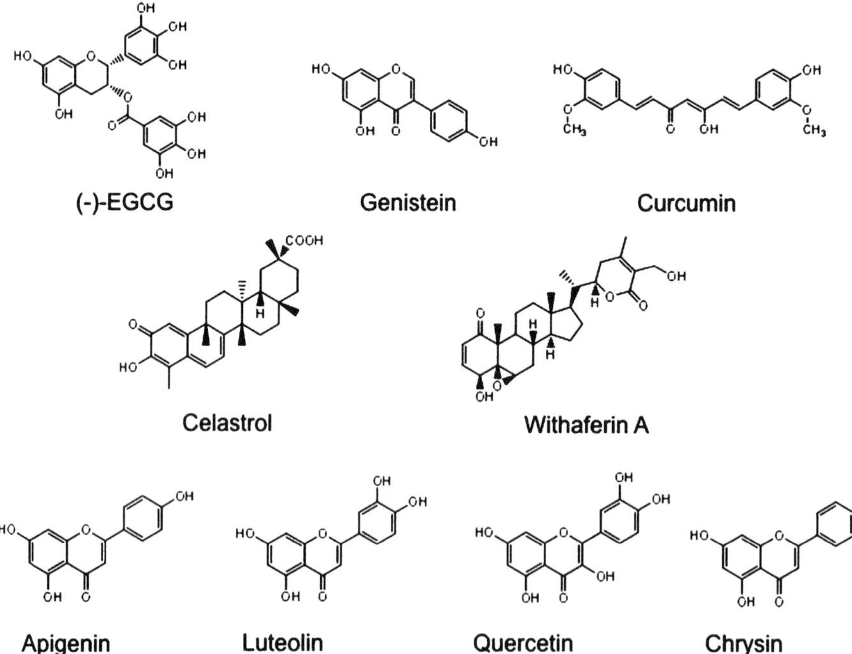

Fig. 6.2 Chemical structures of nutritional compounds

most abundant and most biologically active anticancer catechin in several human cancers (Kemberling et al. 2003; Shimizu et al. 2005).

Numerous anticancer activities and molecular targets of (-)- EGCG have been well described. In fact, (-)-EGCG inhibits the MAPK pathway and activator protein-1 (AP-1) activity in human colon cancer cells (Shimizu et al. 2005), PI3K in the mouse TRAMP model (Adhami et al. 2004), angiogenesis through VEGF phosphorylation (Neuhaus et al. 2004; Lee et al. 2005), and potentially, urokinase-plasminogen activator (uPA) activity (Jankun et al. 1997). Additionally, (-)-EGCG was found to inhibit telomerase activity in mice bearing telomerase-positive colon tumors (HCT-L2), which induced a 50% reduction in tumor size (Naasani et al. 1998). (-)-EGCG also inhibits DNA methyltransferase in HT29 colon and PC-3 prostate cancer cells leading to re-activation of the tumor suppressor gene p16INK4a (Fang et al. 2003) and inhibits dihydrofolate reductase (DHFR) causing reduced lymphoma cell growth, G_0/G_1 phase arrest of the cell cycle, and the induction of apoptosis (Navarro-Peran et al. 2005). Finally, ester bond- containing tea polyphenols [e.g., (-)-EGCG] potently and specifically inhibit the proteasomal chymotrypsin-like (β5) and PGPH-like (β1), but not trypsin-like (β2), activities of the proteasome (Nam et al. 2001). Therefore, (-)-EGCG can target and inhibit multiple pathways involved in cancer cell survival.

In the biological setting, (-)-EGCG exhibits strong inhibitory activity against a purified 20S proteasome (IC50 = 86–194 nM), and a 26S proteasome in intact tumor cells (1–10 μM). These inhibitory concentrations are similar to those found in the serum of green tea drinkers (Landis-Piwowar et al. 2006). (-)-EGCG-induced proteasome inhibition in whole cells stimulates accumulation of the natural proteasome substrates p27 and IkB-a as well as inducing arrest of tumor cells in the G1 phase and/or apoptosis, while having little to no effect on normal, non-transformed cells (Nam et al. 2001; Kuhn et al. 2005; Landis-Piwowar et al. 2005). An *in silico* docking method indicates that inhibition of the chymotrypsin activity of the 20S protea- some may be due to acylation of the β5-subunit's catalytic N-terminal threonine (Thr 1) (Smith et al. 2004). Furthermore, (-)-EGCG appears to bind the chymotrypsin site in an orientation and conformation that is suitable for a nucleophilic attack by Thr 1. The *in silico* model has been corroborated by comparing the predicted and actual activities of several (-)-EGCG analogs. Based on previous studies, the cancer-preventive properties of green tea could be attributed, at least in part, to its ability to inhibit proteasomal activity and the low toxicity of (-)-EGCG points to its potential use as an adjuvant to current anticancer drugs.

Genistein

Genistein (4′,5,7-trihydroxyisoflavone) is the predominant isoflavone with biological activity in soybeans and soy products. Its antitumor activity is associated with inhibiting cell proliferation and angiogenesis and inducing apoptosis (Sarkar and Li 2002). *In silico* computational docking suggests that genistein acts as a proteasome inhibitor and 1 μM inhibits approximately 30% of the chymotrypsin-like activity in purified 20S proteasomes (Kazi et al. 2003). This is consistent with biological data that indicate genistein plasma levels in the range of 0.5–2.5 μM (Watanabe et al. 1998) and that tumor cells exposed to genistein demonstrate reduce NF-kB activity (Sarkar et al. 2006) and cell cycle arrest in breast and prostate cancers (Cappelletti et al. 2000; Choi et al. 2000; Ramos 2007; Yan et al. 2010). Genistein therefore acts, at least in part, as a proteasome inhibitor at physiological concentrations and this proteasome inhibition might contribute to its reported cancer-preventive and anticancer effects.

Curcumin

Curcumin (diferuloylmethane, Fig. 6.2) is the major active ingredient of turmeric, commonly found in South Asian cuisine, and is isolated from the root of Curcuma longa. Anti-tumor effects of curcumin are linked to inhibition of cell proliferation, invasion, angiogenesis, metastasis, and osteoclastogenesis and multiple cellular targets have been identified including NF-κB and COX-2 (Kunnumakkara et al. 2008; von Metzler et al. 2009). *In silico* modeling has determined that curcumin is susceptible to nucleophilic attack by Thr 1 within the β5 subunit of the proteasome, suggesting that curcumin binds to Thr 1 with high predictability and biologically, curcumin inhibits the CT-like activity of a purified 20S proteasome (Milacic et al. 2008). In fact, curcumin inhibits proteasomal activities at all three β-subunits, with its most potent effects against the β5, chymotrypsin-like, activity. This has been associated with induction of cell death in nude mice human colon cancer tumor xenografts (Milacic et al. 2008). Bioavailability of curcumin after oral administration is low (Garcea et al. 2004; Dhillon et al. 2008) yet, it is apparent that curcumin has proteasome inhibitory activity.

Celastrol

Celastrol (3- hydroxy- 9β, 13α- dimethyl- 2- oxo- 24, 25, 26- trinoroleana- 1(10), 3, 5, 7- tetraen- 29- oic acid, Fig. 6.2) is a quinone methide triterpene isolated from *Tripterygium wilfordii* and has been used as a natural medicine in China for centuries. Nucleophilic susceptibility of Celastrol suggests that the conjugated ketone carbons C_2 and C_6 are sites of high nucleophilic susceptibility within the β5 proteasome subunit and may contribute to its proteasome-inhibitory potency (Yang et al. 2006). In fact celastrol inhibits the chymotrypsin-like activity of a purified 20S proteasome ($IC_{50} = 2.5$ μmol/L) and 26S proteasome in androgen-independent PC-3 (androgen receptor-negative) and androgen-dependent LNCaP (androgen receptor-positive) prostate cancer cells at 1–5 μM, resulting in the accumulation of ubiquitinated proteins and proteasome substrates (IκB-α, Bax, and p27), and suppression of androgen receptor protein expression. Furthermore, proteasome inhibition induces apoptotic cell death and Celastrol (1–3 mg/kg/day, i.p., for 31 days) treated nude mice bearing human prostate cell tumors results in significant tumor growth inhibition and massive apoptosis induction, associated with *in vivo* proteasome inhibition and androgen receptor suppression (Yang et al. 2006). Therefore, Celastrol is a proteasome-targeting agent, inhibiting human tumor cell growth, and may be a potent chemopreventing agent.

Withaferin A

Withaferin A (WA) (Fig. 6.2) is derived from the medicinal plant *Withania somnifera*, and has been used for centuries in Ayurvedic medicine, the traditional medical system in India, as a remedy for a variety of musculoskeletal conditions and as a tonic to improve the overall health (Mishra et al. 2000). Its root extract has been accepted as a dietary supplement in the United States (Jayaprakasam et al. 2003) and numerous reports suggest its broad medical application with anti-inflammation, antitumor, cardioprotection, neuroprotection, and immunomodulation properties (Devi et al. 1992; Agarwal et al. 1999; Gupta et al. 2004; Ahmad et al. 2005; Owais et al. 2005; Rasool and Varalakshmi 2006). WA contains two conjugated ketone bonds at C_1 and C_{24} and the nucleophilic susceptibility and in silico docking studies predict that these carbons are highly susceptible to nucleophilic attack by the N-terminal threonine of the proteasomal β5 subunit (Yang et al. 2007). Indeed, WA inhibits the chymotrypsin-like activity of a purified 20S proteasome and 26S proteasome in cultured prostate cancer cells and tumors along with accumulation of the proteasome target proteins Bax, IκB-α, and $p27^{Kip1}$ and induction of apoptosis. Cells treated with a reduced form of WA, results in significant decrease in proteasome inhibition and apoptosis induction. In vivo analysis of human prostate PC-3 xenografts with WA for 24 days indicates a dramatic (70%) inhibition of tumor growth and a 56% decrease in tumor proteasomal chymotrypsin-like activity (Yang et al. 2007). WA therefore appears to act as a natural proteasomal inhibitor in vitro and in vivo and may also possess chemopreventive properties.

Flavonoids

Interest in the potential cancer chemopreventive and therapeutic properties of diet-derived compounds such as plant polyphenols has developed in recent years. Flavonoids are a sub- group of polyphenols containing a flavone backbone with hydroxy- lations at various positions. These compounds can be found in a number of fruits and vegetables including celery, apples, onion, parsley, and capsicum pepper, among others (Ramos 2007), and have been shown to possess anti-cancer activities. The mechanisms by which flavonoids impart their anti-cancer effects are varied and may include action through suppressing inflammation (Choi et al. 2004), free radical scavenging (Sim et al. 2007), modulation of survival/proliferation path- ways (Lee et al. 2004) and proteasome inhibition (Chen et al. 2005, 2007). The flavonoids apigenin, luteolin, quercetin, and chrysin are discussed below.

Apigenin

Briefly, apigenin (5,7,4-trihydroxyflavone, Fig. 6.2), present in parsley, oranges, onions, chamomile tea, etc. (Lepley et al. 1996), is a non- toxic, antimutagen, with antioxidant potential (Lepley et al. 1996; Birt et al. 1997; Romanova et al. 2001). As a proteasome inhibitor, apigenin potently inhibits chymotrypsin-like activity as shown by various methods (Chen et al. 2005). An *in silico* docking method revealed that the carbonyl carbon of apigenin was a site of nucleophilic susceptibility and could bind to the chymotrypsin-like site in an orientation and conformation that is suitable for a nucleophilic attack by Thr 1 (Chen et al. 2005). Furthermore, biological analysis of apigenin indicates strong inhibitory activity against a purified 20S proteasome (IC50 = 1.8–2.3 μM), and 26S proteasome in intact leukemia Jurkat cells (1–10 μM). Accumulation of the proteasome substrates Bax and IkB-a and induction of apoptotic PARP cleavage and caspase-3 activation indicated that proteasome inhibition is closely correlated with apoptosis induction in leukemia Jurkat and prostate PC-3 cells treated with apigenin. A final indicator of apigenin's potential value as a therapeutic proteasome inhibitor was the lack of toxicity in normal, non-transformed cells (Chen et al. 2005).

Apigenin's role as an anti-cancer agent likely exists in categories beyond proteasome inhibition. Apigenin inhibits the serine/threonine kinase CK2 that, in turn, leads to apoptosis in acute myeloid leukemia (AML) cells derived from human patients (Kim et al. 2007). The apoptosis inducing effect of apigenin was AML cell specific and innocuous to normal bone marrow cells. Furthermore, inhibition of carcinogen-induced growth, and induction of involucrin, an early marker of differentiation, have been observed in carcinogen-exposed normal skin keratinocytes simultaneously exposed to apigenin (Elmore et al. 2005).

Luteolin

The flavonoid luteolin (3′,4′,5,7-Tetrahydroxyflavone, Fig. 6.2) can be found in celery, green pepper, chamomile tea, etc. (Selvendiran et al. 2006). Proteasome inhibition by luteolin has been indicated by inhibitory activity against a purified 20S proteasome (IC50 = 1.5 μM), and 26S proteasome in intact tumor cells (1.3 μM) (Chen et al. 2005). Accumulation of the proteasome substrates Bax (Cai et al. 2001) and IkB-a and induction of apoptotic PARP cleavage and caspase-3 activation in a dose- and time-dependent manner showed that proteasome inhibition in leukemia Jurkat, prostate PC-3, and numerous other cell lines (Cai et al. 2001) treated with luteolin led to apoptotic cell death while normal, non-transformed cells were unaffected. In addition to the proteasome inhibitory activity of luteolin, antiproliferative activity in a number of human cancer cell lines including stomach, cervical, lung, and bladder has been observed (Cherng et al. 2007). A decrease in cell proliferation could be due to proteasome inhibition as well as a number of other cellular changes. In fact, apoptosis occurred in hepatoma cells *via* inhibition of signal transducer and activator of transcription 3 (STAT3)/Fas signaling (Selvendiran et al. 2006). All together the chemopreventive activities of luteolin are likely to extend at least in part from its proteasome inhibitory activities.

Quercetin

Quercetin (3,3′,4′,5,7-Pentahydroxyflavone, Fig. 6.2) is one of the most abundant flavonoids found in fruits and vegetables with the highest concentrations in onions, apples, and red wine (Hertog et al. 1993). The potential for quercetin to act as a proteasome inhibitor is strongly suggested by its inhibitory activity against a purified 20S proteasome (IC50 = 3.5 μM), and 26S proteasome in intact tumor cells (2 μM) (Chen et al. 2005). Again, *in silico* docking analysis demonstrated that the carbonyl carbon acted as a site of nucleophilic susceptibility and could bind to the chymotrypsin site in an orientation and conformation suitable for a nucleophilic attack by Thr 1 (Chen et al. 2005). The proteasome substrates Bax and IkBa accumulated and apoptotic PARP cleavage and caspase-3 activation were dose- and time- dependent (Chen et al. 2005). While leukemia Jurkat cells were subject to proteasome inhibition and apoptosis induction, normal, non-transformed cells were unaffected (Chen et al. 2005). While quercetin appears to be chemopreventive, it may also be cardioprotective via proteasome inhibition (Dosenko et al. 2006).

Chrysin

Chrysin (5,7-dihydroxyflavone, Fig. 6.2) is a flavonoid found in various fruits and vegetables, but predominantly in honey (Weng et al. 2005). Chrysin possesses proteasome inhibitory activity against a purified 20S proteasome (IC50 = 4.9 μM), and 26S proteasome in intact tumor cells (6.1 μM) (Chen et al. 2005). Likewise, accumulation of IkB-a and ubiquitinated proteins and the presence of PARP cleavage and caspase-3 activation indicated that proteasome inhibition was associated with apoptosis induction in Jurkat and PC-3 cells treated with chrysin while normal, non-transformed cells were resistant to apoptosis induced by chrysin (Chen et al. 2005; Phan et al. 2011). Finally, hepatocarcinoma cells exposed to chrysin have been shown to decrease signaling by NF-κB (Khan et al. 2011) which may be due to the proteasome inhibitory effects of chrysin.

While flavonoids seemingly impart toxicity in multiple pathways, their ability to inhibit proteasomal activity in tumor cells strongly contributes to their cancer-preventive and therapeutic potentials. In addition, the low toxicity of flavonoids signifies their plausible uses as chemopreventive agents.

Limitations of Nutritional Compounds

Natural compounds such as green tea polyphenols and flavonoids are less potent than the synthetic compound bortezomib as proteasome inhibitors in whole cells (Kane et al. 2006). Therefore, an understanding of proteasome inhibition in whole cells by natural compounds and an investigation of additional proteasome inhibitors with fewer or no toxic side-effects compared to bortezomib is warranted.

The numerous studies mentioned above indicate positive and promising anticancer effects of nutritional compounds. On the other hand, polyphenols exhibit poor oral bioavailability *in vivo* possibly due to their inability to pass intact through the gut into the circulation. Biochemically, the efficacy of ingested tea polyphenols and flavonoids may be limited due to conjugation of the free hydroxyl groups surrounding the molecules (Lu et al. 2003; Manach and Donovan 2004). In fact, the green tea polyphenol (-)-EGCG is relatively unstable under neutral or alkaline conditions and could be rapidly degraded, involving deprotonation of hydroxyl (–OH) groups on the phenol rings (Chen et al. 2001). Furthermore, these –OH groups can be modified through major biotransformation reactions, including methylation, glucuronidation, and sulfonation, resulting in reduced biological activities of (-)-EGCG *in vivo* (Lu et al. 2003). Likewise, a similar decrease in the bioavailability of apigenin, luteolin (Manach et al. 2004), chrysin (Walle et al. 2001), and quercetin (Walle et al. 2001; Manach and Donovan 2004) has been shown. Generally speaking, the anticancer effects of polyphenols depend on their susceptibility to biotransformation reactions.

Epidemiological Data

Epidemiologic studies that distinguish populations based on dietary composition and physiological metabolic variations yield meaningful information when considering natural compounds as chemopreventive agents in regard to cancer rates. Predominating the research involving naturally occurring chemopreventive agents is that of green tea polyphenols and soy isoflavones. Empirical evidence showcases the information that can be attained through epidemiology, as well as some of the challenges in understanding how dietary intake of foods with known chemopreventive properties relates to cancer rates.

Green Tea

Green Tea and Prostate Cancer

Green tea is an abundant source of dietary antioxidants and known to have anticarcinogenic properties. In fact, a significant reduction in the incidence of prostate cancer (3% incidence among green tea-treated subjects compared with 30% incidence among placebo-treated subjects) with no significant side effects have been observed (Bettuzzi et al. 2006). A number of case-control studies have indicated that general tea consumption is associated with a decreased risk of prostate cancer (Jain et al. 1998, 2004; Sonoda et al. 2004) and a recent large prospective study conducted in Japan, showed that green tea consumption was associated with a decrease risk of advanced prostate cancer, but not localized prostate cancer (Kurahashi et al. 2008). However, other case-control and prospective studies have concluded otherwise (Allen et al. 2004; Kikuchi et al. 2006).

Green Tea and Breast Cancer

While some studies indicate no risk reducing benefit of breast cancer in tea drinkers (Seely et al. 2005; Sun et al. 2006; Iwasaki et al. 2010), numerous studies indicate quite the opposite. In fact, drinking green tea green tea is associated with a decreased risk for breast cancer compared to non-drinkers (Zhang et al. 2009) and breast cancer risk was reduced in association with years of green tea drinking and with the amount of tea consumed per month (Shrubsole et al. 2009). Likewise, a low risk of breast cancer among women with higher green tea intake and the low-activity genotype of angiotensin-converting enzyme gene was observed among Singapore Chinese women (Yuan et al. 2005) and regular consumption of green tea has been associated with improved prognosis of breast cancer at early stages (I and II) (Nakachi et al. 1998; Inoue et al. 2001). It should be noted that epidemiological studies have led to disparaging data between Asian and non-Asian populations as to the protective nature of green tea consumption in disease such as breast cancer; with Asian populations showing better response than Western populations (Wu et al. 2003).

Green Tea and Gastrointestinal Cancer

Consuming green tea may also be protective against the development of colon cancer and gastric cancer. A reduced risk of gastric cancer was observed in women whose intake was greater than or equal to five cups a day (Inoue et al. 2009). However, esophageal precancerous lesions were not diminished in individuals consuming decaffeinated green tea for one year (Wang and Bachrach 2002). Furthermore, green tea consumption is shown to have little to no chemopreventive activity in reducing the risk of stomach cancers (Myung et al. 2009).

For each of the various types of cancers described above some controversy exists for risk reduction in association with green tea consumption. Some insights have been made into the role of green tea consumption and the prevention of cancer, but questions like the role of other dietary compounds, lifestyle (Luo et al. 2010), dosage and bioavailability (Wu et al. 2003) are but a few areas of ongoing study.

Soy Isoflavones

Soy isoflavones are widely studied for their role in anti-proliferative and anticarcinogenic properties, and illustrate the complexity the relationship between natural chemopreventive agents and cancer. Some data shows a direct relationship between isoflavones intake and decreased cancer risk (Yamamoto et al. 2003) and while no increased risk of cancer with soy isoflavone intake has been established in humans, epidemiologic studies remain inconsistent (Trock et al. 2006). Epidemiologic studies of soy isoflavones shed light on the importance of the dietary source when evaluating a chemopreventive agent's efficacy. In Japan, for example, most soy is consumed in fermented, tofu or paste form; where as in America, soy intake is both lower and typically used as a flower or protein additive to other foods (Nagata 2010). Differences in dietary source may pose a challenge to assessing this, and other nutritional chemopreventive agents, but recognizing and addressing this issue could lead to more efficacious use and development of such compounds.

Green tea polyphenols and soy isoflavones provide excellent examples of both the challenges and the meaningful data that can be extracted from epidemiological study. Many other factors play a role in how dietary intake and subsequent metabolism of potential and known chemopreventive agents affect a given population. There is still much to be learned from epidemiological assessment of natural chemopreventive agents, and continued research in this arena is essential for using such compounds to their full potential.

Clinical Trials

Clinical use of nutritional compounds as chemopreventive agents is not widely practiced or biologically understood, and yet, some clinical studies have led to improved treatment regimens and potential future applications. The use of dietary and naturally derived compounds in combination with traditional chemotherapy methods has shown encouraging results in several clinical trials. Compounds such as genistine, disulfiram and green tea extracts have reached phase II clinical trials (Landis-Piwowar et al. 2006). Other compounds like resveratrol (Landis-Piwowar et al. 2006), shikonin and an array of flavonoids have shown promise in early trials (Yang et al. 2009).

As understanding of how nutritional compounds act as chemopreventive agents expands, so does the clinical application of such agents. With continued clinical trials, the role of such natural compounds could play an important role in cancer prevention and treatment regimens in the future.

Concluding Remarks

The consumption of natural nutritional compounds from plant material in the diet or in purified synthetic forms may be essential chemopreventive or therapeutic agents. The relevance of plant polyphenols in the prevention and treatment of chronic diseases such as cancer is well-established, yet, understanding the mechanisms of polyphenolic biotransformation and molecular activity is central to defining their benefits for humans. The studies presented in this chapter expand the knowledge of plant polyphenols as proteasome inhibitors with application to cancer prevention and therapeutics.

References

Adhami VM, Siddiqui IA et al (2004) Oral consumption of green tea polyphenols inhibits insulin-like growth factor-I-induced signaling in an autochthonous mouse model of prostate cancer. Cancer Res 64(23):8715–8722

Agarwal R, Diwanay S et al (1999) Studies on immunomodulatory activity of Withania somnifera (Ashwagandha) extracts in experimental immune inflammation. J Ethnopharmacol 67(1):27–35

Ahmad M, Saleem S et al (2005) Neuroprotective effects of Withania somnifera on 6-hydroxydopamine induced Parkinsonism in rats. Hum Exp Toxicol 24(3):137–147

Allen NE, Sauvaget C et al (2004) A prospective study of diet and prostate cancer in Japanese men. Cancer Causes & Control: CCC 15(9):911–920

An B, Goldfarb RH et al (1998) Novel dipeptidyl proteasome inhibitors overcome Bcl-2 protective function and selectively accumulate the cyclin-dependent kinase inhibitor p27 and induce apoptosis in transformed, but not normal, human fibroblasts. Cell Death Differ 5(12):1062–1075

Bendell J, Goldberg RM (2007) Targeted agents in the treatment of pancreatic cancer: history and lessons learned. Curr Opin Oncol 19(4):390–395

Bettuzzi S, Brausi M et al (2006) Chemoprevention of human prostate cancer by oral administration of green tea catechins in volunteers with high-grade prostate intraepithelial neoplasia: a preliminary report from a one-year proof-of-principle study. Cancer Res 66(2):1234–1240

Birt DF, Mitchell D et al (1997) Inhibition of ultraviolet light induced skin carcinogenesis in SKH-1 mice by apigenin, a plant flavonoid. Anticancer Res 17(1A):85–91

Blagosklonny MV (2002) P53: an ubiquitous target of anticancer drugs. Int J Cancer 98(2):161–166

Cai X, Ye T et al (2001) Luteolin induced G2 phase cell cycle arrest and apoptosis on non-small cell lung cancer cells. Toxicol In Vitro 25(7):1385–1391

Cappelletti V, Fioravanti L et al (2000) Genistein blocks breast cancer cells in the G(2)M phase of the cell cycle. J Cell Biochem 79(4):594–600

Carver JR, Shapiro CL et al (2007) American Society of Clinical Oncology clinical evidence review on the ongoing care of adult cancer survivors: cardiac and pulmonary late effects. J Clin Oncol 25(25):3991–4008

Chen Z, Zhu QY et al (2001) Degradation of green tea catechins in tea drinks. J Agric Food Chem 49(1):477–482

Chen W, Lee J et al (2004) Proteasome-mediated destruction of the cyclin a/cyclin-dependent kinase 2 complex suppresses tumor cell growth in vitro and in vivo. Cancer Res 64(11):3949–3957

Chen D, Daniel KG et al (2005) Dietary flavonoids as proteasome inhibitors and apoptosis inducers in human leukemia cells. Biochem Pharmacol 69(10):1421–1432

Chen D, Chen MS et al (2007) Structure-proteasome-inhibitory activity relationships of dietary flavonoids in human cancer cells. Front Biosci 12:1935–1945

Cherng JM, Shieh DE et al (2007) Chemopreventive effects of minor dietary constituents in common foods on human cancer cells. Biosci Biotechnol Biochem 71(6):1500–1504

Choi YH, Lee WH et al (2000) p53-independent induction of p21 (WAF1/CIP1), reduction of cyclin B1 and G2/M arrest by the isoflavone genistein in human prostate carcinoma cells. Jap J Cancer Res: Gann 91(2):164–173

Choi JS, Choi YJ et al (2004) Flavones mitigate tumor necrosis factor-alpha-induced adhesion molecule upregulation in cultured human endothelial cells: role of nuclear factor-kappa B. J Nutr 134(5):1013–1019

Ciechanover A (1998) The ubiquitin-proteasome pathway: on protein death and cell life. EMBO J 17(24):7151–7160

Ciechanover A, Orian A et al (2000a) Ubiquitin-mediated proteolysis: biological regulation via destruction. BioEssays 22(5):442–451

Ciechanover A, Orian A et al (2000b) The ubiquitin-mediated proteolytic pathway: mode of action and clinical implications. J Cell Biochem Suppl 34:40–51

Deng C, Zhang P et al (1995) Mice lacking p21CIP1/WAF1 undergo normal development, but are defective in G1 checkpoint control. Cell 82(4):675–684

Devi PU, Sharada AC et al (1992) In vivo growth inhibitory effect of Withania somnifera (Ashwagandha) on a transplantable mouse tumor, Sarcoma 180. Indian J Exp Biol 30(3):169–172

Dhillon N, Aggarwal BB et al (2008) Phase II trial of curcumin in patients with advanced pancreatic cancer. Clin Cancer Res 14(14):4491–4499

Diehl JA, Zindy F et al (1997) Inhibition of cyclin D1 phosphorylation on threonine-286 prevents its rapid degradation via the ubiquitin-proteasome pathway. Genes Dev 11(8):957–972

Dosenko VE, Nagibin VS et al (2006) The influence of quercetin on the activity of purified 20S, 26S proteasome and proteasomal activity in isolated cardiomyocytes. Biomed Khim 52(2):138–145

Drexler HC (1997) Activation of the cell death program by inhibition of proteasome function. Proc Natl Acad Sci USA 94(3):855–860

Drexler HC, Risau W et al (2000) Inhibition of proteasome function induces programmed cell death in proliferating endothelial cells. FASEB J 14(1):65–77

Elmore E, Siddiqui S et al (2005) Correlation of in vitro chemopreventive efficacy data from the human epidermal cell assay with animal efficacy data and clinical trial plasma levels. J Cell Biochem 95(3):571–588

Fang MZ, Wang Y et al (2003) Tea polyphenol (-)-epigallocatechin-3-gallate inhibits DNA methyltransferase and reactivates methylation-silenced genes in cancer cell lines. Cancer Res 63(22):7563–7570

Garcea G, Jones DJ et al (2004) Detection of curcumin and its metabolites in hepatic tissue and portal blood of patients following oral administration. Br J Cancer 90(5):1011–1015

Garg AK, Buchholz TA et al (2005) Chemosensitization and radiosensitization of tumors by plant polyphenols. Antioxid Redox Signal 7(11–12):1630–1647

Glotzer M, Murray AW et al (1991) Cyclin is degraded by the ubiquitin pathway. Nature 349(6305):132–138

Green DR, Reed JC (1998) Mitochondria and apoptosis. Science 281(5381):1309–1312

Groll M, Heinemeyer W et al (1999) The catalytic sites of 20S proteasomes and their role in subunit maturation: a mutational and crystallographic study. Proc Natl Acad Sci USA 96(20):10976–10983

Gupta S, Hussain T et al (2003) Molecular pathway for (-)-epigallocatechin-3-gallate-induced cell cycle arrest and apoptosis of human prostate carcinoma cells. Arch Biochem Biophys 410(1):177–185

Gupta SK, Mohanty I et al (2004) Cardioprotection from ischemia and reperfusion injury by Withania somnifera: a hemodynamic, biochemical and histopathological assessment. Mol Cell Biochem 260(1–2):39–47

Hertog MG, Hollman PC et al (1993) Intake of potentially anticarcinogenic flavonoids and their determinants in adults in The Netherlands. Nutr Cancer 20(1):21–29

Inoue M, Tajima K et al (2001) Regular consumption of green tea and the risk of breast cancer recurrence: follow-up study from the Hospital-based Epidemiologic Research Program at Aichi Cancer Center (HERPACC), Japan. Cancer Lett 167(2):175–182

Inoue M, Sasazuki S et al (2009) Green tea consumption and gastric cancer in Japanese: a pooled analysis of six cohort studies. Gut 58(10):1323–1332

Iwasaki M, Inoue M et al (2010) Green tea drinking and subsequent risk of breast cancer in a population to based cohort of Japanese women. Breast Cancer Res 12(5):R88

Jain MG, Hislop GT et al (1998) Alcohol and other beverage use and prostate cancer risk among Canadian men. Int J Cancer 78(6):707–711

Jankun J, Selman SH et al (1997) Why drinking green tea could prevent cancer. Nature 387(6633):561

Jayaprakasam B, Zhang Y et al (2003) Growth inhibition of human tumor cell lines by withanolides from Withania somnifera leaves. Life Sci 74(1):125–132

Jemal A, Siegel R et al (2010) Cancer statistics, 2010. CA Cancer J Clin 60(5):277–300

Jian L, Xie LP et al (2004) Protective effect of green tea against prostate cancer: a case-control study in southeast China. Int J Cancer 108(1):130–135

Kane RC, Farrell AT et al (2006) United States Food and Drug Administration approval summary: bortezomib for the treatment of progressive multiple myeloma after one prior therapy. Clin Cancer Res 12(10):2955–2960

Katayose Y, Kim M et al (1997) Promoting apoptosis: a novel activity associated with the cyclin-dependent kinase inhibitor p27. Cancer Res 57(24):5441–5445

Kazi A, Daniel KG et al (2003) Inhibition of the proteasome activity, a novel mechanism associated with the tumor cell apoptosis-inducing ability of genistein. Biochem Pharmacol 66(6):965–976

Kemberling JK, Hampton JA et al (2003) Inhibition of bladder tumor growth by the green tea derivative epigallocatechin-3-gallate. J Urol 170(3):773–776

Khan MS, Halagowder D et al (2011) Methylated chrysin induces co-ordinated attenuation of the canonical Wnt and NF-kB signaling pathway and upregulates apoptotic gene expression in the early hepatocarcinogenesis rat model. Chem Biol Interact 193(1):12–21

Kikuchi N, Ohmori K et al (2006) No association between green tea and prostate cancer risk in Japanese men: the Ohsaki Cohort Study. Br J Cancer 95(3):371–373

Kim JS, Eom JI et al (2007) Protein kinase CK2alpha as an unfavorable prognostic marker and novel therapeutic target in acute myeloid leukemia. Clin Cancer Res 13(3):1019–1028

Kuhn D, Lam WH et al (2005) Synthetic peracetate tea polyphenols as potent proteasome inhibitors and apoptosis inducers in human cancer cells. Front Biosci 10:1010–1023

Kunnumakkara AB, Anand P et al (2008) Curcumin inhibits proliferation, invasion, angiogenesis and metastasis of different cancers through interaction with multiple cell signaling proteins. Cancer Lett 269(2):199–225

Kurahashi N, Sasazuki S et al (2008) Green tea consumption and prostate cancer risk in Japanese men: a prospective study. Am J Epidemiol 167(1):71–77

Landis-Piwowar KR, Kuhn DJ et al (2005) Evaluation of proteasome-inhibitory and apoptosis-inducing potencies of novel (-)-EGCG analogs and their prodrugs. Int J Mol Med 15(4):735–742

Landis-Piwowar KR, Milacic V et al (2006) The proteasome as a potential target for novel anticancer drugs and chemosensitizers. Drug Resist Updat 9(6):263–273

Landis-Piwowar KR, Huo C et al (2007) A novel prodrug of the green tea polyphenol (-)-epigallocatechin-3-gallate as a potential anticancer agent. Cancer Res 67(9):4303–4310

Lee LT, Huang YT et al (2004) Transinactivation of the epidermal growth factor receptor tyrosine kinase and focal adhesion kinase phosphorylation by dietary flavonoids: effect on invasive potential of human carcinoma cells. Biochem Pharmacol 67(11):2103–2114

Lee HJ, Wang CJ et al (2005) Induction apoptosis of luteolin in human hepatoma HepG2 cells involving mitochondria translocation of Bax/Bak and activation of JNK. Toxicol Appl Pharmacol 203(2):124–131

Lepley DM, Li B et al (1996) The chemopreventive flavonoid apigenin induces G2/M arrest in keratinocytes. Carcinogenesis 17(11):2367–2375
Li B, Dou QP (2000) Bax degradation by the ubiquitin/proteasome-dependent pathway: involvement in tumor survival and progression. Proc Natl Acad Sci USA 97(8):3850–3855
Lu H, Meng X et al (2003) Enzymology of methylation of tea catechins and inhibition of catechol-O-methyltransferase by (-)-epigallocatechin gallate. Drug Metab Dispos 31(5):572–579
Luo J, Gao YT et al (2010) Urinary polyphenols and breast cancer risk: results from the Shanghai Women's Health Study. Breast Cancer Res Treat 120(3):693–702
Manach C, Donovan JL (2004) Pharmacokinetics and metabolism of dietary flavonoids in humans. Free Radic Res 38(8):771–785
Manach C, Scalbert A et al (2004) Polyphenols: food sources and bioavailability. Am J Clin Nutr 79(5):727–747
Milacic V, Banerjee S et al (2008) Curcumin inhibits the proteasome activity in human colon cancer cells in vitro and in vivo. Cancer Res 68(18):7283–7292
Mishra LC, Singh BB et al (2000) Scientific basis for the therapeutic use of Withania somnifera (ashwagandha): a review. Altern Med Rev 5(4):334–346
Myung SK, Bae WK et al (2009) Green tea consumption and risk of stomach cancer: a meta-analysis of epidemiologic studies. Int J Cancer 124(3):670–677
Naasani I, Seimiya H et al (1998) Telomerase inhibition, telomere shortening, and senescence of cancer cells by tea catechins. Biochem Biophys Res Commun 249(2):391–396
Nagata C (2010) Factors to consider in the association between soy isoflavone intake and breast cancer risk. J Epidemiol 20(2):83–89
Nakachi K, Suemasu K et al (1998) Influence of drinking green tea on breast cancer malignancy among Japanese patients. Jap J Cancer Res: Gann 89(3):254–261
Nam S, Smith DM et al (2001) Ester bond-containing tea polyphenols potently inhibit proteasome activity in vitro and in vivo. J Biol Chem 276(16):13322–13330
Navarro-Peran E, Cabezas-Herrera J et al (2005) The antifolate activity of tea catechins. Cancer Res 65(6):2059–2064
Neuhaus T, Pabst S et al (2004) Inhibition of the vascular-endothelial growth factor-induced intracellular signaling and mitogenesis of human endothelial cells by epigallocatechin-3 gallate. Eur J Pharmacol 483(2–3):223–227
Orlowski RZ, Eswara JR et al (1998) Tumor growth inhibition induced in a murine model of human Burkitt's lymphoma by a proteasome inhibitor. Cancer Res 58(19):4342–4348
Owais M, Sharad KS et al (2005) Antibacterial efficacy of Withania somnifera (ashwagandha) an indigenous medicinal plant against experimental murine salmonellosis. Phytomedicine 12(3):229–235
Perkins ND (2000) The Rel/NF-kappa B family: friend and foe. Trends Biochem Sci 25(9):434–440
Phan T, Yu XM et al (2011) Antiproliferative effect of chrysin on anaplastic thyroid cancer. J Surg Res 170(1):84–88
Polyak K, Kato JY et al (1994) p27Kip1, a cyclin-Cdk inhibitor, links transforming growth factor-beta and contact inhibition to cell cycle arrest. Genes Dev 8(1):9–22
Ramos S (2007) Effects of dietary flavonoids on apoptotic pathways related to cancer chemoprevention. J Nutr Biochem 18(7):427–442
Rasool M, Varalakshmi P (2006) Immunomodulatory role of Withania somnifera root powder on experimental induced inflammation: an in vivo and in vitro study. Vascul Pharmacol 44(6):406–410
Richardson PG, Sonneveld P et al (2005) Bortezomib or high-dose dexamethasone for relapsed multiple myeloma. N Engl J Med 352(24):2487–2498
Romanova D, Vachalkova A et al (2001) Study of antioxidant effect of apigenin, luteolin and quercetin by DNA protective method. Neoplasma 48(2):104–107
Ruschak AM, Slassi M et al (2011) Novel proteasome inhibitors to overcome bortezomib resistance. J Natl Cancer Inst 103(13):1007–1017

Russo GL (2007) Ins and outs of dietary phytochemicals in cancer chemoprevention. Biochem Pharmacol 74(4):533–544

Sarkar FH, Li Y (2002) Mechanisms of cancer chemoprevention by soy isoflavone genistein. Cancer Metastasis Rev 21(3–4):265–280

Sarkar FH, Adsule S et al (2006) The role of genistein and synthetic derivatives of isoflavone in cancer prevention and therapy. Mini Rev Med Chem 6(4):401–407

Seely D, Mills EJ et al (2005) The effects of green tea consumption on incidence of breast cancer and recurrence of breast cancer: a systematic review and meta-analysis. Integr Cancer Ther 4(2):144–155

Selvendiran K, Koga H et al (2006) Luteolin promotes degradation in signal transducer and activator of transcription 3 in human hepatoma cells: an implication for the antitumor potential of flavonoids. Cancer Res 66(9):4826–4834

Sherr CJ, Roberts JM (1995) Inhibitors of mammalian G1 cyclin-dependent kinases. Genes Dev 9(10):1149–1163

Sherr CJ, Roberts JM (1999) CDK inhibitors: positive and negative regulators of G1-phase progression. Genes Dev 13(12):1501–1512

Shimizu M, Deguchi A et al (2005) (-)-Epigallocatechin gallate and polyphenon E inhibit growth and activation of the epidermal growth factor receptor and human epidermal growth factor receptor-2 signaling pathways in human colon cancer cells. Clin Cancer Res 11(7):2735–2746

Shrubsole MJ, Lu W et al (2009) Drinking green tea modestly reduces breast cancer risk. J Nutr 139(2):310–316

Sim GS, Lee BC et al (2007) Structure activity relationship of antioxidative property of flavonoids and inhibitory effect on matrix metalloproteinase activity in UVA-irradiated human dermal fibroblast. Arch Pharm Res 30(3):290–298

Smith DM, Daniel KG et al (2004) Docking studies and model development of tea polyphenol proteasome inhibitors: applications to rational drug design. Proteins 54(1):58–70

Soligo D, Servida F et al (2001) The apoptogenic response of human myeloid leukaemia cell lines and of normal and malignant haematopoietic progenitor cells to the proteasome inhibitor PSI. Br J Haematol 113(1):126–135

Sonoda T, Nagata Y et al (2004) A case-control study of diet and prostate cancer in Japan: possible protective effect of traditional Japanese diet. Cancer Sci 95(3):238–242

Sun J, Nam S et al (2001) CEP1612, a dipeptidyl proteasome inhibitor, induces p21WAF1 and p27KIP1 expression and apoptosis and inhibits the growth of the human lung adenocarcinoma A-549 in nude mice. Cancer Res 61(4):1280–1284

Sun CL, Yuan JM et al (2006) Green tea, black tea and breast cancer risk: a meta-analysis of epidemiological studies. Carcinogenesis 27(7):1310–1315

Trock BJ, Hilakivi-Clarke L et al (2006) Meta-analysis of soy intake and breast cancer risk. J Natl Cancer Inst 98(7):459–471

von Metzler I, Krebbel H et al (2009) Curcumin diminishes human osteoclastogenesis by inhibition of the signalosome-associated I kappaB kinase. J Cancer Res Clin Oncol 135(2):173–179

Walle T, Otake Y et al (2001) Disposition and metabolism of the flavonoid chrysin in normal volunteers. Br J Clin Pharmacol 51(2):143–146

Wang YC, Bachrach U (2002) The specific anti-cancer activity of green tea (-)-epigallocatechin-3-gallate (EGCG). Amino Acids 22(2):131–143

Watanabe S, Yamaguchi M et al (1998) Pharmacokinetics of soybean isoflavones in plasma, urine and feces of men after ingestion of 60 g baked soybean powder (kinako). J Nutr 128(10):1710–1715

Weng MS, Ho YS et al (2005) Chrysin induces G1 phase cell cycle arrest in C6 glioma cells through inducing p21Waf1/Cip1 expression: involvement of p38 mitogen-activated protein kinase. Biochem Pharmacol 69(12):1815–1827

Won KA, Reed SI (1996) Activation of cyclin E/CDK2 is coupled to site-specific autophosphorylation and ubiquitin-dependent degradation of cyclin E. EMBO J 15(16):4182–4193

Wu AH, Yu MC et al (2003) Green tea and risk of breast cancer in Asian Americans. Int J Cancer 106(4):574–579

Yamamoto S, Sobue T et al (2003) Soy, isoflavones, and breast cancer risk in Japan. J Natl Cancer Inst 95(12):906–913
Yan GR, Xiao CL et al (2010) Global phosphoproteomic effects of natural tyrosine kinase inhibitor, genistein, on signaling pathways. Proteomics 10(5):976–986
Yang H, Chen D et al (2006) Celastrol, a triterpene extracted from the Chinese "Thunder of God Vine," is a potent proteasome inhibitor and suppresses human prostate cancer growth in nude mice. Cancer Res 66(9):4758–4765
Yang H, Shi G et al (2007) The tumor proteasome is a primary target for the natural anticancer compound Withaferin A isolated from "Indian winter cherry". Mol Pharmacol 71(2):426–437
Yang H, Zonder JA et al (2009) Clinical development of novel proteasome inhibitors for cancer treatment. Expert Opin Investig Drugs 18(7):957–971
Yuan JM, Koh WP et al (2005) Green tea intake, ACE gene polymorphism and breast cancer risk among Chinese women in Singapore. Carcinogenesis 26(8):1389–1394
Zhang M, Huang J et al (2009) Dietary intakes of mushrooms and green tea combine to reduce the risk of breast cancer in Chinese women. Int J Cancer 124(6):1404–1408

Chapter 7
STAT Signaling in Cancer Prevention

Su-Ni Tang, Sharmila Shankar, and Rakesh K. Srivastava

Contents

Abstract Members of the signal transducer and activator of transcription (STAT) family of transcription factors are potential targets for the treatment and prevention of cancers. STAT proteins can be phosphorylated and activated by diverse upstream kinases including cytokine receptors and tyrosine kinases. STATs have been associated with inflammation, cellular transformation, survival, proliferation,

S.-N. Tang • R.K. Srivastava (✉)
Department of Pharmacology, Toxicology and Therapeutics, and Medicine, The University of Kansas Cancer Center, The University of Kansas Medical Center, 3901 Rainbow Boulevard, Kansas City, KS 66160, USA
e-mail: stang@kumc.edu; rsrivastava@kumc.edu

S. Shankar
Department of Pathology and Laboratory Medicine,
The University of Kansas Cancer Center, The University of Kansas Medical Center, 3901 Rainbow Boulevard, Kansas City, KS 66160, USA
e-mail: sshankar@kumc.edu

S. Shankar and R.K. Srivastava (eds.), *Nutrition, Diet and Cancer*,
DOI 10.1007/978-94-007-2923-0_7,

invasion, angiogenesis, and metastasis of cancer. Various types of carcinogens, growth factors, oncogenes, radiation, viruses, and inflammatory cytokines have been found to activate STATs. Most STATs are constitutively active in cancer cells but not in normal cells. Phosphorylation of STATs causes dimerization, nuclear translocation, DNA binding, and gene transcription. STATs regulate the expression of genes that mediate cell survival, proliferation, invasion, and angiogenesis. STATs activation has also been associated with both radioresistance and chemoresistance. Furthermore, STATs have been shown to interact, directly or indirectly, with other transcription factors such as hypoxia-inducible factor-1, nuclear factor-kappa B, and peroxisome proliferator activated receptor-gamma. Several small molecule inhibitors, peptides and natural products are being developed for the prevention and treatment of cancer. Some chemopreventive agents have been shown to inhibit the IL6R-JAK/STAT pathway that is crucial for cell proliferation, survival, and inflammation. This suggests that chemopreventive agents might be candidates for cancer prevention because they reduce inflammation and prevent tumor growth, metastasis and angiogenesis. This review discusses the roles of various STATs in cancer prevention.

STAT Family Member

Signal transduction and activators of transcription (Stat) proteins is a family of cytoplasmic transcription factors. Since Stat1 and 2 were discovered as key mediators in the interferon signaling pathways, seven Stat family members (Stat1, 2, 3, 4, 5a, 5b, and 6) have been identified in mammalian cells (Darnell 1997). All seven members of Stats share several common features. Several conserved structural and functional domains have been identified (Fig. 7.1). The most important and conserved domain is SRC homology 2 domain (SH2), which plays three important roles. It could recognize specific phosphotyrosine motifs and induce the recruitments of Stats to activated receptor complex (Heim et al. 1995). It is also essential for the association of Stats to Janus protein-tyrosine kinases. Furthermore, it is required for Stats homo- or heterodimerization (Shuai et al. 1994). DNA binding domain is a β-barrel located in the middle and confers specificity of binding to palindromic sites within promoter regions of sequences. The function of N-terminal domain is to stabilize the interaction between Stat2 and interferon-γ activated sequence sites. The highly divergent carboxyl-terminal is required for transcription activation and account for unique transcriptional activities of different Stats. The phosphorylation of tyrosine residue is required for DNA binding of Stats, while the phosphorylation of Serine residue located can enhance the transcriptional activities in some Stats (Cho et al. 1996). Additionally, the coiled-coil domain is involved interaction with regulatory proteins, tyrosine phosphorylation, and nuclear export (Ma et al. 2003; Zhang et al. 2000).

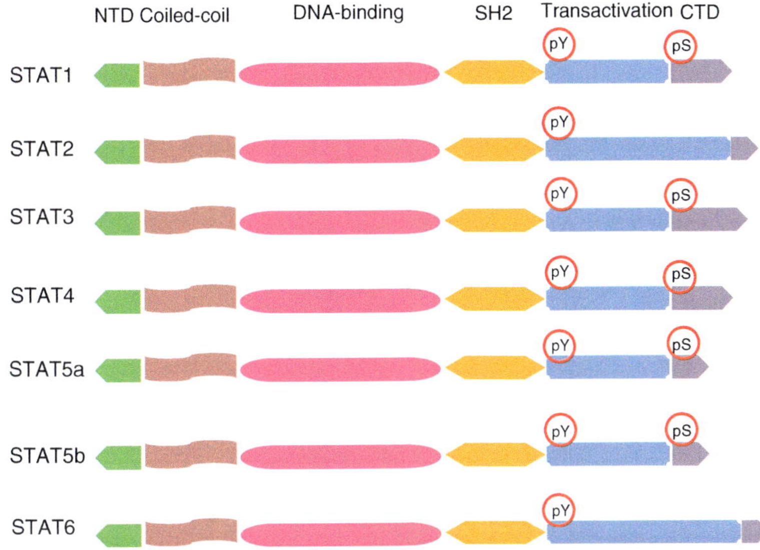

Fig. 7.1 The structures of STAT family proteins. The functional domains of STAT family proteins are shown. These domains include a N-terminal domain (*NTD*), a coiled-coil domain (*Coiled-coil*), the DNA-binding domain (*DNA-binding*), the SRC-homology 2 domain (*SH2*), the transactivation domain (*Transactivation*), a C-terminal domain (*CTD*). The phosphotyrosine residue is important for the interaction between STAT and DNA. The site of serine phosphorylation is able to modulate the transcription activity in STAT

STAT Signaling Pathways

Stats are initially present in inactive forms. They are stimulated by the binding signaling peptides, such as cytokines or hormones, which results in dimerization of their cognate receptors and activation of tyrosine kinases such as Jaks, e.g., Jak1, Jak2, Jak3, and Tyk2. The activated tyrosine kinases could subsequently phosphorylate the cytoplasmic domains of receptors to provide recognition sites for non-phosphorylated Stats monomers. Inactivate Stats are recruited to activated receptor complex through interaction of SH2 domains. Once Stats are phosphorylated by activated tyrosine kinases after binding, they will form homo- or heterodimers via their SH2 domain and rapidly migrate into the nucleus, where the dimers bind to specific DNA-response elements within the promoters of target genes and induce the relevant transcriptions (Darnell et al. 1994; Schindler and Darnell 1995). Stats are also activated by growth-factor receptors (GFR) with intrinsic tyrosine kinase activity such as platelet-derived growth-factor receptor (PDGFR) and epidermal growth-factor receptor (EGFR). The activated GFRs could directly phosphorylated Stats through a mechanism similar to the cytokine receptors (Bromberg et al. 1998; Sartor et al. 1997). Additionally, some non-receptor tyrosine kinases (Jak, Src,

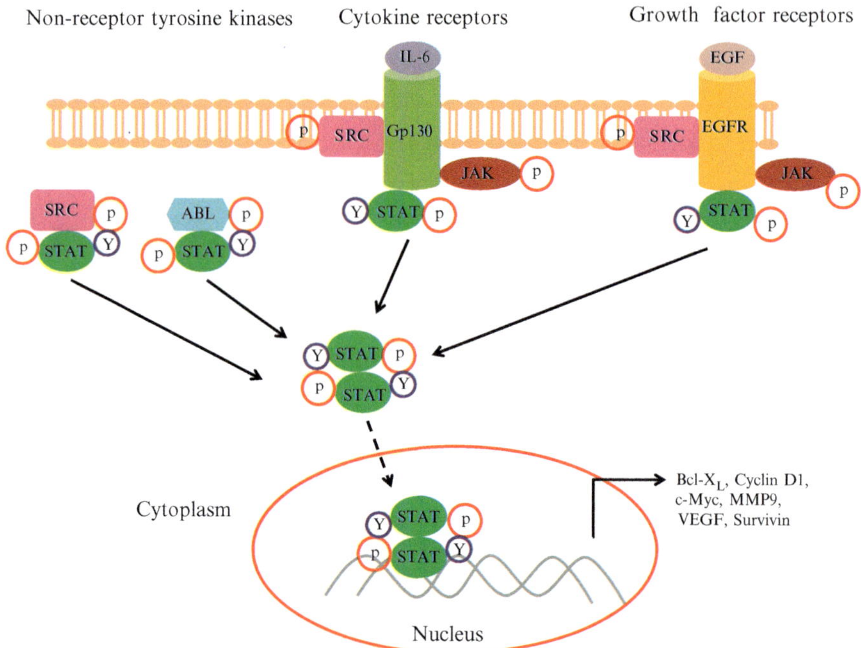

Fig. 7.2 STATs signaling pathways. The mechanisms of activation of STATs by non-receptor tyrosine kinases, cytokine receptors and growth factor receptors are shown. Cytokines (e.g. IL-6) can bind to their receptors (e.g. Gp130), which induce the phosphorylation and activation of SRC tyrosine kinases or Janus kinase (*JAK*). The activated SRC or JAK subsequently phosphorylate monomeric STATs and the STATs form dimers. Growth factors (e.g. EGF) interact with their receptors (e.g. *EGFR*) also resulting in the phosphorylation and activation of SRC or JAK, which induce the formation of dimeric STATs. Moreover, SRC and Abelson leukaemia protein (*ABL*) can phosphorylate themselves without receptor tyrosine kinases, and then activate STATs. The STAT dimers are supposed to translocate to nucleus and activate the expression of target genes

and Abl family kinases) can recruit and phosphorylated Stats independently or in coordinate with the activities of GFRs (Fig. 7.2) (Chai et al. 1997; Chaturvedi et al. 1998).

Biology of STATs

Numerous experiments have demonstrated that normal physical functions of Stats are critical in regulating many aspects of cellular proliferation, differentiation, migration, and survival. Each Stat gene has been deleted to investigate the phenotypes of single-knockout mice and unveil the biological functions of Stats under normal conditions. For example, Stat1 deficient mice became more susceptible to microbial infections and transplanted tumor for its primary roles in regulating response to interferon (IFN) -α and IFN-γ signaling (Bromberg et al. 1996); or Stat5a deficiency mice show impaired mammary gland development (Liu et al. 1997) while Stat5b gene disruption leads to the loss of sexually dimorphic growth patterns (Udy et al. 1997). These gene-targeting experiments exhibit non-redundant in modulating various host immune responses and non-immune responses.

STAT1

Stat1 was initially identified as a component of IFN-γ-activated transcription factor, IFN-stimulated gene factor 3 (ISGF-3), and further found to be responsible for DNA binding in the form of dimer (Schindler et al. 1992; Shuai et al. 1994). STAT1 is present in various dimer conformations, whose abundance is determined by tyrosine phosphorylation (Wenta et al. 2008).

Stat1 plays a pivotal role in the response of both Type I (IFN-α and β) and Type II (IFN-γ) IFNs (Durbin et al. 1996; Meraz et al. 1996; Nguyen et al. 2000). STAT1-deficient mice show a complete lack of biological responsiveness to either IFN-α, β or γ, although Type I and II IFNs are recruiting different Jaks to activates Stats (Platanias 2005). Type I IFNs could trigger Stat1 and Stat2 cascades through Jak1 and Tyk2, while Type II IFNs activate Stat1 by recruiting Jak1 and 2. Cytokines from IL-6 family can activate Jak1, Jak2 or Tyk2 through dimerization of specific receptors, e.g. gp130 and/or LIFR, and leads to the transient phosphorylation of Stat1. Additionally, the activation of Jak2 through growth factor receptors could also leads to transient phosphorylation and activation of Stat1 (Bromberg et al. 1998). Importantly, in IFN- γ signaling pathway, the gamma-interferon-activating sequence activated by Stat1 homodimers could provide binding sites for other activated Stats, e.g. Stat1 and Stat3 heterodimers, Stat3 homodimers, Stat4, Stat5, and Stat6 (Akira et al. 1994; Kotanides and Reich 1993; Mui et al. 1995; Wakao et al. 1994; Zhong et al. 1994).

Consistent with the roles of IFNs in cell growth regulation and antiviral and immune defense, both human and mice expressing Stat1 mutants exhibit highly sensitive to viral and bacterial infections (Dupuis et al. 2001, 2003; Durbin et al. 1996). Stat1 mediates the antiviral and antibacterial effect of IFNs through the transcription of inflammatory genes and the induction of immune effectors such IL-12, CD40, CD80, inducible nitric oxide synthase and several caspases. Intriguingly, Stat1 also exhibits the potential to restrain the response of innate immunity. The $STAT1^{-/-}$ mice is more susceptible to the development of experimental autoimmune encephalomyelitis (EAE) because the dysequilibrium of IFN-γ and IL-10 interferes with Th1 cell development and effector functions (Bettelli et al. 2004). These two opposite roles of Stat1 could contribute to maintain a homeostatic in immune activation. Importantly, Stat1 is also involved in host antitumor effects through modulating IFN-α pathway (Lesinski et al. 2003). Additionally, Ser^{727} of Stat1 can be phosphorylated through interferon regulatory factor-1 or tumor necrosis factor-α (TNF-α) receptor stimulations in the absence of Stat tyrosine kinase. Ser^{727} phosphorylation can enhance cooperate the IFN-γ-induced activation of macrophages (Kovarik et al. 1998). Further studies indicate that Ser^{727} phosphorylation is required by some Stat1-dependant apoptosis (Stephanou et al. 2001). Besides its role in modulating immune responses, Stat1 also participate into other biological activities, such as bone remodeling under both normal and pathologic disorders conditions (Lievens and Liboi 2003; Sahni et al. 2001).

STAT2

Stat2 is the largest protein, 850 amino-acids-long in man and 925 in mouse, among Stats family members (Veals et al. 1992). It was also initially identified as a subunit of ISGF-3, in which Stat1and the protein interferon regulatory factor 9 (IRF-9) are essential for DNA binding and Stat2 provide a carboxyl-terminal transcription activation domain (TAD) (Fu et al. 1992; Li et al. 1996). Stat2 shares about 40% homology with Stat1α, one of two alternatively spliced forms of Stat1 (Shuai et al. 1994) and can be activated by IFN-α, β, and λ (Duncan et al. 1997; Kotenko et al. 2003; Leung et al. 1995).

Although both Stat1 and 2 plays a pivotal role in mediating Type-1 IFNs response in a wide variety of cell types (Park et al. 2000), genetic studies have revealed that Stat2 are indispensable for IFN-α and β responses, such as the antiviral response, and has more potent than Stat1. Stat2 deficient mice are more susceptible to viral infections (Park et al. 2000). Cells lacking f Stat2 don't response at all to IFN-α signaling (Leung et al. 1995). Stat2 and Stat1 heterodimer plays a major role in transcriptional activation of Type-1interferon-stimulated genes (ISG), although Stat1 homodimers could induce IFN-α response (Bromberg et al. 1996). Stat2 could form stable homodimers which could interact IRF-9 and activate IFN-α ISG (Bluyssen and Levy 1997). It has been reported that the un-phosphorylated Stat2 and IRF-9 complex dynamically shuttles between nuclear and cytoplasmic compartments (Banninger and Reich 2004), which provides an alternative pathway modulating the activation of ISG and recapitulate antiviral response independently of Stat1 (Lou et al. 2009). Recent studies indicates that the role of Stat2 in regulating ISG expression is independent of its phosphorylation status and the phosphorylated Stat2 is involved in the transcriptional repression of ISG (Testoni et al. 2011). Additionally, IFN-α activated Stat2 can form an ISGF-3 like complex with Stat6 and p48, a non-Stat protein, in B cells. This complex might be required for the activation of ISG15 gene (Gupta et al. 1999).

STAT3

Stat3 was initially identified as an acute phase response factor in IL-6 signaling pathway (Akira et al. 1994). It is ubiquitously expressed in most tissues (Duncan et al. 1997). Biochemical and genetic studies indicate that Stat3 is pleiotropic and can be activated by IL-6 (IL-6, 11, 31, leukemia inhibitory factor, oncostatin M, neuropoietin, ciliary neurotrophic factor, and cardiotrophin-1) and IL10 (IL-10, 19, 20, 22, 24, and 26) families of cytokines, as well as IL-7, 21, 27, leptin, granulocyte colony-stimulating factor (G-CSF), and epidermal growth factor (EGF) (Finbloom and Winestock 1995; Kotenko 2002; Lin et al. 1995; Tian et al. 1994; Vaisse et al. 1996; Yamauchi-Takihara and Kishimoto 2000; Zhong et al. 1994).

Because germ-line gene targeting has revealed that Stat3 is essential to vital development of mouse embryos (Takeda et al. 1997), conditional gene targeting has been employed to investigate the role of Stat3 in various organs and tissues. The function of Stat3 is cell-type dependent, and Stat may exhibit opposite effects in different cells. The tissue specific knockouts suggest that Stat3 plays an important anti-inflammatory role in myeloid cells. In T cells, Stat3 plays an important role in suppression of apoptosis through IL-6 responses and promote proliferation through upregulating the IL-2 Receptor α (Akaishi et al. 1998). Deletion of Stat3 in macrophages and neutrophils results in hyperactive phenotype, suggesting its role in modulating IL-10 responses (Finbloom and Winestock 1995). Stat-deficient mammary glands exhibit a delay of apoptosis of epithelial cells which is critical to cyclical mammary gland involution (Chapman et al. 1999). Moreover, deleting Stat3 in keratinocytes suggests that it is essential for migration, skin remodeling and wound healing (Sano et al. 1999). Therefore, Stat3 promote proliferative effects in T cells, fibroblasts, hepatocytes, and motor neurons but induce apoptosis in keratinocytes, epithelial cells, endothelial cells, mammary gland and myeloid cells.

Stat3 is most often related to oncogenesis among all Stat family members. A constitutively activated status of Stat3 has been detected in many cancers including multiple myeloma, head and neck, mammary, prostate cancer, renal carcinoma, colorectal carcinoma, pancreatic cancer, and other solid and hematological malignancies. The importance of STAT3 in malignancy is also confirmed through various genetic and biochemical method, e.g. RNA interfere, genetic ablation, and antisense oligonucleotide (Ni et al. 2000; Welte et al. 2003). Sata3 direct the expression of anti-apoptotic and proliferative genes. Additional studies suggest that the activated form of Stat3 is responsible to the invasion and migration of cancer cells, metastasis, and angiogenesis.

STAT4

Stat4 was first identified and cloned in myeloid cells of mice by using degenerative-PCR through its homology to Stat1 and Stat2. It is 52% and 69% identical to Stat1 in the AA sequence and SH2 domain, respectively (Yamamoto et al. 1994). Stat4 expression is restricted in myeloid cells and spermatogonia (Zhong et al. 1994).

Biochemical and genetics studies reveal that Stat4 is activated by IL-12 and IL-23 through similar receptors and also activated by IFN-α receptors through indirect recruitment by interaction with activated Stat2 (Farrar et al. 2000). IL-12 and IFN-α phosphorylate both tyrosine and serine residues of Stat4 (Cho et al. 1996). Additionally, Stat4 can be phosphorylated through Jak1 and Tyk2 induced by IFN-λ1 in human T lymphoma cells (Dumoutier et al. 2004).

The functional analysis of Stat4 suggests it plays a major role in differentiation the differentiation of naive $CD4^+$ T cells to Th1 cells. Its non-redundancy role in IL-12 signaling pathway has been exhibited in many studies. $Stat4^{-/-}$ mice are viable and fertile but deficient in most IL-12 mediated responses, including the induction of IFN-γ, cytolysis function of NK cells, and T helper cells differentiation (Kaplan et al. 1996; Thierfelder et al. 1996). Consequently, Abrogation of STAT4 signaling significantly prevents the development of lymphocytic choriomeningitis virus-mediated autoimmune diabetes (Holz et al. 1999). $Stat4^{-/-}$ mice are resistant to various autoimmune diseases, e.g. experimental autoimmune myocarditis or EAE, mediated by Th1 cells (Chitnis et al. 2001). However, further reports indicate there exists an alternative pathway for Th1 differentiation suppressed by Th1 cytokines because Stat4 and Stat6 double knockout mice are able to mount a Th1 cell–mediated delayed-type hypersensitivity response (Kaplan et al. 1998). Additionally, it is not clear how Stat4 contribute to IL-23-mediated autoimmune inflammation (Huber et al. 2008).

STAT5

Stat5 was initially identified as mammary gland factor in ovine mammary gland tissue and can be activated through Jak2 in prolactin (PRL) signaling pathway (Wakao et al. 1994). Two Stat5 isoforms, which are termed as Stat5a and 5b, were isolated from murine mammary tissue and sequenced at a later time (Liu et al. 1995). Biochemical and genetics studies have showed that the activations of Stat5a and 5b could be induced by IL-3 (IL-3, IL-5 and granulocyte-macrophage colony-stimulating factor), γ chain (IL-2, IL-4, IL-7, IL-13, and IL-15), and single chain (GH, PRL, and EPO) family of ligands (Lin et al. 1995; Mui et al. 1995; Rolling et al. 1996; Schindler and Darnell 1995).

Stat5a and 5b are 96% identical to each other at the AA level and are able bind to GAS sites after inducing cells with relevant cytokines. However, they may execute overlapping functions but also display specificity in signaling characteristics. The responses to PRL and GH favor Stat5a and Stat5b, respectively. The mRNA level of Stat5a is high in mammy gland and Stat5b high in muscle. Mammary gland development is greatly impaired in Stat5-deficient mice but not in Stat5b-deficient ones (Liu et al. 1997). Stat5a-null mice exhibit defectively mammopoietic and lactogenic signaling while Stat5b-defecient mice display a loss of sexual dimorphic growth indicating its key role in mediating GH responses (Liu et al. 1997; Udy et al. 1997). Moreover, stat5b is essential for proliferation and cytolytic activity. Consistent with the phenotypes of Stat5a and 5b single deficient mice, the double-knockout mice exhibit defective development of mammary glands, impaired peripheral T lymphocyte proliferations, and decreased number of NK cells, and developed splenomegaly (Matsumoto et al. 1999). Additionally, recent studies indicate that Stat5 genes play a similar role in early B lymphopoiesis as its known role in during T cell development. (Malin et al. 2010; Yao et al. 2006).

STAT6

In the beginning Stat6 was called as IL-4 Stat because it was found in the course of investigating IL-4-mediated activation of Th2 cells (Hou et al. 1994). Subsequently it is termed as Stat6 after it is identified from database of human genes by using the expressed sequence tag method (Quelle et al. 1995). The murine Stat6 is also identified through the same method and its AA sequence is 83 identical to the human sequence. Stat6 can exist in different isoforms which may benefit the modification of signaling of Stat6 by the abundance of these functionally distinct isoforms (Patel et al. 1998).

Stat6 is activated primarily by Jak1 and 3 via the ligation of the IL-4 (Hou et al. 1994). IL-13 is also able to activate Stat6 vid phosphorylated Tyk2 and induce many similar biological functions as IL-4 in B cells (Murata and Puri 1997). Moreover, it can be activated by IL-3, IL-15 and INF-α under certain circumstances (Gupta et al. 1999; Liu et al. 1995; Masuda et al. 2000).

Like Stat2, Stat6 also have a relatively large TAD, which primarily binds to IL-4 responsive promoters and regulates the transcription of numerous ISR genes including C ε, Sγ3, MHC II, CD23, CD40, and Bcl-x_L (Boothby et al. 1988; Kohler and Rieber 1993; Kotanides and Reich 1993; Masuda et al. 2001; Richards and Katz 1994; Schaffer et al. 1999). Additionally, Stat6 homodimers is also able to bind the GAS site like most Stats but at a low affinity.

IL-4 and IL-13 are cytokines that regulate the gene expression, proliferation, and polarization of naive $CD4^+$ lymphocytes into Th2 effectors Consistent with the functions of IL-4 and IL-13 responses, genetic studies have confirmed that Stat6 plays a key role in TH2 polarization of the immune system. Stat6-deficient mice display defective Th2 response with diminished Th2 differentiation, lack of expression of CD23 and MHC II, diminished IgE switching, diminished proliferative responses to IL-4, and more susceptible to autoimmune diseases (Chitnis et al. 2001; Shimoda et al. 1996). Interestingly, some recent reports indicate that Stat5a may provide an alternative and redundant pathway for Stat6-mediated Th2 cell differentiation (Kagami et al. 2001; Takatori et al. 2005). Furthermore, it has been reported that IL-13 is more important than IL-4 in parasite expulsion through Stat6 activation. Additionally, recent studies suggest that the transient Stat6 activation induced by IL-15 could prevent the apoptosis of mast cells through the expression of Bcl-X_L (Masuda et al. 2001).

Stats and Oncogenesis

As discussed above, the Stats signaling pathways are responsible for modulating the proliferation, differentiation, and apoptosis of cells, angiogenesis, and cellular immune response. Although Stats don't directly regulate cell cycle checkpoint or DNA repair, they are related to oncogenesis through their important roles in mediating cell fates and immune surveillance.

Among all the STAT family members, Stat3 is the most intimately linked to tumorigenesis because its important effects in tumor cell invasion, metastasis and angiogenesis. Stat3 is widely expressed in most tissues and is considered as a potential oncogene. Numerous experiments show that the constitutive activation of Stat3 is detected in 70% of solid and hematological tumors (Kortylewski et al. 2005). STAT3 can be activated by multiple cytokines, including IL-6, IL-11, ciliary neurotrophic factor, and leukemia inhibitory factor, which all use gp130-type receptors. In tumor cells, the constitutive activation of Stat3 generally results from defective or overexpressed GFR (Campbell et al. 2001), the continuous binding of ligand due to autocrine or paracrine (Blume-Jensen and Hunter 2001), and/or the constitutive activation of non-receptor tyrosine kinases, e.g. Abl or Src (Chai et al. 1997). Gene-targeting experiments have showed that Stat3 is required for several tumor-derived cell lines to maintain transformed phenotype (Spiekermann et al. 2002). Stat3 could also initiate angiogenesis by binding and transactivating the VEGF promoter. Further, Stat3 is involved in epithelial-mesenchymal transition and cell migration. Additionally, Stat3 can induce the transcription of many potential oncogenes including those encoding Bcl-X_L, Mcl-1, Cyclin D1, and Myc.

In addition to Stat3, Stat5 is also found to be constitutively activated in several cancer cell lines and tumor tissues, e.g. leukemias, lymphomas, and breast cancer. Stat5 is required to support malignant transformation in hematopoietic cells (Spiekermann et al. 2002). Stat5 can promote the proliferation through upregualting the expression of IL-2Rα (Campbell et al. 2001). Additionally, some Stat5-regualted genes are implicated in anti-apoptotic or pro-survival response, which include bcl-2, bcl-x_L, Mcl-1, and pim-1 (Li et al. 2010a; Soldaini et al. 2000; Takatori et al. 2005).

In contrast to Sta3 and Stat5 Stat1 plays an opposite role in tumorigenesis and be considered as tumor suppressor. It induces various pro-apoptotic and anti-proliferative genes including Fas, Caspases 1, 3, 7 and 8, and NO (Choi et al. 2003; Tomita et al. 2003), inhibits angiogenesis (Battle et al. 2006), and enhances immune responses. Interestingly, both Stat1 and Stat3 are activated by several similar cytokine, e.g. Type-1 IFNs and IL-6 families, and response in opposite manners, which may suggest an effort to achieve a more balanced response.

STATs are thought by many researchers as suitable therapeutic targets for malignancy drug discovery because of constitutive activation of STATs are extensively detected in most cancer cells and tumor tissues, the modulation of STATs signaling could suppress and reverse the development of relevant disease, and the molecular mechanism of tumorigenesis caused by STATs signaling pathways have been well defined. Therefore, the understanding of molecular mechanisms of Stats and elucidating the signaling networks is an obligatory step towards the design of rational clinical treatments.

STATS and Cancer Prevention

A number of anti-inflammatory plant secondary metabolites have been shown to suppress gene activation of members of the STAT family in tumor cells. Polyphenols from green tea inhibit STAT3 expression and cancer growth, and induce apoptosis in various cancers (Aalinkeel et al. 2010; Siddiqui et al. 2008; Singh et al. 2011). In Hodgkins lymphoma cells, curcumin induces cell arrest and apoptosis in association with the inhibition of the constitutively active NF-κB and STAT3 pathways. Its expression in the human chronic myelogenous leukemia cell line K562 also induces a decrease of nuclear STAT3, 5a and -5b, without affecting either STAT1 expression or the phosphorylation states of STAT1, 3 or −5 (Mackenzie et al. 2008). Most interestingly, the decrease of nuclear STAT5a and -5b after curcumin treatment was accompanied by an increase of the truncated STAT5 isoforms, indicating that curcumin is able to induce the cleavage of STAT5 into its dominant negative variants lacking the STAT5 C-terminal region (Blasius et al. 2006). Luteolin, a flavonoid from celery and green pepper, promotes degradation of STAT3 in human hepatoma cells, leading to a downregulation of the targeted downstream gene products such as cyclin D1, survivin, and Bcl-X_L (Selvendiran et al. 2006). Resveratrol modulates IL-6-induced intercellular adhesion molecule-1 (ICAM-1) gene expression by suppressing STAT3 phosphorylation (Wung et al. 2005). Several other chemopreventive agents including kaempferol, found in broccoli and tea, significantly inhibit STAT1 and NF-κB activation in LPS-activated murine macrophage J774 cells (Hamalainen et al. 2007). Silibinin, a flavonolignan in milk thistle extract, inhibits the activation of STAT3 in human prostate and lung cancer cells and suppresses tumor growth both in vitro and in vivo (Agarwal et al. 2007; Li et al. 2010c; Singh et al. 2009; Tyagi et al. 2009). Silibinin robustly decreases the protein expression and nuclear localization of survivin, as well as its secretion from tumor into plasma in the mouse, but it also increases the levels of p53 and cleaved caspase 3 in test tumors (Agarwal et al. 2007; Singh et al. 2009). Cytokine mixture (TNFα + IFNγ) also activated Erk1/2 and caused an increase in both COX2 and iNOS levels. Pretreatment of cells with a MEK, NFκB, and/or EGFR inhibitor inhibited cytokine mixture-induced activation of Erk1/2, NFκB, or EGFR, respectively, and strongly decreased phosphorylation of STAT3 and STAT1 and expression of COX2 and iNOS. Furthermore, JAK1 and JAK2 inhibitors specifically decreased cytokine-induced iNOS expression, suggesting possible roles of JAK1, JAK2, Erk1/2, NFκB, and EGFR in cytokine mixture-caused induction of COX2 and iNOS expression via STAT3/STAT1 activation in LM2 cells (Tyagi et al. 2011). Interestingly, silibinin pretreatment inhibited cytokine mixture-induced phosphorylation of STAT3, STAT1, and Erk1/2, NFκB- DNA binding, and expression of COX2, iNOS, MMP2, and MMP9, which was mediated through impairment of STAT3 and STAT1 nuclear localization (Tyagi et al. 2011). These findings suggest that immunomodulatory and anti-inflammatory plant natural products target the STAT-signaling pathways, and can result in effective suppression of tumor growth, metastasis and angiogenesis.

Triptolide, a diterpenoid triepoxide from the traditional Chinese medicinal herb Tripterygium wilfordii Hook, is a potential treatment for autoimmune diseases as well a possible anti-tumor agent. It inhibits proliferation of colorectal cancer cells in vitro and in vivo (Li et al. 2010b, d; Zhao et al. 2010; Zhu et al. 2010). Treatment of mice with triptolide decreased the incidence of colon cancer formation in nude mice, and increased survival rate. In vitro, triptolide inhibited the proliferation, migration and colony formation of colon cancer cells. Triptolide inhibited the expression of JAK1, IL6R and phosphorylated STAT3 and the secretion of IL6. Triptolide inhibited Rac1 activity and blocked cyclin D1 and CDK4 expression, leading to G1 arrest. Furthermore, triptolide interrupted the IL6R-JAK/STAT pathway that is crucial for cell proliferation, survival, and inflammation. These data suggests that triptolide might be a candidate for prevention of colitis induced colon cancer because it reduces inflammation and prevents tumor formation and development.

The herbal compound 1,2,3,4,6-penta-O-galloyl-beta-D-glucose (PGG) inhibited the growth and metastasis of triple-negative breast cancer (TNBC) xenograft by targeting JAK-STAT 3-signaling axis (Lee et al. 2011). Daily oral gavage of 10 mg PGG/kg body wt decreased MDA-MB-231 xenograft weight by 49.3% at 40 days postinoculation. PGG treatment also decreased the incidence of lung metastasis. PGG also inhibited cell proliferation (Ki-67) and angiogenesis (CD34 staining), and induced apoptosis (TUNEL staining). PGG decreased pSTAT3 and its downstream target proteins, decreased its upstream kinase pJAK1 and induced the expression of SHP1, a JAK1 upstream tyrosine phosphatase, in MDA-MB-231 cells. Oral administration of PGG can inhibit TNBC growth and metastasis, probably through anti-angiogenesis, antiproliferation and apoptosis induction. Mechanistically, PGG-induced inhibition of JAK1-STAT3 axis may contribute to the in vivo efficacy and the effects on the cellular processes.

Future Prospects

In recent decades, a rapid increase in the costs of health care has increased the importance of naturally occurring phytochemicals in plants for the prevention and treatment of human diseases, including obesity. The modulation of signal transduction pathways by plant-derived dietary agents has recently been extended to elucidate the molecular basis for obesity and cancer. Current knowledge suggests that the potential complementary effect of natural products may occur through several mechanisms including suppression of inflammatory proteins, metastasis and angiogenesis, and induction of apoptosis.

Numerous studies confirm the potential roles of dietary and plant products in vitro and in animals, yet further human studies, in particular clinical trials, are required to confirm the therapeutic nature of these agents in obesity, insulin resistance, and cancer prevention. Expanded use of molecular technologies such as DNA microarrays and proteomics will help to identify newly molecular targets of dietary agents and individuals at high risk of cancer and metabolic diseases. Future trials should also include suitably planned pharmacodynamic studies, because the effective dose required for modulating these metabolic responses is unclear. At present, there is not sufficient data to support recommending long-term, safe usage for the prevention and treatment of obesity and cancer. Future translational and clinical research with the aim to unravel the role of natural dietary agents in cancer prevention and obesity is highly warranted. On behalf of such studies, one might be able to gain insights into their mechanisms at a clinical level and assess, within a short period, the potential success or failure of long-term interventions.

Acknowledgements This work was supported in part by the grants from the National Institutes of Health (R01CA125262, RO1CA114469 and RO1CA125262-02S1), Susan G. Komen Breast Cancer Foundation, and Kansas Bioscience Authority.

References

Aalinkeel R, Hu Z, Nair BB, Sykes DE, Reynolds JL, Mahajan SD, Schwartz SA (2010) Genomic analysis highlights the role of the JAK-STAT signaling in the anti-proliferative effects of dietary flavonoid-'Ashwagandha' in prostate cancer cells. Evid Based Complement Altern Med 7:177–187

Agarwal C, Tyagi A, Kaur M, Agarwal R (2007) Silibinin inhibits constitutive activation of Stat3, and causes caspase activation and apoptotic death of human prostate carcinoma DU145 cells. Carcinogenesis 28:1463–1470

Akaishi H, Takeda K, Kaisho T, Shineha R, Satomi S, Takeda J, Akira S (1998) Defective IL-2-mediated IL-2 receptor alpha chain expression in Stat3-deficient T lymphocytes. Int Immunol 10:1747–1751

Akira S, Nishio Y, Inoue M, Wang X-J, We S, Matsusaka T, Yoshida K, Sudo T, Naruto M, Kishimoto T (1994) Molecular cloning of APRF, a novel IFN-stimulated gene factor 3 p91-related transcription factor involved in the gp130-mediated signaling pathway. Cell 77:63–71

Banninger G, Reich NC (2004) STAT2 nuclear trafficking. J Biol Chem 279:39199–39206

Battle TE, Lynch RA, Frank DA (2006) Signal transducer and activator of transcription 1 activation in endothelial cells Is a negative regulator of angiogenesis. Cancer Res 66:3649–3657

Bettelli E, Sullivan B, Szabo SJ, Sobel RA, Glimcher LH, Kuchroo VK (2004) Loss of T-bet, but not STAT1, prevents the development of experimental autoimmune encephalomyelitis. J Exp Med 200:79–87

Blasius R, Reuter S, Henry E, Dicato M, Diederich M (2006) Curcumin regulates signal transducer and activator of transcription (STAT) expression in K562 cells. Biochem Pharmacol 72:1547–1554

Blume-Jensen P, Hunter T (2001) Oncogenic kinase signalling. Nature 411:355–365

Bluyssen HAR, Levy DE (1997) Stat2 is a transcriptional activator that requires sequence-specific contacts provided by Stat1 and p48 for stable interaction with DNA. J Biol Chem 272:4600–4605

Boothby M, Gravallese E, Liou HC, Glimcher LH (1988) A DNA binding protein regulated by IL-4 and by differentiation in B cells. Science 242:1559–1562

Bromberg JF, Horvath CM, Wen Z, Schreiber RD, Darnell JE (1996) Transcriptionally active Stat1 is required for the antiproliferative effects of both interferon alpha and interferon gamma. Proc Natl Acad Sci USA 93:7673–7678

Bromberg J, Fan Z, Brown C, Mendelsohn J, Darnell J Jr (1998) Epidermal growth factor-induced growth inhibition requires Stat1 activation. Cell Growth Differ 9:505–512

Campbell CL, Jiang Z, Savarese DMF, Savarese TM (2001) Increased expression of the interleukin-11 receptor and evidence of STAT3 activation in prostate carcinoma. Am J Pathol 158:25–32

Chai S, Nichols G, Rothman P (1997) Constitutive activation of JAKs and STATs in BCR-Abl-expressing cell lines and peripheral blood cells derived from leukemic patients. J Immunol 159:4720–4728

Chapman RS, Lourenco PC, Tonner E, Flint DJ, Selbert S, Takeda K, Akira S, Clarke AR, Watson CJ (1999) Suppression of epithelial apoptosis and delayed mammary gland involution in mice with a conditional knockout of Stat3. Genes Dev 13:2604–2616

Chaturvedi P, Reddy MR, Reddy EP (1998) Src kinases and not JAKs activate STATs during IL-3 induced myeloid cell proliferation. Nature Publishing Group, Basingstoke

Chitnis T, Najafian N, Benou C, Salama AD, Grusby MJ, Sayegh MH, Khoury SJ (2001) Effect of targeted disruption of STAT4 and STAT6 on the induction of experimental autoimmune encephalomyelitis. J Clin Invest 108:739–747

Cho S, Bacon C, Sudarshan C, Rees R, Finbloom D, Pine R, O'Shea J (1996) Activation of STAT4 by IL-12 and IFN-alpha: evidence for the involvement of ligand-induced tyrosine and serine phosphorylation. J Immunol 157:4781–4789

Choi EA, Lei H, Maron DJ, Wilson JM, Barsoum J, Fraker DL, El-Deiry WS, Spitz FR (2003) Stat1-dependent induction of tumor necrosis factor-related apoptosis-inducing ligand and the cell-surface death signaling pathway by interferon β in human cancer cells. Cancer Res 63:5299–5307

Darnell JE (1997) STATs and gene regulation. Science 277:1630–1635

Darnell J, Kerr I, Stark G (1994) Jak-STAT pathways and transcriptional activation in response to IFNs and other extracellular signaling proteins. Science 264:1415–1421

Dumoutier L, Tounsi A, Michiels T, Sommereyns C, Kotenko SV, Renauld J-C (2004) Role of the interleukin (IL)-28 receptor tyrosine residues for antiviral and antiproliferative activity of IL-29/interferon-λ1. J Biol Chem 279:32269–32274

Duncan SA, Zhong Z, Wen Z, Darnell JE (1997) STAT signaling is active during early mammalian development. Dev Dyn 208:190–198

Dupuis S, Dargemont C, Fieschi C, Thomassin N, Rosenzweig S, Harris J, Holland SM, Schreiber RD, Casanova J-L (2001) Impairment of mycobacterial but not viral immunity by a germline human STAT1 mutation. Science 293:300–303

Dupuis S, Jouanguy E, Al-Hajjar S, Fieschi C, Al-Mohsen IZ, Al-Jumaah S, Yang K, Chapgier A, Eidenschenk C, Eid P, Ghonaium AA, Tufenkeji H, Frayha H, Al-Gazlan S, Al-Rayes H, Schreiber RD, Gresser I, Casanova J-L (2003) Impaired response to interferon-[alpha]/[beta] and lethal viral disease in human STAT1 deficiency. Nat Genet 33:388–391

Durbin JE, Hackenmiller R, Simon MC, Levy DE (1996) Targeted disruption of the mouse Stat1 gene results in compromised innate immunity to viral disease. Cell 84:443–450

Farrar JD, Smith JD, Murphy TL, Murphy KM (2000) Recruitment of Stat4 to the human interferon-alpha/beta receptor requires activated Stat2. J Biol Chem 275:2693–2697

Finbloom D, Winestock K (1995) IL-10 induces the tyrosine phosphorylation of tyk2 and Jak1 and the differential assembly of STAT1 alpha and STAT3 complexes in human T cells and monocytes. J Immunol 155:1079–1090

Fu XY, Schindler C, Improta T, Aebersold R, Darnell JE (1992) The proteins of ISGF-3, the interferon alpha-induced transcriptional activator, define a gene family involved in signal transduction. Proc Natl Acad Sci 89:7840–7843

Gupta S, Jiang M, Pernis AB (1999) IFN-α activates stat6 and leads to the formation of Stat2:Stat6 complexes in B cells. J Immunol 163:3834–3841

Hamalainen M, Nieminen R, Vuorela P, Heinonen M, Moilanen E (2007) Anti-inflammatory effects of flavonoids: genistein, kaempferol, quercetin, and daidzein inhibit STAT-1 and NF-kappaB activations, whereas flavone, isorhamnetin, naringenin, and pelargonidin inhibit only NF-kappaB activation along with their inhibitory effect on iNOS expression and NO production in activated macrophages. Mediators Inflamm 2007:45673

Heim M, Kerr I, Stark G, Darnell J (1995) Contribution of STAT SH2 groups to specific interferon signaling by the Jak-STAT pathway. Science 267:1347–1349

Holz A, Bot A, Coon B, Wolfe T, Grusby MJ, von Herrath MG (1999) Disruption of the STAT4 signaling pathway protects from autoimmune diabetes while retaining antiviral immune competence. J Immunol 163:5374–5382

Hou J, Schindler U, Henzel W, Ho T, Brasseur M, McKnight S (1994) An interleukin-4-induced transcription factor: IL-4 Stat. Science 265:1701–1706

Huber AK, Jacobson EM, Jazdzewski K, Concepcion ES, Tomer Y (2008) Interleukin (IL)-23 receptor is a major susceptibility gene for Graves' ophthalmopathy: the IL-23/T-helper 17 axis extends to thyroid autoimmunity. J Clin Endocrinol Metabol 93:1077–1081

Kagami S, Nakajima H, Suto A, Hirose K, Suzuki K, Morita S, Kato I, Saito Y, Kitamura T, Iwamoto I (2001) Stat5a regulates T helper cell differentiation by several distinct mechanisms. Blood 97:2358–2365

Kaplan MH, Sun Y-L, Hoey T, Grusby MJ (1996) Impaired IL-12 responses and enhanced development of Th2 cells in Stat4-deficient mice. Nature 382:174–177

Kaplan MH, Wurster AL, Grusby MJ (1998) A signal transducer and activator of transcription (Stat)4-independent pathway for the development of T helper type 1 cells. J Exp Med 188:1191–1196

Kohler I, Rieber EP (1993) Allergy-associated Iε and Fcε receptor II (CD23b) genes activated via binding of an interleukin-4-induced transcription factor to a novel responsive element. Eur J Immunol 23:3066–3071

Kortylewski M, Jove R, Yu H (2005) Targeting STAT3 affects melanoma on multiple fronts. Cancer Metastasis Rev 24:315–327

Kotanides H, Reich N (1993) Requirement of tyrosine phosphorylation for rapid activation of a DNA binding factor by IL-4. Science 262:1265–1267

Kotenko SV (2002) The family of IL-10-related cytokines and their receptors: related, but to what extent? Cytokine Growth Factor Rev 13:223–240

Kotenko SV, Gallagher G, Baurin VV, Lewis-Antes A, Shen M, Shah NK, Langer JA, Sheikh F, Dickensheets H, Donnelly RP (2003) IFN-[lambda]s mediate antiviral protection through a distinct class II cytokine receptor complex. Nat Immunol 4:69–77

Kovarik P, Stoiber D, Novy M, Decker T (1998) Stat1 combines signals derived from IFN-[gamma] and LPS receptors during macrophage activation. EMBO J 17:3660–3668

Lee HJ, Seo NJ, Jeong SJ, Park Y, Jung DB, Koh W, Lee EO, Ahn KS, Lu J, Kim SH (2011) Oral administration of penta-O-galloyl-beta-D-glucose suppresses triple-negative breast cancer xenograft growth and metastasis in strong association with JAK1-STAT3 inhibition. Carcinogenesis 32:804–811

Lesinski GB, Anghelina M, Zimmerer J, Bakalakos T, Badgwell B, Parihar R, Hu Y, Becknell B, Abood G, Chaudhury AR, Magro C, Durbin J, Carson WE (2003) The antitumor effects of IFN-α are abrogated in a STAT1-deficient mouse. J Clin Invest 112:170–180

Leung S, Qureshi S, Kerr I, Darnell J Jr, Stark G (1995) Role of STAT2 in the alpha interferon signaling pathway. Mol Cell Biol 15:1312–1317

Li X, Leung S, Qureshi S, Darnell JE, Stark GR (1996) Formation of STAT1-STAT2 heterodimers and their role in the activation of IRF-1 gene transcription by interferon. J Biol Chem 271:5790–5794

Li G, Miskimen KL, Wang Z, Xie XY, Brenzovich J, Ryan JJ, Tse W, Moriggl R, Bunting KD (2010a) STAT5 requires the N-domain for suppression of miR15/16, induction of bcl-2, and survival signaling in myeloproliferative disease. Blood 115:1416–1424

Li H, Takai N, Yuge A, Furukawa Y, Tsuno A, Tsukamoto Y, Kong S, Moriyama M, Narahara H (2010b) Novel target genes responsive to the anti-growth activity of triptolide in endometrial and ovarian cancer cells. Cancer Lett 297:198–206

Li L, Zeng J, Gao Y, He D (2010c) Targeting silibinin in the antiproliferative pathway. Expert Opin Investig Drugs 19:243–255

Li Y, Yu C, Zhu WM, Xie Y, Qi X, Li N, Li JS (2010d) Triptolide ameliorates IL-10-deficient mice colitis by mechanisms involving suppression of IL-6/STAT3 signaling pathway and down-regulation of IL-17. Mol Immunol 47:2467–2474

Lievens PM-J, Liboi E (2003) The thanatophoric dysplasia type II mutation hampers complete maturation of Fibroblast Growth Factor Receptor 3 (FGFR3), which activates signal transducer and activator of transcription 1 (STAT1) from the endoplasmic reticulum. J Biol Chem 278:17344–17349

Lin J-X, Migone T-S, Tseng M, Friedmann M, Weatherbee JA, Zhou L, Yamauchi A, Bloom ET, Mietz J, John S, Leonard WJ (1995) The role of shared receptor motifs and common stat proteins in the generation of cytokine pleiotropy and redundancy by IL-2, IL-4, IL-7, IL-13, and IL-15. Immunity 2:331–339

Liu X, Robinson GW, Gouilleux F, Groner B, Hennighausen L (1995) Cloning and expression of Stat5 and an additional homologue (Stat5b) involved in prolactin signal transduction in mouse mammary tissue. Proc Natl Acad Sci 92:8831–8835

Liu X, Robinson GW, Wagner KU, Garrett L, Wynshaw-Boris A, Hennighausen L (1997) Stat5a is mandatory for adult mammary gland development and lactogenesis. Genes Dev 11:179–186

Lou Y-J, Pan X-R, Jia P-M, Li D, Xiao S, Zhang Z-L, Chen S-J, Chen Z, Tong J-H (2009) IFR-9/STAT2 functional interaction drives retinoic acid–induced gene G expression independently of STAT1. Cancer Res 69:3673–3680

Ma J, Zhang T, Novotny-Diermayr V, Tan ALC, Cao X (2003) A Novel sequence in the coiled-coil domain of Stat3 essential for its nuclear translocation. J Biol Chem 278:29252–29260

Mackenzie GG, Queisser N, Wolfson ML, Fraga CG, Adamo AM, Oteiza PI (2008) Curcumin induces cell-arrest and apoptosis in association with the inhibition of constitutively active NF-kappaB and STAT3 pathways in Hodgkin's lymphoma cells. Int J Cancer 123:56–65

Malin S, McManus S, Busslinger M (2010) STAT5 in B cell development and leukemia. Curr Opin Immunol 22:168–176

Masuda A, Matsuguchi T, Yamaki K, Hayakawa T, Kubo M, Larochelle WJ, Yoshikai Y (2000) Interleukin-15 induces rapid tyrosine phosphorylation of STAT6 and the expression of interleukin-4 in mouse mast cells. J Biol Chem 275:29331–29337

Masuda A, Matsuguchi T, Yamaki K, Hayakawa T, Yoshikai Y (2001) Interleukin-15 prevents mouse mast cell apoptosis through STAT6-mediated Bcl-xL expression. J Biol Chem 276:26107–26113

Matsumoto A, Seki Y, Kubo M, Ohtsuka S, Suzuki A, Hayashi I, Tsuji K, Nakahata T, Okabe M, Yamada S, Yoshimura A (1999) Suppression of STAT5 functions in liver, mammary glands, and T cells in cytokine-inducible SH2-containing protein 1 transgenic mice. Mol Cell Biol 19:6396–6407

Meraz MA, White JM, Sheehan KCF, Bach EA, Rodig SJ, Dighe AS, Kaplan DH, Riley JK, Greenlund AC, Campbell D, Carver-Moore K, DuBois RN, Clark R, Aguet M, Schreiber RD (1996) Targeted disruption of the Stat1 gene in mice reveals unexpected physiologic specificity in the JAK-STAT signaling pathway. Cell 84:431–442

Mui A, Wakao H, Harada N, O'Farrell A, Miyajima A (1995) Interleukin-3, granulocyte-macrophage colony-stimulating factor, and interleukin-5 transduce signals through two forms of STAT5. J Leukoc Biol 57:799–803

Murata T, Puri RK (1997) Comparison of IL-13- and IL-4-induced signaling in EBV-immortalized human B cells. Cell Immunol 175:33–40

Nguyen KB, Cousens LP, Doughty LA, Pien GC, Durbin JE, Biron CA (2000) Interferon [alpha]/[beta]-mediated inhibition and promotion of interferon [gamma]: STAT1 resolves a paradox. Nat Immunol 1:70–76

Ni Z, Lou W, Leman ES, Gao AC (2000) Inhibition of constitutively activated Stat3 signaling pathway suppresses growth of prostate cancer cells. Cancer Res 60:1225–1228

Park C, Li S, Cha E, Schindler C (2000) Immune response in Stat2 knockout mice. Immunity 13:795–804

Patel BK, Keck CL, Leary RSO, Popescu NC, LaRochelle WJ (1998) Localization of the human stat6 gene to chromosome 12q13.3-q14.1, a region implicated in multiple solid tumors. Genomics 52:192–200

Platanias LC (2005) Mechanisms of type-I- and type-II-interferon-mediated signalling. Nat Rev Immunol 5:375–386

Quelle F, Shimoda K, Thierfelder W, Fischer C, Kim A, Ruben S, Cleveland J, Pierce J, Keegan A, Nelms K (1995) Cloning of murine Stat6 and human Stat6, Stat proteins that are tyrosine phosphorylated in responses to IL-4 and IL-3 but are not required for mitogenesis. Mol Cell Biol 15:3336–3343

Richards M, Katz D (1994) Regulation of the murine Fc epsilon RII (CD23) gene. Functional characterization of an IL-4 enhancer element. J Immunol 152:3453–3466

Rolling C, Treton D, Pellegrini S, Galanaud P, Richard Y (1996) IL4 and IL13 receptors share the [gamma]c chain and activate STAT6, STAT3 and STAT5 proteins in normal human B cells. FEBS Lett 393:53–56

Sahni M, Raz R, Coffin JD, Levy D, Basilico C (2001) STAT1 mediates the increased apoptosis and reduced chondrocyte proliferation in mice overexpressing FGF2. Development 128:2119–2129

Sano S, Itami S, Takeda K, Tarutani M, Yamaguchi Y, Miura H, Yoshikawa K, Akira S, Takeda J (1999) Keratinocyte-specific ablation of Stat3 exhibits impaired skin remodeling, but does not affect skin morphogenesis. EMBO J 18:4657–4668

Sartor CI, Dziubinski ML, Yu C-L, Jove R, Ethier SP (1997) Role of epidermal growth factor receptor and STAT-3 activation in autonomous proliferation of SUM-102PT human breast cancer cells. Cancer Res 57:978–987

Schaffer A, Cerutti A, Shah S, Zan H, Casali P (1999) The evolutionarily conserved sequence upstream of the human Ig heavy chain Sγ3 region is an inducible promoter: synergistic activation by CD40 ligand and IL-4 via cooperative NF-κB and STAT-6 binding sites. J Immunol 162:5327–5336

Schindler C, Darnell JE (1995) Transcriptional responses to polypeptide ligands: the JAK-STAT pathway. Annu Rev Biochem 64:621–652

Schindler C, Shuai K, Prezioso V, Darnell J (1992) Interferon-dependent tyrosine phosphorylation of a latent cytoplasmic transcription factor. Science 257:809–813

Selvendiran K, Koga H, Ueno T, Yoshida T, Maeyama M, Torimura T, Yano H, Kojiro M, Sata M (2006) Luteolin promotes degradation in signal transducer and activator of transcription 3 in human hepatoma cells: an implication for the antitumor potential of flavonoids. Cancer Res 66:4826–4834

Shimoda K, van Deursent J, Sangster MY, Sarawar SR, Carson RT, Tripp RA, Chu C, Quelle FW, Nosaka T, Vignali DAA, Doherty PC, Grosveld G, Paul WE, Ihle JN (1996) Lack of IL-4-induced Th2 response and IgE class switching in mice with disrupted State6 gene. Nature 380.630–633

Shuai K, Horvath CM, Huang LHT, Qureshi SA, Cowburn D, Darnell JE (1994) Interferon activation of the transcription factor Stat91 involves dimerization through SH2-phosphotyrosyl peptide interactions. Cell 76:821–828

Siddiqui IA, Shukla Y, Adhami VM, Sarfaraz S, Asim M, Hafeez BB, Mukhtar H (2008) Suppression of NFkappaB and its regulated gene products by oral administration of green tea polyphenols in an autochthonous mouse prostate cancer model. Pharm Res 25:2135–2142

Singh RP, Raina K, Deep G, Chan D, Agarwal R (2009) Silibinin suppresses growth of human prostate carcinoma PC-3 orthotopic xenograft via activation of extracellular signal-regulated kinase 1/2 and inhibition of signal transducers and activators of transcription signaling. Clin Cancer Res 15:613–621

Singh BN, Shankar S, Srivastava RK (2011) Green tea catechin, epigallocatechin-3-gallate (EGCG): mechanisms, perspectives and clinical applications. Biochem Pharmacol 82(12):1807–1821

Soldaini E, John S, Moro S, Bollenbacher J, Schindler U, Leonard WJ (2000) DNA binding site selection of dimeric and tetrameric Stat5 proteins reveals a large repertoire of divergent tetrameric Stat5a binding sites. Mol Cell Biol 20:389–401

Spiekermann K, Pau M, Schwab R, Schmieja K, Franzrahe S, Hiddemann W (2002) Constitutive activation of STAT3 and STAT5 is induced by leukemic fusion proteins with protein tyrosine kinase activity and is sufficient for transformation of hematopoietic precursor cells. Exp Hematol 30:262–271

Stephanou A, Scarabelli TM, Brar BK, Nakanishi Y, Matsumura M, Knight RA, Latchman DS (2001) Induction of apoptosis and fas receptor/fas ligand expression by ischemia/reperfusion in cardiac myocytes requires serine 727 of the STAT-1 transcription factor but not tyrosine 701. J Biol Chem 276:28340–28347

Takatori H, Nakajima H, Hirose K, Kagami S, Tamachi T, Suto A, Suzuki K, Saito Y, Iwamoto I (2005) Indispensable role of Stat5a in Stat6-independent Th2 cell differentiation and allergic airway inflammation. J Immunol 174:3734–3740

Takeda K, Noguchi K, Shi W, Tanaka T, Matsumoto M, Yoshida N, Kishimoto T, Akira S (1997) Targeted disruption of the mouse Stat3 gene leads to early embryonic lethality. Proc Natl Acad Sci 94:3801–3804

Testoni B, Völlenkle C, Guerrieri F, Gerbal-Chaloin S, Blandino G, Levrero M (2011) Chromatin dynamics of gene activation and repression in response to Interferon α (IFNα) reveal new roles for phosphorylated and unphosphorylated forms of the transcription factor STAT2. J Biol Chem 286:20217–20227

Thierfelder WE, van Deursen JM, Yamamoto K, Tripp RA, Sarawar SR, Carson RT, Sangster MY, Vignali DAA, Doherty PC, Grosveld GC, Ihle JN (1996) Requirement for Stat4 in interleukin-12-mediated responses of natural killer and T cells. Nature 382:171–174

Tian S, Lamb P, Seidel H, Stein R, Rosen J (1994) Rapid activation of the STAT3 transcription factor by granulocyte colony-stimulating factor. Blood 84:1760–1764

Tomita Y, Bilim V, Hara N, Kasahara T, Takahashi K (2003) Role of IRF-1 and caspase-7 in IFN-γ enhancement of Fas-mediated apoptosis in ACHN renal cell carcinoma cells. Int J Cancer 104:400–408

Tyagi A, Singh RP, Ramasamy K, Raina K, Redente EF, Dwyer-Nield LD, Radcliffe RA, Malkinson AM, Agarwal R (2009) Growth inhibition and regression of lung tumors by silibinin: modulation of angiogenesis by macrophage-associated cytokines and nuclear factor-kappaB and signal transducers and activators of transcription 3. Cancer Prev Res (Phila) 2:74–83

Tyagi A, Agarwal C, Dwyer-Nield LD, Singh RP, Malkinson AM, Agarwal R (2011) Silibinin modulates TNF-alpha and IFN-gamma mediated signaling to regulate COX2 and iNOS expression in tumorigenic mouse lung epithelial LM2 cells. Mol Carcinog. doi:10.1002/mc.20851

Udy GB, Towers RP, Snell RG, Wilkins RJ, Park S-H, Ram PA, Waxman DJ, Davey HW (1997) Requirement of STAT5b for sexual dimorphism of body growth rates and liver gene expression. Proc Natl Acad Sci USA 94:7239–7244

Vaisse C, Halaas JL, Horvath CM, Darnell JE, Stoffel M, Friedman JM (1996) Leptin activation of Stat3 in the hypothalamus of wild-type and ob/ob mice but not db/db mice. Nat Genet 14:95–97

Veals SA, Schindler C, Leonard D, Fu XY, Aebersold R, Darnell JE Jr, Levy DE (1992) Subunit of an alpha-interferon-responsive transcription factor is related to interferon regulatory factor and Myb families of DNA-binding proteins. Mol Cell Biol 12:3315–3324

Wakao H, Gouilleux F, Groner B (1994) Mammary gland factor (MGF) is a novel member of the cytokine regulated transcription factor gene family and confers the prolactin response. EMBO J 13:2182–2191

Welte T, Zhang SSM, Wang T, Zhang Z, Hesslein DGT, Yin Z, Kano A, Iwamoto Y, Li E, Craft JE, Bothwell ALM, Fikrig E, Koni PA, Flavell RA, Fu X-Y (2003) STAT3 deletion during hematopoiesis causes Crohn's disease-like pathogenesis and lethality: A critical role of STAT3 in innate immunity. Proc Natl Acad Sci USA 100:1879–1884

Wenta N, Strauss H, Meyer S, Vinkemeier U (2008) Tyrosine phosphorylation regulates the partitioning of STAT1 between different dimer conformations. Proc Natl Acad Sci 105:9238–9243

Wung BS, Hsu MC, Wu CC, Hsieh CW (2005) Resveratrol suppresses IL-6-induced ICAM-1 gene expression in endothelial cells: effects on the inhibition of STAT3 phosphorylation. Life Sci 78:389–397

Yamamoto K, Quelle FW, Thierfelder WE, Kreider BL, Gilbert DJ, Jenkins NA, Copeland NG, Silvennoinen O, Ihle JN (1994) Stat4, a novel gamma interferon activation site-binding protein expressed in early myeloid differentiation. Mol Cell Biol 14:4342–4349

Yamauchi-Takihara K, Kishimoto T (2000) A novel role for STAT3 in cardiac remodeling. Trends Cardiovasc Med 10:298–303

Yao Z, Cui Y, Watford WT, Bream JH, Yamaoka K, Hissong BD, Li D, Durum SK, Jiang Q, Bhandoola A, Hennighausen L, O'Shea JJ (2006) Stat5a/b are essential for normal lymphoid development and differentiation. Proc Natl Acad Sci USA 103:1000–1005

Zhang T, Kee WH, Seow KT, Fung W, Cao X (2000) The coiled-coil domain of Stat3 is essential for its SH2 domain-mediated receptor binding and subsequent activation induced by epidermal growth factor and interleukin-6. Mol Cell Biol 20:7132–7139

Zhao F, Chen Y, Li R, Liu Y, Wen L, Zhang C (2010) Triptolide alters histone H3K9 and H3K27 methylation state and induces G0/G1 arrest and caspase-dependent apoptosis in multiple myeloma in vitro. Toxicology 267:70–79

Zhong Z, Wen Z, Darnell J (1994) Stat3: a STAT family member activated by tyrosine phosphorylation in response to epidermal growth factor and interleukin-6. Science 264:95–98

Zhu W, He S, Li Y, Qiu P, Shu M, Ou Y, Zhou Y, Leng T, Xie J, Zheng X, Xu D, Su X, Yan G (2010) Anti-angiogenic activity of triptolide in anaplastic thyroid carcinoma is mediated by targeting vascular endothelial and tumor cells. Vascul Pharmacol 52:46–54

Chapter 8
$\gamma\delta$ T Cells, Tea and Cancer

Jingwei Lu, Vincent J. Pompili, and Hiranmoy Das

Contents

Abstract Environmental factors play an important role in the development of cancer. Tea, one of the most popular beverages in the world, has shown to have anti-cancer effects as well as have protective effects against cancer development. Recent studies have shown that components present in tea could activate the immune system, particularly $\gamma\delta$ T cells, which is an important component of both innate and adaptive immune system. As a first line of defense against tumors, the activation of immune system is important to provide necessary preventive measures against tumor. In this chapter, we focus on the mechanism of $\gamma\delta$ T cell-mediated recognition of antigens, and delineate the mechanisms, by which tea product can activate $\gamma\delta$ T cells to facilitate cancer prevention activities.

J. Lu • V.J. Pompili • H. Das (✉)
Cardiovascular Stem Cell Research Laboratory, The Dorothy M. Davis Heart and Lung Research Institute, The Ohio State University Medical Center, 460 W. 12th Avenue, BRT 382, Columbus, OH 43210, USA
e-mail: hiranmoy.das@osumc.edu

S. Shankar and R.K. Srivastava (eds.), *Nutrition, Diet and Cancer*,
DOI 10.1007/978-94-007-2923-0_8,

Introduction

Cancer is a class of diseases characterized by uncontrolled growth of a group of cells that invade and destroy adjacent cells as well as tissues of an organism. Even though genetics has significant influence on cancer development, environmental factors play a primary role in development of cancer. Among the common environmental factors leading to cancer are tobacco, diet, obesity, infections, radiation, lack of physical activity, and environmental pollutants. It has been shown decades ago that natural dietary agents such as fruits and vegetables have protective effect against cancer (Block et al. 1992). It is proposed that one third of all cancer death in US can be prevented by dietary modifications (Doll and Peto 1981). Tea, the second most popular beverage following water, is consumed by two third of the population worldwide (Odegaard et al. 2008), and was suggested that the drinking green tea prevents development of cancer (Khan et al. 2008). Recently it was found that immune system plays a critical role in resisting or eradicating formation and progression of tumors (Hanahan and Weinberg 2011). A specific population of immune cells, more specifically, a subset of T cells named γδ T cells has attracted lots of attention due to its cytotoxic effects towards invading virus, bacteria and tumors. In various types of cancers, γδ T cells have been consistently identified and isolated from the lymphocytes that infiltrated within the tumors (Kabelitz et al. 2007). The γδ T cells isolated from patients with primary or metastatic colorectal cancer exhibited specific recognition towards autologous or allogenic colorectal cancer cells, renal cancer and pancreatic cancer and showed high level of cytolytic T cell response (Maeurer et al. 1996). Phosphate antigen activated γδ T cells were shown to display a selective lytic potential toward autologous metastatic primary renal tumor cells, which are inherently resistant to conventional treatment (Viey et al. 2005). The γδ T cell infiltration has also been found in ovarian cancer tissues in many patients. It was shown that such infiltration is correlated with higher; 5 year overall survival rate (Zhang et al. 2003). A brief disease-free interval was reported to correlate with γδ T cells in advanced ovarian carcinomas (Raspollini et al. 2005). All of these evidences support a strong role of γδ T cells in cancer survival. In this chapter we shall focus on the mechanisms of γδ T cell-mediated recognition of antigens and recognition of tea products. Emphasis will also be given to unveil detailed mechanisms by which γδ T cells recognizes cancer cells, and the role of key components in this recognition, such as T cell receptor (TCR) and second signaling pathway.

γδ T Cells: A Bridge Between Innate and Adaptive Immunity

T lymphocytes belong to a group of white blood cells and play a central role in cell-mediated immunity. T cell functionality depends on the recognition of antigens. The T cell receptors (TCR) expressed on the surface of these cells are responsible for recognition of antigens, which are presented by professional antigen presenting cells

(APCs) such as dendritic cells, macrophages and B cells or other non-professional APCs. Upon recognition of antigens, T cells get stimulated and results in various functional activities, such as cytotoxicity or regulatory and secret various cytokines or factors depending on the subpopulation of these T cells.

TCR molecules are composed of heterodimeric glycoprotein chains. The majority of the T cells possess α and β chains. In γδ T cells, the TCR is composed of one γ chain and one δ chain. Compare to αβ T cells, γδ T cells only compose 2–5% of the total T cell population in primates. The highest abundance of γδ T cells were found in the gut mucosa (Holtmeier and Kabelitz 2005). Like CD4+ and CD8+ αβ T cells in the adaptive immune system γδ T cells, which are mostly CD8+ also rearrange TCR genes via V(D)J recombination, which provides junctional diversity and develop a memory phenotype (Bukowski et al. 1999). This junctional diversity provides an advantage of various antigen recognitions via TCR. The antigen recognition of γδ TCR requires cell-cell contact, which is very common in T cell-mediated antigen recognition (Green et al. 2004). This antigen recognition process is necessary for T cell activation.

The γδ T cells demonstrate an innate immune response towards variety of microbial infections. This innate immune response is associated with the recognition of various antigen molecules by TCR. Structural analysis has shown that some of the intraepithelial γδ T cells express invariant or semi-invariant TCR. Rather than relying on the antigen recognition, the recognition pattern seems to be predetermined during the developmental process, which enables those γδ T cells to recognize a class of antigens. This provides an advantage for quick recognition of variety of antigens from multiple bacteria or virus, and ligand specific innate immune response by γδ T cells (Nishimura et al. 2004). It has been shown that the complementary-determining region 3 (CDR3) of γδ T cells presented in δ chain, play an important role in the diversity of γδ TCRs and in the recognition of antigens (Adams et al. 2005). By analyzing the TCR sequences of natural γδ T cells population specific for the major histocompatibility complex class IB molecule T22, it was shown that the sequence diversity around CDR3 modulates TCR ligand binding activities rather than specificity. The V gene is correlated mainly with the origin of tissues, which limits the number of antigens that γδ T cells recognize (Shin et al. 2005). γδ T cells also share some similarity with Natural Killer (NK) cells, which is essential for innate immune response. NK cells, γδ T cells and CD8+ αβ T cells express a common activating receptor, NKG2D, which was initially discovered in NK cells. However, in γδ T cells and CD8+ αβ T cells, NKG2D acts as a co stimulatory receptor in the TCR dependent activation (Das et al. 2001a; Groh et al. 2001). Recently, it was shown that culturing of PBMC with immobilized NKG2D ligand MHC class I related protein A (MICA) induces partial activation of γδ T cells but not CD8+ αβ T cells, indicating γδ T cells have certain similarity with the NK cells, which is also a member of innate immune system (Rincon-Orozco et al. 2005). Despite providing antigen-specific adaptive immunity, antigen-presenting cells also process antigens to present to the T cells for their activation. It was reported that γδ T cells could serve as an antigen presenting cells in some special conditions. Upon activation, human Vγ2Vδ2 T cells efficiently

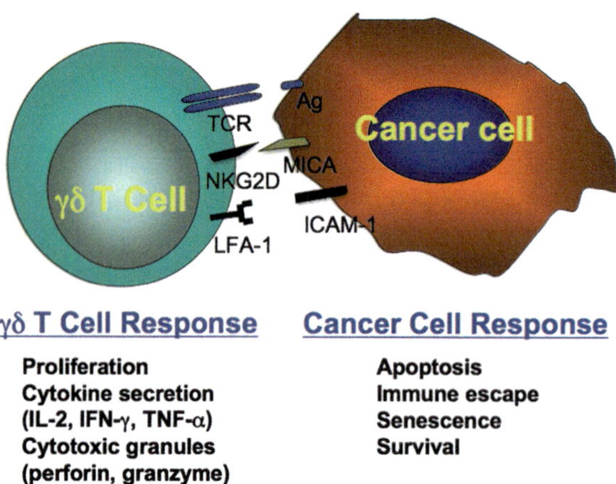

Fig. 8.1 Interaction between γδ T cells and cancer cells for antigen recognition, activation and cellular response. *TCR* T cell receptor, *Ag* antigen, *NKG2D* natural killer cell activating receptor, *MICA* MHC class-I chain linked molecule A, *LFA-1* leukocyte function-associated antigen-1, *ICAM-1* intracellular adhesion molecule-1, *IL-2* interleukin-2, *IFN-γ* interferon-γ, *TNF-α* tumor necrosis factor-α

process and display antigens and provide co-stimulatory signals to the naive αβ T cells for their proliferation and differentiation as a highly effective APCs (Born et al. 2006; Brandes et al. 2005).

Other than types of antigens and recognition of antigens, there are no major differences in mechanism of cytotoxic lysis between γδ T cells and CD8+ αβ T cells, which are mediated by the release of various cytokines and granzyme/perforin molecules (Fig. 8.1). It has been shown that as early as in 2 h after antigen exposure, human Vγ2Vδ2 T cells produce IFN-γ and TNF-α, which are important for innate immune response and induce apoptotic cell death to the target cells (Wang et al. 2001). The γδ T cells also release cytotoxic granules containing perforin molecules for lysis of tumor cells (Narazaki et al. 2003).

γδ T Cell Receptor

The T cell receptor (TCR), expressed on the surface of T cells, is responsible for recognizing antigens bound to major histocompatibility complex (MHC) presented by antigen presenting cells. When the TCR engages with antigen and MHC molecule, the T lymphocyte is activated through a series of biochemical events mediated by associated enzymes, co-receptors, specialized accessory molecules, and activated or released transcription factors. In αβ T cells, the T cell receptor contain V (variable), D (diverse) and J (joining) gene segments in their α (V and J gene) and β (V, D, J gene) chains, which contribute to the diversity of TCR through a process called V(D)J recombination. The basic organization of γδ TCR loci is similar to that of the αβ TCR, whereas γ chain contains VJ recombination and δ chain contains V(D)J recombination. The variable domain of TCR has three hypervariable regions called the complementarity determining region (CDRs), which are responsible for antigen recognition (Li et al. 1998). CDR1 and CDR2 were encoded in V gene segments while CDR3 regions are encoded in V(D)J junctions and bear the most length and sequence heterogeneity (Chien and Konigshofer 2007). Through analyzing the rearrangement of the TCR γ and δ chain loci in progenies of individual γδ thymocytes have revealed that fewer V genes are involved in generating γδ TCR than αβ TCRs. Moreover, individual TCR γ chain only pair efficiently with a variable number of TCR δ, which further reduces the diversity (Pereira and Boucontet 2004). Unlike αβ T cells, there are only eight Vγ and eight Vδ gene segments (McVay and Carding 1999). Despite the limited variety formed by CDR1 and CDR2 in γδ TCR compared with αβ TCR, it is believed that the diversity CDR3 formed by V(D)J recombination is the key determinant of specificity in antigen recognition by TCR (Xu and Davis 2000). By considering all elements that contribute to the variability of the CDR3 region, it was shown that the diversity of CDR3 in γδ T cells is much higher than in αβ T cells. This higher diversity of CDR3 contribute to the capability of recognizing a variety of antigens by γδ T cells (Chien et al. 1996). Further analysis has shown that compare to TCR α and β, the length distribution of γ and δ chains are more similar to immunoglobulins (Ig), indicate that γδ T cells act more similar to immunoglobulins in their recognitions. It was shown that Ig H and TCR δ are most variable in size and significantly longer than that of Ig L and γ chain. In contrast, TCR α and β chain showed a highly constrained distribution. This similarity in length and distribution of γδ TCR and Ig is also consistent with its ability to recognize a variety of pathogens (Rock et al. 1994).

Antigen Recognition by γδ T Cells

As discussed above, the two most important receptor-ligand interactions contribute to γδ T cells activation is TCRs and natural killer receptors (NKRs). TCRs are mainly contribute to the antigen recognition, while natural killer receptors such as NKG2D, act as a co-receptors that fine tune the activation threshold (Thedrez et al. 2007).

Phosphates

There are mainly three classes of small non-peptide antigen that activate Vγ2Vδ2 T cells in a TCR-dependent manner: pyrophosphomonoesters, nitrogen-containing bisphosphonates (N-BPs), and alkylamines (Fig. 8.2). The isoprenoid biosynthesis

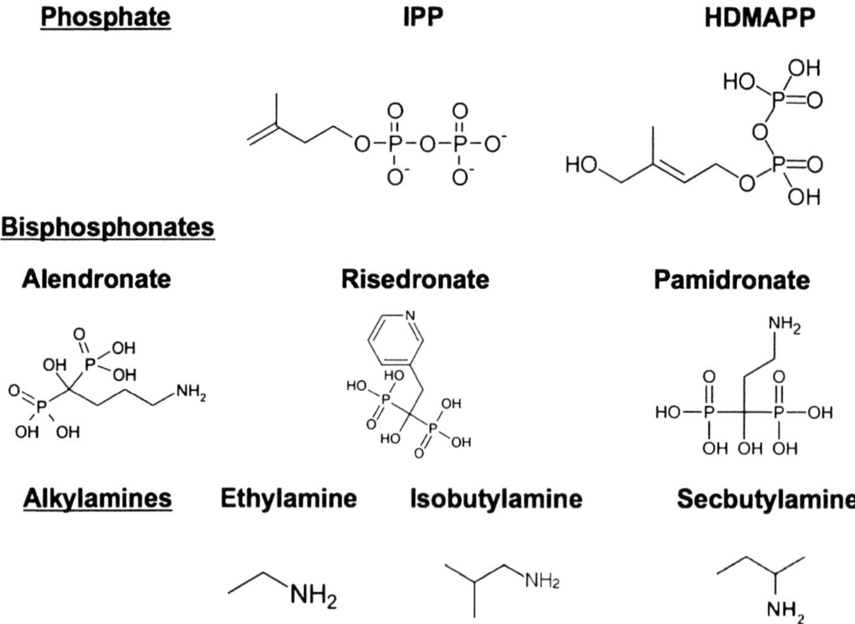

Fig. 8.2 Molecular structures of various non-peptide antigens of γδ T cells

pathway plays a key role in the activation of Vγ2Vδ2 T cells. One of the critical metabolites in this pathway is isopentenyl pyrophosphate (IPP). The accumulated IPP could be directly presented to the cell surface and could be recognized by Vγ2Vδ2 T cells in a TCR-depended manner (Bonneville and Scotet 2006). In mammalian cells and in some bacteria, IPP is an intermediate of the mevalonate (MVA) pathway. It was shown that the increased amount of mevalonate metabolites is accumulated in tumor cells, which is recognized by Vγ2Vδ2 T cells, and induced T cells activation. The blocking of this pathway prevents accumulation of mevalonate metabolites and as a result reduced activation of Vγ2Vδ2 T cells. Since, in many tumor cells, the level of expression and function of hydroxy-methylglutaryl-CoA reductase (HMCR), the rate limiting enzyme in the mevalonate pathway is significantly upregulated as a result accumulation of IPP takes place, that mediates γδ T cells activation rather than normal cells (Gober et al. 2003). In microorganisms, even though extracts from bacteria can stimulate Vγ2Vδ2 T cells, the amount of IPP present are not sufficient to induce Vγ2Vδ2 T cells activation. It was found that hydroxy-dimethyl-allyl-pyrophosphate (HDMAPP), an intermediates of 1-deoxy-D-xylulose-5-phosphate (DOXP) pathway, are responsible for the activation of γδ T cells, and provide a much more potent agonist than IPP (Begley et al. 2004; Jomaa et al. 1999).

Bisphosphonates

Bisphosphonates are synthetic compounds commonly used to inhibit bone resorption in osteoporosis, Paget's disease (Hosking 2006) and tumor bone metastasis diseases (Perry and Figgitt 2004). Nitrogen-containing bisphosphonates, such as alendronate and risedronate were found to activate Vγ2Vδ2 T cells. Patients treated with pamidronate as the sole therapy for increased bone resorption has shown an expansion of Vγ2Vδ2 T cells population (Kunzmann et al. 1999). Recognition of bisphosphonates by Vγ2Vδ2 T cells requires TCR, the pretreatment of various cancer cells with bisphosphonates enhanced Vγ2Vδ2 TCR recognition and increased cytotoxic effect on various cancer cells (Das et al. 2001b; Kato et al. 2003). However, rather than direct activation, it was shown that N-containing biophosphonates inhibit the isoprenoid biosynthesis pathway and target farnesyl pyrophosphate synthase (FPPS), an enzyme acting downstream of IPP synthesis of the MVA pathway. This inhibition resulted in accumulation of IPP, which in turn activate Vγ2Vδ2 T cells, rather than direct engagement (Bergstrom et al. 2000). Chemically, bisphosphonates are characterized by a phosphate-carbon-phosphate group and function as synthetic analogs of inorganic pyrophosphate for FPPS binding. The length of the aliphatic carbon chain and the hydroxyl group to the carbon atom at position 1 is important. Other structures such as the amino group at the end of the side chain and the nitrogen atom can further increase the potency of the bisphosphonates. Of those, cyclic genimal bisphosphonates such as risedronate and zoledronate are very potent and among the most active compounds (Fleisch 2002). By analyzing 45 different compounds, it was shown that there is a strong correlation between the stimulation of Vγ2Vδ2 T cells and FPPS inhibition by bisphosphonates, and modifying the structure of biophosphonate resulted in losing activation of Vγ2Vδ2 T cell and bone resorption (Morita et al. 2007; Sanders et al. 2004). Crystallographic analysis has shown that risedronate inhibits FPPS by binding to the dimethylallyl/geranyl pyrophosphate ligand pocket, which competes out the binding of DMAPP. The interaction between nitrogen in the n-containing bisphosphonate with Thr-201 and Lys-200 further enhances the potency by positioning the nitrogen in the carbonation-binding site (Kavanagh et al. 2006).

Alkylamines

Alkylamines is the other group of antigens recognized by Vγ2Vδ2 T cells. Amine antigens are small compounds present in tumor cells, bacteria, parasites, fungi, and are also found in plant products such as tea, apples, mushrooms and wine. It was shown that alkylamines could be synthesized by drinking tea, which stimulates Vγ2Vδ2 T cells in a TCR-dependent manner (Bukowski et al. 1999; Kamath et al.

2003). Alkylamines is a class of amines, where an alkyl group replaces hydrogen atoms of ammonia. Chemically they are distinct from prenyl pyrophosphates and bisphosphonates, since they contain positively charged amine group rather than negatively charged phosphonate or phosphate group (Morita et al. 2007). Like N-containing bisphosphonates, alkylamines was also recently shown to activate Vγ2Vδ2 T cells in a similar fashion. It was shown that alkylamines is a weak inhibitor of FPPS, which lead to accumulation of IPP, that could be recognized by Vγ2Vδ2 T cells (Thompson et al. 2006).

Among other compounds, a complex formed by apolipoprotein (apo) A1 and F-1 adenosine triphosphatase (ATPase), which were expressed on the surface of some tumor cells, were found to selectively activate Vγ2Vδ2 T cells. This raised a possible relationship between Vγ2Vδ2 T cell recognition and lipid metabolites (Scotet et al. 2005). Later it was shown that F-1 ATPase demonstrated characteristic properties of antigen presenting molecules rather than antigen for Vγ2Vδ2 T cells. T cells contact with F-1-ATPase bound on polystyrene beads can partially replace the APCs in phospho antigen-mediated responses. Moreover, derivative of IPP can bind to F-1-ATPase beads and promote TCR aggregation and cytotoxic activities (Mookerjee-Basu et al. 2010). It is now evident that certain density of membrane bound phospho antigen is required to induce efficient TCR signaling, and this may be achieved by antigen presenting molecules and by other adhesion molecules (Gomes et al. 2010). However, it is still under investigation how the mitochondrion F-1 ATPase translocates to the cell surface. It was proposed that during apoptosis, the inner membrane of mitochondria is disrupted and fused with the plasma membrane. This mechanism allows Vγ2Vδ2 T cells to recognize and clear the stressed and pre-apoptotic cells (Thedrez et al. 2007). However, the above mechanisms seem to be only applied to Vγ2Vδ2 T cells. Non-Vδ2 T cells may be activated through other antigens, which are yet to be defined.

NKG2D: Co-stimulatory Receptor of γδ T Cells

One of the common natural killer cell receptors, NKG2D, is found on both Vδ2 and non-Vδ2 γδ T cells are designated as a co-stimulatory receptor. NKG2D is a type II trans-membrane protein with an extra cellular C-type (Ca^{2+} dependent) lectin-like domain. However, rather than recognition of Ca^{2+}, NKG2D recognizes protein ligands and lacks the Ca^{2+} binding site (Raulet 2003). In γδ T cells NKG2D acts as a co-stimulatory receptor and fine-tunes the activation threshold of γδ T cells (Fisch et al. 2000; Halary et al. 1999; Thedrez et al. 2007). It was reported that NKG2D is recruited to the contact area between γδ T cells and tumor cells, which is called immunological synapse (IS) and promote recognition between γδ T cells and tumor cells together with phosphor-tyrosine, CD2, γδ TCR and CD94 (Favier et al. 2003). NKG2D also plays important role in mediating activation of δ1 T cells, where microbial components were presented by dendritic cells. It was shown that pre-incubation of Vδ1 T cells with blocking NKG2D monoclonal antibody significantly inhibit the proliferation of Vδ1 T cells upon activation (Das et al. 2004).

Various ligands has been identified for NKG2D, including major histocompatibility complex (MHC) class I chain-related molecule A/B (MICA/B) (Bahram et al. 1994), RAET1 (Cosman et al. 2001; Kubin et al. 2001), Rae-1 (Ogawa et al. 2011) and H-60 (Bui et al. 2006). MICA/B is a stress related protein, expressed on various cell types and up-regulated upon stress. The high expression of MICA/B was found in leukemia, gliomas, neuroblastomas, melanomas and various carcinomas such as breast, lung, colon, ovary and prostate (Castriconi et al. 2007; Friese et al. 2003; Groh et al. 1998, 1999; Pende et al. 2002; Salih et al. 2003; Vetter et al. 2002; Watson et al. 2006). Structurally, MICA/B is similar to MHC-I molecule, which is highly polymorphic and contains α1, α2 and α3 domains. However, MICA/B is not associated with β2-microglobulin and doesn't exhibit conventional type of class I peptide binding (Cao and He 2005). It was found that fibroblasts and endothelial cells showed increased MIC expression infected by cytomegalovirus (CMV), which augmented T cell antigen receptor-dependent cytolytic and cytokine responses through engagement of NKG2D (Groh et al. 2001). MICA/B has been proposed as an important tumor antigen recognized by both Vδ1 T cells and Vδ2 T cells (Das et al. 2001a, 2004). MICA/B can be recognized by subsets of Vδ1 γδ T cells through both TCR and NKG2D, as blocking either of the receptors will reduce the T cell activity (Wu et al. 2002). It was shown that MICA/B were able to deliver both the TCR-dependent signal and NKG2D-dependent co-stimulatory signal, a dual function of MICA/B in activation of Vδ1 γδ T cells (Wu et al. 2002). Vδ1 single polypeptide chain of TCR can specifically bind to immobilized MICA molecule through α1and α2 domains are responsible for the interaction (Zhao et al. 2006). However, doubts has have been raised about the functional relevance of MICA/B recognition by Vδ1 TCRs (Thedrez et al. 2007). In Vδ2 T cells, it was shown that MICA engagement occurs through NKG2D, which result in substantial enhancement of the TCR-dependent activation of Vγ2Vδ2 T cells by non-peptide antigens (Das et al. 2001a).

Recently, RAET1 proteins, initially named as UL16 binding protein (ULBPs), were identified as a novel ligand for NKG2D. ULBPs have a structure similarity to MICA/B molecules, but only contain α1 and α2 domain (Strong 2002). Ten members of this gene family are currently identified and six of them were shown to be expressed as functional proteins (Nausch and Cerwenka 2008). The RAET1 protein was found to be expressed by various tumors, including leukemia, gliomas and melanomas (Friese et al. 2003; Pende et al. 2002; Salih et al. 2003). It has been shown that Vδ1 T cells were able to lyse autologous chronic lymphocytic leukemia of B-cell type, when ULBP3 expression was up-regulated. It was also shown that higher expression of ULBP3 was related with reduced progression of disease in some patients with chronic lymphocytic leukemia (Poggi et al. 2004).

Tea and γδ T Cells

There are mainly six classes of tea, such as white, yellow, green, oolong, black and post-fermented tea. All of them contain alkylamine antigens at various degrees. L-theanine, that resembles with the non-peptide antigens of bacteria is enriched in black tea, were shown to prime γδ T cells, which lead to enhance innate immune response to bacteria and tumors (Kamath et al. 2003). This finding leads to define a new mechanism, by which tea may provide defense against cancer development (Fig. 8.3). It was reported that green tea consumption is associated with the reduced risk of breast, colorectum, lung, prostate, ovarian and pancreatic cancer, and antioxidant as well as priming of γδ T cell effect may contribute to the reduction of cancer risks (Percival et al. 2008). L-theanine, an amino acid derivative commonly found in tea has been proposed to be important as a dietary supplement to protect against cancer. L-theanine exists in green tea, white tea and in black tea in a significant amount. The product of L-theanine after catabolized produces ethylamine, which act as an antigenic alkylamines and activate Vγ2Vδ2 T cells, and expand the Vγ2Vδ2 T cell population by up to 15-fold in a TCR-dependent manner (Bukowski et al. 1999). Ethylamine also inhibits the mevalonate pathway and accumulates the Vγ2Vδ2 T cells antigen IPP (Bukowski and Percival 2008). The conversion of L-theanine into ethylamine can happen within 2 h after

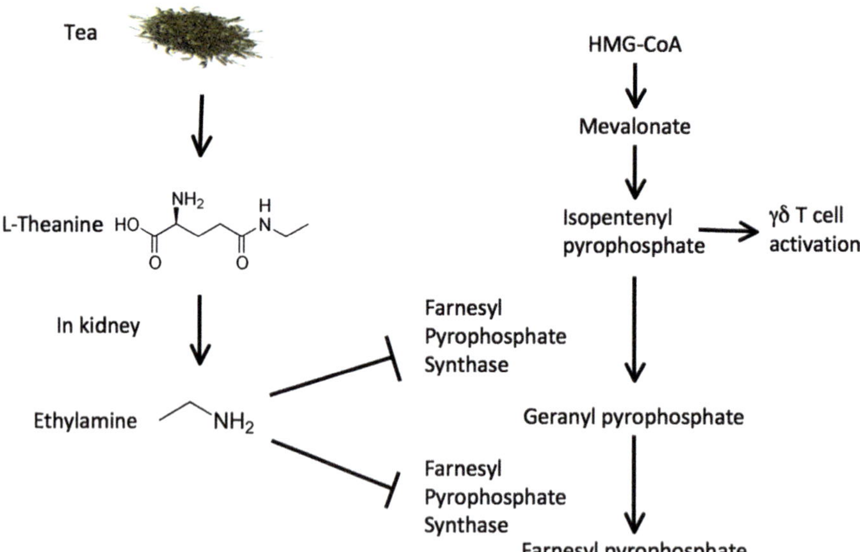

Fig. 8.3 Interaction between tea breakdown products, mevalonate (MVA) pathway and γδ T cells. Ethylamine, a breakdown product of tea inhibits various steps in the mevalonate (MVA) pathway, results in accumulation of isopentenyl pyrophosphate (IPP), which activates γδ T cells. HMG-CoA; 3-hydroxy-3-methyl-glutaryl-CoA

administration through breakdown metabolism in kidney (Percival et al. 2008; Tsuge et al. 2003). Indeed, drinking tea has shown to increase the urinary ethylamine level (Mitchell et al. 2000). One of the clinical studies was performed by analyzing blood sample from healthy non-tea drinkers before and 1–4 weeks after they drank black tea (600 ml/day containing 2.2 mM L-theanine) or coffee (no L-theanine) has shown that tea drinking had no effect on the absolute numbers of γδ T cells in blood. However, in response to bacteria antigen as well as synthetic organophosphate antigen, the capability of producing IFN-γ was increased twofold to threefold in the γδ T cells isolated from the blood sample of subjects drinking tea compared to the control (did not drink tea). Enhanced γδ T cell response were also seen in exposure to whole bacteria after drinking tea. Thus, ingestion of tea could prime γδ T cells for an augmented response to γδ TCR-dependent antigen (Kamath et al. 2003). In a randomized, double-blinded, placebo-controlled clinical study showed that the individuals taking a specific formulation of *camellia sinensis* (tea) has significantly reduced symptoms due to cold and flu compared to the controls. It has been shown that in the treated patients, γδ T cells proliferated 28% more and secreted 26% more IFN-γ in response to γδ T cell antigens compared to control group. These findings indicated that the tea product could enhance γδ T cell function and improve patients resistant to foreign bacteria (Rowe et al. 2007). It has also been shown that the apple polyphenols (APP), a key component of tea can stimulate CD11b expression in γδ T cells. APP treated γδ T cells showed an enhanced adherence to the plastic and also an elevated expression of cytokines. This finding indicated that polyphenols, which is also a key component of tea, may have a pro-inflammatory effects and enhance the migration and function of γδ T cells (Graff and Jutila 2007). Moreover, in murine model, it was reported that mice fed with traditional botanical supplement-101 (TBS-101), which contains extract from green tea, showed a significant inhibition of tumor growth and invasion compared to the control group (Evans et al. 2009). It was also shown that soy combined with tea components significantly reduced final tumor weight in mice (Zhou et al. 2003). In a phase II randomized, placebo-controlled trial in patients with high-risk oral premalignant lesions, it was shown that uptake of green tea extract helped in preventing oral cancer in a dose dependent manner (Tsao et al. 2009). Using a highly metastatic tumor cell line it was shown that the combination of polyphenol epigallocatechin 3 gallate (EGCG, the most abundant catechin in tea) with doxorubicin (Dox) exhibited a synergistic activity in blocking tumor cell growth *in vivo* (Stearns et al. 2010). Overall, it seems that tea component has various inhibitory effect on the metastasis of skin, prostate, breast, liver, colon, pancreatic and lung cancer (Khan and Mukhtar 2010).

Overall, uptake of tea has multiple beneficial effects such as anti-inflammatory, anti-oxidant, anti-microbial and anti-neoplastic. As tea products can potentially stimulate γδ T cells, it is likely that the beneficial effects of tea are partly associated with the priming of γδ T cells. Once, γδ T cells are activated they provide necessary innate defensive response towards any microbial attack and neoplastic diseases by secreting cytokines and cytotoxic granules.

Conclusions

Immunosurveillance plays an important role in cancer prevention. $\gamma\delta$ T cells, acting both as innate and adaptive immune cells, provide the first line of defense against various infections and neoplastic diseases. Priming $\gamma\delta$ T cells can enhance the responses towards microbial and neoplastic diseases. Tea, as one of the most popular beverage, has been shown to be able to prime $\gamma\delta$ T cells through its various chemical components, which could serve as antigens for Vγ2Vδ2 T cells. By using simple dietary supplement, or by consumption of tea is a convenient way to prevent development of tumor. Studies need to further address the efficacy of $\gamma\delta$ T cells in preventing cancer cells in the context of tea products.

Acknowledgements This work was supported in part by National Institutes of Health grants, K01 AR054114 (NIAMS), SBIR R44 HL092706-01 (NHLBI), R21 CA143787 (NCI) and The Ohio State University start-up fund. The funders had no role in study design, data collection and analysis, decision to publish or preparation of the manuscript.

References

Adams EJ, Chien YH, Garcia KC (2005) Structure of a gamma delta T cell receptor in complex with the nonclassical MHC T22. Science 308:227–231

Bahram S, Bresnahan M, Geraghty DE, Spies T (1994) A second lineage of mammalian major histocompatibility complex class I genes. Proc Natl Acad Sci U S A 91:6259–6263

Begley M, Gahan CGM, Kollas AK, Hintz M, Hill C, Jomaa H, Eberl M (2004) The interplay between classical and alternative isoprenoid biosynthesis controls gamma delta T cell bioactivity of Listeria monocytogenes. FEBS Lett 561:99–104

Bergstrom JD, Bostedor RG, Masarachia PJ, Reszka AA, Rodan G (2000) Alendronate is a specific, nanomolar inhibitor of farnesyl diphosphate synthase. Arch Biochem Biophys 373:231–241

Block G, Patterson B, Subar A (1992) Fruit, vegetables, and cancer prevention: a review of the epidemiological evidence. Nutr Cancer 18:1–29

Bonneville M, Scotet E (2006) Human Vgamma9Vdelta2 T cells: promising new leads for immunotherapy of infections and tumors. Curr Opin Immunol 18:539–546

Born WK, Reardon CL, O'Brien RL (2006) The function of gammadelta T cells in innate immunity. Curr Opin Immunol 18:31–38

Brandes M, Willimann K, Moser B (2005) Professional antigen-presentation function by human gammadelta T Cells. Science 309:264–268

Bui JD, Carayannopoulos LN, Lanier LL, Yokoyama WM, Schreiber RD (2006) IFN-dependent down-regulation of the NKG2D ligand H60 on tumors. J Immunol 176:905–913

Bukowski JF, Percival SS (2008) L-theanine intervention enhances human gammadeltaT lymphocyte function. Nutr Rev 66:96–102

Bukowski JF, Morita CT, Brenner MB (1999) Human gamma delta T cells recognize alkylamines derived from microbes, edible plants, and tea: implications for innate immunity. Immunity 11:57–65

Cao W, He W (2005) The recognition pattern of gammadelta T cells. Front Biosci 10:2676–2700

Castriconi R, Dondero A, Negri F, Bellora F, Nozza P, Carnemolla B, Raso A, Moretta L, Moretta A, Bottino C (2007) Both CD133(+) and CD133(−) medulloblastoma cell lines express ligands for triggering NK receptors and are susceptible to NK-mediated cytotoxicity. Eur J Immunol 37:3190–3196

Chien YH, Konigshofer Y (2007) Antigen recognition by gammadelta T cells. Immunol Rev 215:46–58

Chien YH, Jores R, Crowley MP (1996) Recognition by gamma/delta T cells. Annu Rev Immunol 14:511–532

Cosman D, Mullberg J, Sutherland CL, Chin W, Armitage R, Fanslow W, Kubin M, Chalupny NJ (2001) ULBPs, novel MHC class I-related molecules, bind to CMV glycoprotein UL16 and stimulate NK cytotoxicity through the NKG2D receptor. Immunity 14:123–133

Das H, Groh V, Kuijl C, Sugita M, Morita CT, Spies T, Bukowski JF (2001a) MICA engagement by human Vgamma2Vdelta2 T cells enhances their antigen-dependent effector function. Immunity 15:83–93

Das H, Wang L, Kamath A, Bukowski JF (2001b) Vgamma2Vdelta2 T-cell receptor-mediated recognition of aminobisphosphonates. Blood 98:1616–1618

Das H, Sugita M, Brenner MB (2004) Mechanisms of Vdelta1 gammadelta T cell activation by microbial components. J Immunol 172:6578–6586

Doll R, Peto R (1981) The causes of cancer: quantitative estimates of avoidable risks of cancer in the United States today. J Natl Cancer Inst 66:1191–1308

Evans S, Dizeyi N, Abrahamsson PA, Persson J (2009) The effect of a novel botanical agent TBS-101 on invasive prostate cancer in animal models. Anticancer Res 29:3917–3924

Favier B, Espinosa E, Tabiasco J, Dos Santos C, Bonneville M, Valitutti S, Fournie JJ (2003) Uncoupling between immunological synapse formation and functional outcome in human gamma delta T lymphocytes. J Immunol 171:5027–5033

Fisch P, Moris A, Rammensee HG, Handgretinger R (2000) Inhibitory MHC class I receptors on gammadelta T cells in tumour immunity and autoimmunity. Immunol Today 21:187–191

Fleisch H (2002) Development of bisphosphonates. Breast Cancer Res 4:30–34

Friese MA, Platten M, Lutz SZ, Naumann U, Aulwurm S, Bischof F, Buhring HJ, Dichgans J, Rammensee HG, Steinle A et al (2003) MICA/NKG2D-mediated immunogene therapy of experimental gliomas. Cancer Res 63:8996–9006

Gober HJ, Kistowska M, Angman L, Jeno P, Mori L, De Libero G (2003) Human T cell receptor gammadelta cells recognize endogenous mevalonate metabolites in tumor cells. J Exp Med 197:163–168

Gomes AQ, Martins DS, Silva-Santos B (2010) Targeting gammadelta T lymphocytes for cancer immunotherapy: from novel mechanistic insight to clinical application. Cancer Res 70:10024–10027

Graff JC, Jutila MA (2007) Differential regulation of CD11b on gammadelta T cells and monocytes in response to unripe apple polyphenols. J Leukoc Biol 82:603–607

Green AE, Lissina A, Hutchinson SL, Hewitt RE, Temple B, James D, Boulter JM, Price DA, Sewell AK (2004) Recognition of nonpeptide antigens by human V gamma 9 V delta 2 T cells requires contact with cells of human origin. Clin Exp Immunol 136:472–482

Groh V, Steinle A, Bauer S, Spies T (1998) Recognition of stress-induced MHC molecules by intestinal epithelial gammadelta T cells. Science 279:1737–1740

Groh V, Rhinehart R, Secrist H, Bauer S, Grabstein KH, Spies T (1999) Broad tumor-associated expression and recognition by tumor-derived gamma delta T cells of MICA and MICB. Proc Natl Acad Sci U S A 96:6879–6884

Groh V, Rhinehart R, Randolph-Habecker J, Topp MS, Riddell SR, Spies T (2001) Costimulation of CD8alphabeta T cells by NKG2D via engagement by MIC induced on virus-infected cells. Nat Immunol 2:255–260

Halary F, Fournie JJ, Bonneville M (1999) Activation and control of self-reactive gammadelta T cells. Microbes Infect 1:247–253

Hanahan D, Weinberg RA (2011) Hallmarks of cancer: the next generation. Cell 144:646–674

Holtmeier W, Kabelitz D (2005) gammadelta T cells link innate and adaptive immune responses. Chem Immunol Allergy 86:151–183

Hosking D (2006) Pharmacological therapy of Paget's and other metabolic bone diseases. Bone 38:S3–S7

Jomaa H, Feurle J, Luhs K, Kunzmann V, Tony HP, Herderich M, Wilhelm M (1999) Vgamma9/Vdelta2 T cell activation induced by bacterial low molecular mass compounds depends on the 1-deoxy-D-xylulose 5-phosphate pathway of isoprenoid biosynthesis. FEMS Immunol Med Microbiol 25:371–378

Kabelitz D, Wesch D, He W (2007) Perspectives of gammadelta T cells in tumor immunology. Cancer Res 67:5–8

Kamath AB, Wang L, Das H, Li L, Reinhold VN, Bukowski JF (2003) Antigens in tea-beverage prime human Vgamma 2Vdelta 2T cells in vitro and in vivo for memory and nonmemory antibacterial cytokine responses. Proc Natl Acad Sci U S A 100:6009–6014

Kato Y, Tanaka Y, Tanaka H, Yamashita S, Minato N (2003) Requirement of species-specific interactions for the activation of human gamma delta T cells by pamidronate. J Immunol 170:3608–3613

Kavanagh KL, Guo K, Dunford JE, Wu X, Knapp S, Ebetino FH, Rogers MJ, Russell RG, Oppermann U (2006) The molecular mechanism of nitrogen-containing bisphosphonates as antiosteoporosis drugs. Proc Natl Acad Sci U S A 103:7829–7834

Khan N, Mukhtar H (2010) Cancer and metastasis: prevention and treatment by green tea. Cancer Metastasis Rev 29:435–445

Khan N, Afaq F, Mukhtar H (2008) Cancer chemoprevention through dietary antioxidants: progress and promise. Antioxid Redox Signal 10:475–510

Kubin M, Cassiano L, Chalupny J, Chin W, Cosman D, Fanslow W, Mullberg J, Rousseau AM, Ulrich D, Armitage R (2001) ULBP1, 2, 3: novel MHC class I-related molecules that bind to human cytomegalovirus glycoprotein UL16, activate NK cells. Eur J Immunol 31:1428–1437

Kunzmann V, Bauer E, Wilhelm M (1999) Gamma/delta T-cell stimulation by pamidronate. N Engl J Med 340:737–738

Li H, Lebedeva MI, Llera AS, Fields BA, Brenner MB, Mariuzza RA (1998) Structure of the Vdelta domain of a human gammadelta T-cell antigen receptor. Nature 391:502–506

Maeurer MJ, Martin D, Walter W, Liu K, Zitvogel L, Halusczcak K, Rabinowich H, Duquesnoy R, Storkus W, Lotze MT (1996) Human intestinal Vdelta1+ lymphocytes recognize tumor cells of epithelial origin. J Exp Med 183:1681–1696

McVay LD, Carding SR (1999) Generation of human gammadelta T-cell repertoires. Crit Rev Immunol 19:431–460

Mitchell SC, Zhang AQ, Smith RL (2000) Ethylamine in human urine. Clin Chim Acta 302:69–78

Mookerjee-Basu J, Vantourout P, Martinez LO, Perret B, Collet X, Perigaud C, Peyrottes S, Champagne E (2010) F1-adenosine triphosphatase displays properties characteristic of an antigen presentation molecule for Vgamma9Vdelta2 T cells. J Immunol 184:6920–6928

Morita CT, Jin CG, Sarikonda G, Wang H (2007) Nonpeptide antigens, presentation mechanisms, and immunological memory of human V gamma 2 V delta 2 T cells: discriminating friend from foe through the recognition of prenyl pyrophosphate antigens. Immunol Rev 215:59–76

Narazaki H, Watari E, Shimizu M, Owaki A, Das H, Fukunaga Y, Takahashi H, Sugita M (2003) Perforin-dependent killing of tumor cells by Vgamma1Vdelta1-bearing T-cells. Immunol Lett 86:113–119

Nausch N, Cerwenka A (2008) NKG2D ligands in tumor immunity. Oncogene 27:5944–5958

Nishimura H, Yajima T, Kagimoto Y, Ohata M, Watase T, Kishihara K, Goshima F, Nishiyama Y, Yoshikai Y (2004) Intraepithelial gamma delta T cells may bridge a gap between innate immunity and acquired immunity to herpes simplex virus type. J Virol 78:4927–4930

Odegaard AO, Pereira MA, Koh WP, Arakawa K, Lee HP, Yu MC (2008) Coffee, tea, and incident type 2 diabetes: the Singapore Chinese Health Study. Am J Clin Nutr 88:979–985

Ogawa T, Tsuji-Kawahara S, Yuasa T, Kinoshita S, Chikaishi T, Takamura S, Matsumura H, Seya T, Saga T, Miyazawa M (2011) Natural killer cells recognize friend retrovirus-infected erythroid progenitor cells through NKG2D-RAE-1 interactions in vivo. J Virol 85:5423–5435

Pende D, Rivera P, Marcenaro S, Chang CC, Biassoni R, Conte R, Kubin M, Cosman D, Ferrone S, Moretta L et al (2002) Major histocompatibility complex class I-related chain A and UL16-binding protein expression on tumor cell lines of different histotypes: analysis of tumor susceptibility to NKG2D-dependent natural killer cell cytotoxicity. Cancer Res 62:6178–6186

Percival SS, Bukowski JF, Milner J (2008) Bioactive food components that enhance gammadelta T cell function may play a role in cancer prevention. J Nutr 138:1–4

Pereira P, Boucontet L (2004) Rates of recombination and chain pair biases greatly influence the primary gammadelta TCR repertoire in the thymus of adult mice. J Immunol 173:3261–3270

Perry CM, Figgitt DP (2004) Zoledronic acid – A review of its use in patients with advanced cancer. Drugs 64:1197–1211

Poggi A, Venturino C, Catellani S, Clavio M, Miglino M, Gobbi M, Steinle A, Ghia P, Stella S, Caligaris-Cappio F et al (2004) Vdelta1 T lymphocytes from B-CLL patients recognize ULBP3 expressed on leukemic B cells and up-regulated by trans-retinoic acid. Cancer Res 64:9172–9179

Raspollini MR, Castiglione F, Rossi Degl'innocenti D, Amunni G, Villanucci A, Garbini F, Baroni G, Taddei GL (2005) Tumour-infiltrating gamma/delta T-lymphocytes are correlated with a brief disease-free interval in advanced ovarian serous carcinoma. Ann Oncol 16:590–596

Raulet DH (2003) Roles of the NKG2D immunoreceptor and its ligands. Nat Rev Immunol 3:781–790

Rincon-Orozco B, Kunzmann V, Wrobel P, Kabelitz D, Steinle A, Herrmann T (2005) Activation of V gamma 9V delta 2T cells by NKG2D. J Immunol 175:2144–2151

Rock EP, Sibbald PR, Davis MM, Chien YH (1994) CDR3 length in antigen-specific immune receptors. J Exp Med 179:323–328

Rowe CA, Nantz MP, Bukowski JF, Percival SS (2007) Specific formulation of Camellia sinensis prevents cold and flu symptoms and enhances gamma, delta T cell function: a randomized, double-blind, placebo-controlled study. J Am Coll Nutr 26:445–452

Salih HR, Antropius H, Gieseke F, Lutz SZ, Kanz L, Rammensee HG, Steinle A (2003) Functional expression and release of ligands for the activating immunoreceptor NKG2D in leukemia. Blood 102:1389–1396

Sanders JM, Ghosh S, Chan JM, Meints G, Wang H, Raker AM, Song Y, Colantino A, Burzynska A, Kafarski P et al (2004) Quantitative structure-activity relationships for gammadelta T cell activation by bisphosphonates. J Med Chem 47:375–384

Scotet E, Martinez LO, Grant E, Barbaras R, Jeno P, Guiraud M, Monsarrat B, Saulquin X, Maillet S, Esteve JP et al (2005) Tumor recognition following Vgamma9Vdelta2 T cell receptor interactions with a surface F1-ATPase-related structure and apolipoprotein A-I. Immunity 22:71–80

Shin S, El-Diwany R, Schaffert S, Adams EJ, Garcia KC, Pereira P, Chien YH (2005) Antigen recognition determinants of gamma delta T cell receptors. Science 308:252–255

Stearns ME, Amatangelo MD, Varma D, Sell C, Goodyear SM (2010) Combination therapy with epigallocatechin-3-gallate and doxorubicin in human prostate tumor modeling studies: inhibition of metastatic tumor growth in severe combined immunodeficiency mice. Am J Pathol 177:3169–3179

Strong RK (2002) Asymmetric ligand recognition by the activating natural killer cell receptor NKG2D, a symmetric homodimer. Mol Immunol 38:1029–1037

Thedrez A, Sabourin C, Gertner J, Devilder MC, Allain-Maillet S, Fournie JJ, Scotet E, Bonneville M (2007) Self/non-self discrimination by human gammadelta T cells: simple solutions for a complex issue? Immunol Rev 215:123–135

Thompson K, Rojas-Navea J, Rogers MJ (2006) Alkylamines cause Vgamma9Vdelta2 T-cell activation and proliferation by inhibiting the mevalonate pathway. Blood 107:651–654

Tsao AS, Liu D, Martin J, Tang XM, Lee JJ, El-Naggar AK, Wistuba I, Culotta KS, Mao L, Gillenwater A et al (2009) Phase II randomized, placebo-controlled trial of green tea extract in patients with high-risk oral premalignant lesions. Cancer Prev Res (Phila) 2:931–941

Tsuge H, Sano S, Hayakawa T, Kakuda T, Unno T (2003) Theanine, gamma-glutamylethylamide, is metabolized by renal phosphate-independent glutaminase. Bba-Gen Subj 1620:47–53

Vetter CS, Groh V, thor Straten P, Spies T, Brocker EB, Becker JC (2002) Expression of stress-induced MHC class I related chain molecules on human melanoma. J Invest Dermatol 118: 600–605

Viey E, Fromont G, Escudier B, Morel Y, Da Rocha S, Chouaib S, Caignard A (2005) Phosphostim-activated gamma delta T cells kill autologous metastatic renal cell carcinoma. J Immunol 174:1338–1347

Wang L, Das H, Kamath A, Bukowski JF (2001) Human V gamma 2V delta 2T cells produce IFN-gamma and TNF-alpha with an on/off/on cycling pattern in response to live bacterial products. J Immunol 167:6195–6201

Watson NFS, Spendlovel I, Madjd Z, McGilvray R, Green AR, Ellis IO, Scholefield JH, Durrant LG (2006) Expression of the stress-related MHC class I chain-related protein MICA is an indicator of good prognosis in colorectal cancer patients. Int J Cancer 118:1445–1452

Wu J, Groh V, Spies T (2002) T cell antigen receptor engagement and specificity in the recognition of stress-inducible MHC class I-related chains by human epithelial gamma delta T cells. J Immunol 169:1236–1240

Xu JL, Davis MM (2000) Diversity in the CDR3 region of V(H) is sufficient for most antibody specificities. Immunity 13:37–45

Zhang L, Conejo-Garcia JR, Katsaros D, Gimotty PA, Massobrio M, Regnani G, Makrigiannakis A, Gray H, Schlienger K, Liebman MN et al (2003) Intratumoral T cells, recurrence, and survival in epithelial ovarian cancer. N Engl J Med 348:203–213

Zhao J, Huang J, Chen H, Cui L, He W (2006) Vdelta1 T cell receptor binds specifically to MHC I chain related A: molecular and biochemical evidences. Biochem Biophys Res Commun 339:232–240

Zhou JR, Yu L, Zhong Y, Blackburn GL (2003) Soy phytochemicals and tea bioactive components synergistically inhibit androgen-sensitive human prostate tumors in mice. J Nutr 133:516–521

Chapter 9
Phytochemical Intakes with a Mediterranean Diet: Levels Achievable with an Exchange List Diet and Potential Biomarkers in Blood

Zora Djuric Ph.D.

Contents

Abstract There is substantial epidemiological evidence that a Mediterranean dietary pattern can reduce risks of cardiovascular disease, cancer, diabetes and even aging-associated cognitive decline. A prominent feature of the traditional Greek diet was a high monounsaturated fatty acid (MUFA) intake, stemming largely from the use of olive oil. In addition, there was a high consumption of fruits and vegetables. All of these foods are rich in phytochemicals, and it is the combination of these dietary phytochemicals that might provide the best protection against the major chronic diseases that humans face. With a Mediterranean diet that is achieved using an exchange list approach, total intakes of flavonoids can be increased to about 200 mg/d using foods readily available in the United States. This is much higher

Z. Djuric Ph.D. (✉)
Departments of Family Medicine and Environmental Health Sciences (Nutrition Program), University of Michigan, 1500 E. Hospital Drive, Room 2150 Cancer Center, Ann Arbor, MI 48109-5930, USA
e-mail: zoralong@umich.edu

S. Shankar and R.K. Srivastava (eds.), *Nutrition, Diet and Cancer*, DOI 10.1007/978-94-007-2923-0_9,

than intakes of carotenoids at about 28 mg/day with a Mediterranean exchange list diet. To best capture intakes of the major flavonoid classes, it is proposed that a biomarker panel could comprehensively capture diversity in Mediterranean intakes. Development of such biomarker panels will be critical for evaluating the biological effects phytochemicals when consumed in concert as part of a preventive eating pattern.

Abbreviations

ESI	electrospray ionization
ECD	electrochemical detection
GC	gas chromatography
HPLC	high pressure liquid chromatography
LOD	limit of detection
LC	liquid chromatography
MS	mass spectral

Introduction

Mediterranean eating patterns have been associated with increased longevity and decreased all-cause mortality (de Lorgeril et al. 1999; Knoops et al. 2004; Sofi et al. 2010, 2008; Trichopoulou et al. 2005). This likely stems from the beneficial effects of a Mediterranean diet on multiple health domains. A landmark study done in Europe, the Seven Countries Study, initially described the lower risk of coronary heart disease in Crete, despite a high fat intake (Keys 1980). Many observational studies have been done since then pointing to the beneficial effects of a Greek-Mediterranean diet. As Western populations have drifted away from traditional eating patterns, and disease risks have increased, an interest in developing Mediterranean interventions has grown. These interventions have been instituted to target several chronic disease groups (Lairon 2007). The interventions developed range from using a single component of the Mediterranean diet to multi-faceted interventions involving dietary counseling over many years of time.

A large, randomized intervention trial of a Mediterranean diet in patients with a prior myocardial infarct was the Lyon Heart Study which used dietitian-led counseling and a spread high in mono-unsaturated fats. There was a 50–70% reduction in the risk of further coronary events during 4 years of follow-up in persons randomized to the Mediterranean intervention (de Lorgeril et al. 1999). In a more recent randomized trial of persons at increased cardiovascular risks, incidence of diabetes was reduced by 51–52% over 4 years of follow-up using counseling for a Mediterranean diet supplemented with either olive oil or nuts (Salas-Salvado et al. 2010). Epidemiological evidence also points to the substantial protective effects of a Greek-Mediterranean diet on risks of several cancers (La Vecchia 2009; Simopoulos

2004; Verberne et al. 2010). In other studies, protective effects of a Mediterranean diet on Alzheimer's disease and cognitive decline with aging have been established (Feart et al. 2009; Scarmeas et al. 2009; Sofi et al. 2008).

A prominent feature of the traditional Greek diet was a high monounsaturated fatty acid (MUFA) intake, stemming largely from the use of olive oil (Kafatos et al. 1993; Trichopoulou et al. 1993). Relative to the American diet, a Greek-Mediterranean diet has lower n-6/n-3 fatty acid ratios, lower polyunsaturated fatty acid (PUFA) intake, lower red meat intake, much higher intakes of monounsaturated fatty acids (MUFA) and increased amount and variety of plant-based foods. The traditional Greek diet had a high consumption of fruit and vegetables in a wide variety (Renaud et al. 1995; Trichopoulou 1989, 1993). In addition, legumes, as well as whole grains, are thought to be important contributors to the health effects of Mediterranean eating patterns (Aranceta 2001; Bosetti et al. 2009; Gallus et al. 2004; La Vecchia 2004; Perez Rodrigo and Ruiz Vadillo 2004).

All of these plant-based foods in a Mediterranean diet contain many phytochemicals with antioxidant and anticancer properties (Khan et al. 2008; Sotiroudis and Kyrtopoulos 2008). As summarized by DeLorgeril and Salen, "many micro- and macronutrients characteristic of the Mediterranean diet interact in a synergistic way to induce states of resistance to chronic diseases" (de Lorgeril and Salen 2008). The goal of this chapter is to identify the phytochemical intakes that could be increased by a Mediterranean diet. Many of these appear to be consumed in sufficient quantity to be potentially useful as biomarkers of a Mediterranean eating pattern.

Mediterranean Eating Patterns and Dietary Interventions

In epidemiological studies several scores have been developed to facilitate research on the health effects of Mediterranean dietary patterns as whole. The most widely used is that of Trichopoulou et al. (2003). This score has a range of 0–9 points for dietary intakes that are either below of above the median for a population. One point is added for each of six dietary intakes that are above the median, namely olive oil, fruits and nuts, fish and seafood, vegetables, the monounsaturated to saturated fat ratio and cereals, and one point is added for each two intakes that are below the median, namely meat and meat products, milk and dairy products (Trichopoulou et al. 2003). In addition, a point is scored for a moderate intake of alcohol. Since typical energy intakes are higher in men, the score is calculated using a different energy adjustment for men and women. With use of a median value for food intakes as a cut-point for assigning a score, the actual value of the score will be different in different populations. Variations of this score have been used by other groups. An alternate Mediterranean score was also developed by Fung et al., and this excluded potatoes from vegetable intakes, eliminated the diary group, included only processed meats in the meat group and included whole grains only instead of all cereals (Fung et al. 2005; Panagiotakos et al. 2009a; Rumawas et al. 2009). Several other groups used similar scores, but in each case there are no subcategories for fruit nor for vegetables (Benitez-Arciniega et al. 2011; Panagiotakos et al. 2009b).

Since all fruits and vegetables are lumped into one or two categories, these Mediterranean scores then do not reflect diversity of fruit and vegetable intakes. In dietary interventions that have targeted a Mediterranean pattern, often the specifics of the counseling approach have not been provided, making it difficult to evaluate how increases in fruits and vegetables were achieved. In general, intake of olive oil is encouraged, or a high monounsaturated fat spread is provided by the study in addition to counseling to encourage use of legumes, fruit, and vegetables, and discourage use of other fats and red meat. In one study, a Mediterranean exchange list diet was developed (Djuric et al. 2009, 2008. With the exchange list, foods are listed in defined categories and each individual has a goal to consume a certain number of servings (i.e. exchanges) from each category. There are eight categories of fruits and vegetables in the Mediterranean exchange list to ensure variety of intakes. A caveat of this approach, however, is that it is not all that well known which fruits and vegetables could be classified as "Mediterranean". In addition, the foods consumed in one geographic area would likely be different than in other areas were availability of fruits and vegetables differs.

The 1960s diet of Crete included more than 700 g/day of fruits and vegetables, which would roughly translate to about 8–9 servings/day of fruits and vegetables (Renaud et al. 1995; Trichopoulou 1989). Importantly, the Greek diet included a wide assortment of fruits and vegetables, including dark green vegetables and herbs that are low in most American diets (Djuric et al. 2002; Fortes et al. 1995; Hakim 1998). Intake of wild greens in Greece was estimated to be 20 g/day (Trichopoulou et al. 2001), and wild greens are not commonly consumed in industrialized countries. It is therefore difficult to replicate this diet. Increased intake of other lutein-rich, dark-green vegetables is, however, possible. Dark green vegetables are rich in lutein and other nutrients such as folate (Ribaya-Mercado and Blumberg 2004). Chlorophyll, which is often over-looked, also has been shown to inhibit formation toxic heme products that may increase colorectal cancer risk (de Vogel et al. 2005).

To target both increased amount and variety of fruit and vegetable intakes, two different fruit and vegetable exchange lists have been developed. The University of Minnesota developed a botanical classification scheme for fruits and vegetables, which was successful for increasing carotenoid intakes (Martini et al. 1995; Smith et al. 1995). Another exchange list approach targeted 9-a-day intake of fruits and vegetables using carotenoid content to guide the classification of foods (Le Marchand et al. 1994).This latter method formed the basis of the Mediterranean exchange list, but it was modified to include categories for green culinary herbs and allium vegetables. The food lists also were modified to include fruits and vegetables that can be obtained in the Midwestern United States. To complete the Mediterranean profile, exchanges in other food groups to target fat and whole grain intakes were added (Djuric et al. 2009). Compliance to this intervention was quite good, and the intervention resulted in decreased intakes of polyunsaturated fats and carbohydrates from grains and sugars, while intakes of monounsaturated fats and carbohydrates from fruits and vegetables increased (Djuric et al. 2008). In that study, blood carotenoid levels increased, but flavonoids were not measured (Djuric et al. 2009).

Dietary Intakes of Phytochemicals with a Mediterranean Exchange List Diet

The Mediterranean exchange list utilized by Djuric et al. has eight categories of fruits and vegetables (Djuric et al. 2008). These are: (1) Dark green vegetables, (2) Red vegetables and fruits, (3) Orange and yellow vegetables, (4) Allium vegetables, (5) Other vegetables (the listed first four vegetable categories can be used to substitute for the "other" vegetable category but not vice-versa), (6) Green culinary herbs, (7) Vitamin C fruits, and (8) Other fruit. In addition, there are lists for whole grains (three or more whole grains are required each day), high omega three foods (twice a week) and individualized daily fat, protein and milk exchange goals that depend on usual energy intakes (selected from lists that guide low-fat choices).

Dietary intakes of flavonoids that could be expected with the Mediterranean diet were calculated using example menus created for study participants. Seven days of menus at the 2000 kcal/day level are shown in Table 9.1. For the calculation of flavonoid intakes, we used the USDA flavonoids database (release 2.1 containing about 230 foods) and supplemented that with other published data (Arabbi et al. 2004; D'Archivio et al. 2007; Erlund 2004; Franke et al. 2004; Gattuso et al. 2007; Kodera et al. 2002; Koponen et al. 2007; Kuhnle et al. 2008; Kulawinek et al. 2008; Landberg et al. 2006; Lawson and Gardner 2005; Nutrient Data Laboratory and Food Composition Laboratory 2007; Ovaskainen et al. 2008; Peterson et al. 2006; Ross et al. 2003; Song et al. 2005; Steinbrecher and Linseisen 2009; Thompson et al. 2006; Vanamala et al. 2005; Wu et al. 2006). The averaged phytochemical content of the diet over for a 7-day menu at the 2,000 kcal/day level, excluding tea, is shown in Table 9.2. These example menus might under-estimate flavonoid intakes since they did not have many foods high in malvidin such as red grapes, black beans and blueberries. Despite this, the flavonoids combined came to a total daily intake of 198 mg/day for the example menus in Table 9.1. By comparison, intakes of total carotenoids averaged 28 mg/day with the Mediterranean diet (Djuric et al. 2009). The distribution of flavonoids was flavanones 36%, flavonols 26%, anthocyanidins 23%, flavones 9% and flavan-3-ols 5%. Additional photochemical intakes were calculated to be 9 mg/day of indoles, 16 mg/day of glucosinolates and 8 mg/day of alkyl resorcinol 19:0.

These non-tea intakes of flavonoids with the Mediterranean exchange list diet of about 200 mg/day are about 6-fold higher than flavonoid intakes for the typical diet in the United States. For non-consumers of tea in the National Health and Nutrition Evaluation Survey 1999–2002, flavonoid intake was estimated to be 32 mg/day distributed in four main classes (excluding tea intake): flavanones 45%, flavonols 22%, anthocyanidins 10%, flavones 5% and flavanols 16% (Chun et al. 2007). It is important to note, however, that estimates of flavonoids intakes in various studies have varied widely (Chun et al. 2007). In a modern-day Greek population recruited to the European Prospective Investigation into Cancer and Nutrition in the late 1990s, total median flavonoid intake was about 92 mg/day, with an additional 75 mg from proanthocyanidins from fruits and wine (Dilis and

Table 9.1 One week of example menus for a 2,000 kcal/day Mediterranean diet at 30% of energy from fat

Meal	Monday	Tuesday	Wednesday	Thursday	Friday	Saturday	Sunday
Breakfast	1 c bran flakes, 2 T dried apricot, ½ c skim milk, 1 med. orange, 2 sl. whole wheat toast, 2 T jam, Coffee	1 lg multi-grain bagel, 6 oz. nonfat yogurt, 1 T hazelnuts, ½ pink grapefruit	1 c oatmeal cooked in 1 c skim milk, 1T almonds, 1 c strawberries	2 eggs, 1 t olive oil, 1 oz Canadian bacon, 2 sl. whole wheat English muffins, 1 orange, coffee	1 c bran flakes, ½ c skim milk, 1 med. banana, 1 T hazelnuts, Coffee	1½ c Special K cereal, 2 T dry cherries, 1 c low-fat milk, 1 med banana, 1 T hazelnuts, 1 sl whole wheat bread, 1 T jam	1 multi-grain bagel, 1 T jam, 1 T light cream cheese, ½ pink grapefruit, ½ c skim milk, with coffee
Snack	1 small banana	1 c green grapes	1 small apple	8 oz. nonfat yogurt, 3 T hazelnuts, 1 med banana	8 oz. nonfat yogurt, 3 T hazelnuts, 2 T raisins	1 med pear	½ mango
Lunch	2 sl. whole wheat bread, 3 oz ham, ½ oz cheese, 1 tsp. mustard, 1 c watermelon, 2 c salad, 1 t olive oil, 1 t vinegar	2 sl Rye bread, 4 oz. roast beef, ¾ c coleslaw with olive oil vinaigrette and 1 t dried herbs, 10 baby carrots, 1 med apple	1 c beans with, 2 t olive oil, 1 t chopped onion, 3 c tossed greens, 1 T herbs, ½ can water-pack tuna with, 2 t olive oil, 1 t vinegar	1 chicken breast, 1 t olive oil, Whole wheat bun, 1 T barbecue sauce, 1 c broccoli, 10 baby carrots, 3 T fat free ranch with ½ t dill, ½ t garlic powder, 1 nectarine	½ can tuna in water with ½ c tomato and 1 c yellow peppers, ½ c shredded lettuce, ½ c beans, 1 t olive oil, 1 t herbs, 1 c apple juice	1 whole wheat flour tortilla, ½ c low-fat refried beans, 1 med tomato, 1 c broccoli, 10 black olives, 10 baby carrots, 1 Cappuccino with 4 oz. skim milk	1 large pita, 2 oz. deli turkey, 1 T pesto, 2 leaf lettuce, 2 sl tomato, 1 c spinach sauteed with 2 T onion and 1 t olive oil, ½ c orange juice

Dinner	1 c acorn squash with 1T olive oil for sautéing, 5 oz. chicken breast with 1 tsp olive oil, 1T parsley and oregano, ½ c peas, ½ c zucchini with 1 t olive oil, 1T hazelnuts	Oven fries from 2 potatoes with paprika and 1 T olive oil, 1 c broccoli, 5 oz. baked catfish, 8 oz. skim milk	1 c brown rice pilaf with 1 t olive oil, ½ cup carrots, ½ c green beans roasted in 1 t olive oil, 4 oz. pork loin, 3T cranberry sauce, iced tea	2 corn tortillas, 2 t olive oil, 1 oz. avocado, 10 black olives, ½ c fat free refried beans, ½ t garlic powder, ¼ c tomato, ½ c lettuce, 1 ½ oz. cheese, ¼ c salsa	1 c spaghetti, ½ c tomato sauce, 1 t chopped onion, 2 oz. lean meat, 2 c green salad, ½ c cucumber, 2 t olive oil, 1 t vinegar, 1 t herbs, 2 sl French bread, 1 t olive oil, 3 T parmesan	1 c brown rice pilaf with 1 t olive oil, 6 oz. salmon with 1 t olive oil, 1 c roasted mixed vegetables with 1 t olive oil, 1 t dried herbs, 1 clove garlic, 1 c cantaloupe	Grilled chicken Caesar salad: 3 oz. chicken, 1 t olive oil, 2 T fat free dressing, 2 t olive oil, 4 T Parmesan, 4 c Romaine, 9 cherry tomato, 1 whole grain roll, 2 T tapenade, 1 Cappuccino
Snack	6 oz. low-fat vanilla pudding, 2 T raisins, 2 T hazelnuts	¼ c trail mix made with Macadamia nuts	¼ c trail mix, ¼ c dried cherries	1 pear, 1 c mint tea	4 c low-fat popcorn, 1T Parmesan cheese, 1 c orange juice	¼ c trail mix, 8 oz. nonfat yogurt	1 c Brown rice pudding made with non-fat milk and honey, 2 T hazelnuts, 4 dried apricots

c cup, *lg* large, *med* medium, *sl* slice, *T* tablespoon, *t* teaspoon

Table 9.2 The calculated average daily phytochemical content of a 2,000 kcal/day Mediterranean menu using an exchange list diet

Compound	Estimated daily intake (mg)
Quercetin	8.5
Naringenin	46.4
Hesperitin	25.7
Cyanidin	39.5
Malvidin	0.02
Delphinidin	6.6
Luteolin	12.2
Apigenin	4.9
Epicatechin	10.3
Glucobrassicin	9.32
Total glucosinolates	15.8
Alkylresorcinol (19:0)	8.5
Hydroxytyrosol	2
S-allyl cysteine	1.3

Trichopoulou 2010). The distribution of flavonoids in that Greek population was flavanones 29%, flavonols 30%, anthocyanidins 11%, flavones 8% and flavan-3-ols 15% (Dilis and Trichopoulou 2010).

Detection of Mediterranean Phytochemical Biomarkers in Blood

Blood-based biomarkers of diet might have an advantage for capturing dietary intakes versus self-report of diet. For example, fruit and vegetable intakes have had inconsistent relationships to breast cancer risk, but in three large prospective studies blood levels of carotenoids, the relative risk of breast cancer was 57–24% lower in women who had relatively higher levels of blood carotenoids (Sato et al. 2002; Tamimi et al. 2005; Toniolo et al. 2001). A profile of phytochemical levels in blood should capture the complexity of the Mediterranean eating pattern better than carotenoid analyses alone. An example selection of phytochemicals is shown in Table 9.3: hydroxytyrosol, quercetin, anthocyanidins, hesperitin, naringenin, 3,3′-diindolylmethane, luteolin, 19:0 alkylresorcinol, S-allycysteine, and carotenoids. These phytochemicals could serve as markers of olives, olive oil, a wide variety of fruits and vegetables (including allium vegetables and green herbs) and whole grains. Since many of these compounds occur in the diet as glycosides, and most are metabolized to glucuronides and sulfates, samples must be hydrolyzed before quantifying levels of each phytochemical.

It is recognized that no biomarker will be a perfect indicator of dietary intakes due to the complexities of absorption, metabolism and analysis (Jenab et al. 2009), but these phytochemicals should be increased in blood when consuming a complex Mediterranean type of diet. Indeed, many flavonoids can be combined in one

Table 9.3 Summary of phytochemicals that could serve as biomarkers of a Mediterranean eating pattern

Food group	Biomarkers	Increases that have been observed with diet in the literature
High MUFA fats	Fatty acids, MUFA to PUFA and MUFA to SFA ratios	13% increase in MUFA and 62% increase in MUFA:SFA ratio with a Mediterranean exchange list diet (Djuric et al. 2009)
Olives and olive oil	Hydroxytyrosol	1.8 (SD 0.6) increases to 3.15 (SD 0.34) μg/ml after 20 olives, n = 8 (Kountouri et al. 2007)
Fish and flax	n3:n6 fatty acid ratios, long-chain n3 fatty acids	33% increase in n3/n6 ratio, 20% increase in fish oil n3 fatty acids with a Mediterranean exchange list diet (Djuric, the Healthy Eating Study for Colon Cancer Prevention, unpublished data)
Dark green vegetables	Lutein	Lutein increases 41% with a Mediterranean diet (Djuric et al. 2009)
	5-methyl Tetrahydrofolate	5methyl-tetrahydrofolate increased 112% after high fruit-vegetable diet (Kawashima et al. 2007)
Red Vegetables	Lycopene	Increases 24% with a Mediterranean diet (Djuric et al. 2009)
Orange-yellow vegetables	α-Carotene	Increases 248% with a Mediterranean diet (Djuric et al. 2009)
Allium vegetables	Quercetin	Quercetin increased from 28 (SD 1.9) to 248 ng/ml after 225 g fried onions, n = 5 (McAnlis et al. 1999)
	S-allyl cysteine	18 ng/ml (SD 6, n = 3) after consuming ~0.7 mg (Kodera et al. 2002)
Green Herbs	Lutein	Lutein see above
	Luteolin	Luteolin – detected in humans but level not reported (Shimoi et al. 1998)
Other vegetables	Quercetin	Quercetin see above
	β-Carotene	Increases 175% with a Mediterranean diet (Djuric et al. 2009)
Cruciferous	3.3′-diindolylmethane (DIM)	DIM increases from 0 to 18 ng/ml after a 50 mg dose and to 32 ng/ml (SD 4, n = 3) after a 100 mg dose, with cruciferous-free diet at baseline (Reed et al. 2008)
	Total isothiocyanates (ITC)	ITC went from 0.20 to 0.39 μM after 10 days of 200 g/day broccoli (Riso et al. 2009)

(continued)

Table 9.3 (continued)

Food group	Biomarkers	Increases that have been observed with diet in the literature
Fruit	β-Cryptoxanthin, Zeaxanthin	β-cryptoxanthin increases 92% and zeaxanthin increases 31% with a Mediterranean diet (Djuric et al. 2009)
Grapes, berries, apple	Epicatechin	6–10-fold increases with consumption of 40–200 mg amounts (Loke et al. 2009; Rein et al. 2000)
Pear, apricot		
Berries	Cyanidin, Delphinidin, Malvidin	Dietary intakes increase from 3–12 mg/day to 46 mg/day with a Mediterranean diet (Djuric, the Healthy Eating Study for Colon Cancer Prevention, unpublished data)
Vitamin C fruit	Hesperitin, Naringenin	Hesperitin (baseline 3.2 nmol/l, SE 2.6, n = 13) increases 1016% and naringenin (baseline 7.3, SE 2.5 nmol/l, n = 13) increases 612% in fasting plasma 1 week after 24 oz/day orange juice (Franke et al. 2005)
Legumes	Cyanidin, Delphinidin, Folate	See above
Whole grain wheat and rye	1,3-Dihydroxy-5-nonadecylbenzene alkylresorcinol (19:0)	Increases 26% in fasting blood after "low dose" rye bran flakes for 1 week, from 44 ng/m to 56 ng/ml (Landberg et al. 2009b)

chromatographic analysis, making profiling of flavonoids possible (Mennen et al. 2008; Neilson et al. 2007; Urpi-Sarda et al. 2009). In one intervention study, urinary total flavonoids (as a sum of six species) were significantly correlated with fruit and vegetables intakes, and change in flavonoid excretion was also correlated with increases in fruit and vegetable consumption (Johannot and Somerset 2006; Nielsen et al. 2002). Urine has been shown to be useful for measuring flavonoid profiles in other studies as well (Baranowska and Magiera 2011; Johannot and Somerset 2006; Krogholm et al. 2004; Loke et al. 2009; Magiera et al. 2011; Mennen et al. 2006; Mikkelsen et al. 2007; Nielsen et al. 2002). In many studies, however, urine is not available. The data on potential blood-based biomarkers of Mediterranean foods is reviewed here.

Biomarkers of Olives and Olive Oil

Hydroxytyrosol is the main phenolic found in most varieties of olives (Rodriguez et al. 2009). There is good evidence that hydroxytyrosol would be a good biomarker of olive or olive oil intakes. The levels of hydroxytyrosol in human plasma were about a 20-fold higher than tyrosol after consuming olives (Kountouri et al. 2007). Another study found 2-fold higher levels of hydroxytyrosol than tyrosol in LDL, and sulfate conjugates predominated, making it important to hydrolyze the samples before analysis (de la Torre-Carbot et al. 2007). Phenolics in olive oil do vary in different types of olive oil, but hydroxytyrosol levels in urine were increased after consuming only 25 ml (five teaspoons) olive oil that was very low in total phenolics (Weinbrenner et al. 2004).

Levels of hydroxytyrosol in plasma of Greek subjects before and after consuming 20 olives were 1.8 and 3.15 μg/ml, respectively, which should be easily detectable (Kountouri et al. 2007). The measures were performed after hydrolysis of plasma with 100 units β-glucuronidase for 2 h, sep-pak purification by applying acidified plasma to a reverse phase sep-pak and eluting phenolics with methanol. The dried phenols were converted to trimethyl silyl derivatives and analyzed by gas chromatography with mass spectral detection (GC-MS) (Kountouri et al. 2007). Using HPLC-MS-MS and detection of negative ions, one study achieved a limit of detection (LOD) of 0.32 ng/ml for hydroxytyrosol (de la Torre-Carbot et al. 2007). Since levels of this compound can be expected to be in the low μg/ml range with a Mediterranean diet, HPLC with UV detection may be adequate. Another study was able to achieve a LOD of 37 ng/ml in plasma with HPLC detection performed by UV at 280 nm (Ruiz-Gutierrez et al. 2000).

Biomarkers of a Wide Variety of Fruits and Vegetables

Many fruits and vegetables are not high in carotenoids such as onion, beans, apple, berries and citrus fruits (Holden et al. 1999). That is why carotenoids intakes are not sufficient to capture variety of fruit and vegetable intakes. Interestingly many of the flavonoids might not only be biomarkers of intakes but can also work to decrease pro-inflammatory states via a variety of mechanisms. For example, flavones can occupy the active site of COX1 and COX2 to decrease activity thereby resulting in an anti-inflammatory effect (Cai et al. 2009). It would be ideal to analyze for at least one compound in each of the following classes: anthocyanins (cyanidin, delphinidin, malvidin), flavanones (hesperitin, naringenin), flavonol (quercetin), flavones (luteolin) and flavanols (epicatechin). These have a relatively high abundance in foods, maximizing the likelihood that detectable levels could be achieved with a Mediterranean diet. Levels of quercetin, kaempferol, naringenin, and hesperitin in fasting plasma have been shown to be reasonable biomarkers of recent dietary intakes (Radtke et al. 2002).

Quercetin is widely distributed in many fruits and vegetables and has been reported to account for about 75% of typical U.S. intakes of flavonoids (Sampson et al. 2002). Quercetin, which is in the flavonol chemical class, therefore might be a good biomarker of fruit and vegetable intakes. Main dietary contributors have been identified as tea, onions and apples with skin (Hertog et al. 1993; Sampson et al. 2002). Allium vegetables also are good sources of quercetin (Gorinstein et al. 2008; Miean and Mohamed 2001). Other food sources of quercetin are berries, cucumber, sweet potato, cruciferous vegetables, beans, fruits and even some herbs such as sage, rosemary and oregano (Beecher 2003; Exarchou et al. 2002; Hakkinen et al. 1999; Koli et al. 2010; Miean and Mohamed 2001). Importantly, quercetin levels may capture intakes that are poorly represented by fiber, vitamin C, β-carotene and folate since correlations between dietary intakes of these and quercetin were quite poor with $r = 0.3–0.2$ (Sampson et al. 2002). In plasma of un-supplemented individuals, levels of quercetin have ranged 25–1,500 ng/ml, and this is readily detectable by HPLC (Cao et al. 2010; Paganga and Rice-Evans 1997; Soleas et al. 2001). Quercetin accumulates in the plasma mainly as conjugates, and incubation of plasma with β-glucuronidase and sulfatase is needed, with short incubations of 50 min being sufficient (Moon et al. 2000). Since tea intake is not addressed by the Mediterranean diet, increases in quercetin with a Mediterranean intervention would most likely be due to onions and other vegetables and herbs rather than tea.

Anthocyanins would be excellent candidate biomarkers of fruit and vegetable as well since they are fairly widely distributed, including many kinds of berries, red leaf lettuce, red onion, red beans, kidney beans, black beans, broadbeans, cowpeas, pistachios, apricots, apples, red grapes and hazelnuts (Cooke et al. 2006; Giordano et al. 2007; Kay et al. 2004; Nutrient Data Laboratory and Food Composition Laboratory 2007; Wu et al. 2006). Intake of anthocyanins recently has been estimated to be 12.5 mg/day in the United States, with cyanidin, delphinidin and malvidin contributing 85% of that intake (Wu et al. 2006). Cyanidin is metabolized, but levels of metabolites are much lower than that of the parent compound (Kay et al. 2004). Sensitive methods have been developed for analysis of the glucosides, termed anthocyanins, and their metabolites but analyzing for the anthocyanidin aglycones may offer some advantages (Garcia-Alonso et al. 2009; Kay et al. 2005; Milbury et al. 2010; Thomasset et al. 2009; Zhang et al. 2004). To maximize sensitivity for detecting consumption of foods containing anthocyanins, it may be prudent to hydrolyze blood samples with a mixture of β-glucuronidase, sulfatase, β-glycosidase and β-glucosidase to release anthocyanidins, or acid hydrolysis can be used. In the gut, microbial hydrolysis of glucosides can also occur, making analysis of intact glucosides problematic as a biomarker of intake (Liu et al. 2003).

From the flavonol class of compounds, catechin and epicatechin are generally found together in foods and in most foods epicatechin is more abundant, making it perhaps a better biomarker choice (Nutrient Data Laboratory and Food Composition Laboratory 2007). There is sparse data on levels of catechins in plasma, but in one study, fasting plasma levels of catechin were more than 3-fold higher (about 450 ng/ml versus 150 ng/ml) in persons who consumed fruits and vegetables the day before at their evening meal versus in those who did not (Ruidavets et al. 2000). Epicatechin in plasma increased 10-fold after consuming 137 mg epicatechin in a chocolate preparation and 6-fold (from about 0.5 μM to 3 μM) after consuming 200 mg pure epicatechin (Loke et al. 2009; Rein et al. 2000). Similar to other phytochemicals, epicatechin is metabolically conjugated and should be hydrolyzed before analysis (Richelle et al. 1999; Zimmermann et al. 2009). Alternatively, the major metabolite of epicatechin can be measured. This metabolite increased from 20 to 100 ng/ml in plasma after consumption of 40 mg epicatechin in cocoa for 4 weeks, namely 5-(3′,4′-dihydroxyphenyl)-γ-valerolactone (Urpi-Sarda et al. 2009). A major caveat with epicatechin as a biomarker is that consumption of chocolate and tea can obscure increases with fruits and vegetables.

Biomarkers of Garlic

Although quercetin can be a biomarker of allium vegetable intake, garlic intake may be better assessed though S-allylcysteine levels. S-Allylcysteine is a non-volatile component of garlic that has been detected in blood of persons consuming aged garlic or a garlic supplement (Kodera et al. 2002; Rosen et al. 2000). S-Allycysteine is thought to be formed from ingestion of gamma-glutamyl-S-allyl-l-cysteine, and the N-acetyl derivative of S-allyl cysteine is excreted in urine after consumption of garlic (de Rooij et al. 1996; Verhagen et al. 2001). This particular pathway has been of interest as a biomarker of garlic intake because of the preventive properties of S-allyl cysteine (Verhagen et al. 2001). S-allyl cysteine was detected in plasma after one dose of aged garlic, but quercetin was not (Rosen et al. 2001). In human plasma, levels of 12–25 ng/ml S-ally cysteine can be reached after consuming a 0.67 mg S-ally cysteine supplement and it had a relatively long half-life (8 ng/ml in plasma 24 h after dosing), excellent bioavailability and good stability (Kodera et al. 2002). The compound was also detected in individuals following their own usual diet, but not when avoiding allium-containing foods (Kodera et al. 2002). Consuming 1–2 cloves of garlic per week would result in an average S-allyl cysteine intake of 3 mg/day, using content data of Lawson (Lawson and Gardner 2005).

Biomarkers of Dark Green Vegetables and Beans

As a biomarker of dark green vegetables and legumes, folate may be important. Leafy green vegetables, fruits (including citrus fruits and juices), dried beans and peas are all natural sources of folate (Nutrient Data Laboratory and Food Composition Laboratory 2007). Bean intakes tend to be increased with Mediterranean diets since it is low-fat source of protein, and consumption of low-fat proteins is an important goal of the Mediterranean diet to accommodate an increase in olive oil. Total serum folate increased 174% after a 28-day fruit-vegetable juice intervention (Kawashima et al. 2007). In blood, 5-methyl tetrahydrofolate (mTHF) is the predominant species that can be measured as a result of metabolism of folate by dihydrofolate reductase, and mTHF accounts for more than 86% of the total folate and folate metabolites (Hannisdal et al. 2009). Significant free serum folate is typically only found with supplement use and would thus not be relevant biomarker for assessing dietary change. The levels of mTHF are fairly high in blood (6 μg/ml), and sensitivity should not be an issue for its detection (Hannisdal et al. 2009).

Biomarkers of Cruciferous Vegetables

For cruciferous vegetables, glucosinolates should be considered. Glucosinolates are converted to isothiocyanates and indoles either upon chopping, chewing or cutting, which stimulates the myrosinase present in the plant, or upon hydrolysis by gut microflora. Different kinds of glucosinolates are present in the commonly consumed cruciferous vegetables, and it is important to select a compound that is widely present across these foods. Isothiocyanates that are present in high levels in broccoli were much lower in cabbage and cauliflower (Kushad et al. 1999). Only glucobrassicin, which is hydrolyzed to indole-3-carbinol, was shown to be present in similar levels in cauliflower, broccoli, cabbage, kale and Brussels sprouts (Higdon et al. 2007; Kushad et al. 1999). The glucobrassicin product indole-3-carbinol therefore should represent intakes of cruciferous vegetables more evenly. Indole-3-carbinol also has been suggested to have a role as a chemopreventive agent (Rogan 2006). In the acid environment of the stomach, indole-3-carbinol is converted to 3,3′-diindoylylmethane (DIM), and DIM is the only compound detected after supplementation of humans with indole-3-carbinol (Reed et al. 2006). It also may be useful to consider quantifying total isothiocyanates (ITC) (Liebes et al. 2001). After consuming a broccoli diet for 10 days (200 g/day), total ITC levels increased from 0.20 to 0.39 μM in plasma (Riso et al. 2009).

Biomarkers of Fruit

A variety of compounds could be used as biomarkers of fruit intakes. Vitamin C is an obvious candidate. For the determination of vitamin C, however, serum must be frozen mixed with m-phosphoric acid. In many studies, this is not available. Levels of hesperitin and naringenin, which are flavanones present in citrus fruits, may therefore be a better biomarker for citrus fruits. Among the non-citrus fruits, quercetin is present in many fruits as is β-carotene and β-cryptoxanthin. To better capture intakes of berries and cherries, measuring the three major anthocyanidins could be useful. Epicatechin from the flavanol family could be included, and it is high in grapes, berries, apricots, apples and some kinds of beans. Catechin and epicatechin are generally found together in foods and in most epicatechin is more abundant, making it the better biomarker choice (Nutrient Data Laboratory and Food Composition Laboratory 2007).

After consumption of 1 cup orange juice three times a day, levels of various phytochemicals increased in fasting, hydrolyzed, plasma: lutein by 29–32%, total carotenoids by 20–22%, beta-cryptoxanthin by 56–94%, ascorbic acid by 62–59%, folic acid by 44–46%, hesperitin by 1,016–657% and naringenin by 612–974% after 1 and 3 weeks, respectively (Franke et al. 2005). In that same study, levels of naringenin and hesperitin at baseline were about 1–1.9 ng/ml in plasma, and levels after orange juice intervention were about 1 μg/ml. Levels of these two flavanones also were much higher in fasting plasma of persons following a high versus a low fruit and vegetable diet (50–2,708%) (Erlund et al. 2002). The relatively large changes in the flavanones with the most commonly consumed citrus fruit juice, namely orange juice, make them a desirable marker of citrus intake, and one would expect an increase even with more modest intakes.

Biomarkers of Green Culinary Herbs

Green culinary herbs were included in the Mediterranean exchange list to mimic as much as possible the wild herbs such as pursulane consumed in the Cretan diet. Herbs are known to contain a large variety of phytochemicals, many of which are responsible for the distinctive flavors of herbs. This makes it difficult to select a biomarker that would capture intake of herbs broadly. Green culinary herbs, however, are good sources of lutein, and some are also known to contain luteolin (parsley, rosemary, thyme, oregano, sage, peppermint) (Karakaya and El 1999; Lopez-Lazaro 2009; Miean and Mohamed 2001; Nutrient Data Laboratory and Food Composition Laboratory 2007). Luteolin is present in a larger number of foods than apigenin, making it an attractive biomarker for the flavone class of flavonoids, although apigenin might also be considered since the literature is very sparse on levels of these compounds in humans (Nutrient Data Laboratory and Food Composition Laboratory 2007). Luteolin is the major metabolite of apigenin, and levels of luteolin are quite a bit higher in serum (Cao et al. 2010; Gradolatto et al. 2004). Luteolin, like many other flavonoids, is extensively glucuronidated, and this can occur in the colonocytes immediately after absorption (Shimoi et al. 1998). Interestingly, neutrophils have been indicated to have beta-glucuronidase activity which can liberate free luteolin at the site of inflammation, making conjugates biologically available (Goldstein et al. 1975; Shimoi et al. 1998).

Biomarkers of Whole Grains

Gas chromatographic methods have been developed for analysis of alkylresorcinols in plasma, and alkylresorcinols have been shown to be a dose-dependent marker of whole grain wheat and rye dietary intakes (Landberg et al. 2009a). The gas chromatographic method with mass spectral detection has excellent sensitivity, and fasting blood samples were suggested to be ideal to reflect usual intakes (Landberg et al. 2009b, c). The other alkylresorcinols can also be quantified in the same analysis, but 1,3-dihydroxy-5-nonadecyl-benzene alkylresorcinol 19:0 is generally the most abundant one and is not as sensitive to type of grain ingested as 17:0 and 21:0 are (Landberg et al. 2009a). Levels of alkylresorcinol 19:0 in un-supplemented individuals have been reported to be 12–50 ng/ml (Linko et al. 2002; Soderholm et al. 2009). The maximum concentration was reached 6 h after consumption and there was a very slow turn-over (Landberg et al. 2009b). Both gas chromatography (GC) and high pressure liquid chromatography (HPLC) have been used for detection of alkylresorcinol after hydrolysis of plasma (Koskela et al. 2008; Landberg et al. 2009c; Linko et al. 2002). A limitation is that this marker will not capture intakes of whole grain oats, rice or maize (Ross et al. 2003). The alkylresorcinols should, however, represent the major grain in the U.S. diet from cereals and breads, which is wheat (Bachman et al. 2008; Economic Research Service 2009). In two European studies, plasma alkylresorcinols correlated with self-reported intakes of whole grains well $r = 0.57-0.58$, and dose/response profiles with dietary whole grains were excellent (Landberg et al. 2009a, b).

Conclusions

There is substantial epidemiological evidence that a Mediterranean dietary pattern can reduce risks of cardiovascular disease, cancer, diabetes and even aging-associated cognitive decline (Sofi et al. 2008). To identify a Mediterranean diet pattern, several Mediterranean indices or scores have been developed. These generally use food frequency questionnaires to score consumption of foods, giving negative or no points for typical Western intakes and positive points for increased consumption of Mediterranean foods (Fung et al. 2005; Panagiotakos et al. 2009a; Rumawas et al. 2009; Trichopoulou et al. 2003). These indices are useful and can capture overall eating patterns, but they do not capture diversity in fruit and vegetable intakes. Different fruits and vegetables all contain differing levels of phytochemicals. It is the combination of these dietary phytochemicals that might provide the best protection against the major chronic diseases that humans face. This highlights a need for using biomarkers of a Mediterranean diet since these might have an even stronger association with health outcomes than self-reported total amount of fruit and vegetable intake.

With a Mediterranean diet that is achieved using an exchange list approach, increased variety of fruit and vegetable intakes is targeted with specific goals for sub-categories of fruits and vegetables. With this kind of approach, total intakes of flavonoids can be increased to about 200 mg/day using foods readily available in the United States. This was estimated using menus constructed to meet Mediterranean exchange goals for a 2,000 kcal/day diet. To capture intakes of the major flavonoid classes that are consumed with a Mediterranean diet, it is possible to analyze select biomarkers of each flavonoid class in blood: flavanones, flavonols, anthocyanidins, and flavanols. Analysis of flavonoid biomarkers can help capture intakes of fruits and vegetables which are not particularly high in carotenoids. Other potentially useful biomarkers of a Mediterranean diet are folate, S-allylcysteine, hydroxytyrosol, alkyl resorcinol, indole-3-carbinol, and total isothiocyanates (Table 9.3). Such a biomarker panel could comprehensively capture diversity in Mediterranean intakes and be useful for evaluating the biological effects phytochemicals in concert versus singly.

Acknowledgements This work was supported by NIH grants RO1 CA120381, PO1 CA130810 and Cancer Center Support grant P30 CA046592.

References

Arabbi PR, Genovese MI, Lajolo FM (2004) Flavonoids in vegetable foods commonly consumed in Brazil and estimated ingestion by the Brazilian population. J Agric Food Chem 52:1124–1131

Aranceta J (2001) Spanish food patterns. Public Health Nutr 4:1399–1402

Bachman JL, Reedy J, Subar AF, Krebs-Smith SM (2008) Sources of food group intakes among the US population, 2001–2002. J Am Diet Assoc 108:804–814

Baranowska I, Magiera S (2011) Analysis of isoflavones and flavonoids in human urine by UHPLC. Anal Bioanal Chem 399:3211–3219

Beecher GR (2003) Overview of dietary flavonoids: nomenclature, occurrence and intake. J Nutr 133:3248S–3254S

Benitez-Arciniega AA, Mendez MA, Baena-Diez JM, Rovira Martori MA, Soler C, Marrugat J, Covas MI, Sanz H, Llopis A, Schroder H (2011) Concurrent and construct validity of Mediterranean diet scores as assessed by an FFQ. Public Health Nutr 14(11):2015–2021

Bosetti C, Pelucchi C, La Vecchia C (2009) Diet and cancer in Mediterranean countries: carbohydrates and fats. Public Health Nutr 12:1595–1600

Cai H, Sale S, Schmid R, Britton RG, Brown K, Steward WP, Gescher AJ (2009) Flavones as colorectal cancer chemopreventive agents–phenol-o-methylation enhances efficacy. Cancer Prev Res (Phila Pa) 2:743–750

Cao J, Zhang Y, Chen W, Zhao X (2010) The relationship between fasting plasma concentrations of selected flavonoids and their ordinary dietary intake. Br J Nutr 103:249–255

Chun OK, Chung SJ, Song WO (2007) Estimated dietary flavonoid intake and major food sources of U.S. adults. J Nutr 137:1244–1252

Cooke DN, Thomasset S, Boocock DJ, Schwarz M, Winterhalter P, Steward WP, Gescher AJ, Marczylo TH (2006) Development of analyses by high-performance liquid chromatography and liquid chromatography/tandem mass spectrometry of bilberry (Vaccinium myrtilus) anthocyanins in human plasma and urine. J Agric Food Chem 54:7009–7013

D'Archivio M, Filesi C, Di Benedetto R, Gargiulo R, Giovannini C, Masella R (2007) Polyphenols, dietary sources and bioavailability. Ann Ist Super Sanita 43:348–361

de la Torre-Carbot K, Chavez-Servin JL, Jauregui O, Castellote AI, Lamuela-Raventos RM, Fito M, Covas MI, Munoz-Aguayo D, Lopez-Sabater MC (2007) Presence of virgin olive oil phenolic metabolites in human low density lipoprotein fraction: determination by high-performance liquid chromatography-electrospray ionization tandem mass spectrometry. Anal Chim Acta 583:402–410

de Lorgeril M, Salen P (2008) The Mediterranean diet: rationale and evidence for its benefit. Curr Atheroscler Rep 10:518–522

de Lorgeril M, Salen P, Martin JL, Monjaud I, Delaye J, Mamelle N (1999) Mediterranean diet, traditional risk factors, and the rate of cardiovascular complications after myocardial infarction: final report of the Lyon Diet Heart Study. Circulation 99:779–785

de Rooij BM, Boogaard PJ, Rijksen DA, Commandeur JN, Vermeulen NP (1996) Urinary excretion of N-acetyl-S-allyl-L-cysteine upon garlic consumption by human volunteers. Arch Toxicol 70:635–639

de Vogel J, Jonker-Termont DS, van Lieshout EM, Katan MB, van der Meer R (2005) Green vegetables, red meat and colon cancer: chlorophyll prevents the cytotoxic and hyperproliferative effects of haem in rat colon. Carcinogenesis 26:387–393

Dilis V, Trichopoulou A (2010) Antioxidant intakes and food sources in Greek adults. J Nutr 140:1274–1279

Djuric Z, Poore KM, Depper JB, Uhley VE, Lababidi S, Covington C, Klurfeld DM, Simon MS, Kucuk O, Heilbrun LK (2002) Methods to increase fruit and vegetable intake with and without a decrease in fat intake: compliance and effects on body weight in the nutrition and breast health study. Nutr Cancer 43:141–151

Djuric Z, VanLoon G, Radakovich K, DiLaura NM, Heilbrun LK, Sen A (2008) Design of a Mediterranean exchange list diet that can be implemented by telephone counseling. J Am Diet Assoc 208:2059–2065

Djuric Z, Ren J, Blythe J, VanLoon G, Sen A (2009) A Mediterranean dietary intervention in healthy American women changes plasma carotenoids and fatty acids in distinct clusters. Nutr Res 29:156–163

Economic Research Service (2009) Loss-adjusted food availability data, vol 2009. USDA, Washington, DC

Erlund I (2004) Review of the flavonoids quercetin, hesperetin, and naringenin. Dietary sources, bioactivities, bioavailability, and epidemiology. Nutr Res 24:851–874

Erlund I, Silaste ML, Alfthan G, Rantala M, Kesaniemi YA, Aro A (2002) Plasma concentrations of the flavonoids hesperetin, naringenin and quercetin in human subjects following their habitual diets, and diets high or low in fruit and vegetables. Eur J Clin Nutr 56:891–898

Exarchou V, Nenadis N, Tsimidou M, Gerothanassis IP, Troganis A, Boskou D (2002) Antioxidant activities and phenolic composition of extracts from Greek oregano, Greek sage, and summer savory. J Agric Food Chem 50:5294–5299

Feart C, Samieri C, Rondeau V, Amieva H, Portet F, Dartigues JF, Scarmeas N, Barberger-Gateau P (2009) Adherence to a Mediterranean diet, cognitive decline, and risk of dementia. JAMA 302:638–648

Fortes C, Forastiere F, Anatra F, Schmid G (1995) Re: Consumption of olive oil and specific food groups in relation to breast cancer risk in Greece. J Natl Cancer Inst 87:1020–1022

Franke AA, Custer LJ, Arakaki C, Murphy SP (2004) Vitamin C and flavonoid levels of fruits and vegetables consumed in Hawaii. J Food Compos Anal 17:1–35

Franke AA, Cooney RV, Henning SM, Custer LJ (2005) Bioavailability and antioxidant effects of orange juice components in humans. J Agric Food Chem 53:5170–5178

Fung TT, McCullough ML, Newby PK, Manson JE, Meigs JB, Rifai N, Willett WC, Hu FB (2005) Diet-quality scores and plasma concentrations of markers of inflammation and endothelial dysfunction. Am J Clin Nutr 82:163–173

Gallus S, Bosetti C, La Vecchia C (2004) Mediterranean diet and cancer risk. Eur J Cancer Prev 13:447–452

Garcia-Alonso M, Minihane AM, Rimbach G, Rivas-Gonzalo JC, de Pascual-Teresa S (2009) Red wine anthocyanins are rapidly absorbed in humans and affect monocyte chemoattractant protein 1 levels and antioxidant capacity of plasma. J Nutr Biochem 20:521–529

Gattuso G, Barreca D, Gargiulli C, Leuzzi U, Caristi C (2007) Flavonoid composition of Citrus juices. Molecules 12:1641–1673

Giordano L, Coletta W, Rapisarda P, Donati MB, Rotilio D (2007) Development and validation of an LC-MS/MS analysis for simultaneous determination of delphinidin-3-glucoside, cyanidin-3-glucoside and cyanidin-3-(6-malonylglucoside) in human plasma and urine after blood orange juice administration. J Sep Sci 30:3127–3136

Goldstein IM, Hoffstein ST, Weissmann G (1975) Mechanisms of lysosomal enzyme release from human polymorphonuclear leukocytes. Effects of phorbol myristate acetate. J Cell Biol 66:647–652

Gorinstein S, Leontowicz H, Leontowicz M, Namiesnik J, Najman K, Drzewiecki J, Cvikrova M, Martincova O, Katrich E, Trakhtenberg S (2008) Comparison of the main bioactive compounds and antioxidant activities in garlic and white and red onions after treatment protocols. J Agric Food Chem 56:4418–4426

Gradolatto A, Canivenc-Lavier MC, Basly JP, Siess MH, Teyssier C (2004) Metabolism of apigenin by rat liver phase I and phase ii enzymes and by isolated perfused rat liver. Drug Metab Dispos 32:58–65

Hakim I (1998) Mediterranean diets and cancer prevention. Arch Intern Med 158:1169–1170

Hakkinen SH, Karenlampi SO, Heinonen IM, Mykkanen HM, Torronen AR (1999) Content of the flavonols quercetin, myricetin, and kaempferol in 25 edible berries. J Agric Food Chem 47:2274–2279

Hannisdal R, Ueland PM, Svardal A (2009) Liquid chromatography-tandem mass spectrometry analysis of folate and folate catabolites in human serum. Clin Chem 55:1147–1154

Hertog MG, Hollman PC, Katan MB, Kromhout D (1993) Intake of potentially anticarcinogenic flavonoids and their determinants in adults in The Netherlands. Nutr Cancer 20:21–29

Higdon JV, Delage B, Williams DE, Dashwood RH (2007) Cruciferous vegetables and human cancer risk: epidemiologic evidence and mechanistic basis. Pharmacol Res 55:224–236

Holden JM, Eldridge AL, Beecher GR, Buzzard IM, Bhagwat SA, Davis CS, Douglass LW, Gebhardt SE, Haytowitz DB, Schakel S (1999) Carotenoid content of U.S. foods: an update of the database. J Food Compos Anal 12:169–196

Jenab M, Slimani N, Bictash M, Ferrari P, Bingham SA (2009) Biomarkers in nutritional epidemiology: applications, needs and new horizons. Hum Genet 125:507–525

Johannot L, Somerset SM (2006) Age-related variations in flavonoid intake and sources in the Australian population. Public Health Nutr 9:1045–1054

Kafatos A, Diacatou A, Labadarios D, Kounali D, Apostolaki J, Vlachonikolis J, Mamalakis G, Megremis S (1993) Nutrition status of the elderly in Anogia, Crete, Greece. J Am Coll Nutr 12:685–692

Karakaya S, El SN (1999) Quercetin, luteolin, apigenin and kaempferol content of soem foods. Food Chem 66:289–292

Kawashima A, Madarame T, Koike H, Komatsu Y, Wise JA (2007) Four week supplementation with mixed fruit and vegetable juice concentrates increased protective serum antioxidants and folate and decreased plasma homocysteine in Japanese subjects. Asia Pac J Clin Nutr 16:411–421

Kay CD, Mazza G, Holub BJ, Wang J (2004) Anthocyanin metabolites in human urine and serum. Br J Nutr 91:933–942

Kay CD, Mazza GJ, Holub BJ (2005) Anthocyanins exist in the circulation primarily as metabolites in adult men. J Nutr 135:2582–2588

Keys A (1980) Seven countries: a multivariate analysis of death and coronary heart disease. Harvard University Press, Cambridge

Khan N, Afaq F, Mukhtar H (2008) Cancer chemoprevention through dietary antioxidants: progress and promise. Antioxid Redox Signal 10:475–510

Knoops KT, de Groot LC, Kromhout D, Perrin AE, Moreiras-Varela O, Menotti A, van Staveren WA (2004) Mediterranean diet, lifestyle factors, and 10-year mortality in elderly European men and women: the HALE project. JAMA 292:1433–1439

Kodera Y, Suzuki A, Imada O, Kasuga S, Sumioka I, Kanezawa A, Taru N, Fujikawa M, Nagae S, Masamoto K, Maeshige K, Ono K (2002) Physical, chemical, and biological properties of s-allylcysteine, an amino acid derived from garlic. J Agric Food Chem 50:622–632

Koli R, Erlund I, Jula A, Marniemi J, Mattila P, Alfthan G (2010) Bioavailability of various polyphenols from a diet containing moderate amounts of berries. J Agric Food Chem 58:3927–3932

Koponen JM, Happonen AM, Mattila PH, Torronen AR (2007) Contents of anthocyanins and ellagitannins in selected foods consumed in Finland. J Agric Food Chem 55:1612–1619

Koskela A, Samaletdin A, Aubertin-Leheudre M, Adlercreutz H (2008) Quantification of alkylresorcinol metabolites in plasma by high-performance liquid chromatography with coulometric electrode array detection. J Agric Food Chem 56:7678–7681

Kountouri AM, Mylona A, Kaliora AC, Andrikopoulos NK (2007) Bioavailability of the phenolic compounds of the fruits (drupes) of Olea europaea (olives): impact on plasma antioxidant status in humans. Phytomedicine 14:659–667

Krogholm KS, Haraldsdottir J, Knuthsen P, Rasmussen SE (2004) Urinary total flavonoid excretion but not 4-pyridoxic acid or potassium can be used as a biomarker for the intake of fruits and vegetables. J Nutr 134:445–451

Kuhnle GG, Dell'Aquila C, Aspinall SM, Runswick SA, Mulligan AA, Bingham SA (2008) Phytoestrogen content of beverages, nuts, seeds, and oils. J Agric Food Chem 56:7311–7315

Kulawinek M, Jaromin A, Kozubek A, Zarnowski R (2008) Alkylresorcinols in selected Polish rye and wheat cereals and whole-grain cereal products. J Agric Food Chem 56:7236–7242

Kushad MM, Brown AF, Kurilich AC, Juvik JA, Klein BP, Wallig MA, Jeffery EH (1999) Variation of glucosinolates in vegetable crops of Brassica oleracea. J Agric Food Chem 47:1541–1548

La Vecchia C (2004) Mediterranean diet and cancer. Public Health Nutr 7:965–968

La Vecchia C (2009) Association between Mediterranean dietary patterns and cancer risk. Nutr Rev 67(Suppl 1):S126–S129

Lairon D (2007) Intervention studies on Mediterranean diet and cardiovascular risk. Mol Nutr Food Res 51:1209–1214

Landberg R, Kamal-Eldin A, Andersson R, Aman P (2006) Alkylresorcinol content and homologue composition in durum wheat (Triticum durum) kernels and pasta products. J Agric Food Chem 54:3012–3014

Landberg R, Aman P, Friberg LE, Vessby B, Adlercreutz H, Kamal-Eldin A (2009a) Dose response of whole-grain biomarkers: alkylresorcinols in human plasma and their metabolites in urine in relation to intake. Am J Clin Nutr 89:290–296

Landberg R, Kamal-Eldin A, Andersson SO, Johansson JE, Zhang JX, Hallmans G, Aman P (2009b) Reproducibility of plasma alkylresorcinols during a 6-week rye intervention study in men with prostate cancer. J Nutr 139:975–980

Landberg R, Man P, Kamal-Eldin A (2009c) A rapid gas chromatography-mass spectrometry method for quantification of alkylresorcinols in human plasma. Anal Biochem 385:7–12

Lawson LD, Gardner CD (2005) Composition, stability, and bioavailability of garlic products used in a clinical trial. J Agric Food Chem 53:6254–6261

Le Marchand L, Hankin JH, Carter FS, Essling C, Luffey D, Franke AA, Wilkens LR, Cooney RV, Kolonel LN (1994) A pilot study on the use of plasma carotenoids and ascorbic acid as markers of compliance to a high fruit and vegetable dietary intervention. Cancer Epidemiol Biomarkers Prev 3:245–251

Liebes L, Conaway CC, Hochster H, Mendoza S, Hecht SS, Crowell J, Chung FL (2001) High-performance liquid chromatography-based determination of total isothiocyanate levels in human plasma: application to studies with 2-phenethyl isothiocyanate. Anal Biochem 291:279–289

Linko AM, Parikka K, Wahala K, Adlercreutz H (2002) Gas chromatographic-mass spectrometric method for the determination of alkylresorcinols in human plasma. Anal Biochem 308:307–313

Liu Y, Dai Y, Xun L, Hu M (2003) Enteric disposition and recycling of flavonoids and ginkgo flavonoids. J Altern Complement Med 9:631–640

Loke WM, Jenner AM, Proudfoot JM, McKinley AJ, Hodgson JM, Halliwell B, Croft KD (2009) A metabolite profiling approach to identify biomarkers of flavonoid intake in humans. J Nutr 139:2309–2314

Lopez-Lazaro M (2009) Distribution and biological activities of the flavonoid luteolin. Mini Rev Med Chem 9:31–59

Magiera S, Uhlschmied C, Rainer M, Huck Ch W, Baranowska I, Bonn GK (2011) GC-MS method for the simultaneous determination of beta-blockers, flavonoids, isoflavones and their metabolites in human urine. J Pharm Biomed Anal 56:93–102

Martini MC, Campbell DR, Gross MD, Grandits GA, Potter JD, Slavin JL (1995) Plasma carotenoids as biomarkers of vegetable intake: the University of Minnesota Cancer Prevention Research Unit Feeding Studies. Cancer Epidemiol Biomarkers Prev 4:491–496

McAnlis GT, McEneny J, Pearce J, Young IS (1999) Absorption and antioxidant effects of quercetin from onions, in man. Eur J Clin Nutr 53:92–96

Mennen LI, Sapinho D, Ito H, Bertrais S, Galan P, Hercberg S, Scalbert A (2006) Urinary flavonoids and phenolic acids as biomarkers of intake for polyphenol-rich foods. Br J Nutr 96:191–198

Mennen LI, Sapinho D, Ito H, Galan P, Hercberg S, Scalbert A (2008) Urinary excretion of 13 dietary flavonoids and phenolic acids in free-living healthy subjects – variability and possible use as biomarkers of polyphenol intake. Eur J Clin Nutr 62:519–525

Miean KH, Mohamed S (2001) Flavonoid (myricetin, quercetin, kaempferol, luteolin, and apigenin) content of edible tropical plants. J Agric Food Chem 49:3106–3112

Mikkelsen TB, Olsen SF, Rasmussen SE, Osler M (2007) Relative validity of fruit and vegetable intake estimated by the food frequency questionnaire used in the Danish National Birth Cohort. Scand J Public Health 35:172–179

Milbury PE, Vita JA, Blumberg JB (2010) Anthocyanins are bioavailable in humans following an acute dose of cranberry juice. J Nutr 140:1099–1104

Moon JH, Nakata R, Oshima S, Inakuma T, Terao J (2000) Accumulation of quercetin conjugates in blood plasma after the short-term ingestion of onion by women. Am J Physiol Regul Integr Comp Physiol 279:R461–R467

Neilson AP, Hopf AS, Cooper BR, Pereira MA, Bomser JA, Ferruzzi MG (2007) Catechin degradation with concurrent formation of homo- and heterocatechin dimers during in vitro digestion. J Agric Food Chem 55:8941–8949

Nielsen SE, Freese R, Kleemola P, Mutanen M (2002) Flavonoids in human urine as biomarkers for intake of fruits and vegetables. Cancer Epidemiol Biomarkers Prev 11:459–466

Nutrient Data Laboratory, Food Composition Laboratory (2007) USDA Database for the Flavonoid Content of Selected Foods, Release 2.1. In: Agricultural Research Service (ed). U.S. Department of Agriculture, Beltsville

Ovaskainen ML, Torronen R, Koponen JM, Sinkko H, Hellstrom J, Reinivuo H, Mattila P (2008) Dietary intake and major food sources of polyphenols in Finnish adults. J Nutr 138:562–566

Paganga G, Rice-Evans CA (1997) The identification of flavonoids as glycosides in human plasma. FEBS Lett 401:78–82

Panagiotakos D, Kalogeropoulos N, Pitsavos C, Roussinou G, Palliou K, Chrysohoou C, Stefanadis C (2009a) Validation of the MedDietScore via the determination of plasma fatty acids. Int J Food Sci Nutr 60(Suppl 5):168–180

Panagiotakos DB, Dimakopoulou K, Katsouyanni K, Bellander T, Grau M, Koenig W, Lanki T, Pistelli R, Schneider A, Peters A, Group AS (2009b) Mediterranean diet and inflammatory response in myocardial infarction survivors. Int J Epidemiol 38:856–866

Perez Rodrigo C, Ruiz Vadillo V (2004) Wheat, bread and pasta in Mediterranean diets. Arch Latinoam Nutr 54:52–58

Peterson JJ, Beecher GR, Bhagwat SA, Dwyer JT, Gebhard SE, Haytowitz DB, Holden JM (2006) Flavanones in grapefruit, lemons, and limes: a compilation and review of the data from the analytical literature. J Food Compos Anal 19:S74–S80

Radtke J, Linseisen J, Wolfram G (2002) Fasting plasma concentrations of selected flavonoids as markers of their ordinary dietary intake. Eur J Nutr 41:203–209

Reed GA, Arneson DW, Putnam WC, Smith HJ, Gray JC, Sullivan DK, Mayo MS, Crowell JA, Hurwitz A (2006) Single-dose and multiple-dose administration of indole-3-carbinol to women: pharmacokinetics based on 3,3′-diindolylmethane. Cancer Epidemiol Biomarkers Prev 15:2477–2481

Reed GA, Sunega JM, Sullivan DK, Gray JC, Mayo MS, Crowell JA, Hurwitz A (2008) Single-dose pharmacokinetics and tolerability of absorption-enhanced 3,3′-diindolylmethane in healthy subjects. Cancer Epidemiol Biomarkers Prev 17:2619–2624

Rein D, Lotito S, Holt RR, Keen CL, Schmitz HH, Fraga CG (2000) Epicatechin in human plasma: in vivo determination and effect of chocolate consumption on plasma oxidation status. J Nutr 130:2109S–2114S

Renaud S, de Lorgeril M, Delaye J, Guidollet J, Jacquard F, Mamelle N, Martin JL, Monjaud I, Salen P, Toubol P (1995) Cretan Mediterranean diet for prevention of coronary heart disease. Am J Clin Nutr 61:1360S–1367S

Ribaya-Mercado JD, Blumberg JB (2004) Lutein and zeaxanthin and their potential roles in disease prevention. J Am Coll Nutr 23:567S–587S

Richelle M, Tavazzi I, Enslen M, Offord EA (1999) Plasma kinetics in man of epicatechin from black chocolate. Eur J Clin Nutr 53:22–26

Riso P, Brusamolino A, Moro M, Porrini M (2009) Absorption of bioactive compounds from steamed broccoli and their effect on plasma glutathione S-transferase activity. Int J Food Sci Nutr 60(Suppl 1):56–71

Rodriguez G, Lama A, Jaramillo S, Fuentes-Alventosa JM, Guillen R, Jimenez-Araujo A, Rodriguez-Arcos R, Fernandez-Bolanos J (2009) 3,4-Dihydroxyphenylglycol (DHPG): an important phenolic compound present in natural table olives. J Agric Food Chem 57:6298–6304

Rogan EG (2006) The natural chemopreventive compound indole-3-carbinol: state of the science. In Vivo 20:221–228

Rosen RT, Hiserodt RD, Fukuda EK, Ruiz RJ, Zhou Z, Lech J, Rosen SL, Hartman TG (2000) The determination of metabolites of garlic preparations in breath and human plasma. Biofactors 13:241–249

Rosen RT, Hiserodt RD, Fukuda EK, Ruiz RJ, Zhou Z, Lech J, Rosen SL, Hartman TG (2001) Determination of allicin, S-allylcysteine and volatile metabolites of garlic in breath, plasma or simulated gastric fluids. J Nutr 131:968S–971S

Ross AB, Shepherd MJ, Schupphaus M, Sinclair V, Alfaro B, Kamal-Eldin A, Aman P (2003) Alkylresorcinols in cereals and cereal products. J Agric Food Chem 51:4111–4118

Ruidavets J, Teissedre P, Ferrieres J, Carando S, Bougard G, Cabanis J (2000) Catechin in the Mediterranean diet: vegetable, fruit or wine? Atherosclerosis 153:107–117

Ruiz-Gutierrez V, Juan ME, Cert A, Planas JM (2000) Determination of hydroxytyrosol in plasma by HPLC. Anal Chem 72:4458–4461

Rumawas ME, Dwyer JT, McKeown NM, Meigs JB, Rogers G, Jacques PF (2009) The development of the Mediterranean-style dietary pattern score and its application to the American diet in the Framingham Offspring Cohort. J Nutr 139:1150–1156

Salas-Salvado J, Bullo M, Babio N, Martinez-Gonzalez MA, Ibarrola-Jurado N, Basora J, Estruch R, Covas MI, Corella D, Aros F, Ruiz-Gutierrez V, Ros E (2010) Reduction in the incidence of type 2 diabetes with the Mediterranean diet: results of the PREDIMED-Reus nutrition intervention randomized trial. Diabetes Care 34:14–19

Sampson L, Rimm E, Hollman PC, de Vries JH, Katan MB (2002) Flavonol and flavone intakes in US health professionals. J Am Diet Assoc 102:1414–1420

Sato R, Helzlsouer KJ, Alberg AJ, Hoffman SC, Norkus EP, Comstock GW (2002) Prospective study of carotenoids, tocopherols, and retinoid concentrations and the risk of breast cancer. Cancer Epidemiol Biomarkers Prev 11:451–457

Scarmeas N, Luchsinger JA, Schupf N, Brickman AM, Cosentino S, Tang MX, Stern Y (2009) Physical activity, diet, and risk of Alzheimer disease. JAMA 302:627–637

Shimoi K, Okada H, Furugori M, Goda T, Takase S, Suzuki M, Hara Y, Yamamoto H, Kinae N (1998) Intestinal absorption of luteolin and luteolin 7-O-beta-glucoside in rats and humans. FEBS Lett 438:220–224

Simopoulos AP (2004) The traditional diet of Greece and cancer. Eur J Cancer Prev 13:219–230

Smith SA, Campbell DR, Elmer PJ, Martini MC, Slavin JL, Potter JD (1995) The University of Minnesota Cancer Prevention Research Unit vegetable and fruit classification scheme (United States). Cancer Causes Control 6:292–302

Soderholm P, Koskela AH, Lundin JE, Tikkanen MJ, Adlercreutz HC (2009) Plasma pharmacokinetics of alkylresorcinol metabolites: new candidate biomarkers for whole-grain rye and wheat intake. Am J Clin Nutr 90(5):1167–1171

Sofi F, Cesari F, Abbate R, Gensini GF, Casini A (2008) Adherence to Mediterranean diet and health status: meta-analysis. BMJ 337:a1344

Sofi F, Abbate R, Gensini GF, Casini A (2010) Accruing evidence on benefits of adherence to the Mediterranean diet on health: an updated systematic review and meta-analysis. Am J Clin Nutr 92:1189–1196

Soleas GJ, Yan J, Goldberg DM (2001) Ultrasensitive assay for three polyphenols (catechin, quercetin and resveratrol) and their conjugates in biological fluids utilizing gas chromatography with mass selective detection. J Chromatogr B Biomed Sci Appl 757:161–172

Song L, Morrison JJ, Botting NP, Thornalley PJ (2005) Analysis of glucosinolates, isothiocyanates, and amine degradation products in vegetable extracts and blood plasma by LC-MS/MS. Anal Biochem 347:234–243

Sotiroudis TG, Kyrtopoulos SA (2008) Anticarcinogenic compounds of olive oil and related biomarkers. Eur J Nutr 47(Suppl 2):69–72

Steinbrecher A, Linseisen J (2009) Dietary intake of individual glucosinolates in participants of the EPIC-Heidelberg cohort study. Ann Nutr Metab 54:87–96

Tamimi RM, Hankinson SE, Campos H, Spiegelman D, Zhang S, Colditz GA, Willett WC, Hunter DJ (2005) Plasma carotenoids, retinol, and tocopherols and risk of breast cancer. Am J Epidemiol 161:153–160

Thomasset S, Berry DP, Cai H, West K, Marczylo TH, Marsden D, Brown K, Dennison A, Garcea G, Miller A, Hemingway D, Steward WP, Gescher AJ (2009) Pilot study of oral anthocyanins for colorectal cancer chemoprevention. Cancer Prev Res (Phila Pa) 2:625–633

Thompson LU, Boucher BA, Liu Z, Cotterchio M, Kreiger N (2006) Phytoestrogen content of foods consumed in Canada, including isoflavones, lignans, and coumestan. Nutr Cancer 54:184–201

Toniolo P, Van Kappel AL, Akhmedkhanov A, Ferrari P, Kato I, Shore RE, Riboli E (2001) Serum carotenoids and breast cancer. Am J Epidemiol 153:1142–1147

Trichopoulou A (1989) Nutrition policy in Greece. Eur J Clin Nutr 43:79–82

Trichopoulou A, Katsouyanni K, Gnardellis C (1993) The traditional Greek diet. Eur J Clin Nutr 47:S76–S81

Trichopoulou A, Naska A, Vasilopoulou E (2001) Guidelines for the intake of vegetables and fruit: the Mediterranean approach. Int J Vitam Nutr Res 71:149–153

Trichopoulou A, Costacou T, Bamia C, Trichopoulos D (2003) Adherence to a Mediterranean diet and survival in a Greek population. N Engl J Med 348:2599–2608

Trichopoulou A, Orfanos P, Norat T, Bueno-de-Mesquita B, Ocke MC, Peeters PH, van der Schouw YT, Boeing H, Hoffmann K, Boffetta P, Nagel G, Masala G, Krogh V, Panico S, Tumino R, Vineis P, Bamia C, Naska A, Benetou V, Ferrari P, Slimani N, Pera G, Martinez-Garcia C, Navarro C, Rodriguez-Barranco M, Dorronsoro M, Spencer EA, Key TJ, Bingham S,

Khaw KT, Kesse E, Clavel-Chapelon F, Boutron-Ruault MC, Berglund G, Wirfalt E, Hallmans G, Johansson I, Tjonneland A, Olsen A, Overvad K, Hundborg HH, Riboli E, Trichopoulos D (2005) Modified Mediterranean diet and survival: EPIC-elderly prospective cohort study. BMJ 330:991–998

Urpi-Sarda M, Monagas M, Khan N, Lamuela-Raventos RM, Santos-Buelga C, Sacanella E, Castell M, Permanyer J, Andres-Lacueva C (2009) Epicatechin, procyanidins, and phenolic microbial metabolites after cocoa intake in humans and rats. Anal Bioanal Chem 394:1545–1556

Vanamala J, Cobb G, Turner ND, Lupton JR, Yoo KS, Pike LM, Patil BS (2005) Bioactive compounds of grapefruit (Citrus paradisi Cv. Rio Red) respond differently to postharvest irradiation, storage, and freeze drying. J Agric Food Chem 53:3980–3985

Verberne L, Bach-Faig A, Buckland G, Serra-Majem L (2010) Association between the Mediterranean diet and cancer risk: a review of observational studies. Nutr Cancer 62:860–870

Verhagen H, Hageman GJ, Rauma AL, Versluis-de Haan G, van Herwijnen MH, de Groot J, Torronen R, Mykkanen H (2001) Biomonitoring the intake of garlic via urinary excretion of allyl mercapturic acid. Br J Nutr 86(Suppl 1):S111–S114

Weinbrenner T, Fito M, Farre Albaladejo M, Saez GT, Rijken P, Tormos C, Coolen S, De La Torre R, Covas MI (2004) Bioavailability of phenolic compounds from olive oil and oxidative/antioxidant status at postprandial state in healthy humans. Drugs Exp Clin Res 30:207–212

Wu X, Beecher GR, Holden JM, Haytowitz DB, Gebhardt SE, Prior RL (2006) Concentrations of anthocyanins in common foods in the United States and estimation of normal consumption. J Agric Food Chem 54:4069–4075

Zhang Z, Kou X, Fugal K, McLaughlin J (2004) Comparison of HPLC methods for determination of anthocyanins and anthocyanidins in bilberry extracts. J Agric Food Chem 52:688–691

Zimmermann BF, Papagiannopoulos M, Brachmann S, Lorenz M, Stangl V, Galensa R (2009) A shortcut from plasma to chromatographic analysis: straightforward and fast sample preparation for analysis of green tea catechins in human plasma. J Chromatogr B Analyt Technol Biomed Life Sci 877:823–826

Chapter 10
Plant Polyphenols and Their Role in Cancer Prevention and Chemotherapy

Sharmila Shankar, Brahma N. Singh, and Rakesh K. Srivastava

Contents

Abstract Chemoprevention has been proposed as the good tool to target these high-risk cancer patients. Among various identified chemopreventive agents, plant polyphenols (PPs) have been shown to be safe and highly effective in inhibiting of carcinogen-induced mutagenesis and tumorigenesis in bioassays and animal models for different target organ sites. The compounds derived from the plants are of considerable interest among oncologists. PPs have been studied for their chemopreventive and chemotherapeutic properties against human cancer, including green tea polyphenols, genistein (found in soy), apigenin (celery, parsley), luteolin (broccoli), quercetin (onions), kaempferol (broccoli, grapefruits), curcumin (turmeric), etc. Whilst such naturally occurring polyphenols have been the subject of numerous mechanistic studies in cells, information on their clinical properties, which might

S. Shankar
Department of Pathology and Laboratory Medicine, The University of Kansas Cancer Center, The University of Kansas Medical Center, 3901 Rainbow Boulevard, Kansas City, KS 66160, USA
e-mail: sshankar@kumc.edu

B.N. Singh • R.K. Srivastava (✉)
Department of Pharmacology, Toxicology and Therapeutics, and Medicine, The University of Kansas Cancer Center, The University of Kansas Medical Center, 3901 Rainbow Boulevard, Kansas City, KS 66160, USA
e-mail: bsingh@kumc.edu; rsrivastava@kumc.edu

S. Shankar and R.K. Srivastava (eds.), *Nutrition, Diet and Cancer*,
DOI 10.1007/978-94-007-2923-0_10, © Springer Science+Business Media B.V. 2012

help assess their promise as human cancer chemopreventive agents, is scarce. The more we discuss their molecular mechanisms and cellular targets, the better we could utilize these "natural gifts" for the prevention and treatment of human cancers. The abundance of flavonoids and related phenolics in the plant kingdom makes it possible that several hitherto uncharacterised agents with cancer preventive potential are still to be identified, which may constitute attractive alternatives to currently used chemopreventive drugs. In this article, the effective PPs against human cancers will also be discussed, with more emphases on the basic conceptions of phenolics with strong antioxidant activity.

Introduction

Chemoprevention of cancer through the use of naturally occurring dietary agents recently has received an increasing interest, and plant polyphenols (PPs) have become not only important potential chemopreventive agents, but also therapeutic, and natural antioxidants (Aggarwal and Shishodia 2006). Chemoprevention, by definition, is a means of the therapy of precancerous lesions, which are called preinvasive neoplasia, dysplasia, or intraepithelial neoplasia, depending on the organ system. One misconception about chemoprevention is the thinking for complete prevention of cancer, an unachievable goal. Since the mechanism of cancer development is carcinogenesis, we believe that our key aim should be to prevent or retard carcinogenesis process, which in turn will lead to lower cancer burden. We, therefore, define chemoprevention as *slowing the process of carcinogenesis*, a goal that can be met (Korkina et al. 2009; Singh et al. 2009a). PPs have been demonstrated to act on multiple key elements in intracellular signal transduction pathways related to cell proliferation, differentiation, apoptosis, inflammation, angiogenesis and metastasis; however, these molecular mechanisms of action are not completely characterized and many features remain to be elucidated (Stoner and Morse 1997). Among all the PPs, green tea and soy polyphenols have especially received considerable attention because of demonstrated chemoprevention efficacy against a variety of human malignances. The cancer chemopreventive effects of PPs may be the result of decreased cell transformation and proliferation or increased cell cycle arrest and apoptosis (Stoner and Mukhtar 1995). *In vitro*, polyphenols have been shown to cause growth inhibition and apoptosis in a number of human cancer cell lines including leukemia, melanoma, breast, pancreatic, prostate, brain, lung, and colon cancers (Coates et al. 2007; D'Archivio et al. 2008; Duthie et al. 2000). These effects have been extensively studied *in vitro* to try to elucidate the potential mechanism(s) of action of PPs. Moreover, these chemopreventive effects have been observed *in vivo* in certain animal models, but no clear and fully understandable mechanism(s) has been reported for PPs (Gorlach et al. 2011).

In addition to many essential nutritional components, plants contain PPs, a large and heterogeneous group of biologically active non-nutrients. Flavonoids are divided into many categories, including flavonols, flavones, catechins, proanthocyanidins, anthocyanidins and isoflavonoids. Phenolic acids present in plants are hydroxylated derivatives of benzoic and cinnamic acids (Kampa et al. 2000). Flavonoids and phenolic acids have many functions in plants. They act as cell wall support materials and as colourful attractants for birds and insects helping seed dispersal and pollination. PPs are also important in the defence mechanisms of plants under different environmental stress conditions such as wounding, infection, and excessive light or UV irradiation (Kuhnau 1976).

The biological potency of secondary PPs was found empirically already by our ancestors; phenolics are not only unsavoury or poisonous, but also of possible pharmacological value (Gorlach et al. 2011). Flavonoids have long been recognised to possess anticancer, anti-inflammatory, antiviral and antiproliferative activities (Bennani et al. 2007; D'Alessandro et al. 2003; Dai et al. 2008). Flavonoids and phenolic acids also have antioxidative and anticarcinogenic effects. Inverse relationships between the intake of flavonoids (flavonols and flavones) and the risk of liver and stomach cancer have been shown in epidemiological studies (Beltz et al. 2006). PPs including quercetin protocatechuic acid (Lin et al. 2011), ellagic acid (Edderkaoui et al. 2008), gallic acid (You et al. 2011), and caffeic acid (Hung et al. 2003) are natural antioxidants, which decrease oxidation of biomolecules essential for life. They are also having anti-carcinogenic and anti-tumorigenic activities against several chemically-induced hepatocarcinogenesis.

Many so-called secondary products can act as potent bio-antimutagens. Anticancer action of PPs has been studied, for which many compounds seems to be most responsible (Dashwood 2007; Gorlach et al. 2011). Therefore, there is currently a strong interest in the study of natural compounds with free radical scavenger capacity and their role in human health and nutrition (Prakash et al. 2007). Dietary polyphenols may contribute to the decrease of cancer disease by reduction of free radical formation as well as oxidative stress in general, by protection of low density lipoprotein (LDL) oxidation and platelet aggregation and by inhibiting synthesis of proinflammatory cytokines (Singh et al. 2009a). In this article, for the sake of better understanding, the effective PPs against various cancers will be discussed, with more emphases on the basic conceptions of phenolics with strong antioxidant activity (Singh et al. 2009b; Wang et al. 2000).

Plant Polyphenols (PPs)

The term polyphenols or phenolics refer precisely to those chemical compounds, which have an aromatic ring with hydroxyl substituent(s), including their derivatives like esters, methyl ethers and glycosides (Augustin et al. 2008; Singh et al. 2010). On the basis of chemical structure, they can be classified into phenolic acids, flavonoids, stilbenes and lignans. A 'recommended' human diet contains significant quantities of polyphenolics, as they have long been assumed to be 'antioxidants' that scavenge excessive, damaging, free radicals arising from normal metabolic processes (Ivanova et al. 2005). There is recent evidence that polyphenolics also have 'indirect' antioxidant effects through induction of endogenous protective

Table 10.1 The major classes of PPs in plants

No. of C atoms	Basic skeleton	Class	Example
6	C6	Simple phenols – benzoquinones	Catechol, hydroquinone2, 6-dimethoxybenzoquinone
7	C6–C1	Phenolics acids	p-hydroxybenzoic, salicylic, Gallic acid, Syringic acid
8	C6–C2	Acetophenones phenylacetic acid	3-Acetyi-6-methoxybenzaldehyde, p-Hydroxyphenylacetic acid
9	C6–C3	Hydroxycinnamic acids coumarin, isocoumarin, chromones	Caffieic, ferulic myristicin, eugenol umbelliferone, aesculetin, bergenin, eugenin
10	C6–C4	Napthoquinone,	Juglone, plumbagin
13	C6–C1–C6	Xanthones	Mangiferin
14	C6–C2–C6	Stilbenes, anthraquinone	Lunularic acid, emodin
15	C6–C3–C6	Flavonoids, isoflavonoids	Quercitin, cyaniding, genistein
18	$(C6–C3)_2$	Lignans, neolignans	Pinoresinol eusiderin
30	$(C6–C-3–C6)_2$	Biflavonoids	Amentoflavone
N	$(C6\text{-}3)n(C6)_6$ (C6–C3–C6) n	Lignins, catechol, melanins, flavolans (condensed tannins)	

enzymes (Bennani et al. 2007; Singh et al. 2009a). There is also increasing evidence for many potential benefits through polyphenolic mediated regulation of cellular processes such as inflammation and cancer.

Some classes of polyphenol, such as the condensed tannins, have many catechol and phloroglucinol groups in their structure. A purely chemical definition of a PP, however is not entirely satisfactory, since it would mean including some compounds such as the phenolic carotinoid or the phenolic female sex hormone orstrone, which are principally terpinoid in origin. For this reason a biogenetic definition is preferable. The natural PP arises biogenetically from two main pathways. The Shikimate pathway which is directly provides phenylpropanoids such as hydroxycinnamic and coumarins and the polyketide pathway (acetate) which can produce simple phenols and also many quinines. Major classes of phenolics have been described in Table 10.1 and Fig. 10.1 (Harborne and Williams 2001).

PPs are the most abundantly occurring polyphenols in plants, of which flavonoids and phenolic acids accounts for about 60% and 30% of total dietary phenols, respectively (Nichenametla et al. 2006). Antioxidant activity and biological properties of PPs from berries, red wine, ginkgo, onions, apples, grapes, chamomile, citrus, dandelion, green tea, hawthorn, licorice, rosemary, thyme, fruits, vegetables and beverages have been studied. They are rich sources of phenols that can enhance the efficacy of vitamin C, reduce the risk of cancer, act against allergies, ulcers, tumors, platelet aggregation and are also effective in controlling hypertension (Monde et al. 2011).

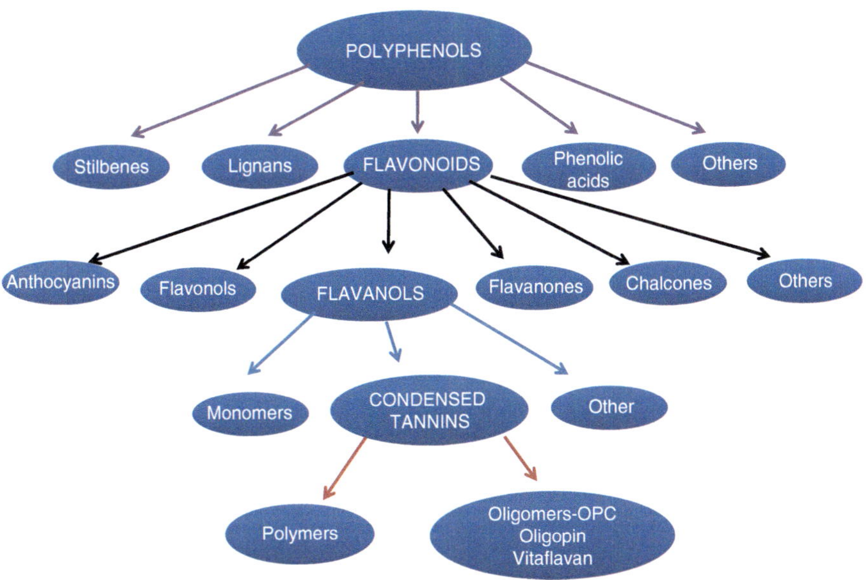

Fig. 10.1 Typical classes of polyphenols found in plants

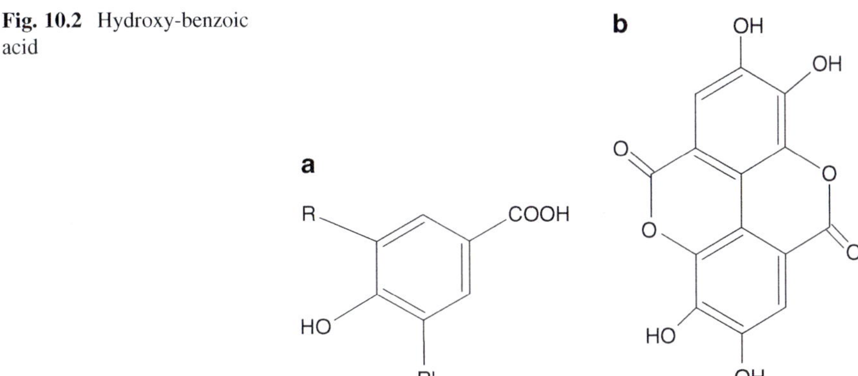

Fig. 10.2 Hydroxy-benzoic acid

Classification of PPs

Hydroxy-benzoic Acid

Hydroxybenzoic acids have a general structure of C6–C1 derived directly from benzoic acid (Fig 10.2). Variations in the structures of individual hydroxybenzoic acids lie in the hydroxylations and methylations of the aromatic ring. Four acids occur commonly: p-hydroxybenzoic, vanillic, syringic, and protocatechuic acid (Starke and Herrmann 1976).

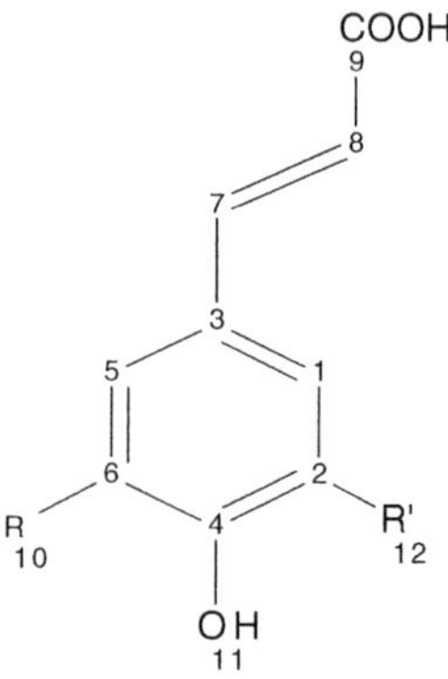

Fig. 10.3 Hydroxy-cinnamic acids

Protocatechuic acid	(R=OH, R′=H)
Gallic acid	(R=R′=OH)
Syringic acid	(R=R′=OMe)
p-Hydroxybenzoic acid	(R=R′=H)
Vanillic acid	(R=OMe, R′=H)

Hydroxy-cinnamic Acids

The four most widely distributed hydroxycinnamic acids in fruits are *p*-coumaric, caffeic, ferulic and sinapic acids (Fig. 10.3) (Inglett and Chen 2011; Starke and Herrmann 1976).

p-Coumaric acid	(R=R′=H)
Caffeic acid	(R=OH, R′=H)
Ferulic acid	(R=OMe, R′=H)
Sinapic acid	(R=R′=OMe)

Flavonoids

Flavonoids are formed in plants from the aromatic amino acids phenylalanine and tyrosine, and malonate. The structural basis of all flavonoids is flavone nucleus (2 phenyl-benzo-ϒ-pyrone) (Fig. 10.4) but, depending on the classification method, the flavonoids group can be divided into several categories on the basis of hydroxylation of flavonoids nucleus and linked sugar (Harborne and Sherratt 1961).

	R	C_2–C_3
Flavone	H	Double bond
Flavonol	OH	Double bond
Flavanone	H	Single bond
Flavanol	OH	Single bond

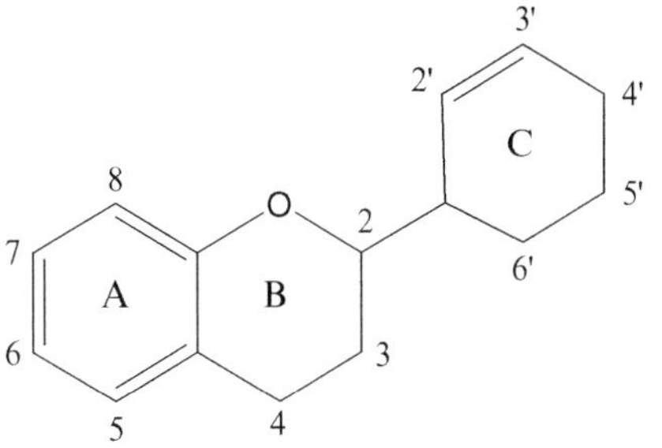

Fig. 10.4 Flavone nucleus (2 phenyl-benzo-ϒ-pyrone)

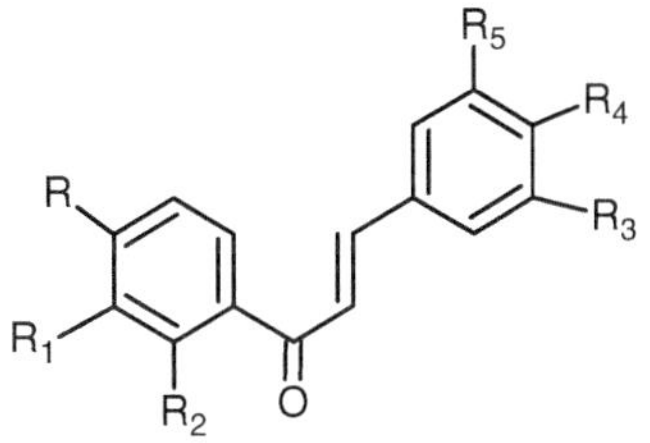

Fig. 10.5 Chalcones

	R	R_1	R_2	R_3	R_4	R_5
Butein	OH	H	OH	H	OH	OH
Isoquirtigenin	OH	H	OH	H	OH	H

Flavonoids and their relatives are derived biosynthetically from the Shikimate pathway. They share a three-ring structure of two aromatic centers, ring A and B and a central oxygenated heterocycle moiety, ring C (Fig. 10.4). They have a flavone nucleus (2 phenyl-benzo-γ-pyrone) and on the basis of variation in the heterocyclic C ring may be classified into flavones, flavonols, flavanones, flavanols, isoflavones, anthocyanidins and proanthocyanidins. Chalcones such as butein, and isoquirtigenin (Fig. 10.5) are considered to be members of the flavonoids, despite of lacking heterocycle ring C (Harborne and Sherratt 1961). Flavones and flavonols have a double bond between C-2 and C-3 (Figs. 10.6 and 10.7). Flavonols have a hydroxy group at the C-3 position that is lacking in flavones. Flavanones and flavanols are characterized by the presence of a saturated three-carbon chain. Flavanols differ from flavanones by having a hydroxyl group at C-3 position (Figs. 10.8 and 10.9). Isoflavones (Fig. 10.10) are derived by cyclization of chalcones in such a way that the B ring is located at C-3 position. Anthocyanins (Fig. 10.11) are composed of aglycon called anthocynidins and sugar moiety(ies). Proanthocyanidins are condensed tannins or polymeric flavonols, which are generally formed as a result of coupling between electrophilic and nucleophilic flavanyl units (Harborne and Sherratt 1961; Seyoum et al. 2006).

	R	R_1	R_2	R_3	R_4	R_5	R_6
Apigenin	OH	H	OH	H	OH	H	H
Vitexin	OH	H	OH	H	OH	H	O-Glucose
Isovitexin	OH	O-Glucose	OH	H	OH	H	H
Luteolin	OH	H	OH	H	OH	OH	H

Fig. 10.6 Flavones

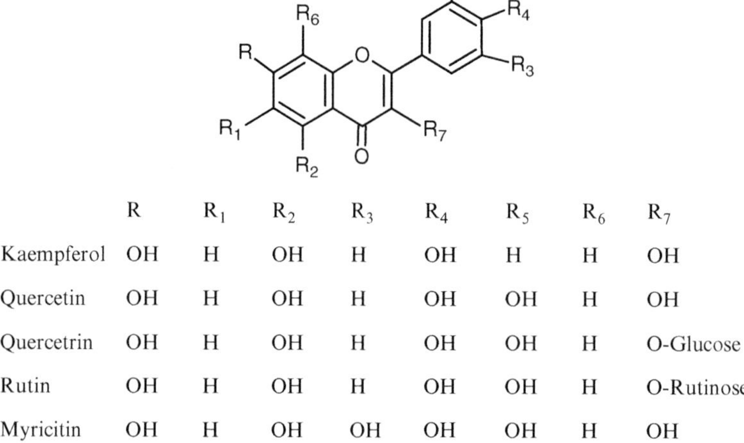

	R	R_1	R_2	R_3	R_4	R_5	R_6	R_7
Kaempferol	OH	H	OH	H	OH	H	H	OH
Quercetin	OH	H	OH	H	OH	OH	H	OH
Quercetrin	OH	H	OH	H	OH	OH	H	O-Glucose
Rutin	OH	H	OH	H	OH	OH	H	O-Rutinose
Myricitin	OH	H	OH	OH	OH	OH	H	OH

Fig. 10.7 Flavonol

Antioxidant Activity of PPs

Flavonoids possess ideal structure for free radicals scavenging activity and have been found to be more effective cancer preventive agents *in vitro* than tocopherols and ascorbates. They are efficient reducing agents that can stabilize the polyphenols derived radicals and delocalise the unpaired electrons. It has been reported that flavonoids with strong antioxidant activity are excellent hydrogen donors and have a 3′, 4′-dihydroxy configuration (Seyoum et al. 2006). Interestingly the hydroxyl groups on the chromane ring do not appear to participate directly in the redox

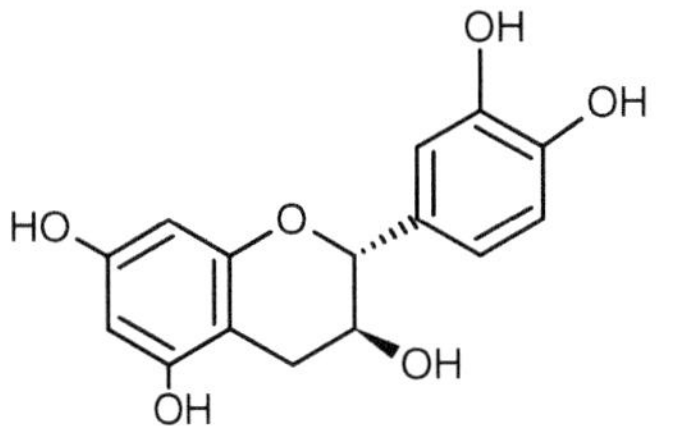

Catechin

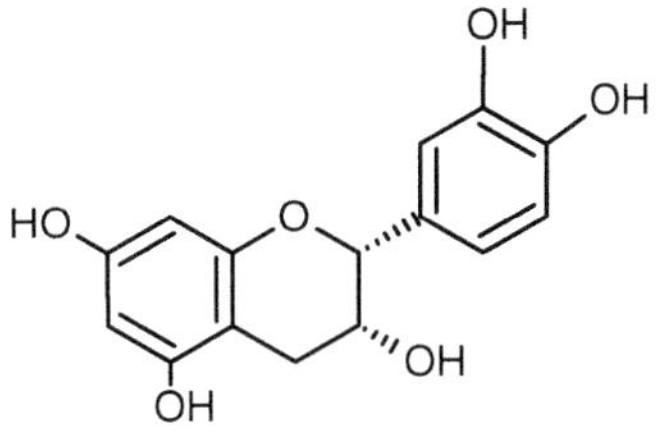

Epicatechin

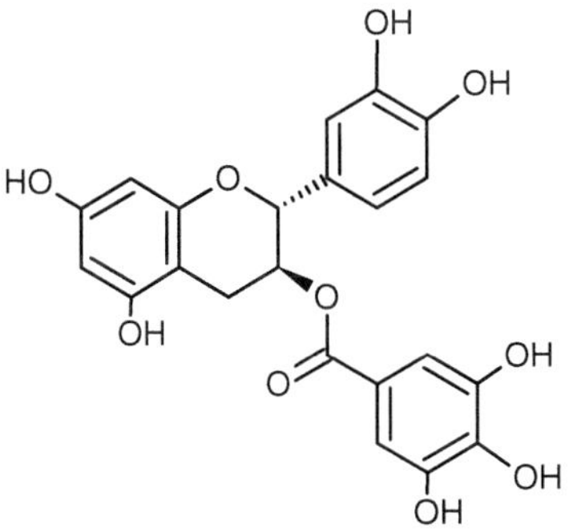

Catechin gallate

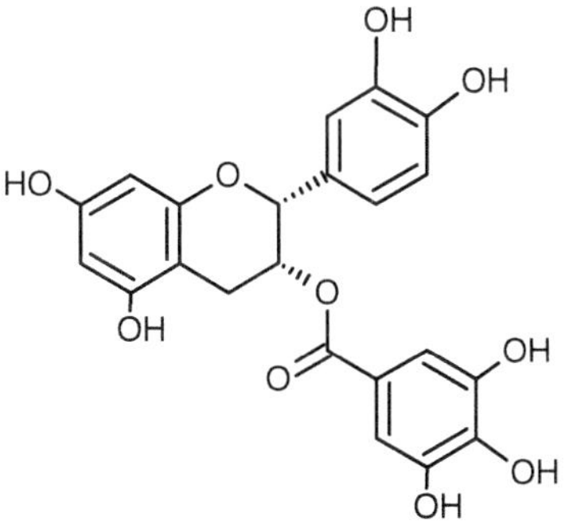

Epicatechin-3-gallate (EGCG)

Fig. 10.8 Flavanol (Flavan-3-ols)

Fig. 10.9 Flavanone

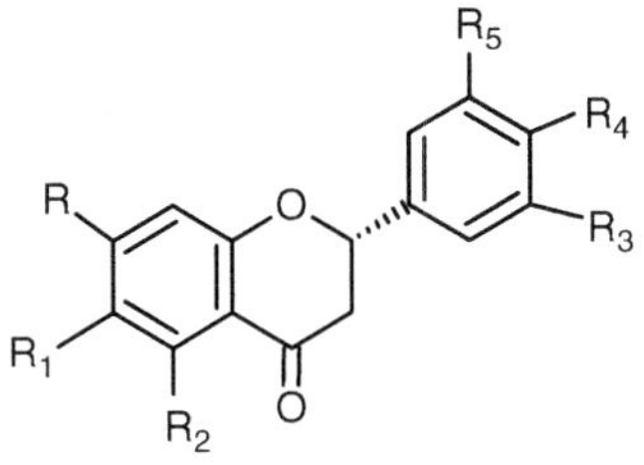

	R	R_1	R_2	R_3	R_4	R_5
Naringenin	OH	H	OH	H	OH	H
Hesperitin	OH	H	OH	H	OCH_3	H

chemistry. Instead it is the hydroxyl group of catechol moiety present in the B ring that donates or accepts hydrogen. However, while the flavonoids nucleus does not undergo direct redox modification, it does affect redox behaviour of substituents on B ring. Therefore, flavonoids containing catechol structure can exert a powerful radical scavenging activity. The position and number of hydroxyl groups also plays an important role in antioxidant activity. For example in apigenin (Fig. 10.6), the three-hydroxyl groups at position 5, 7, 4′ were associated with a small but definite

Fig. 10.10 Isoflavones

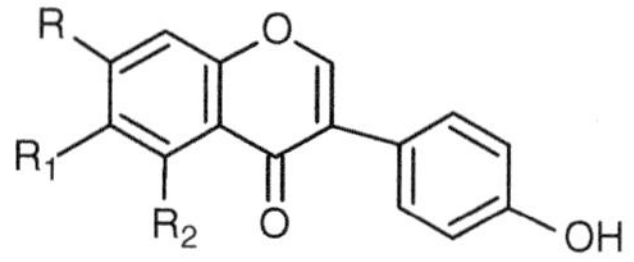

	R	R_1	R_2
Daidzein	OH	H	OH
Genistein	OH	H	H

Fig. 10.11 Anthocyanin

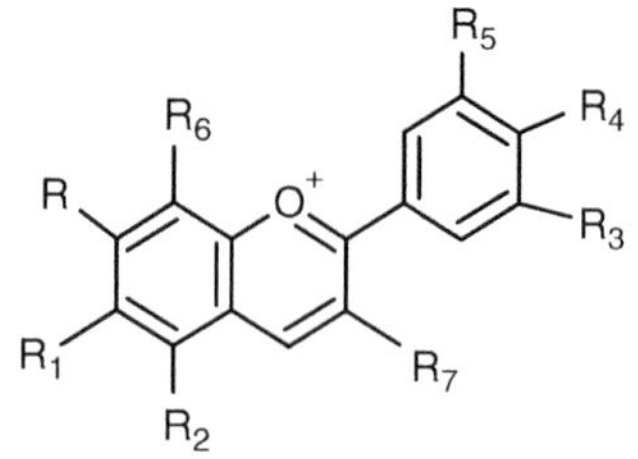

	R	R_1	R_2	R_3	R_4	R_5	R_6
Pelargonidin	OH	H	OH	H	OH	H	H
Cyanidin	OH	H	OH	H	OH	OH	H
Delphinidin	OH	H	OH	OH	OH	OH	H

antioxidant effect, while kaempferol (Fig. 10.7) with an additional hydroxyl at position 3 was more potent than apigenin. Quercetin with additional hydroxyl group at 3′ and myrcetin at 3′, 5′ positions (Fig. 10.7) were still more effective (Priego et al. 2008; Ranilla et al. 2007; Seyoum et al. 2006). Flavonoids can also generate H_2O_2 by donating a hydrogen atom from their pyrogallol or catechol structure to oxygen, through a superoxide anion radical. The pyrogallol-type compounds generate more H_2O_2 than that of catechol. H_2O_2 has been reported to raise levels of intracellular Ca^{2+}, activate transcription factors, repress expression of certain genes, promote or inhibit cell proliferation, be cytotoxic, activate or suppress certain signal transduction pathways, promote or suppress apoptosis (Rizvi et al. 2010; Singh et al. 2009a; Stoner and Morse 1997; Tedesco et al. 2000).

More than 4,000 flavonoids have been identified in plants, which are responsible for the color of vegetables, fruits, grains, seeds, leaves, flowers, bark and products derived from them (Terao et al. 2008). Luteolin, kaempferol, quercetin, quercitrin, rutin, myricetin and vitamin C are powerful antioxidants that inhibit the oxidation of LDL, a major factor in the promotion of atherosclerosis, which is the plaque build up in arteries that can lead to heart attack or stroke (Covas et al. 2006; Duthie et al. 2000). In general, the aglycones were found with greater antioxidant potential than their glycosides. Use of comet assay to assess DNA damage during oxidative stress showed that quercetin was more potent antioxidant as compared to rutin and vitamin C (Delgado et al. 2008; Katiyar et al. 2010). Isoflavones like genestein and daidzein found abundantly in legumes such as lentils, chickpeas and soybeans, have nutraceutical properties against tumor growth and cancer and they form one of the main classes of oestrogenic substances in plants (Fig. 10.10). Anthocyanins, another major group of flavonoids play a significant role in collagen protein synthesis and sport medicines (Fig. 10.11). Athletes who exercise a lot produce free radicals that can be tackled by anthocyanidins (Noda et al. 2002; Yue and Xu 2008).

PPs and Molecular Targets for Prevention and Therapy of Cancer

Fruits, vegetables, and spices have drawn a great deal of attention from both the scientific community and the general public owing to their demonstrated ability to suppress cancers. The questions that remain to be answered are which component of these dietary agents is responsible for the anti-cancer effects and what is the mechanism by which they suppress cancer? Dietary agents consist of a wide variety of biologically active compounds that are ubiquitous in plants, many of which have been used in traditional medicines for thousands of years. As early as 2,500 years ago, Hippocrates recognized and professed the importance of various foods both natural.

Fruits and vegetables are excellent sources of polyphenols, but they also contain components like fiber, vitamins, and minerals, terpenes, and alkaloids that may provide substantial health benefits beyond basic nutrition (Monde et al. 2011; Starke and Herrmann 1976; Terao et al. 2008). Research over the last decade has shown that several micronutrients in fruits and vegetables reduce cancer (10; Table 10.2). The active components of dietary phytochemicals that most often appear to be protective against cancer are curcumin, genistein, resveratrol, ellagic acid, quercetin, rutin, morin, diallyl sulfide, *S*-allyl, lycopene, ellagic acid, epicatechin gallate, gallic acid, silymarin, catechins, isothiocyanates, isoflavones, Vitamin C, lutein, Vitamin E, and flavonoids (Aggarwal and Shishodia 2006; Araujo et al. 2011). These dietary polyphenols are believed to suppress the inflammatory processes that lead to transformation, hyperproliferation, and initiation of carcinogenesis (Araujo et al. 2011). Their inhibitory influences may ultimately suppress the final steps of carcinogenesis as well as angiogenesis and metastasis (Fig. 10.12).

Tumorigenesis is a multistep process that can be activated by any of various environmental carcinogens (such as cigarette smoke, industrial emissions, gasoline vapors), inflammatory agents (such as tumor necrosis factor (TNF) and H_2O_2), and tumor promoters (such as phorbol esters and okadaic acid). These carcinogens are known to modulate the transcription factors (e.g., NF-kB, AP-1, STAT3), anti-apoptotic proteins (e.g., Akt, Bcl-2, Bcl-X_L), proapoptotic proteins (e.g., caspases, PARP), protein kinases (e.g., AKT, IKK, JNK, ERK), cell cycle proteins (e.g., cyclins, cyclin-dependent kinases), cell adhesion molecules, COX-2, and growth

Table 10.2 Molecular targets of PPs for prevention and therapy of cancer

PPs	Plant name	Molecular target
Resveratrol	Grapes (*Vitis vinifera*)	↓COX-2, ↓iNOS, ↓JNK, ↓MEK, ↓AP-1, ↓NF-κB, ↑P21 Cip1/WAF1, ↑p53, ↑Bax, ↑caspases, ↑TNF, ↓survivin, ↓cyclin D1, ↓cyclin E, ↓Bcl-2, ↓Bcl-xL, ↓CIAP, ↓Egr-1, ↓PKC, ↓PKD, ↓casein kinase II, ↓5-LOX, ↓VEGF, ↓IL-1, ↓IL-6, ↓IL-8, ↓AR, ↓PSA, ↓CYP1A1, ↓TypeII-Ptdlns-4kinase, ↓Cdc2-tyr15[a], ↑HO-1, ↑Nrf2, ↓endothelin-1
Caffeoylquinic acids	Quince (*Cydonia oblonga*)	↓IFN-γ, ↓IL-2, ↓ERK1/2, ↓AKT, ↓NF-κB, ↓NO, ↓iNOS
Ellagic acid	Pomegranate (*Punica granatum*)	↓NF-κB, ↓COX-2, ↓cyclin D1, ↓MMP-9, ↓PDGF, ↓VEGF, ↑GST, ↑p21/WAF1, ↑p53
Genistein	Soyabean (*Glycine max*)	↓NF-κB, ↑caspase-12, ↑p21/WAF1, ↑glutathione peroxidase
Flavonoids, catechins	Tea (*Camellia sinensis*)	↓NF-κB, ↓AP-1, ↓JNK, ↓COX-2, ↓cyclin D1, ↓MMP-9, ↑HO-1, ↓IL-6, ↓VEGF, ↓IGF, ↑p53, ↓Bcl-2, ↑p21/WAF1
Quercetin	Citrus fruits, apple (*Citrus* sp.)	NF-κB, ↑Bax, ↓ Bcl-2, ↓cyclin D1, ↑caspase, ↑PARP, ↑Gadd 45
Silymarin	*Silybum marianum*	↓NF-kB, ↓AP-1, ↓JNK, ↓COX-2, ↓cyclin D1, ↓MMP-9

AR androgen receptor, *NF-κB* nuclear factor kappa B, *NO* nitric oxide, *PGE* prostaglandin, *iNOS* inducible nitric oxide synthase, *COX-2* cyclooxygenase-2, *IL* interleukin, *MAP* mitogen-activated protein, *TNF* tumor necrosis factor, *CYP7A1* cholesterol 7alpha-hydroxylase, *CYP* cytochrome p450, *HO* heme oxygenase, *IAP* inhibitor-of-apoptosis protein, *PKC* protein kinase C, *PKD* protein kinase D, *LOX* lipoxygenase, *VEGF* vascular endothelial growth factor, *PSA* prostate-specific antigen, molecules, *GST* glutathione *S*-transferase, *MMP* matrix metalloprotease

factor signaling pathways (Aggarwal and Shishodia 2006; Beltz et al. 2006; Dashwood 2007; Nichenametla et al. 2006). In the recent years, many studies have showed that molecular targets of polyphenols for not only prevention but also for therapy of cancers (Fig. 10.13). NF-κB is a family of closely related protein dimers that bind to a common sequence motif in DNA called the κB site (Aggarwal 2004; Shishodia and Aggarwal 2004b). The identification of the p50 subunit of NF-κB as a member of the reticuloendotheliosis (REL) family of viruses provided the first evidence that NF-κB is linked to cancer. Under resting condition, the NF-κB dimers reside in the cytoplasm. NF-κB is activated by free radicals, inflammatory stimuli, cytokines, carcinogens, tumor promoters, endotoxins, γ-radiation, ultraviolet (UV) light, and X-rays (Shishodia and Aggarwal 2004b; Zheng et al. 2004). Upon activation, it is translocated to the nucleus, where it induces the expression of more than 200 genes that have been shown to suppress apoptosis and induce cellular transformation, proliferation, invasion, metastasis, chemo-resistance, radio-resistance, and inflammation (Shishodia and Aggarwal 2004a). Many of the target

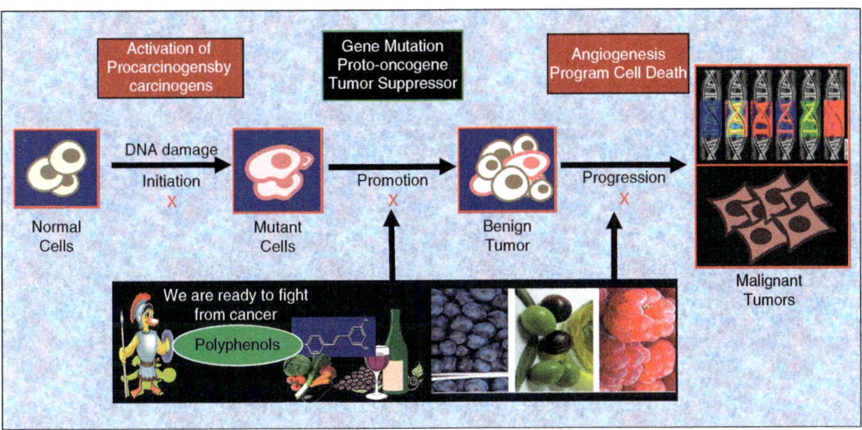

Fig. 10.12 Preventive effects of dietary polyphenols by inhibiting various stages of tumorigenesis

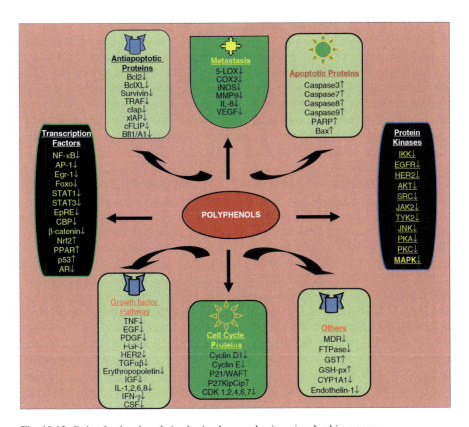

Fig. 10.13 Role of polypohenols in altering key mechanisms involved in cancer

genes that are activated are critical to the establishment of the early and late stages of aggressive cancers, including expression of cyclin D1, apoptosis suppressor proteins such as Bcl-2 and Bcl-X_L and those required for metastasis and angiogenesis, such as matrix metalloproteases (MMP) and vascular endothelial growth factor (VEGF).

Several dietary agents like curcumin (Singh and Aggarwal 1995), resveratrol (Manna et al. 2000), ellagic acid (Chainy et al. 2000), green tea catechins (Augustin et al. 2008) are natural chemopreventive agents that have been found to be potent inhibitors of NF-κB (Table 10.2). How these agents suppress NF-κB activation is becoming increasingly apparent. These inhibitors may block any one or more steps in the NF-κB signaling pathway such as the signals that activate the NF-κB signaling cascade, translocation of NF-κB into the nucleus, DNA binding of the dimers, or interactions with the basal transcriptional machinery. To investigate the inhibitory and apoptosis-inducing effects of flavonoids from oil-removed seeds *of Hippophae rhamnoides* (FSH) on liver cancer cell line BEL-7402. FSH has potent inhibitive effect on BEL-7402 cell line in a concentration-dependent manner. BEL-7402 cells exhibit typical morphological alteration of apoptosis when sub-Gl peak can be seen. FSH exerts its inhibitory effect on BEL-7402 cells by inducing apoptosis (Sun et al. 2003). AP-1 was originally identified by its binding to a DNA sequence in the SV40 enhancer [125]. Many stimuli, most notably serum, growth factors, and oncoproteins, are potent inducers of AP-1 activity; it is also induced by TNF and Interleukin 1 (IL-1), as well as by a variety of environmental stresses, such as UV radiation (Eferl and Wagner 2003). AP-1 has been implicated in regulation of genes involved in apoptosis and proliferation and may promote cell proliferation by activating the *cyclin D1* gene, and repressing tumor-suppressor genes, such as p53, p21cip1/waf1 and p16.

Several polyphenols such as green tea catechins (Dong 2000), quercetin (Lagarrigue et al. 1995; Srivastava et al. 2011; Tang et al. 2010), and resveratrol (Manna et al. 2000), have been shown to suppress the AP-1 activation process. Epicatechin-3-gallate (EGCG) and theaflavins inhibit TPA- and epidermal growth factor-induced transformation of JB6 mouse epidermal cells (Chen et al. 1999). This finding correlates with the inhibition of AP-1 DNA binding and transcriptional activity. The inhibition of AP-1 activity by EGCG was associated with inhibition of JNK activation but not ERK activation. Interestingly, in another study where EGCG blocked the UVB-induced c-Fos activation in a human keratinocyte cell line HaCaT, inhibition of p38 activation was suggested as the major mechanism underlying the effects of EGCG (Chen et al. 1999; Chung et al. 2001). The role of MAPK pathways in the regulation of AP-1 activity by EGCG has been further investigated (Chung et al. 2001). Treatment of Ha-ras-transformed human bronchial cells with EGCG has been shown to inhibit c-Jun and ERK1/2 phosphorylation as well as the phosphorylation of ELK1 and MEK1/2 (Yang et al. 2000). In contrast to these reports, EGCG has been shown to markedly increase AP-1 factor-associated responses through a MAPK signaling mechanism in normal human keratinocytes, suggesting that the signaling mechanism of EGCG action could be markedly different in different cell types (Balasubramanian et al. 2002). Lagarrigue et al. showed that the flavonoid quercetin could inhibit the transformation of the rat liver epithelial cell line overexpressing c-Fos, suggesting that regulation of c-Fos/AP-1 complexes might be involved in the antitransforming mechanism of quercetin (Wadsworth et al. 2001). Pretreatment of RAW 264.7 macrophages with quercetin blocked LPS-induced TNF transcription. This effect of quercetin was mediated by inhibiting the phosphorylation and activation of JNK/stress-activated protein kinase, by suppressing AP-1 DNA binding, and by down-regulating TNF transcription (Wadsworth et al. 2001). Resveratrol has been shown to inhibit the activity of AP-1 as demonstrated by several studies. We have found that resveratrol inhibits TNF-dependent AP-1 activation in U-937 cells, and that pretreatment with resveratrol strongly attenuates TNF-activated JNK and MEK kinases (Singh and Aggarwal 1995).

Cyclin D1, a component subunit of cyclin-dependent kinase (Cdk)-4 and Cdk6, is a rate-limiting factor in progression of cells through the first gap (G1) phase of the cell cycle (Baldin et al. 1993). Dysregulation of the cell cycle check points and overexpression of growth-promoting cell cycle factors such as cyclin D1 and cyclin-dependent kinases (CDK) are associated with tumorigenesis (Sikkema et al. 2011). Several dietary agents including resveratrol, genistein, apigenin, and silibinin have been shown to block the deregulated cell cycle in cancers (Aggarwal and Shishodia 2006; Araujo et al. 2011). The green tea component EGCG causes cell cycle arrest and promotes apoptosis via a dose- and time-dependent up-regulation of p21/Cip1/Waf1, p27Kip1, and p16/INK4A, and down-regulation of proteins such as cyclin D1, cyclin E, Cdk2, and Cdk4 (Gupta et al. 2000).

In liver cancer cells (HepG2), EGCG has been shown to induce apoptosis and block cell cycle progression at G1 (Kuo and Lin 2003). These effects were accompanied by increased expression of p53 and p21/WAF1 proteins and proapoptotic Fas and Bax proteins. The serine/threonine protein kinase Akt/PKB is the cellular homologue of the viral oncogene v-Akt and is activated by various growth and survival factors. Activated Akt promotes cell survival by activating the NF-κB signaling pathway and by inhibiting apoptosis through inactivation of several proapoptotic factors including Bad, Forkhead transcription factors, Foxo and caspase-9 (Brunet et al. 1999; Ozes et al. 1999). Several phytochemicals including genistein, and EGCG are known to suppress the activation of Akt (Li and Sarkar 2002; Shi et al. 2006).

p53 is a tumor-suppressor and transcription factor. It is a critical regulator in many cellular processes including cell signal transduction, cellular response to DNA-damage, genomic stability, cell cycle control, and apoptosis. The protein activates the transcription of downstream genes such as p21/WAF1 and Bax to induce the apoptotic process, inhibiting the growth of cells with damaged DNA or cancer cells (el-Deiry et al. 1993). Some of the polyphenols that are known to modulate p53 activity are resveratrol (Huang et al. 1999), EGCG (Kuo and Lin 2003), and silibinin (Gu et al. 2005). Apoptosis and the expression of the non-steroidal anti-inflammatory drug-activated gene-1 (NAG-1), a member of the TGFβ superfamily that has been associated with proapoptotic and antitumorigenic activities, is induced by resveratrol-induced NAG-1 expression through an increase in the expression of p53 (Baek et al. 2002). In a human liver cancer cell line, EGCG also significantly increased the expression of p53 and p21WAF1 protein, and this contributed to cell cycle arrest (Kuo and Lin 2003). Several studies examined the potential effects of PPs on the proliferation and induction of apoptosis in human prostate cancer cell lines with different p53 status. They found that induction of apoptosis by I3C was p53-independent (Nachshon-Kedmi et al. 2003), and induction of p21WAF1 expression by DIM was independent of estrogen-receptor signaling and p53 (Chen et al. 2001a). Growth factors are proteins such as epidermal growth factor (EGF), platelet-derived growth factor (PDGF), fibroblast growth factors (FGFs), transforming growth factors (TGF)-α and -β, erythropoietin (Epo), insulin-like growth factor (IGF), interleukin (IL)-1, 2, 6, 8, tumor necrosis factor (TNF), interferon-γ (INF-γ) and colony-stimulating factors (CSFs) that bind to receptors on the cell surface, with the primary result of activating cellular proliferation and/or differentiation. Several chemopreventive phytochemicals including genistein, resveratrol, and catechins have been shown to be potent inhibitors of several growth factor signaling pathways.

TNF, initially discovered as a result of its antitumor activity, has now been shown to mediate tumor initiation, promotion, and metastasis (Aggarwal 2003). In agreement with these observations, mice deficient in TNF have been shown to be resistant to skin carcinogenesis (Moore et al. 1999). The induction of proinflammatory genes by TNF has been linked to most diseases. Phytochemicals such as green tea polyphenols (Yang et al. 1998), resveratrol, kaempferol and apigenin (Kowalski et al. 2005) have been shown to suppress TNF production. Green tea polyphenols are potent antioxidants that demonstrate both anti-cancer and anti-inflammatory effects. EGCG, the major green tea polyphenol, have been shown to down-regulate LPS-induced TNF production in a dose-dependent fashion (Yang et al. 1998). Flavonoids have been reported to bring benefits in lowering inflammation and oxidative stress and exert positive effects in cancer and cardiovascular and chronic inflammatory diseases. Apigenin, kaempferol, and resveratrol, which are present in fruits, vegetables, and grains, exert inhibitory effects on the expression of TNF (Kowalski et al. 2005).

Cyclooxygenases are prostaglandin H synthase, which convert arachidonic acid released by membrane phospholipids into prostaglandins. Two isoforms of prostaglandin H synthase, COX-1 and COX-2, have been identified. COX-1 is constitutively expressed in many tissues, but the expression of COX-2 is regulated by mitogens, tumor promoters, cytokines, and growth factors. COX-2 is overexpressed in practically every premalignant and malignant condition involving the colon, liver, pancreas, breast, lung, bladder, skin, stomach, head and neck, and esophagus (Subbaramaiah and Dannenberg 2003). Several dietary components including galangin, luteolin (Baumann et al. 1980), apigenin (Landolfi et al. 1984), 6-hydroxykaempferol, quercetagenin (Williams et al. 1999), genistein (Mutoh et al. 2000), wogonin (Chen et al. 2001b), green tea catechins (Gerhauser et al. 2003), and resveratrol (Subbaramaiah et al. 1998) have been shown to suppress COX-2. LOXs are the enzymes responsible for generating leukotrienes (LT) from arachidonic acid. There are three types of LOX isozymes depending upon the different cells and tissues they affect. 15-LOX synthesizes anti-inflammatory 15-HETE; 12-LOX is involved in provoking inflammatory/allergic disorders; and 5-LOX produces 5-HETE and LTs, which are potent chemoattractants and lead to the development of asthma. Aberrant arachidonic acid metabolism is involved in the inflammatory and carcinogenic processes. Several dietary agents known to suppress LOX are green and black tea polyphenols (Hong et al. 2001), resveratrol (MacCarrone et al. 1999), and flavonols (Laughton et al. 1991). Flavonols, including kaempferol, quercetin, morin, and myricetin, were found to be potent inhibitors of 5-LOX (Laughton et al. 1991).

The concept of cancer prevention using naturally occurring substances that could be included in the diet has gained increased attention. After water, tea is the most popular beverage worldwide and is grown in about 30 countries. All types of tea, including black, green and red (oolong), contain polyphenols with antioxidant properties (Mukhtar and Ahmad 1999). Green tea is the least processed and most of the polyphenols in green tea are flavanols, commonly known as catechins. The main catechins in green tea are epicatechin, and EGCG. During fermentation of green tea, the polyphenols are oxidized to theaflavins and thearubigins, which are the main polyphenols of black tea (Yanagida et al. 2006). Several epidemiological and experimental studies have shown the preventive effects of tea consumption against various diseases including atherosclerosis (Zaveri 2006), cardiovascular diseases, and neurological diseases (Dryden et al. 2006; Shankar et al. 2008; Tang et al. 2010). There are also abundant data, from several laboratories and epidemiological studies performed during the past 10 years, that provide strong evidences that polyphenolic antioxidants present in tea reduce the risk of cancer in many animal-tumor bioassay system esophagus, liver (Zaveri 2006) cancers induced by chemical carcinogens. Green and black teas have shown cancer chemopreventive activity against ultraviolet light irradiation, as well as in chemically induced and genetic models of cancer, such as cancer of the skin, lung, prostate, bladder, liver, colon, oral cavity, esophagus, stomach, small intestine, and pancreas (Lambert and Yang 2003). The antidotal capability of rats' livers can be significantly improved after long-term consumption of tea polyphenols. There are differences in changes of drug-metabolizing enzymes between the sexes induced by tea polyphenols and normal condition (Liu et al. 2003). EGCG and theaflavins are responsible for most cancer chemopreventive properties of tea (Mukhtar and Ahmad 1999). A significant reduction in the number of proliferating cells (Mu et al. 2003) and an increased number of apoptotic cells was found after treatment with the aflavins and EGCG in benzo(a) pyrene (B(a)P)-exposed mice (Banerjee et al. 2005). A study on animals and human cell lines demonstrated tea polyphenols ability to modulate signaling pathways, which have an important role in the prevention of cancer. Studies in rat liver have shown that tea polyphenols inhibit the production of mitochondrial ROS induced by chemical carcinogens, thereby preventing oxidative damage in the liver (Lambert and Yang 2003). As bioactivation of the precarcinogens and detoxification of carcinogens are mainly performed by hepatic metabolizing enzymes, and previous studies investigated modulation of enzyme activities after tea consumption in animal models (Kalra et al. 2005). It was shown that tea consumption provides protection by modulating the expression of both phase I and phase II hepatic drug metabolizing enzymes in Wistar rats (Maliakal et al. 2001). Cytochrome P450 (CYPs) are mainly expressed in the liver, except CYP1A1 and CYP1B1, which are extrahepatic isoenzymes in humans. Polyphenols' beneficial effects have been also attributed to their competitive inhibition of enzymes such as CYPs. Indeed, black tea polyphenols have been reported to inhibit the benzo(a)pyrene-induced activity and levels of cytochrome P4501A1 and 1A2 in mouse liver and lungs (Krishnan et al. 2005).

A cross-sectional study in Japanese men showed that increased consumption of green tea may also protect against liver disorders by reducing concentrations of hepatological markers in the serum (Imai and Nakachi 1995). Tea catechins, black tea extract and oolong tea extract (0.05% or 0.1%) significantly decreased the number and area of preneoplastic glutathione-S-transferase placental form (GST-P)-positive foci in the hepatocarcinogenesis model induced by NDEA in the male F344 rat liver. demonstrated the protective role of tea polyphenols on the development of DEN-induced altered hepatic foci (AHF) in a rat medium-term bioassay has been demonstrated, indicating that polyphenols may prevent cancer at an early stage of rat liver carcinogenesis (Srivastava et al. 2008). These results also indicate that GTP is more effective than BTP in modulation of NDEA + 2-acetyl aminofluorene (2-AAF)-induced AHF at the tested doses. Dietary administration of black tea polyphenols effectively suppressed ρ-dimethylaminoazobenzene (DAB)-induced hepatocarcinogenesis, as evidenced by reduced preneoplastic and neoplastic lesions, modulation of xenobiotic-metabolizing enzymes and amelioration of oxidative stress (Srivastava et al. 2008). Thus, it can be concluded that black tea polyphenols acts as an effective chemopreventive agent by modulating xenobiotic-metabolizing enzymes and mitigating oxidative stress in an *in vivo* model of hepatocarcinogenesis.

Few studies have evaluated the chemopreventive effects of resveratrol against liver cancer. Carbo et al. (1999) demonstrated that resveratrol administration to rats inoculated with a fast growing tumour (the Yoshida AH-130 ascites hepatoma) caused a very significant decrease (25%) in the tumor cell content. This effect was found to be associated with an increase in the number of cells in the G2/M phase of the cell cycle. Interestingly, flow cytometric analysis of the tumor cell population revealed the existence of an aneuploid peak (representing 28% of total), which suggested that resveratrol causes apoptosis in the tumor cell population resulting in a decreased cell number. Resveratrol inhibited the growth of hepatoma cells line H22 in a dose- and time-dependent manner via the induction of apoptosis (Sun et al. 2002). Some studied have shown that *trans*-resveratrol decreased hepatocyte growth factor-induced cell scattering and invasion (De Ledinghen et al. 2001). However, *trans*-resveratrol did not: (i), decrease the level of the hepatocyte growth factor receptor c-met; (ii), impede the hepatocyte growth factor induced increase in c-met precursor synthesis; (iii), decrease hepatocyte growth factor-induced c-met autophosphorylation, or Akt-1 or extracellular-regulated kinases-1 and -2 activation; (iv), decrease urokinase expression; and (v), block the catalytic activity of urokinase. It was also demonstrated that *trans*resveratrol decreases hepatocyte growth factor-induced HepG2 cell invasion by an as yet unidentified post-receptor mechanism (Kozuki et al. 2001). Resveratrol suppressed the invasion of the hepatoma cells even at low concentrations. Sera from rats orally given resveratrol restrained only the invasion of AH109A cells.

Resveratrol and resveratrol-loaded rat serum suppressed reactive oxygen species-mediated invasive capacity. The antiinvasive activity of resveratrol was found to be independent of the anti-proliferative activity (Chen et al. 2010; Ganapathy et al. 2010; Kozuki et al. 2001; Shankar et al. 2007a, b, c, 2011; Srivastava et al. 2010). Ciolino and Yeh (2001) examined the effect of resveratrol on the function of the aryl hydrocarbon receptor (AHR) and the transcription of CYP1A1 in human HepG2 hepatoma cells. Resveratrol was found to inhibit the increase in CYP1A1 mRNA caused by the AHR ligand 2,3,7,8-tetrachlorodibenzo-p-dioxin (TCDD) in a concentration-dependent fashion. The induction of transcription of an aryl hydrocarbon-responsive reporter vector containing the CYP1A1 promoter by TCDD was also inhibited by resveratrol (Beedanagari et al. 2009). Resveratrol was also found to inhibit the constitutive level of CYP1A1 mRNA and reporter vector transcription in HepG2 cells. The increase in CYP1A1 enzyme activity induced by TCDD was inhibited by resveratrol. Further, resveratrol was found to prevent TCDD-induced transformation of the cytosolic AHR to its nuclear DNA binding form (Beedanagari et al. 2009). These data demonstrated that resveratrol inhibits CYP1A1 expression *in vitro*, by preventing the binding of the AHR to promoter sequences that regulate CYP1A1 transcription (Beedanagari et al. 2009). This activity was suggested to be important for the chemopreventive activity of resveratrol. Ciolino et al. (1998) also investigated the effect of resveratrol, on the carcinogen activation pathway regulated by the aryl hydrocarbon receptor.

Resveratrol inhibited the metabolism of the environmental aryl hydrocarbon benzo[a]pyrene (B[a]P) catalyzed by microsomes isolated from B[a]P-treated human hepatoma HepG2 cells (Chang et al. 2001). Resveratrol was found to inhibit, in a concentration-dependent manner, the activity of CYP1A1/CYP1A2 in microsomes and intact HepG2 cells. Resveratrol inhibited the B[a]P-induced expression of the CYP1A1 gene, as measured at the mRNA and transcriptional levels. Resveratrol also abolished the binding of B[a]P-activated nuclear aryl hydrocarbon receptor to the xenobiotic-responsive element of the CYP1A1 promoter but did not bind to the receptor (Chang et al. 2001). These data demonstrated that resveratrol inhibits aryl hydrocarbon-induced CYP1A activity *in vitro* by directly inhibiting CYP1A1/CYP1A2 enzyme activity and by inhibiting the signal transduction pathway that up-regulates the expression of carcinogen activating enzymes (Chang et al. 2001).

Conclusion

From this discussion it is clear that numerous PPs in fruits, vegetables, herbs and medicinal plants can interfere with multiple cell-signaling pathways. These compounds with strong antioxidant activity can be used either in their natural form for the prevention and perhaps in their pure form for the therapy for liver cancer, where large doses may be needed. While these PPs are pharmacologically safe in most situations, one of the concerns commonly expressed is the lack of bioavailability. Experience again indicates that these agents exhibit bioresponse at serum concentrations that are insufficient to demonstrate in vitro response; thus suggesting that their bioavailability should not be evaluated in the same manner as synthetic compounds. Most modern medicines currently available for treating liver cancers are very expensive, toxic, and less effective in treating the disease. Thus, one must investigate further in detail the agents derived from natural sources, described traditionally, for the prevention and treatment of liver cancer and disease. More clinical trials are also needed to validate the usefulness of these agents either alone or in combination with existing therapy.

Acknowledgements This work was supported in part by the grants from the National Institutes of Health (R01CA125262, RO1CA114469 and RO1CA125262-02S1) and Kansas Bioscience Authority.

References

Aggarwal BB (2003) Signalling pathways of the TNF superfamily: a double-edged sword. Nat Rev Immunol 3:745–756

Aggarwal BB (2004) Nuclear factor-kappaB: the enemy within. Cancer Cell 6:203–208

Aggarwal BB, Shishodia S (2006) Molecular targets of dietary agents for prevention and therapy of cancer. Biochem Pharmacol 71:1397–1421

Araujo JR, Goncalves P, Martel F (2011) Chemopreventive effect of dietary polyphenols in colorectal cancer cell lines. Nutr Res 31:77–87

Augustin K, Blank R, Boesch-Saadatmandi C, Frank J, Wolffram S, Rimbach G (2008) Dietary green tea polyphenols do not affect vitamin E status, antioxidant capacity and meat quality of growing pigs. J Anim Physiol Anim Nutr (Berl) 92:705–711

Baek SJ, Wilson LC, Eling TE (2002) Resveratrol enhances the expression of non-steroidal anti-inflammatory drug-activated gene (NAG-1) by increasing the expression of p53. Carcinogenesis 23:425–434

Balasubramanian S, Efimova T, Eckert RL (2002) Green tea polyphenol stimulates a Ras, MEKK1, MEK3, and p38 cascade to increase activator protein 1 factor-dependent involucrin gene expression in normal human keratinocytes. J Biol Chem 277:1828–1836

Baldin V, Lukas J, Marcote MJ, Pagano M, Draetta G (1993) Cyclin D1 is a nuclear protein required for cell cycle progression in G1. Genes Dev 7:812–821

Banerjee S, Manna S, Saha P, Panda CK, Das S (2005) Black tea polyphenols suppress cell proliferation and induce apoptosis during benzo(a)pyrene-induced lung carcinogenesis. Eur J Cancer Prev 14:215–221

Baumann J, von Bruchhausen F, Wurm G (1980) Flavonoids and related compounds as inhibition of arachidonic acid peroxidation. Prostaglandins 20:627–639

Beedanagari SR, Bebenek I, Bui P, Hankinson O (2009) Resveratrol inhibits dioxin-induced expression of human CYP1A1 and CYP1B1 by inhibiting recruitment of the aryl hydrocarbon receptor complex and RNA polymerase II to the regulatory regions of the corresponding genes. Toxicol Sci 110:61–67

Beltz LA, Bayer DK, Moss AL, Simet IM (2006) Mechanisms of cancer prevention by green and black tea polyphenols. Anticancer Agents Med Chem 6:389–406

Bennani H, Drissi A, Giton F, Kheuang L, Fiet J, Adlouni A (2007) Antiproliferative effect of polyphenols and sterols of virgin argan oil on human prostate cancer cell lines. Cancer Detect Prev 31:64–69

Brunet A, Bonni A, Zigmond MJ, Lin MZ, Juo P, Hu LS, Anderson MJ, Arden KC, Blenis J, Greenberg ME (1999) Akt promotes cell survival by phosphorylating and inhibiting a Forkhead transcription factor. Cell 96:857–868

Carbo N, Costelli P, Baccino FM, Lopez-Soriano FJ, Argiles JM (1999) Resveratrol, a natural product present in wine, decreases tumour growth in a rat tumour model. Biochem Biophys Res Commun 254:739–743

Chainy GB, Manna SK, Chaturvedi MM, Aggarwal BB (2000) Anethole blocks both early and late cellular responses transduced by tumor necrosis factor: effect on NF-kappaB, AP-1, JNK, MAPKK and apoptosis. Oncogene 19:2943–2950

Chang TK, Chen J, Lee WB (2001) Differential inhibition and inactivation of human CYP1 enzymes by trans-resveratrol: evidence for mechanism-based inactivation of CYP1A2. J Pharmacol Exp Ther 299:874–882

Chen W, Dong Z, Valcic S, Timmermann BN, Bowden GT (1999) Inhibition of ultraviolet B–induced c-fos gene expression and p38 mitogen-activated protein kinase activation by (-)-epigallocatechin gallate in a human keratinocyte cell line. Mol Carcinog 24:79–84

Chen DZ, Qi M, Auborn KJ, Carter TH (2001a) Indole-3-carbinol and diindolylmethane induce apoptosis of human cervical cancer cells and in murine HPV16-transgenic preneoplastic cervical epithelium. J Nutr 131:3294–3302

Chen YC, Shen SC, Chen LG, Lee TJ, Yang LL (2001b) Wogonin, baicalin, and baicalein inhibition of inducible nitric oxide synthase and cyclooxygenase-2 gene expressions induced by nitric oxide synthase inhibitors and lipopolysaccharide. Biochem Pharmacol 61:1417–1427

Chen Q, Ganapathy S, Singh KP, Shankar S, Srivastava RK (2010) Resveratrol induces growth arrest and apoptosis through activation of FOXO transcription factors in prostate cancer cells. PLoS One 5:e15288

Chung JY, Park JO, Phyu H, Dong Z, Yang CS (2001) Mechanisms of inhibition of the Ras-MAP kinase signaling pathway in 30.7b Ras 12 cells by tea polyphenols (-)-epigallocatechin-3-gallate and theaflavin-3,3′-digallate. FASEB J 15:2022–2024

Ciolino HP, Yeh GC (2001) The effects of resveratrol on CYP1A1 expression and aryl hydrocarbon receptor function in vitro. Adv Exp Med Biol 492:183–193

Ciolino HP, Daschner PJ, Yeh GC (1998) Resveratrol inhibits transcription of CYP1A1 in vitro by preventing activation of the aryl hydrocarbon receptor. Cancer Res 58:5707–5712

Coates EM, Popa G, Gill CI, McCann MJ, McDougall GJ, Stewart D, Rowland I (2007) Colon-available raspberry polyphenols exhibit anti-cancer effects on in vitro models of colon cancer. J Carcinog 6:4

Covas MI, Nyyssonen K, Poulsen HE, Kaikkonen J, Zunft HJ, Kiesewetter H, Gaddi A, de la Torre R, Mursu J, Baumler H, Nascetti S, Salonen JT, Fito M, Virtanen J, Marrugat J (2006) The effect of polyphenols in olive oil on heart disease risk factors: a randomized trial. Ann Intern Med 145:333–341

D'Alessandro T, Prasain J, Benton MR, Botting N, Moore R, Darley-Usmar V, Patel R, Barnes S (2003) Polyphenols, inflammatory response, and cancer prevention: chlorination of isoflavones by human neutrophils. J Nutr 133:3773S–3777S

D'Archivio M, Santangelo C, Scazzocchio B, Vari R, Filesi C, Masella R, Giovannini C (2008) Modulatory effects of polyphenols on apoptosis induction: relevance for cancer prevention. Int J Mol Sci 9:213–228

Dai GJ, Jin HY, Ding YJ, Xia JG, Liu XF, Liu F, Tan XZ, Geng JX (2008) Anticancer effects of tea polyphenols on colorectal cancer with microsatellite instability in nude mice. Zhong Xi Yi Jie He Xue Bao 6:1263–1266

Dashwood RH (2007) Frontiers in polyphenols and cancer prevention. J Nutr 137:267S–269S

De Ledinghen V, Monvoisin A, Neaud V, Krisa S, Payrastre B, Bedin C, Desmouliere A, Bioulac-Sage P, Rosenbaum J (2001) Trans-resveratrol, a grapevine-derived polyphenol, blocks hepatocyte growth factor-induced invasion of hepatocellular carcinoma cells. Int J Oncol 19:83–88

Delgado ME, Haza AI, Arranz N, Garcia A, Morales P (2008) Dietary polyphenols protect against N-nitrosamines and benzo(a)pyrene-induced DNA damage (strand breaks and oxidized purines/pyrimidines) in HepG2 human hepatoma cells. Eur J Nutr 47:479–490

Dong Z (2000) Effects of food factors on signal transduction pathways. Biofactors 12:17–28

Dryden GW, Song M, McClain C (2006) Polyphenols and gastrointestinal diseases. Curr Opin Gastroenterol 22:165–170

Duthie GG, Duthie SJ, Kyle JA (2000) Plant polyphenols in cancer and heart disease: implications as nutritional antioxidants. Nutr Res Rev 13:79–106

Edderkaoui M, Odinokova I, Ohno I, Gukovsky I, Go VL, Pandol SJ, Gukovskaya AS (2008) Ellagic acid induces apoptosis through inhibition of nuclear factor kappa B in pancreatic cancer cells. World J Gastroenterol 14:3672–3680

Eferl R, Wagner EF (2003) AP-1: a double-edged sword in tumorigenesis. Nat Rev Cancer 3: 859–868

el-Deiry WS, Tokino T, Velculescu VE, Levy DB, Parsons R, Trent JM, Lin D, Mercer WE, Kinzler KW, Vogelstein B (1993) WAF1, a potential mediator of p53 tumor suppression. Cell 75: 817–825

Ganapathy S, Chen Q, Singh KP, Shankar S, Srivastava RK (2010) Resveratrol enhances antitumor activity of TRAIL in prostate cancer xenografts through activation of FOXO transcription factor. PLoS One 5:e15627

Gerhauser C, Klimo K, Heiss E, Neumann I, Gamal-Eldeen A, Knauft J, Liu GY, Sitthimonchai S, Frank N (2003) Mechanism-based in vitro screening of potential cancer chemopreventive agents. Mutat Res 523–524:163–172

Gorlach S, Wagner W, Podsedek A, Sosnowska D, Dastych J, Koziolkiewicz M (2011) Polyphenols from Evening Primrose (Oenothera paradoxa) Defatted Seeds Induce Apoptosis in Human Colon Cancer Caco-2 Cells. J Agric Food Chem 59(13):6985–6997

Gu M, Dhanalakshmi S, Mohan S, Singh RP, Agarwal R (2005) Silibinin inhibits ultraviolet B radiation-induced mitogenic and survival signaling, and associated biological responses in SKH-1 mouse skin. Carcinogenesis 26:1404–1413

Gupta S, Ahmad N, Nieminen AL, Mukhtar H (2000) Growth inhibition, cell-cycle dysregulation, and induction of apoptosis by green tea constituent (-)-epigallocatechin-3-gallate in androgen-sensitive and androgen-insensitive human prostate carcinoma cells. Toxicol Appl Pharmacol 164:82–90

Harborne JB, Sherratt HS (1961) Plant polyphenols. 3. Flavonoids in genotypes of Primula sinensis. Biochem J 78:298–306

Harborne JB, Williams CA (2001) Anthocyanins and other flavonoids. Nat Prod Rep 18:310–333

Hong J, Smith TJ, Ho CT, August DA, Yang CS (2001) Effects of purified green and black tea polyphenols on cyclooxygenase- and lipoxygenase-dependent metabolism of arachidonic acid in human colon mucosa and colon tumor tissues. Biochem Pharmacol 62:1175–1183

Huang C, Ma WY, Goranson A, Dong Z (1999) Resveratrol suppresses cell transformation and induces apoptosis through a p53-dependent pathway. Carcinogenesis 20:237–242

Hung MW, Shiao MS, Tsai LC, Chang GG, Chang TC (2003) Apoptotic effect of caffeic acid phenethyl ester and its ester and amide analogues in human cervical cancer ME180 cells. Anticancer Res 23:4773–4780

Imai K, Nakachi K (1995) Cross sectional study of effects of drinking green tea on cardiovascular and liver diseases. BMJ 310:693–696

Inglett GE, Chen D (2011) Contents of phenolics and flavonoids and antioxidant activities in skin, pulp, and seeds of miracle fruit. J Food Sci 76:C479–C482

Ivanova D, Gerova D, Chervenkov T, Yankova T (2005) Polyphenols and antioxidant capacity of Bulgarian medicinal plants. J Ethnopharmacol 96:145–150

Kalra N, Prasad S, Shukla Y (2005) Antioxidant potential of black tea against 7,12-dimethylbenz(a)anthracene- induced oxidative stress in Swiss albino mice. J Environ Pathol Toxicol Oncol 24:105–114

Kampa M, Hatzoglou A, Notas G, Damianaki A, Bakogeorgou E, Gemetzi C, Kouroumalis E, Martin PM, Castanas E (2000) Wine antioxidant polyphenols inhibit the proliferation of human prostate cancer cell lines. Nutr Cancer 37:223–233

Katiyar SK, Vaid M, van Steeg H, Meeran SM (2010) Green tea polyphenols prevent UV-induced immunosuppression by rapid repair of DNA damage and enhancement of nucleotide excision repair genes. Cancer Prev Res (Phila) 3:179–189

Korkina LG, De Luca C, Kostyuk VA, Pastore S (2009) Plant polyphenols and tumors: from mechanisms to therapies, prevention, and protection against toxicity of anti-cancer treatments. Curr Med Chem 16:3943–3965

Kowalski J, Samojedny A, Paul M, Pietsz G, Wilczok T (2005) Effect of apigenin, kaempferol and resveratrol on the expression of interleukin-1beta and tumor necrosis factor-alpha genes in J774.2 macrophages. Pharmacol Rep 57:390–394

Kozuki Y, Miura Y, Yagasaki K (2001) Resveratrol suppresses hepatoma cell invasion independently of its anti-proliferative action. Cancer Lett 167:151–156

Krishnan R, Raghunathan R, Maru GB (2005) Effect of polymeric black tea polyphenols on benzo(a)pyrene [B(a)P]-induced cytochrome P4501A1 and 1A2 in mice. Xenobiotica 35: 671–682

Kuhnau J (1976) The flavonoids. A class of semi-essential food components: their role in human nutrition. World Rev Nutr Diet 24:117–191

Kuo PL, Lin CC (2003) Green tea constituent (-)-epigallocatechin-3-gallate inhibits Hep G2 cell proliferation and induces apoptosis through p53-dependent and Fas-mediated pathways. J Biomed Sci 10:219–227

Lagarrigue S, Chaumontet C, Heberden C, Martel P, Gaillard-Sanchez I (1995) Suppression of oncogene-induced transformation by quercetin and retinoic acid in rat liver epithelial cells. Cell Mol Biol Res 41:551–560

Lambert JD, Yang CS (2003) Mechanisms of cancer prevention by tea constituents. J Nutr 133:3262S–3267S

Landolfi R, Mower RL, Steiner M (1984) Modification of platelet function and arachidonic acid metabolism by bioflavonoids. Structure-activity relations. Biochem Pharmacol 33:1525–1530

Laughton MJ, Evans PJ, Moroney MA, Hoult JR, Halliwell B (1991) Inhibition of mammalian 5-lipoxygenase and cyclo-oxygenase by flavonoids and phenolic dietary additives. Relationship to antioxidant activity and to iron ion-reducing ability. Biochem Pharmacol 42:1673–1681

Li Y, Sarkar FH (2002) Inhibition of nuclear factor kappaB activation in PC3 cells by genistein is mediated via Akt signaling pathway. Clin Cancer Res 8:2369–2377

Lin HH, Chen JH, Chou FP, Wang CJ (2011) Protocatechuic acid inhibits cancer cell metastasis involving the down-regulation of Ras/Akt/NF-kappaB pathway and MMP-2 production by targeting RhoB activation. Br J Pharmacol 162:237–254

Liu TT, Liang NS, Li Y, Yang F, Lu Y, Meng ZQ, Zhang LS (2003) Effects of long-term tea polyphenols consumption on hepatic microsomal drug-metabolizing enzymes and liver function in Wistar rats. World J Gastroenterol 9:2742–2744

MacCarrone M, Lorenzon T, Guerrieri P, Agro AF (1999) Resveratrol prevents apoptosis in K562 cells by inhibiting lipoxygenase and cyclooxygenase activity. Eur J Biochem 265:27–34

Maliakal PP, Coville PF, Wanwimolruk S (2001) Tea consumption modulates hepatic drug metabolizing enzymes in Wistar rats. J Pharm Pharmacol 53:569–577

Manna SK, Mukhopadhyay A, Aggarwal BB (2000) Resveratrol suppresses TNF-induced activation of nuclear transcription factors NF-kappa B, activator protein-1, and apoptosis: potential role of reactive oxygen intermediates and lipid peroxidation. J Immunol 164:6509–6519

Monde A, Carbonneau MA, Michel F, Lauret C, Diabate S, Konan KE, Sess D, Cristol JP (2011) Potential health implication of in vitro human LDL-Vitamin E oxidation modulation by polyphenols deriving from Cote d'Ivoire's oil palm species. J Agric Food Chem 59(17): 9166–9171

Moore RJ, Owens DM, Stamp G, Arnott C, Burke F, East N, Holdsworth H, Turner L, Rollins B, Pasparakis M, Kollias G, Balkwill F (1999) Mice deficient in tumor necrosis factor-alpha are resistant to skin carcinogenesis. Nat Med 5:828–831

Mu LN, Zhou XF, Ding BG, Wang RH, Zhang ZF, Chen CW, Wei GR, Zhou XM, Jiang QW, Yu SZ (2003) A case-control study on drinking green tea and decreasing risk of cancers in the alimentary canal among cigarette smokers and alcohol drinkers. Zhonghua Liu Xing Bing Xue Za Zhi 24:192–195

Mukhtar H, Ahmad N (1999) Green tea in chemoprevention of cancer. Toxicol Sci 52:111–117

Mutoh M, Takahashi M, Fukuda K, Komatsu H, Enya T, Matsushima-Hibiya Y, Mutoh H, Sugimura T, Wakabayashi K (2000) Suppression by flavonoids of cyclooxygenase-2 promoter-dependent transcriptional activity in colon cancer cells: structure-activity relationship. Jpn J Cancer Res 91:686–691

Nachshon-Kedmi M, Yannai S, Haj A, Fares FA (2003) Indole-3-carbinol and 3,3′-diindolylmethane induce apoptosis in human prostate cancer cells. Food Chem Toxicol 41:745–752

Nichenametla SN, Taruscio TG, Barney DL, Exon JH (2006) A review of the effects and mechanisms of polyphenolics in cancer. Crit Rev Food Sci Nutr 46:161–183

Noda Y, Kaneyuki T, Mori A, Packer L (2002) Antioxidant activities of pomegranate fruit extract and its anthocyanidins: delphinidin, cyanidin, and pelargonidin. J Agric Food Chem 50: 166–171

Ozes ON, Mayo LD, Gustin JA, Pfeffer SR, Pfeffer LM, Donner DB (1999) NF-kappaB activation by tumour necrosis factor requires the Akt serine-threonine kinase. Nature 401:82–85

Prakash D, Suri S, Upadhyay G, Singh BN (2007) Total phenol, antioxidant and free radical scavenging activities of some medicinal plants. Int J Food Sci Nutr 58:18–28

Priego S, Feddi F, Ferrer P, Mena S, Benlloch M, Ortega A, Carretero J, Obrador E, Asensi M, Estrela JM (2008) Natural polyphenols facilitate elimination of HT-29 colorectal cancer xenografts by chemoradiotherapy: a Bcl-2- and superoxide dismutase 2-dependent mechanism. Mol Cancer Ther 7:3330–3342

Ranilla LG, Genovese MI, Lajolo FM (2007) Polyphenols and antioxidant capacity of seed coat and cotyledon from Brazilian and Peruvian bean cultivars (Phaseolus vulgaris L.). J Agric Food Chem 55:90–98

Rizvi SI, Jha R, Pandey KB (2010) Activation of erythrocyte plasma membrane redox system provides a useful method to evaluate antioxidant potential of plant polyphenols. Methods Mol Biol 594:341–348

Seyoum A, Asres K, El-Fiky FK (2006) Structure-radical scavenging activity relationships of flavonoids. Phytochemistry 67:2058–2070

Shankar S, Chen Q, Siddiqui I, Sarva K, Srivastava RK (2007a) Sensitization of TRAIL-resistant LNCaP cells by resveratrol (3, 4′, 5 tri-hydroxystilbene): molecular mechanisms and therapeutic potential. J Mol Signal 2:7

Shankar S, Siddiqui I, Srivastava RK (2007b) Molecular mechanisms of resveratrol (3,4,5-trihydroxy-trans-stilbene) and its interaction with TNF-related apoptosis inducing ligand (TRAIL) in androgen-insensitive prostate cancer cells. Mol Cell Biochem 304:273–285

Shankar S, Singh G, Srivastava RK (2007c) Chemoprevention by resveratrol: molecular mechanisms and therapeutic potential. Front Biosci 12:4839–4854

Shankar S, Ganapathy S, Hingorani SR, Srivastava RK (2008) EGCG inhibits growth, invasion, angiogenesis and metastasis of pancreatic cancer. Front Biosci 13:440–452

Shankar S, Nall D, Tang SN, Meeker D, Passarini J, Sharma J, Srivastava RK (2011) Resveratrol inhibits pancreatic cancer stem cell characteristics in human and KrasG12D transgenic mice by inhibiting pluripotency maintaining factors and epithelial-mesenchymal transition. PLoS One 6:e16530

Shi W, Li L, Shi X, Zheng F, Zeng J, Jiang X, Gong F, Zhou M, Li Z (2006) Inhibition of nuclear factor-kappaB activation is essential for membrane-associated TNF-alpha-induced apoptosis in HL-60 cells. Immunol Cell Biol 84:366–373

Shishodia S, Aggarwal BB (2004a) Nuclear factor-kappaB activation mediates cellular transformation, proliferation, invasion angiogenesis and metastasis of cancer. Cancer Treat Res 119:139–173

Shishodia S, Aggarwal BB (2004b) Nuclear factor-kappaB: a friend or a foe in cancer? Biochem Pharmacol 68:1071–1080

Sikkema AH, den Dunnen WF, Diks SH, Peppelenbosch MP, de Bont ES (2011) Optimizing targeted cancer therapy: towards clinical application of systems biology approaches. Crit Rev Oncol Hematol

Singh S, Aggarwal BB (1995) Activation of transcription factor NF-kappa B is suppressed by curcumin (diferuloylmethane) [corrected]. J Biol Chem 270:24995–25000

Singh BN, Singh BR, Sarma BK, Singh HB (2009a) Potential chemoprevention of N-nitrosodiethylamine-induced hepatocarcinogenesis by polyphenolics from Acacia nilotica bark. Chem Biol Interact 181:20–28

Singh BN, Singh BR, Singh RL, Prakash D, Sarma BK, Singh HB (2009b) Antioxidant and anti-quorum sensing activities of green pod of Acacia nilotica L. Food Chem Toxicol 47:778–786

Singh BN, Zhang G, Hwa YL, Li J, Dowdy SC, Jiang SW (2010) Nonhistone protein acetylation as cancer therapy targets. Expert Rev Anticancer Ther 10:935–954

Srivastava S, Singh M, Roy P, Prasad S, George J, Shukla Y (2008) Inhibitory effect of tea polyphenols on hepatic preneoplastic foci in Wistar rats. Invest New Drugs 27(6):526–533

Srivastava RK, Unterman TG, Shankar S (2010) FOXO transcription factors and VEGF neutralizing antibody enhance antiangiogenic effects of resveratrol. Mol Cell Biochem 337:201–212

Srivastava RK, Tang SN, Zhu W, Meeker D, Shankar S (2011) Sulforaphane synergizes with quercetin to inhibit self-renewal capacity of pancreatic cancer stem cells. Front Biosci (Elite Ed) 3:515–528

Starke H, Herrmann K (1976) The phenolics of fruits. VIII. Changes in flavonol concentrations during fruit development (authors transl). Z Lebensm Unters Forsch 161:131–135

Stoner GD, Morse MA (1997) Isothiocyanates and plant polyphenols as inhibitors of lung and esophageal cancer. Cancer Lett 114:113–119

Stoner GD, Mukhtar H (1995) Polyphenols as cancer chemopreventive agents. J Cell Biochem Suppl 22:169–180

Subbaramaiah K, Dannenberg AJ (2003) Cyclooxygenase 2: a molecular target for cancer prevention and treatment. Trends Pharmacol Sci 24:96–102

Subbaramaiah K, Chung WJ, Michaluart P, Telang N, Tanabe T, Inoue H, Jang M, Pezzuto JM, Dannenberg AJ (1998) Resveratrol inhibits cyclooxygenase-2 transcription and activity in phorbol ester-treated human mammary epithelial cells. J Biol Chem 273:21875–21882

Sun ZJ, Pan CE, Liu HS, Wang GJ (2002) Anti-hepatoma activity of resveratrol in vitro. World J Gastroenterol 8:79–81

Sun B, Zhang P, Qu W, Zhang X, Zhuang X, Yang H (2003) Study on effect of flavonoids from oil-removed seeds of Hippophae rhamnoides on inducing apoptosis of human hepatoma cell. Zhong Yao Cai 26:875–877

Tang SN, Singh C, Nall D, Meeker D, Shankar S, Srivastava RK (2010) The dietary bioflavonoid quercetin synergizes with epigallocathechin gallate (EGCG) to inhibit prostate cancer stem cell characteristics, invasion, migration and epithelial-mesenchymal transition. J Mol Signal 5:14

Tedesco I, Russo M, Russo P, Iacomino G, Russo GL, Carraturo A, Faruolo C, Moio L, Palumbo R (2000) Antioxidant effect of red wine polyphenols on red blood cells. J Nutr Biochem 11: 114–119

Terao J, Kawai Y, Murota K (2008) Vegetable flavonoids and cardiovascular disease. Asia Pac J Clin Nutr 17(Suppl 1):291–293

Wadsworth TL, McDonald TL, Koop DR (2001) Effects of Ginkgo biloba extract (EGb 761) and quercetin on lipopolysaccharide-induced signaling pathways involved in the release of tumor necrosis factor-alpha. Biochem Pharmacol 62:963–974

Wang JN, Chen YJ, Hano Y, Nomura T, Tan RX (2000) Antioxidant activity of polyphenols from seeds of Vitis amurensis in vitro. Acta Pharmacol Sin 21:633–636

Williams CA, Harborne JB, Geiger H, Hoult JR (1999) The flavonoids of Tanacetum parthenium and T. vulgare and their anti-inflammatory properties. Phytochemistry 51:417–423

Yanagida A, Shoji A, Shibusawa Y, Shindo H, Tagashira M, Ikeda M, Ito Y (2006) Analytical separation of tea catechins and food-related polyphenols by high-speed counter-current chromatography. J Chromatogr A 1112:195–201

Yang F, de Villiers WJ, McClain CJ, Varilek GW (1998) Green tea polyphenols block endotoxin-induced tumor necrosis factor-production and lethality in a murine model. J Nutr 128: 2334–2340

Yang GY, Liao J, Li C, Chung J, Yurkow EJ, Ho CT, Yang CS (2000) Effect of black and green tea polyphenols on c-jun phosphorylation and H(2)O(2) production in transformed and non-transformed human bronchial cell lines: possible mechanisms of cell growth inhibition and apoptosis induction. Carcinogenesis 21:2035–2039

You BR, Kim SZ, Kim SH, Park WH (2011) Gallic acid-induced lung cancer cell death is accompanied by ROS increase and glutathione depletion. Mol Cell Biochem 357(1–2): 295–303

Yue X, Xu Z (2008) Changes of anthocyanins, anthocyanidins, and antioxidant activity in bilberry extract during dry heating. J Food Sci 73:C494–C499

Zaveri NT (2006) Green tea and its polyphenolic catechins: medicinal uses in cancer and noncancer applications. Life Sci 78:2073–2080

Zheng B, Georgakis GV, Li Y, Bharti A, McConkey D, Aggarwal BB, Younes A (2004) Induction of cell cycle arrest and apoptosis by the proteasome inhibitor PS-341 in Hodgkin disease cell lines is independent of inhibitor of nuclear factor-kappaB mutations or activation of the CD30, CD40, and RANK receptors. Clin Cancer Res 10:3207–3215

Chapter 11
Role of Food Micro-molecules in the Prevention of Cancer

Latha Sabikhi, Alok Jha, Sudhir Kumar Tomer, and Ashish Kumar Singh

Contents

Abstract Diet is now recognized as one of the major factors contributing to the etiology of cancer. Among the several dietary components, micronutrients have attracted much attention of the scientific community worldwide. This chapter deals with the role of food micro-molecules such as dietary fibre, vitamins C, D and E, calcium, iron, folate and carotenoids on cancer. Inclusion of these micronutrients through the diet may protect an individual from the onset and prevention of cancer. Consumption of fruits and vegetables that contain vitamins, fibre and carotenoids and dairy products rich in calcium have the potential to produce folate through fermentations are recommended dietary interventions. Caution should be exercised in the consumption of iron, as excess iron content in blood may prove tumerogenic. In summary, risk of cancer may be decreased by increasing the consumption of fruits and vegetables, whole grains, dairy products, particularly fermented ones and by decreasing the intake of red meat and processed foods.

L. Sabikhi • S.K. Tomer • A.K. Singh
National Dairy Research Institute, Karnal, India

A. Jha (✉)
Centre of Food Science and Technology, Institute of Agricultural Sciences, Banaras Hindu University, Varanasi 221 005, Uttar Pradesh, India
e-mail: alok_ndri@rediffmail.com

S. Shankar and R.K. Srivastava (eds.), *Nutrition, Diet and Cancer*,
DOI 10.1007/978-94-007-2923-0_11, © Springer Science+Business Media B.V. 2012

Introduction

Cancer is predominantly a disease in the area of cell biology, owing to the disordered balance between proliferation, differentiation, and apoptosis. It is the leading cause of death throughout the world. WHO associates cancer with 84 million deaths during the decade of 2005–2015, particularly if left without remedial interventions (Strong et al. 2005). There are only 5–10% of all cancer cases due to genetic defects, the remaining 90–95% attributed to lifestyle factors (smoking, diet, alcohol, physical inactivity, obesity and exposure of sun), infections and environmental pollutants (Anand et al. 2008). The prevalence of the majority of the risk factors increases with age, particularly in women than in men. Diet is reckoned as one of the major factors contributing to the etiology of cancer (Levi et al. 2001). As it dawned that dietary components influence an individuals' vulnerability to cancer, micronutrients have attracted much attention of the scientific community worldwide.

Out of all the cancers, the cancer of alimentary tract is the main cause of morbidity and deaths across the world (Doll and Peto 1981). Of these, diet has been implicated in as many as 90% of colon cancer deaths in the United States (Se-Young et al. 2005). Most findings on the effects of diet on cancer risk have been derived from examination of the associations between dietary patterns and cancer rates in different populations around the world. While early reports register that diets high in animal products, fat and sugar as consumed in the developed Western countries are closely associated with high rates of cancer of the colorectum, breast and prostate, in developing countries with diets based on one or two starchy staple foods, low intakes of animal products, fat and sugar, higher incidences of oesophageal, stomach and liver cancers prevail (Armstrong and Doll 1975). Thus, high energy intake, low energy expenditure and obesity are major risk factors for several types of cancer, including carcinomas of the alimentary tract. Dietary factors related to cancer risk include low intakes of fruit and vegetables, calcium, and antioxidant vitamins, as well as high intakes of animal fat and sugar. Three principal classes of food-related mutagens are the heterocyclic aromatic amines (HAAs) and polycyclic aromatic amines formed during cooking (Goldman and Shields 2003) and nitrosamines formed during food processing and by action of colonic flora digestive residues of meat protein (Bingham 1999). This chapter focuses on the effect of selected micronutrients such as dietary fibre, calcium, vitamins, and some minerals (selenium, iron) on cancer.

Role of Dietary Fibre

Dietary fibre is composed of plant cell walls and components obtained from these walls. It also includes non-starch polysaccharides from sources other than plant cell walls (Harris and Ferguson 1993). Dietary fibre includes several complex materials, though all are not able to protect against cancer to the same extent. More than 95% of dietary fibre in vegetarian diets is contributed by plant cell wall, which is primarily composed of polysaccharides. The cell wall should reach colon intact for their preventive action. Dietary fibre is classified as soluble or insoluble, depending upon its solubility in buffers or water. Insoluble fibre has more significant effect on cancer than soluble ones (Jacobs 1990).

There are very early reports that suggest that the low rates of colorectal cancer in Africa were due to the high consumption of dietary fibre (Burkitt 1969). Fibre can act against cancer directly or indirectly. Direct mechanisms include increasing faecal bulk (diluting carcinogens), increasing transit time through the colon (reducing interactions of carcinogens with mucosal cells), direct binding of carcinogens like aflatoxin B1, HAAs, polycyclic aromatic hydrocarbons (PAHs) etc. (Martinez et al. 1999), which otherwise can alter DNA. Indirect mechanism, attributed to partial or total degradation of dietary fibre, includes modification of the enzyme activities of intestinal bacterial flora and production of short-chain fatty acids (SCFAs) – mainly acetic, butyric and propionic – carbon dioxide, hydrogen, methane and water (Kobayashi and Fleming 2001) and altering the colonic pH (Greenwald et al. 2001).

Butyrate arrests growth by inducing cyclin-dependent kinase inhibitors (e.g. p21WAF1/Cip1), differentiation and apoptosis in colon tumour and breast cancer cell lines. In a comparative study it was reported that fermentation of oat bran produces more butyrate than wheat bran (Zoran et al. 1997). The fermentation of dietary fibre results in reduction of pH up to 6.0–6.5 and acidification of the colonic contents. The low pH increases the availability of calcium for binding to free bile and fatty acids due to the relative solubility of different forms of calcium phosphate. Decrease in pH also results in suppression of production of secondary bile acids (Newmark and Lupton 1990). Several mechanisms have been proposed for butyrate's ability to induce apoptosis, including the stimulation of histone acetylation, which enhances the production of p21WAF1/Cip1, and down-regulation of bcl-2, an oncogene that acts by blocking apoptotic cell death (Lupton 2000). Dietary fibre stimulates activity of GST (Glutathione-S-transferase) in HT29 cells and LT97 cells, thus inhibiting cell survival (Miyanishi et al. 2001). A study revealed that the dietary butyrate inhibited chemically-induced mammary cancer in rats (Belobrajdic and McIntosh 2003). The action of butyrate on cell lines depends critically on the availability of other energy sources. In the absence of glucose and pyruvate, both adenoma and carcinoma cells showed increased apoptosis. But in contrast, the same concentrations of butyrate induced apoptosis under energy-replete conditions (Singh et al. 1997).

Prebiotic fibre encourages the growth of beneficial bacteria in the gut, which reportedly boost the immune system and helps in digesting food. Foods which include prebiotic fibre are onions, garlic, leeks, beans, lentils and oats. Allium compounds in garlic and onions are thought to be particularly effective at preventing bowel cancer (Anonymous 2009). Despite limitations in methodology and variations across studies, convincing evidence exists for inverse risk associations with vegetable and fruit intake for cancers of the mouth and pharynx, oesophagus, lung and stomach (Smith-Warner and Giovannucci 1999). A study conducted in Korea on 270 cases (136 were patients either newly diagnosed with colorectal cancer or with large bowl adenomatous polyps, 134 were control with no such history). Protective associations were observed for fibre on assessment of intakes of nutrients and food groups by a semi-quantitative food frequency questionnaire and analysis by the logistic regression model (Se-Young et al. 2005).

Role of Calcium and Vitamin D

Calcium is present in a variety of foods, including whole grain cereal products, leafy vegetables, legumes, nuts, and abundantly in dairy products such as milk, yoghurt, and cheese (Hegarty et al. 1999). It is reported that calcium has protective effect against the many type of cancers, which includes ovarian, breast and prostate cancers. Relatively high intakes of calcium may reduce the risk for colorectal cancer, perhaps by forming complexes with secondary bile acids in the intestinal lumen (Anonymous 1997) or by inhibiting the hyper-proliferative effects of dietary haem (Sesink et al. 2001). Dietary calcium and ovarian cancer are inversely related according to some studies (Nordin 2000). There is also a contradictory report that there was no relationship between dietary and serum calcium (Jorde et al. 2001). Also the mechanisms of its action is not well known but the plausible pathways are the effects of calcium on apoptosis, cell growth and proliferation (Ramasamy 2006), effects of the calcium receptor (CaR) on cell proliferation and differentiation (McCarty 2000; Rodland 2004) and effects of calcium on down-regulating PTH (parathyroid) production (McCarty 2000).

At the time of bone remodelling, calcium Ca^{2+} is the main inorganic factor which releases from the osseous tissue. It is reported that Ca^{2+} acts on hematopoietic stem cells which directs them to the bone marrow where local Ca^{2+} levels are high, through the activation of the Calcium Sensing Receptor (CaSR) (Adams et al. 2006). The primary physiological role of the CaSR is the control of Ca^{2+} homeostasis by regulating PTH secretion (Brown and MacLeod 2001). It has been hypothesized that PTH may be a tumour promoter acting as a co-mitogen and anti-apoptotic factor (McCarty 2000). It also increases hepatic and osteoblastic synthesis of insulin-like growth factor-1 (IGF-1) (McCarty 2000; Coxam et al. 1992) which has strong mitogenic effects and has been implicated in the pathogenesis of ovarian and other cancers (Lukanova et al. 2002; Renehan et al. 2004). Hence, by down-regulating PTH production, calcium potentially mitigates against the mitogenic and anti-apoptotic effects of PTH.

High extracellular calcium can modulate vitamin D metabolism in favour of increased conversion to 1,25-dihydroxyvitamin D (the active form of vitamin D) which in turn may up-regulate the expression of the calcium receptor and increase intestinal calcium absorption (Peterlik et al. 2009). The decrease in dietary calcium and consumption of dairy products resulting in increased risk of prostate cancer (Grant 1999) may be due to the high circulating levels of 1,25- dihydroxyvitamin D (Giovannucci 1998). On the other hand, in a survey of men with food frequency and cancer risk questionnaires and 6.3 years of follow-up, no association was observed between dietary calcium (or animal product) intake and prostate cancer (Schuurman et al. 1999).

A study carried out to evaluate the combined effect of vitamin D3, calcium and acetyl-salicyclic acid on azoxymethane-induced crypt foci and colorectal tumours in rats revealed that the total number of ACF (aberrant crypt foci) was inversely proportional to calcium. High levels of calcium alone or in combination with 1α,25(OH)2–vitamin D_3 increased the incidence of tumour-bearing animals. 1α,25(OH)2–vitamin D_3 and acetylsalicylic acid at 5,000 ppm calcium also increased the incidence (Molck et al. 2002). Another group (Wactawski-Wende et al. 2006) conducted a randomized, double-blind, placebo-controlled trial involving 36,282 postmenopausal women from 40 Women's Health Initiative centers to study the effect of calcium and vitamin D supplementation on colo-rectal cancer. Of the total test population, 18,176 women received 500 mg of elemental calcium as calcium carbonate with 200 IU of vitamin D3 twice daily (1,000 mg of elemental calcium and 400 IU of vitamin D3) and 18,106 received a matching placebo for an average of 7 years and concluded that the supplementation had no effect on the incidence of colorectal cancer among postmenopausal women.

Role of Vitamin C and Vitamin E

The anti-oxidant action of vitamins C and E and dietary carotenoids are well documented. Although it is difficult to state with certainty that fruits and vegetables containing several of these anti-oxidants have cancer-preventive compounds, reports have suggested that these nutritional antioxidants have a major protective role against the disease owing to their ability to induce programmed cell death or apoptosis (Zimmermann et al. 2001). These antioxidants also have a synergistic effect on the action of one another, as is suggested in Table 11.1 (Borek 1997).

Because of their antioxidant properties, dietary carotenoids and vitamins C and E can neutralize reactive oxygen species, reducing oxidative DNA damage and genetic mutations and may also enhance host immunological functions (Frei 1994; Kelley and Bendich 1996). Studies in cell cultures show that vitamins C and E, along with selenium and some phytochemicals selectively induce apoptosis in cancer cells while sparing normal cells (Sigounas et al. 1997; Borek and Pardo 2002; Taper et al. 2004). All these reactions could help to protect against carcinogenesis.

Table 11.1 Synergistic roles of common dietary anti-oxidants (Borek 1997)

Anti-oxidant	Synergy
Beta carotene	Conversion to vitamin A requires vitamin E
Selenium	Synergistic with vitamin E
Vitamin C	Regenerates active α-tocopherol (vitamin E) by reducing its radical form
Vitamin E	Transport and storage depend on selenium; absorption is reduced when vitamin A and β-carotene levels are high

Epidemiological studies of diets high in vitamin C-containing vegetables and fruits indicate that vitamin C probably decreases risk for stomach, mouth, pharynx, oesophagus, lung, pancreas and cervix cancer (WCRF 1997). A relative risk reduction of 40–60% for gastric cancer (Ekstrom et al. 2000), 66% for oral/pharyngeal cancer (Negri et al. 2000) and 23% in lung cancer was reported in men on high vitamin C intake to that of lowest intake of vitamin C (Voorrips et al. 2000). A study in Linxian (China) was conducted on 29,584 adults to evaluate the effect of vitamin C in conjunction with molybdenum at the concentration of 120 mg and 30 μg respectively and found that relative risk of mortality due to cancer at any site was 0.9–1.2 (Blot et al. 1993). Vitamin C is effective in the detoxification of the pharmaceutical drugs in the liver, which could otherwise lead to liver damage and liver cancer (Rath 2001).

Randomized controlled trials involving 29,133 male smokers aged 50–69 years from south-western Finland have provided substantial, consistent evidence that long-term supplementation with α-tocopherol reduced prostate cancer incidence and mortality in male smokers (Heinonen et al. 1998). After a randomized, placebo-controlled trial involving 35,533 healthy men from 427 participating sites in the USA, Canada and Puerto Rico randomly assigned to four groups (selenium, vitamin E, selenium + vitamin E and placebo) between 2001 and 2004, another group (Lippman et al. 2009) found that selenium or vitamin E, alone or in combination at the doses and formulations used, did not prevent prostate cancer. An epidemiological data concluded that decreased risk for lung and cervical cancers can be possibly whittled down with vitamin E supplementation (WCRF 1997). In another study, it was reported that the high vitamin E intake did not reduce lung cancer risk in men (Voorrips et al. 2000). Vitamin E succinate (VES), a derivative of vitamin E, has been shown to trigger apoptosis of human prostate carcinoma cells *in vitro* (Israel et al. 2000).

In a Women's Health Study conducted between 1992 and 2004 (Lee et al. 2005), 39,876 healthy US women aged at least 45 years were randomly assigned to receive vitamin E or placebo and aspirin or placebo, using a 2 × 2 factorial design, and were followed up for an average of 10.1 years. There was no significant effect on the incidences of total cancer or breast, lung or colon cancers. Cancer deaths also did not differ significantly between groups, resulting in the conclusion that the data do not support recommending vitamin E supplementation for cancer prevention among healthy women. Vitamin E induced apoptosis in human breast and prostate cancer cells as well as leukemia (Sigounas et al. 1997) and glioblastoma cells (Borek and Pardo 2002). Glioblastoma multiforme is the most common and aggressive human brain cancer against which all forms of therapy is ineffective. Vitamin E (α-tocopherol succinate) induced apoptosis in a dose-related manner, in with after 48 h exposure to 50 μmol α-tocopherol succinate resulted in a 15% increase in apoptosis in the glioblastoma cells over controls (Borek and Pardo 2002). α-tocopherol succinate given alone or in combination with ϒ-rays had a growth inhibitory effect on a variety of cancer cells (Prasad et al. 2003). A combined treatment with vitamins E and C inhibited apoptosis in human endothelial cells more effectively than each alone (Haendeler et al. 1996).

Associations between intakes of specific carotenoids, vitamins A, C, and E, consumption of fruits and vegetables, and breast cancer risk were assessed in 83,234 women aged 33–60 years in a Nurses' Health Study conducted between 1980 and 1994 (Zhang et al. 1999). Increasing total vitamin C from foods had strong inverse associations among premenopausal women with a positive family history of breast cancer. A contrary result (Cho et al. 2003) reported no evidence between higher intakes of Vitamin C and E and lower risk of breast cancer.

Role of Folate

Folic acid (also known as folacin), folate (the naturally occurring form), pteroyl-L-glutamic acid, pteroyl-L-glutamate and pteroylmonoglutamic acid are forms of the water-soluble vitamin B9 (Iyer and Tomar 2009). Folic acid is itself not biologically active, but its biological importance is due to tetrahydrofolate and other derivatives after its conversion to dihydrofolic acid in the liver (Bailey and Ayling 2009). Folate is present in high concentrations in dark-green leafy vegetables, legumes, fruits, fermented foods and liver, while folic acid is the synthetic, bioavailable form of the vitamin used in fortification programmes worldwide, as well as in supplements and other fortified foods. Many dairy products are processed using microbial fermentations in which folate can be synthesized, significantly increasing folate concentrations in the final product (Lin and Young 2000; Iyer et al. 2010). Numerous researchers have reported that lactic acid bacteria (LAB), such as *Lactococcus lactis, Streptococcus thermophilus, Leuconostoc species, Bifidobacterium longum* and some strains of *Propionibacteria* have the ability to synthesize folate (Lin and Young 2000; Hugenholtz et al. 2002; Crittenden et al. 2003; Papastoyiannidis et al. 2006) whereas lactobacilli (*L. plantarum* at low levels) utilize folate (Hugenholtz and Kleerebezem 1999; Smid et al. 2001; Sybesma et al. 2003a,b).

Epidemiologic evidences indicate positive effect of higher intakes of dietary folate on reduction in risk of several types of cancer. Folate's possible cancer-preventive properties have been attributed to its function in the *de novo* synthesis of nucleotides that are needed for DNA replication and repair. Furthermore, adequate folate status is important for the production of *S*-adenosylmethionine (SAM), a universal donor of methyl groups for a number of methylation reactions, including DNA methylation. Suppressive effect of folic and tetrahydrofolic acid (THFA) on the DNA alkylation with a spin-labeled (containing nitroxyl radical) hydrazine mustard antitumor agent was demonstrated (Raykov et al. 2004) which led to the conclusion that folate status modulates the risk of developing cancers in several tissues. Folate depletion enhanced carcinogenesis while folate supplementation had a protective effect. They proposed that folate deficiency causes DNA hypomethylation and proto-oncogene activation and induces continuous uracil misincorporation during DNA synthesis leading to a catastrophic DNA repair cycle, DNA stand breakage and chromosome damage. The authors recommended the application of folic acid in pharmacological doses during and after antitumor therapy of cancer patients, for cancer prevention of individuals from the high risk groups and for treatment of all disorders in which the oxidative stress is implicated.

Several reports suggest that the timing and dose of folate supplementation during carcinogenesis are important (Kim 2004; Ulrich and Potter 2006). Although increases in folate before the existence of preneoplastic lesions (such as aberrant crypt foci or polyps in the colon) can prevent tumor development, supplementation with synthetic folic acid may enhance progression once preneoplastic lesions are present. Animal experiments suggest that modest supplementation can reduce carcinogenesis, whereas excessive supplementation may increase tumor growth (Kim 2006). These opposing effects are thought to be attributable to folate's function in nucleotide synthesis, which is needed to support rapidly proliferating tissues. Cancers frequently up-regulate folate receptors to meet their elevated need for nucleotides to support DNA synthesis and growth.

Folate can be looked upon as one of the most promising chemopreventive agents for colorectal carcinogenesis. Alterations in DNA methylation and in particular, a global hypomethylation and a regional hypermethylation, especially of promoters of tumor suppressor genes, have been described in human tumors (Warnecke and Bestor 2000). Researchers from the American Cancer Society investigated the association between folate intake and colorectal cancer among 99,523 participants and reported an association between high folate intake and reduced risk of colorectal cancer. No increased risk of colorectal cancer was found for the highest intake levels, suggesting that the high levels of this vitamin consumed by significant numbers of Americans should not lead to increased incidence rates of this cancer in the population (www.gastro.org/news/articles/2011/07/05/high-folate-intake-may-reduce-risk-of-colorectal-cancer). The proposed mechanism for folic acid's protection against colorectal cancer is the prevention of occurrence of mistakes (inserting uracils into DNA, for example) during DNA replication and repair (Hazra et al. 2010). Contrary to this, some reports show that folic acid supplements intake increases advanced colorectal cancer development (Johansson et al. 2008). Folic acid supplements stimulate the PI3k/Akt signaling cascade, which leads to improved cell survival, but this could be beneficial or harmful for the body because cancer cells may use this pathway to survive. Folic acid may also reduce the levels of PTEN (a tumor suppressor gene), making this relationship even more controversial (Seto et al. 2010).

Most epidemiologic studies suggest diets high in folate are associated with decreased risk of breast cancer, but results are not uniformly consistent (Kim 2006; Ericson et al. 2007; Zhang et al. 2008). A strong inverse association exists between dietary intakes of folate and invasive postmenopausal breast cancer, with risk reductions of more than 40% in the highest compared with the lowest quintile of intake (Ericson et al. 2007). The optimum folate intake for breast cancer prevention is not well defined and depends on genetic factors, alcohol consumption, and detrimental effect of polymorphisms in folate metabolism on its bioavailability (Rohan et al. 2000; Stolzenberg-Solomon et al. 2006).

Although genetic alterations, alcoholism and smoking have usually been associated with pancreatitis, it was recently demonstrated that folate deficiency appeared to be the key factor in hyper-homocysteinemia in chronic pancreatitis patients (Gopalakrishna et al. 2010). Head and neck cancer squamous cell carcinomas (HNSCCs) include SCCs of the oral cavity, pharynx, and larynx. Folate supplementation, whether obtained via the dietary or the pharmacologic approach, could be considered a novel tool for chemoprevention of this ailment (Almadori et al. 2006), which is more prevalent in India, Southeast Asia and Brazil. A study was conducted on 56 controls and 167 patients with oral precancerous conditions (OPC) and 214 head and neck cancer patients, to evaluate the plasma vitamin B12 and folate levels to determine their association with tobacco habits and vegetarianism and several socio-demographic factors (Raval et al. 2002). It was found that the tobacco consumption, lower education and low income were among the risk factors. A decrease in the plasma vitamin B12 and folate levels with respect to tobacco habits, disease progression, and vegetarian diet was also observed.

Folate deficiency has also been identified as a potential risk factor for oral cancers, due to its primary role in dysregulation of DNA synthesis, repair and DNA methylation associated with carcinogenesis. The source of some folate deficiencies can be traced to a common DNA polymorphism in the methylene-tetrahydrofolate reductase (MTHFR) gene, which encodes the enzyme responsible for producing the circulating form of folate (Capaccio et al. 2005). Insufficient dietary folate intake, and poor diet in general, may be responsible for as much as 10–15% of all cases of oral cancer (Pelucchi et al. 2003). Behavioral risk factors for oral cancer, such as tobacco and alcohol use, interfere with folate absorption and increase the rate of folate excretion by the kidney, thereby lowering folate concentrations in serum and tissues (Gabriel et al. 2006).

Folic acid is more bioavailable than folate and, thus, is probably more potent in fostering cancerous growth. On passage through the intestinal wall, folic acid is converted to 5-methyltetrahydrofolate, the naturally circulating form of folate. High oral doses of folic acid may overwhelm this conversion pathway, leading to measurable levels of folic acid in the blood. High levels of folic acid may increase cancer risk because of its role in nucleotide synthesis which is needed by proliferating neoplastic cells (Figueiredo et al. 2010). Unmetabolized folic acid is associated with a reduction in natural killer cell cytotoxicity, which reduces the immune system's ability to defend against malignant cells. While on one hand, the uptake of high doses of folic acid has been associated with reduction in the risk of developing different types of cancers by exerting its beneficial effect on the DNA repair system, thereby preventing the accumulation of mutations and genomic instability, folate has also been identified to promote the growth of tumours in early stages of cancer. Hence more research and caution in developing public health policy and guidance is warranted to determine the effect of folic acid fortification on the incidence of cancer and on DNA methylation. Furthermore, safe and effective amounts of folic acid fortification need to be scientifically determined by using relevant animal, experimental, and clinical models.

Role of Carotenoids

The ability of fruits and vegetables to ward off diseases such as cataract, scurvy, cancer and cardio vascular diseases (CVD) is mainly attributed to the phytochemicals present in minor quantities. These phytochemicals belongs to diverse groups and among them, carotenoids are the major ones. Their role in prevention of different types of cancer and CVD are due to their ability to scavenge the free radicals that are implicated in the onset of cancer and CVD. The free radical scavenging ability of carotenoids check the peroxidation of cell membrane constituents and more specifically damage to DNA molecule (Yahia and Ornelas-Paz 2010).

Carotenoids are major pigments in majority of fruits and vegetables, algae, certain fungi and bacteria. They are responsible for characteristic deep red, yellow or orange colour of foods including tomato, carrots, citrus fruits, egg yolk, cow milk, liver, lobster, salmon etc. Many green coloured plants also contain carotenoids which are masked by the chlorophyll, particularly in green leafy vegetables such as spinach, cabbage, lettuce and mustard leaves. Structurally carotenoids consist of C-40 poly-isoprenoid with an extensive conjugated double bond system. Of the 600 or so carotenoids that have been identified, about 50 serve as precursors for vitamin A. Out of these, 50–60% are typically present in diet and around 18 have been identified in human plasma. These carotenoids are grouped into two major classes namely carotenes (hydrocarbon carotenoids) and xanthophyll (oxygenated carotenoids). The various dietary carotenoids are listed in Table 11.2.

Among the carotenoids mentioned above, β-carotene and lycopene have been thoroughly investigated for their disease-preventing abilities. Carotenes are tissue-specific in their biological activity. β-Carotene, α–carotene and ε-carotene have vitamin A activity. Vitamin A regulates the action of certain genes associated with cellular functions (McGrane 2007). In a critical review (Ziegler 1989) of studies conducted to elucidate the effect of dietary carotenoids and prevalence of cancer in different populations, it is mentioned that low intake of fruits, vegetables, and carotenoids is consistently associated with increased risk of lung cancer in both prospective and retrospective investigations. In addition, low plasma β-carotene levels are associated with subsequent development of lung cancer. However the ability of β-carotene is not related with its provitamin A activity. In another review (Yahia and Ornelas-Paz 2010) the chemistry, stability and biological action of carotenoids, the role of carotenoids in cancer, cardiovascular disease prevention, skin protection and provitamin A activity have been covered in detail. The carotenes, including ϒ-carotene, lycopene and lutien, protect against uterine, prostate, breast,colorectal and lung cancers. They may also protect against risk of digestive tract cancer. There are also strong correlations of lutien, cryptoxanthin, α-carotene and β-carotene, but not of lycopene. The xanthophylls type of carotenoids offer protection to other antioxidants and may exhibit tissue specific protection. Zeaxanthin, cryptoxanthin and astazanthin are members of the xanthophyll group. *In-vitro* and animal model investigations have indicated that β-carotene may protect against several forms of cancer (Finley 2005). During a prospective study on long-term intake of dietary carotenoids, vitamin A, C and E on the incidence of breast

Table 11.2 Carotenoids from dietary sources[a]

Sr. No.	Carotenoids	Occurrence	Remark
1	α-Carotene	Carrot, lemon, watermelon, papaya, banana, pumpkins, squash	Precursor of vitamin A
2	β-Carotene	Apricot, oranges, mango, papaya, pumpkin, carrot, spinach, red pepper, crude palm oil	Pro-vitamin A activity, Anti-oxidant prevent cancer and check conversion of LDL Cholesterol into its atherogenic form
3	Lycopene	Tomato, watermelon, pink guava, red grapefruit, pink papaya	Higher amount in deep red coloured tomatoes, lack vitamin A activity but higher singlet oxygen scavenging activity, prevent cancer
4	Lutein	Spinach, egg yolk, broccoli, green bell pepper	Required for protection of macula in retina, play role in age related macular degeneration (AMD)
5	Cryptoxanthin	Mango, tangerine, orange, papaya, apricot	Possess pro-vitamin A activity and free radical scavenging activity
	Zeaxanthin	Kale, collard, turnip green, spinach, Brussels sprout	Similar function as lutein also assist in prevention of cataract
6	Capsanthin	Paprika, red Chili	Exhibit anti-oxidant activity and act as vitamin A precursor

[a]Compiled from various sources

cancer in a cohort of 83,234 women, it was found that intake of β-carotene from food and supplements, lutein/ zeaxanthin and vitamin A from food were weakly inversely related with breast cancer risk in premenopausal women (Zhang et al. 1999). Strong inverse relationship was observed for α– carotene, β- carotene, lutein/ zeaxanthin, total vitamin C from foods and total vitamin A among premenopausal women with a positive family history of breast cancer.

In vitro investigations have shown that retinoic acid strongly inhibits the proliferation of estrogen receptor (ER)-positive human breast cancer cells through retinoic acid receptors but does not check the growth of ER-negative cells (van der Leede et al. 1995). On the basis of these findings it was suggested that anticancer effects of retinoic acid depends on estrogens for inducing its nuclear receptors. It was observed that hormones may alter the metabolism of the carotenoids (Michaud et al. 1998). Although epidemiological investigations observed strong relationship between β-carotene intake and cancer reduction, the evidence primarily was for β-carotene as component of fruits and vegetables and not as β-carotene alone (Finley 2005). Although there is accumulating evidence from animal studies and *in vitro* investigations regarding role of β-carotene in cancer prevention, but these studies lack desired number and cancer models.

Epidemiological studies indicated the lower incidence of prostate cancer among individuals consuming fruits and vegetables (Giovannucci 1999; Cook et al. 1999). β-carotene supplementation at a concentration of less than 30 μmol/L significantly reduced the growth in three human prostate cancer cell lines i.e. PC-3, DU 145 and LNCaP (Williams et al. 2000). Carotenoids can arrest cell-cycle (Stivara et al. 2000), enhancement of gap junctional communication and inhibit lipid peroxidation (Zhang et al. 1999), induce apoptosis (Bertram et al. 1991) and cell differentiation (Amir et al. 1999). On the basis of an investigation to explore the effect of various carotenoids in lung cancer prevention on Finnish population, it was concluded (Knekt et al. 1999) that α-carotene may be the major anti-carcinogenic factor rather than β-carotene with a reduced risk of cancer. However, they have not ruled out the possibility of other carotenoids like β-cryptoxanthin in the prevention of lung cancers.

Tomatoes with their distinctive nutritional attributes and lycopene content, may play an important role in reducing the risk of cardiovascular and associated disease through their bioactivity in modulating disease process pathway. Lycopene's ability to act as an anti-oxidant and scavenger of free radicals that are often associated with carcinogenesis is potentially a key for mechanism for its beneficial effects on human health (Khachik et al. 1995). Lycopene may prevent carcinogenesis and atherogenesis by interfering passively with oxidative damage to DNA and lipoproteins. Lycopene is the most effective quencher of singlet oxygen in biological system. Consumption of tomato paste (an intake of 40 g tomatoes corresponding to a lycopene dose of approximately 16 mg) for more than 8 weeks reduced ultraviolet light-induced erythema (Rizwan et al. 2011). Cis–isomers of lycopene are more readily absorbed through the intestinal wall into the plasma because of the greater solubility in micelles, preferential incorporation into chylomicrons, less tendency to aggregate and crystallize, more efficient volatilization in lipophilic solutions, and easier transport within cells, across plasma membrane and tissue matrix. The greatest increase in cis-isomer formation occurs when tomato products are heated at very high temperatures (Schierle et al. 1996). Likewise, lycopene bioavailability increases in the presence of oil (Stahl and Sies 1992).

Role of Iron

Iron has always been associated with strength and vitality. In addition, iron deficiency anaemia (IDA), one of the most prevalent causes of micronutrient malnutrition, particularly in developing countries requires iron supplementations in diet or through medicines. The Recommended Dietary Allowance for iron in healthy adults is 10 mg per day for men and 15 mg for premenopausal women (Yee and Shaari 2011). Premenopausal women's need for iron is higher than men because women lose iron during menstruation. However, though iron is a necessary nutrient, when too high an iron intake can cause a wide variety of health problems. Recent research suggests that high levels of iron are associated with an increased risk for cancer, heart disease, and other illnesses such as endocrine problems, arthritis, diabetes, and liver disease (Niederau et al. 1996). Among these, cancer has been considered as the most widespread and potential risk. Iron is carcinogenic because of its catalytic effect on the formation of hydroxyl radicals, suppression of the activity of host defence cells and promotion of cancer cell multiplication (Weinberg 1999).

The amount of iron absorbed from various foods range from 1% to 10% from plant sources (non-heme) and 10–20% from animal sources (heme). Phytates, oxalates, phosphates, tannins and to some extent, fibre inhibit the absorption of iron, whereas vitamin C greatly increases the absorption of non-heme iron. The human body has no mechanism to be rid of the excess iron absorbed through diet. Hemochromatosis, a genetic disorder where individuals absorb more iron than normal can lead to iron stores in the body and eventually, to organ damage. The problem is more serious in men, as women are generally protected from excess iron accumulation through regular iron loss by way of menstrual blood (Sullivan 1981). Iron, being a pro-oxidant promotes oxidative damage that leads to several ailments. Iron promotes cancer by two separate, but mutually dependent mechanisms. It first produces free radicals, and then, feeds the cancer cells. The production of free radicals is directly proportional to the level of iron (Herbert et al. 1994; Stevens et al. 1994). Free radicals are oxygen-containing molecules which oxidize and hence, damage the DNA of cells. Since activities of cells are controlled by DNA, damage to DNA results in cells becoming uncontrollable. These cancer cells that are out of control then replicate and grow rapidly, leading to the inevitable damage of the body's organs. Additionally, cancer cells consume many nutrients, notably iron, resulting in malnutrition and weakness in the host.

One of the best sources of absorbable iron being red meat, subjects who consume red meat are more susceptible to cancer than those who avoid it. It is reported that the incidence of lung cancer was 300% higher in the red meat eaters than non-eaters (Blaylock 2003). As phytates chelate iron, thus preventing the iron from doing harm, including phytates in diets is an excellent way to remove excess iron from the body. Phytates are natural substances found in grains, potatoes and many other foods. Many flavonoids and plant components found in common fruits and vegetables can also chelate iron. Research reports have shown that flavonoids in foods allow just enough iron to be absorbed to prevent anemia. Even though broccoli and spinach contain as much iron as a comparable amount of beef, only a small amount of the iron is absorbed from the vegetables, as compared to the 60–70% iron absorption from beef (Stevens et al. 1988).

The more general tests involving hemoglobin and hematocrit are not sufficient to check the iron levels in the body. Research reports indicate that iron levels which correlate with a serum ferritin value greater than 100 and a transferrin saturation value greater than 35% may influence the development of cancer and other ailments (Sullivan 1981; Stevens et al. 1988; Lauffer 1991; Conrad1993). Others prescribe that the ratio of serum iron to total iron binding capacity (TIBC) should be 16–50% in women and 16–62% in men. Results above and below these norms indicate respectively, excess iron and iron deficiency (www.cancerproject.org/protective_foods/building_strength/iron.php). Several practices that are recommended to lower ingested and inhaled quantities of iron have been reportedly effective in reducing incidences of tumours (Weinberg 1992). Some of these are (a) natural or innate defence mechanisms, (b) medical and pharmaceutical methods and (c) environmental and nutritional interventions (Weinberg 1996). Some nutritional methods recommended to reduce the quantity of ingested iron are:

- reducing the quantity of mammalian meats, ethanol, ascorbic acid and iron supplements, unless one has a correctly diagnosed iron deficiency
- avoiding processed foods that contain or have been contaminated with inorganic iron, blood and
- increasing consumption of tea (tannins chelate iron), whole grains (phytic acid binds iron)

Conclusion

Since cancer may have dormant initiation, factors such as genetics, environment, diet and lifestyle should be considered as potential factors in its etiology. Numerous studies have tested theories of associations between food consumption and cancer risk. But the relationship between them is quite complex. A diet-related carcinogen does not have a single potency for all individuals in a population. Therefore, its contribution to the total tumor incidence in a population cannot be correctly estimated on the basis of an average exposure level and an average carcinogenic potency. It can be concluded that incorporation of micronutrients like calcium, vitamin E, vitamin C and dietary fibre may potentially decrease the cancer risk.

References

Adams GB, Chabner KT, Alley IR, Olson DP et al (2006) Stem cell engraftment at the endosteal niche is specified by the calcium-sensing receptor. Nature 439:599–603

Almadori G, Bussu F, Navarra P, Galli J et al (2006) Pilot Phase IIA Study for evaluation of the efficacy of folic acid in the treatment of laryngeal leucoplaki. Cancer 107:328–336

Amir H, Karas M, Giat J, Denilenko M et al (1999) Lycopene and 1, 25-dihydroxyvitamin D3 cooperate in the inhibition of cell cycle progression and induction of differentiation in HL-60 leukemia cells. Nutr Cancer 33:105–112

Anand P, Kunnumakkara AB, Sundaram C, Harikumar KB et al (2008) Cancer is a preventable disease that requires major lifestyle changes. Pharm Res 25:2097–2116

Anonymous (1997) Food, nutrition and the prevention of cancer: a global perspective. World Cancer Research Fund, American Institute for Cancer Research, Washington, DC, pp 63

Anonymous (2009) Diet, nutrition and bowel cancer http://www.bowelcanceruk.org.uk. Accessed 16 May 2011

Armstrong B, Doll R (1975) Environmental factors and cancer incidence and mortality in different countries, with special reference to dietary practices. Int J Cancer 15:617–631

Bailey SW, Ayling JE (2009) The extremely slow and variable activity of dihydrofolate reductase in human liver and its implications for high folic acid intake. PNAS USA 106(36):15424–15429

Belobrajdic DP, McIntosh GH (2003) Dietary butyrate inhibits NMU induced mammary cancer in rats. Nutr Cancer 36:217–223

Bertram JS, Pung A, Churley M, Kappock TJ IV et al (1991) Diverse carotenoids protect against chemically induced neoplastic transformation. Carcinogenesis 12:671–678

Bingham SA (1999) High-meat diets and cancer risk. Proc Nutr Soc 58:243–248

Blaylock RL (2003) Natural strategies for cancer patients. Kensington Publishing Corp, New York

Blot WJ, Li JY, Taylor PR, Gou W et al (1993) Nutrition intervention trials in Linxian, China: supplementation with specific vitamin/ mineral combinations, cancer incidence, and disease-specific mortality in the general population. J Natl Cancer Inst 85:1483–1492

Borek C (1997) Antioxidants and cancer. Sci Med (Phila) 4:51–62

Borek C, Pardo F (2002) Vitamin E and apoptosis: a dual role. In: Pasquier C (ed) Biennial meeting of the society for free radicals research international, Paris, Bologna, 16–20 July 2002, pp 327–331

Brown EM, MacLeod RJ (2001) Extracellular calcium sensing and extracellular calcium signaling. Physiol Rev 81:239–297

Burkitt DP (1969) Related disease—related cause? Lancet 2:1229–1231

Capaccio P, Ottaviani F, Cuccarini V, Cenzuales S et al (2005) Association between methylenetetrahydrofolate reductase polymorphisms, alcohol intake and oropharyngolaryngeal carcinoma in northern Italy. J Laryngol Otol 119:371–376

Cho E, Spiegelman D, Hunter DJ, Chen WY et al (2003) Premenopausal intakes of vitamins A, C, and E, folate, and carotenoids, and risk of breast cancer. Cancer Epidemiol Biomarkers Prev 12.713–720

Conrad ME (1993) Excess iron and catastrophic illness. Am J Hematol 43:234–236

Cook NR, Stampfer MJ, Ma J, Manson JE et al (1999) β-Carotene supplementation for patients with low baseline level and decreased risks of total prostate carcinoma. Cancer 86:1783–1792

Coxam V, Davicco MJ, Durand D, Bauchart D et al (1992) The influence of parathyroid hormone-related protein on hepatic IGF-1 production. Acta Endocrinol 126:430–433

Crittenden RG, Martinez NR, Playne MJ (2003) Synthesis and utilization of folate by yogurt starter cultures and probiotic bacteria. Int J Food Microbiol 80:217–222

Doll R, Peto R (1981) The cases of cancer: quantitative estimates of avoidable risks of cancer in the United States today. J Natl Cancer Inst 66:1191–1308

Ekstrom AM, Serafini M, Nyren O, Hansson LE et al (2000) Dietary antioxidant intake and the risk of cardia cancer and noncardia cancer of the intestinal and diffuse types: a population- based case–control study in Sweden. Int J Cancer 87:133–140

Ericson U, Sonestedt E, Gullberg B, Olsson H et al (2007) High folate intake is associated with lower breast cancer incidence in postmenopausal women in the Malmö Diet and Cancer cohort. Am J Clin Nutr 86:434–443

Figueiredo JC, Levine AJ, Lee WH, Conti DV et al (2010) Genes involved with folate uptake and distribution and their association with colorectal cancer risk. Cancer Causes Control 21:597–608

Finley WJ (2005) Proposed criteria for assessing the efficacy of cancer reduction by plant foods enriched in carotenoids, glucosinolatesm polyphenols and selenocompounds. Ann Bot 95:1075–1096

Frei B (1994) Reactive oxygen species and antioxidant vitamins: mechanisms of action. Am J Med 97:5–13

Gabriel HE, Crott JW, Ghandour H, Dallal GE et al (2006) Chronic cigarette smoking is associated with diminished folate status, altered folate form distribution, and increased genetic damage in the buccal mucosa of healthy adults. Am J Clin Nutr 83:835–841

Giovannucci E (1998) Dietary influences of 1,25(OH)$_2$ vitamin D in relation to prostate cancer: a hypothesis. Cancer Causes Control 9:567–582

Giovannucci E (1999) Tomatoes, tomato based products, lycopene and cancer: review of the epidemiologic literature. J Natl Cancer Inst 91:317–320

Goldman R, Shields PG (2003) Food mutagens. J Nutr 133:965–973

Gopalakrishna R, Narasimhamurthy BG, Vaidyanathan K, Menon S et al (2010) Folate deficiency in chronic pancreatitis. J Pancreas 11:409–410

Grant WB (1999) An ecologic study of dietary links to prostate cancer. Altern Med Rev 4:162–169

Greenwald P, Clifford CK, Milner JA (2001) Diet and cancer prevention. Eur J Cancer 37:948–965

Haendeler J, Zeiher AM, Dimmeler S (1996) Vitamin C and E prevent lipopolysaccharide-induced apoptosis in human endothelial cells by modulation of Bcl-2 and Bax. Eur J Pharmacol 317(2–3):407–411

Harris PJ, Ferguson LR (1993) Dietary fibre: its composition and role in protection against colorectal cancer. Mutat Res 290:97–110

Hazra A, Selhub J, Chao WH, Ueland PM et al (2010) Uracil misincorporation into DNA and folic acid supplementation. Am J Clin Nutr 91:160–165

Hegarty NJ, Fitzpatrick JM, Ritchie JP, Scardino PT et al (1999) Future prospects in prostate cancer. Prostate 40:261–268

Heinonen OP, Albanes D, Virtamo J, Taylor PR et al (1998) Prostate cancer and supplementation with alpha-tocopherol and beta-carotene: incidence and mortality in a controlled trial. J Natl Cancer Inst 90:440–446

Herbert V, Shaw S, Jayatilleke E, Stopler-Kasdan T (1994) Most free-radical injury is iron-related: it is promoted by iron, hemin, holoferritin and vitamin C, and inhibited by desferoxamine and apoferritin. Stem Cells 12:289–303

Hugenholtz J, Kleerebezem M (1999) Metabolic engineering of lactic acid bacteria: overview of the approaches and results of pathway rerouting involved in food fermentations. Curr Opin Biotechnol 10:492–497

Hugenholtz J, Hunik J, Santos H, Smid E (2002) Nutraceuticals production by propionibacteria. Lait 82:103–111

Israel K, Yu W, Sanders BG, Kline K (2000) Vitamin E, succinate induces apoptosis in human prostate cancer cells: role for FAs in vitamin E, succinate-triggered apoptosis. Nutr Cancer 36:90–100

Iyer R, Tomar SK (2009) Folate: a functional food constituent. J Food Sci 74:114–122

Iyer R, Tomar SK, Kapila S, Mani J et al (2010) Probiotic properties of folate-producing *Streptococcus thermophilus* strains. Food Res Int 43:103–110

Jacobs LR (1990) Influence of soluble fibres on experimental colon carcinogens. In: Kritchevsky D, Bonfield C, Anderson JW (eds) Dietary fibre: chemistry, physiology and health effects. Plenum Press, New York, pp 389–401

Johansson M, Appleby PN, Allen NE, Travis RC et al (2008) Circulating concentrations of folate and vitamin B12 in relation to prostate cancer risk: results from the European prospective investigation into cancer and nutrition study. Cancer Epidemiol Biomarkers Prev 17:279–285

Jorde R, Sundsfjord J, Bønaa KH (2001) Determinants of serum calcium in men and women: the Tromso study. Eur J Epidemiol 17:1117–1123

Kelley DS, Bendich A (1996) Essential nutrients and immunologic functions. Am J Clin Nutr 63:994–996

Khachik F, Carvalho L, Bernstein PS, Muir GJ et al (1995) Carotenoid content of thermally processed tomato-based food products. J Agric Food Chem 43:579–586

Kim YI (2004) Will mandatory folic acid fortification prevent or promote cancer? Am J Clin Nutr 80:1123–1128

Kim YI (2006) Does a high folate intake increase the risk of breast cancer? Nutr Rev 64:468–475

Knekt P, Jarvinen R, Teppo L, Aromaa A et al (1999) Role of various carotenoids in lung cancer prevention. J Natl Cancer Inst 91:182–184

Kobayashi H, Fleming SE (2001) The source of dietary fibre influences-short chain fatty acid production and concentrations in the large bowel. In: Spiller GA (ed) CRC handbook of dietary fibre in human nutrition. CRC Press, Hoboken, pp 287–315

Lauffer RB (1991) Iron and your heart. St. Martin's Press, New York

Lee I-M, Cook NR, Gaziano JM, Gordon D et al (2005) Vitamin E in the primary prevention of cardiovascular disease and cancer. The women's health study: a randomized controlled trial. J Am Med Assoc 294(1):56–65

Levi F, Pasche C, Lucchini F, La-Vecchia C (2001) Dietary intake of selected micronutrients and breast cancer risk. Int J Cancer 91:260–263

Lin MY, Young CM (2000) Folate levels in cultures of lactic acid bacteria. Int Dairy J 10:409–414

Lippman SM, Klein EA, Goodman PJ, Lucia MS et al (2009) Effect of selenium and vitamin E on risk of prostate cancer and other cancers. The selenium and vitamin E cancer prevention trial (SELECT). J Am Med Assoc 301(1):39–51

Lukanova A, Lundin E, Toniola P (2002) Circulating levels of insulin-like growth factor-1 and risk of ovarian cancer. Int J Cancer 10:549–554

Lupton JR (2000) Is fibre protective against colon cancer where the research is leading us? Nutr 16:558–561

Martinez ME, Marshall JR, Alberts DS (1999) Dietary fibre, carbohydrates and cancer. In: Heber D, Blackburn GL, Go LW (eds) Nutritional oncology. Academic, San Diego, pp 185–194

McCarty MF (2000) Parathyroid hormone may be a cancer promoter– an explanation for the decrease in cancer risk associated with ultraviolet light, calcium and vitamin D. Med Hypotheses 54:475–482

McGrane MM (2007) Vitamin A regulation gene expression: molecular mechanism of a prototype gene. J Nutr Biochem 18:497–508

Michaud DS, Giovannucci EL, Ascherio A, Rimm EB et al (1998) Association of plasma carotenoid concentrations and dietary intake of specific carotenoids in samples of two prospective cohort studies using a new carotenoid database. Cancer Epidemiol Biomarkers Prev 7:283–290

Miyanishi K, Takayama T, Ohi M, Hayashi T et al (2001) Glutathione S-transferase-pi over-expression is closely associated with K-ras mutation during human colon carcinogenesis. Gastroenterol 121:865–874

Molck AM, Poulsen M, Meyer O (2002) The combination of 1a,25(OH)2–vitamin D3, calcium and acetylsalicylic acid affects azoxymethane-induced aberrant crypt foci and colorectal tumours in rats. Cancer Lett 186:19–28

Negri E, Franceschi S, Bosetti C, Levi F et al (2000) Selected micronutrients and oral and pharyngeal cancer. Int J Cancer 86:122–127

Newmark HL, Lupton JR (1990) Determinants and consequences of colonic luminal pH: implications for colon cancer. Nutr Cancer 14:161–173

Niederau C, Fischer R, Purschel A, Stremmel W et al (1996) Long-term survival in patients with hereditary hemochromatosis. Gastroenterol 110:1107–1119

Nordin BC (2000) Calcium requirement is a sliding scale. Am J Clin Nutr 71:1381–1383

Papastoyiannidis G, Polychroniadou A, Michaelidou A-M, Alichanidis E (2006) Fermented milks fortified with b-group vitamins: vitamin stability and effect on resulting products. Food Sci Technol Int 12(6):521–529

Pelucchi C, Talamini R, Negri E, Levi F et al (2003) Folate intake and risk of oral and pharyngeal cancer. Ann Oncol 13:1677–1681

Peterlik M, Grant WB, Cross HS (2009) Calcium, vitamin D and cancer. Anticancer Res 29:3687–3698

Prasad KN, Kumar B, Yan XD, Hanson AJ et al (2003) Alpha tocopheryl succinate the most effective form of vitamin E for adjuvant cancer treatment: a review. J Am Coll Nutr 22:108–117

Ramasamy I (2006) Recent advances in physiological calcium homeostasis. Clin Chem Lab Med 44:237–273

Rath M (2001) Cellular health series: cancer. MR Publishing, Inc, Santa Clara, 95054

Raval GN, Sainger RN, Rawal RM, Patel JB et al (2002) Vitamin B12 and folate status in head and neck cancer. Asian Pac J Cancer Prev 3:155–162

Raykov ZZ, Ivanov VA, Raikova ET, Galabov AS (2004) Folic acid role in mutagenesis, carcinogenesis, prevention and treatment of cancer. Biotechnol Biotec Eq 18:125–135

Renehan AG, Zwahlen M, Minder C, Egger M (2004) Insulin-like growth factor (IGF)-1, IGF binding protein-3, and cancer risk: systematic review and meta-regression analysis. Lancet 363:346–353

Rizwan M, Rodriquez-Blanco I, Harbottle A, Birch-Machin MA et al (2011) Tomato paste rich in lycopene protects against cutaneous photodamage in humans in vivo: a randomized controlled trial. Br J Dermatol 164:154–162

Rodland KR (2004) The role of the calcium-sensing receptor in cancer. Cell Calcium 35:291–295

Rohan TE, Jain MG, Howe GR, Miller AB (2000) Dietary folate consumption and breast cancer risk. J Natl Cancer Inst 92:266–269

Schierle J, Bretzel W, Buhler I, Faccin N et al (1996) Content and isomeric ratio of lycopene in food and human blood plasma. Food Chem 59:459–465

Schuurman AG, van den Brandt PA, Dorant E, Goldbohm RA (1999) Animal products, calcium and protein and prostate cancer risk in The Netherlands Cohort Study. Br J Cancer 80:1107–1113

Sesink AL, Termont DS, Kleibeuker JH, van der Meer R (2001) Red meat and colon cancer: dietary haem-induced colonic cytotoxicity and epithelial hyperproliferation are inhibited by calcium. Carcinogenesis 22:1653–1659

Seto SW, Lam TY, Or PM, Lee WY et al (2010) Folic acid consumption reduces resistin level and restores blunted acetylcholine-induced aortic relaxation in obese/diabetic mice. J Nutr Biochem 21:872–880

Se-Young OT, Ji Hyun L, Jangb DK, Heoc SC et al (2005) Relationship of nutrients and food to colorectal cancer risk in Koreans. Nutr Res 25:805–813

Sigounas G, Anagnostu A, Steiner M (1997) Dl-alpha tocopherol induces apoptosis in erythroleukemia, prostate and breast cancer cells. Nutr Cancer 28:30–35

Singh B, Halestrap AP, Paraskeva C (1997) Butyrate can act as a stimulator of growth or inducer of apoptosis in human colonic epithelial cell lines depending on the presence of alternative energy sources. Carcinogenesis 18:1265–1270

Smid EJ, Starrenburg MJC, Mierau I, Sybesma W et al (2001) Increase of folate levels in fermented foods. Innov Food Technol 10:13–15

Smith-Warner SA, Giovannucci E (1999) Fruit and vegetable intake and cancer. In: Heber D, Blackburn GL, Go LW (eds) Nutritional oncology. Academic, San Diego, pp 153–193

Stahl W, Sies H (1992) Uptake of lycopene and its geometrical isomers is greater from heat processed than from unprocessed tomato juice in humans. J Nutr 122:2161–2166

Stevens RG, Jones DY, Micozzi MS, Taylor PR (1988) Body iron stores and the risk of cancer. N Engl J Med 319:1047–1052

Stevens RG, Graubard BI, Micozzi MS, Neriishi K et al (1994) Moderate elevation of body iron level and increased risk of cancer occurrence and death. Int J Cancer 56:364–369

Stivara LA, Savio M, Quarta S, Scotti C et al (2000) The antiproliferative effect of β-carotene requires p21waf1/cip 1 in normal human fibroblasts. Eur J Biochem 267:2290–2296

Stolzenberg-Solomon RZ, Chang SC, Leitzmann MF, Johnson KA et al (2006) Folate intake, alcohol use, and postmenopausal breast cancer risk in the prostate, lung, colorectal, and ovarian cancer screening trial. Am J Clin Nutr 83:895–904

Strong K, Mathers C, Leeder S, Beeglehole R (2005) Preventing chronic disease: how many lives can we save? Lancet 366:1578–1582

Sullivan JL (1981) Iron and the sex difference in heart disease risk. Lancet 1:1293–1294

Sybesma W, Starrenburg M, Kleerebezem M, Mierau I et al (2003a) Increased production of folate by metabolic engineering of Lactococcus lactis. Appl Environ Microbiol 69:3069–3076

Sybesma W, Starrenburg M, Tijsseling L, Hoefnagel MHN et al (2003b) Effects of cultivation conditions on folate production by lactic acid bacteria. Appl Environ Microbiol 69:4542–4548

Taper HS, Jamison JM, Gilloteax J, Summers JL et al (2004) Inhibition of the development of metastases by dietary vitamin C:K3 combination. Life Sci 75:955–967

Ulrich CM, Potter JD (2006) Folate supplementation: too much of a good thing? Cancer Epidemiol Biomarkers Prev 15:189–193

van der Leede BJ, Folkers GE, van den Brink CE, van der Saag PT et al (1995) Retinoic acid receptor α1 isoform is induced by estradiol and confers retinoic acid sensitivity in human breast cancer cells. Mol Cell Endocrinol 109:77–86

Voorrips LE, Goldbohm RA, Brants HA, van Poppel GA et al (2000) A prospective cohort study on antioxidant and folate intake and male lung cancer risk. Cancer Epidemiol Biomarkers Prev 9:357–365

Wactawski-Wende J, Kotchen JM, Anderson GL, Assaf AR et al (2006) Calcium plus vitamin D supplementation and the risk of colorectal cancer. N Engl J Med 354(7):684–696

Warnecke PM, Bestor TH (2000) Cytosine methylation and humancancer. Curr Opin Oncol 12:68–73

WCRF (1997) http://www.wcrf.org/cancer_research/expert_report/index.php. Accessed March 2011

Weinberg ED (1992) Iron depletion: a defence against intracellular infection and neoplasia. Life Sci 50:1289–1297

Weinberg ED (1996) The role of iron in cancer. Eur J Cancer Prev 5:19–36

Weinberg ED (1999) Iron therapy and cancer. Kidney Int 55(Suppl 69):S131–S134

Williams AW, Boileau TW-M, Zhou JR, Clinton SK et al (2000) β-carotene modulates human prostate cancer cell growth and may undergo intracellular metabolism to retinol. J Nutr 130:728–732

www.cancerproject.org/protective_foods/building_strength/iron.php.Accessed 2 July 2011

www.gastro.org/news/articles/2011/07/05/high-folate-intake-may-reduce-risk-of-colorectal-cancer. Accessed 1 July 2011

Yahia ME, Ornelas-Paz JJ (2010) Chemistry, stability, and biological actions of carotenoids. In: de la Rosa LA, Alvarez-Parrilla E, Gonzalez-Aguilar GA (eds) Fruit and vegetable phytochemicals: chemistry, nutritional value and stability. Wiley Blackwell, Ames, pp 177–222

Yee YS, Shaari K (2011) Iron and cancer. http://ejtcm.com/2011/03/18/iron-and-cancer-2/. Accessed 2 July 2011

Zhang S, Hunter DJ, Forman MR, Rosner BA et al (1999) Dietary carotenoids and vitamins A, C and E and risk of breast cancer. J Natl Cancer Inst 91:547–556

Zhang SM, Cook NR, Albert CM, Gaziano JM et al (2008) Effect of combined folic acid, vitamin B6, and vitamin B12 on cancer risk in women: a randomized trial. J Am Med Assoc 300(17):2012–2021

Ziegler RG (1989) A review of epidemiologic evidence that carotenoids reduce the risk of cancer. J Nutr 119:116–122

Zimmermann KC, Bonzon C, Green DR (2001) The machinery of programmed cell death. Pharmacol Ther 92:57–70

Zoran DL, Turner ND, Taddeo SS, Chapkin RS et al (1997) Wheat bran diet reduces tumor incidence in a rat model of colon cancer independent of effects on distal luminal butyrate concentrations. J Nutr 127:2217–2225

Chapter 12
The Protective Role of Zinc in Cancer: A Potential Chemopreventive Agent

Bin Bao M.D., Ph.D., Aamir Ahmad Ph.D., Azfar S Azmi Ph.D., Zhiwei Wang Ph.D., Sanjeev Banerjee Ph.D., and Fazlul H. Sarkar Ph.D.

Contents

Abstract The essentiality of trace mineral element-zinc in human health has been recognized over several decades. Zinc is known to participate in the activation of approximately 300 enzymes and is involved in the regulation of over 2,000

B. Bao M.D., Ph.D. • A. Ahmad Ph.D. • A.S. Azmi Ph.D. • Z. Wang Ph.D. • S. Banerjee Ph.D. • F.H. Sarkar Ph.D. (✉)
Department of Pathology, Barbara Ann Karmanos Cancer Institute, Wayne State University School of Medicine, 740 HWCRC, 4100 John R Street, Detroit, MI 48201, USA
e-mail: baob@karmanos.org; ahmada@karmanos.org; azmia@karmanos.org; zwang6@bidmc.harvard.edu; ar9010@wayne.edu; fsarkar@med.wayne.edu

S. Shankar and R.K. Srivastava (eds.), *Nutrition, Diet and Cancer*,
DOI 10.1007/978-94-007-2923-0_12,

zinc-dependent transcription factors, which are involved in DNA synthesis, protein synthesis, cell division, and other metabolisms. Early evidence suggested that zinc deficiency can cause growth retardation, delayed sexual maturation, depressed immune response, and cause abnormal cognitive functions. A large body of epidemiological and clinical studies demonstrates that zinc deficiency is associated with the increased risk of some cancers, such as prostate, esophageal and oral cancers. The data from *in vitro and in vivo* studies clearly suggest that zinc may play a protective role in the development and progression of cancer; however, the exact mechanism of zinc action in carcinogenesis is not fully understood. A large number of studies have demonstrated that zinc deficiency induces inflammatory cytokines and oxidative stress, apoptosis and cellular dysfunction, disrupts DNA-protein interaction, and depresses the functioning of T cell mediated immune response. Zinc supplementation reverses these adverse effects, suggesting that the anti-tumor effect of zinc could be potentially due to its anti-inflammatory, anti-oxidative, DNA and protein integrity, T-cell immune response, and other properties. Therefore, zinc may be implicated as a chemopreventive agent as summarized in this article.

Introduction

It is well known that zinc participates in the activation of approximately 300 enzymes and it is involved in the regulation of over 2,000 zinc-dependent transcription factors (Prasad 1995), suggesting that zinc may play an important role in a wide range of biological processes. Early evidence suggests that zinc deficiency impairs growth and development, immune, and cognitive functions (Prasad 1995, 1988, 2003; Prasad et al. 1963). Nutritional zinc deficiency is very common in the developing countries. Moreover, it has been estimated that 30–40% of the elderly population has mild to modest zinc deficiency in the USA (Prasad et al. 1993, 2007). Zinc deficiency is also found to be associated with many chronic diseases such as rheumatoid arthritis, diabetes, and cancers, which are associated with chronic inflammation and oxidative stress (Prasad et al. 2004; Prasad 2008). Over the last few decades, zinc deficiency has been recognized to be associated with increased risk of cancer, such as prostate, head and neck, esophageal, and lung cancers. Although the exact mechanism of zinc action in carcinogenesis is not fully understood, emerging evidence suggests that zinc deficiency increases the level of inflammatory cytokines and oxidative stress, induces apoptosis and causes endothelial and epithelial cell dysfunction, and disrupts DNA-protein interaction and immune function. Moreover, recent experimental, clinical, and epidemiological studies have suggested that zinc may have a protective role in the development and progression of tumors, which could in fact be due to its anti-inflammatory, anti-oxidative, DNA and protein integrity, immune response, and other properties (Prasad et al. 2009; Prasad 2009). In the following paragraphs we will summarize the "state-of-our-knowledge" on the biological functions of zinc in human health and diseases.

Physio-Biological Function of Zinc

Zinc is an essential trace element for mammals and plays important roles in various biochemical and physiological functions (Prasad 1995, 1979; Shankar and Prasad 1998). Zinc is well known to participate in the activation of approximately 300 enzymes involved in DNA synthesis, cell division, protein synthesis, and other metabolisms (Prasad 1979, 1995). Zinc is also required to stabilize three dimensional structures of over 2,000 transcription factors such as "the zinc-finger" proteins. These transcription factors are involved in the regulation of gene expression of various growth factors, steroid receptors, and immune response mediators (Prasad 1979, 1995; Shankar and Prasad 1998). Several studies have indicated that the loss of zinc from zinc-dependent enzymes, or mutations in the zinc-finger domain of these proteins, could result in the loss of protein function and may also cause DNA damage (Yan et al. 2008). Zinc deficiency in humans can cause growth and development retardation, anemia, delayed sexual maturation, abnormal immune response to viral, bacterial, and yeast infections, and cognitive dysfunctions. Zinc supplementation to these zinc deficient human subjects can reverse all these adverse effects or symptoms (Prasad 1998, 2007, 2009), which clearly suggest the essentiality of zinc in human health.

Immunological Function of Zinc

Clinical observation, experimental and animal studies have indicated that zinc plays an important role in immune functions. Zinc regulates several functions of lymphocytes, such as mitogenesis, antibody synthesis, the activation of T-cells and natural killer (NK) cells, and more specifically, cellular immunity (Antoniou et al. 1981; Fraker et al. 1986; Prasad et al. 1987, 1988). Increasing evidence suggests that zinc deficiency impairs cellular immune functions, such as decreased T helper 1 (Th1) cytokine production and DNA-binding activity of T-bet, a major transcription factor for Th1 cytokine gene expression (Bao et al. 2011). Dysfunction of cellular immunity due to zinc deficiency in humans induces frequent severe fungi, virus, and bacterial infections, thymic atrophy, anergy, reduced serum lymphocyte proliferative response to mitogens, a selective decrease in T helper cells and reduced thymic hormone (thymulin) activity. Zinc supplementation reverses all of these manifestations (Falchuk 1998, Wellinghausen and Rink 1998). These data clearly suggest that zinc could be an important immune responsive mediator. Moreover, recent studies have shown that zinc possess anti-inflammatory, anti-oxidant, increased T-cell-medicated immune responsive function, and anti-apoptotic effects (Prasad et al. 2007, 2009; Prasad 2008, 2009).

Anti-inflammatory Function of Zinc

Inflammation, Cellular and Tissue Injury, Cancer

Inflammation is a critical biological process responsive to micro-organism infection and other environmental factors, or a combination, which is most often resolve; however, such sustained chronic conditions could lead to cellular or tissue injury. This process is involved through innate and adaptive immune response systems. There are several mechanisms by which inflammation causes cellular injury. These include complement injury involving lytic complex of complement protein (c5b-9) and c5a, a chemo-attractant for neutrophils and macrophages, which release toxic reactive oxygen species (ROS) and proteases as a result of interaction with these complement factors (Ward 1995). Intravascular activation of complement leads to neutrophil activation and oxidant production, up-regulation of the endothelial adhesion molecule P-selectin, rapid adhesion of neutrophils to endothelial cells and endothelial cell injury within a short period of time (Ward 1995). In addition, complement is activated in the vascular compartment by trauma, infection, thermal injury, septicemia, and other factors (Ward 1995).

Immune complexes also have major tissue injuring capacity. With IgG-containing complexes, products of both neutrophils and macrophages are implicated. With complexes containing IgA, macrophage products seem to be exclusively involved. Complement activation products are probably important in immune complex-induced injury. The main role of complement would be to provide products that, along with immune complexes, optimally stimulate macrophages to produce cytokines and oxidants, both of which play critical roles in cell or tissue injury (Ward 1995; De Marzo et al. 2007).

When alveolar macrophages are stimulated by IgG-containing immune complexes and complement, inflammatory cytokine TNF-α is released, along with IL-1β, PAF (platelet activating factor) and other cytokines (Ward 1995; De Marzo et al. 2007). Simultaneously, nitric oxide (NO) and oxygen radicals are released into the alveolar space causing tissue damage which is linked with TNF-α- and IL-1β-induced up-regulation of various leukocyte adhesion molecules (E-selectin, ICAM-1, and VCAM-1) on endothelial surfaces. These molecules interact with targets on leukocytes such as β_2 integrins to facilitate chemotactic migration of neutrophils from circulation to alveolar space. Neutrophils then release proteases and toxic oxygen radicals that interact with NO to generate tissue-damaging derivatives. When the Ig moiety of the immune complex IgA is involved then the reaction is much simpler, involving only macrophages which release nitrogen and oxygen centered radicals. Together, such cellular injury or damage can cause deregulated cell proliferation, which is susceptible to tumorigenesis.

Inflammation has been implicated in the development and progression of various cancers, such as liver, prostate, pancreatic, breast, lung, bladder, esophageal, and colon cancer by several proposed mechanisms such as disruption of cytokine production and regulation, increased oxidative stress from activated phagocytic inflammatory cells, and disruption of cell-mediated anti-tumor immune surveillance system (De Marzo et al. 2007; Sutcliffe and Platz 2007; Zhang and Rigas 2006). Anti-inflammatory drugs such as non-steroid anti-inflammatory drugs (NSAID) have been implicated in the prevention or treatment of certain tumors such as breast cancer, prostate cancer, and colon cancer (Sutcliffe and Platz 2007). Therefore one could only speculate that agents that would function as ant-inflammatory would be useful in the prevention and/or treatment of above mentioned health conditions.

Zinc as Anti-inflammatory Agent

Zinc has been identified to be an immune mediator against infection and inflammation (Prasad 1995, 2008, 2009; Shankar and Prasad 1998). Numerous early studies have demonstrated that zinc deficiency increases the infection of various micro-organisms such as virus, bacteria, and yeasts. Other human subject studies also showed that oral zinc supplementation could decrease the severity of the radiation-induced oropharyngeal mucositis in patients with head and neck cancer (Ertekin et al. 2003, 2004). These data strongly suggest that zinc could act as an anti-inflammatory agent. It has been proposed that zinc contain anti-inflammatory property by down-regulation of inflammatory cytokines and adhesion molecules via inhibition of NF-κB activation, a major transcription factor for inflammatory and immune response (Barnes 1997; Perkins 1997). Plasma zinc has been found to be inversely associated with plasma level of pro-inflammatory cytokine IL-1β in patients with cutaneous leishmaniasis (Kocyigit et al. 2002). Dietary zinc-depletion in normal human volunteers increased the generation of IL-1β in isolated human peripheral blood mononuclear cells (PMNC). Zinc supplementation could correct the increased generation of this cytokine (Prasad et al. 1997). Recent *in vitro* studies have also demonstrated that zinc decreases TNF-α, IL-1β, macrophage chemoattractant protein 1 (MCP-1), vascular cell adhesion molecule-1 (VCAM-1) cytokines and mRNAs, as well as PMA-, or LPS-induced NF-κB activation in HL-60 (a human promyeloycytic leukemia cell line), THP-1 (monocytic leukemia cells), and vascular endothelial cells (HAEC and HUVEC cells) (Prasad et al. 2004, 1997; Bao et al. 2003, 2010). Our recent human subject studies in normal volunteers and sickle cell disease (SCD) patients showed that zinc supplementation could decrease TNF-α and IL-1β mRNAs, as well as TNF-α induced NF-κB activation in isolated PMNC, compared to placebo control group (Prasad et al. 2007; Prasad 2009; Bao et al. 2010, 2008). Normal elderly subjects showed decreased levels of plasma and lymphocyte zinc, and increased levels of TNF-α, IL-1β, VCAM-1, and intercellular adhesion molecule 1 (ICAM-1) as tested in isolated PMNC cells compared to normal young adult. Six months of zinc supplementation to normal elderly subjects increased plasma zinc and *ex vivo* production of IL-2 and interferon (IFN)-γ, and decreased *ex vivo* production of TNF-α and IL-1β, and plasma levels of C-reactive protein (CRP), IL-6, VCAM-1, ICAM, and MCP-1, consistent with decreased incidence of infection, compared to the placebo-supplemented elderly subjects (Prasad et al. 1963, 1988, 1989, 2007; Prasad 2009; Bao et al. 2008, 2010). These data confirmed that zinc decreases the inflammatory markers, suggesting that zinc may have anti-inflammatory effect, which could be useful for maintaining normal health conditions in elderly population who are vulnerable to infections and many other chronic diseases.

Anti-oxidant Function of Zinc

Physiological Role of ROS

Reactive oxygen species (ROS) are produced as intermediates in reduction-oxidation (redox) processes, generated during oxygen to water reactions (Touyz 2004; Fridovich 1997). The univalent reduction of oxygen, in the presence of a free electron (e), yields $^{\cdot}O_2^-$ (superoxide), H_2O_2 (hydrogen peroxide) and $^{\cdot}OH$ (hydroxyl radical). Superoxide has an unpaired electron, which imparts high reactivity and renders it unstable and short-lived (Han et al. 2003; Schafer and Buettner 2001). ROS are produced continuously *in vivo* under aerobic conditions; however, the production of ROS and its elimination is a tightly controlled process for maintaining normal physiology. In eukaryotic cells, the mitochondrial respiratory chain, microsomal cytochrome P450 enzymes, flavoprotein oxidases, and peroxisomal fatty acid metabolism are the most significant intracellular sources of ROS (Castro et al. 1996; Castro and Freeman 2001; Lachance et al. 2001; Landmesser and Harrison 2001). The NADPH oxidases are a group of plasma membrane associated enzymes, which catalyze the production of $^{\cdot}O_2^-$ from oxygen by using NADPH as the electron donor (DeCoursey et al. 2003). ROS are considered as second messengers and have been implicated as important signaling molecules (Touyz 2004). Similar to second messengers, production of ROS is tightly regulated by extra-cellular stimuli such as hypoxia and inflammatory cytokines. Redox signaling involves at least one reaction in which oxidation of a signaling molecule by a ROS occurs, which is reversible (Forman and Torres 2002).

Physiological generation of ROS has been implicated in a variety of biological responses from transcriptional activation to cell proliferation. Under pathological conditions, a disequilibrium between ROS generation and antioxidant protection results in increased bio-availability of ROS leading to a state of oxidative stress (Landmesser and Harrison 2001; Zalba et al. 2001). The pathogenic outcome of oxidative stress is oxidative damage of cells or tissues (Schafer and Buettner 2001), which is a major cause of DNA damage that ultimately leads to genomic instability during the development of many chronic diseases including cancers.

ROS and Cellular or Tissue Injury

ROS reacts with and modifies the structure and function of bio-molecules including proteins, lipids, sugars, and nucleic acids, which contribute to cellular stresses, leading to cellular injury. Increasing oxidative damage to DNA is believed to be an etiologic factor in cancers induced by smoking and chronic inflammatory disease. Oxidative damage to nucleic acids includes adducts of both base and sugar group modifications, single and double strand breaks in the DNA "backbone" and cross-links between DNA and other molecules (Castro and Freeman 2001; Lachance et al. 2001). Proteins represent a diverse spectrum of molecular targets for oxidative damage. Oxidizable prosthetic groups such as metal-sulfur clusters contribute to the sensitivity of proteins to damage by reactive species. A principal target is SH group of cysteine, methionine, histidine, proline, arginine, tyrosine and tryptophan (Castro and Freeman 2001; Bettger 1993; Stadtman 1992). These protein modifications are believed to be in part responsible for the development of chronic diseases such as cancers, suggesting that zinc could be useful in reversing the sustained chronic conditions of oxidative stress, and as such could be useful cancer preventive agent as discussed below.

Zinc as an Anti-oxidant Agent

Accumulating evidence suggests that oxidative stress could be an important contributing factor in causing several chronic human diseases including cancers through oxidation of macro-molecules, such as DNA and proteins, leading to genomic instability (Fleshner and Klotz 1998; Minelli et al. 2009; Khandrika et al. 2009). Thus, dietary anti-oxidants such as zinc could in deed be useful for the prevention of these chronic diseases.

Earlier, *in vitro* and *in vivo* studies showed that zinc functions as an anti-oxidant agent in as a site-specific anti-oxidant in the body by several mechanisms (Bettger 1993; Candan et al. 2002; Demirci et al. 2003; Roussel et al. 2003). First, zinc competes with Fe and Cu ions, which catalyze the production of $^{\cdot}OH$ from H_2O_2, for binding to cell membranes and some proteins, by displacing these redox-active metals. Secondly it binds to SH groups protecting them from oxidation (Bettger 1993). Thirdly, zinc has been shown to increase the activities of GSH, catalase, and SOD (scavengers of ROS), and could decrease the activities of inducible nitric oxide synthase (iNOS) and NADPH oxidase and lipid peroxidation products (Dimitrova et al. 2005; Goel et al. 2005). Finally, zinc is known to induce the expression of metallothionein (MT) protein, which is very rich in cysteine and an excellent scavenger of $^{\cdot}OH$ (Prasad 2008; Kagi and Schaffer 1988).

An *in vitro* study showed that human lung fibroblast cells cultured under zinc deficient conditions not only undergo oxidative stress and DNA damage but also loses the capacity to repair this damage (Ho and Ames 2002; Ho et al. 2003). Thus, adequate zinc levels are necessary for maintaining DNA integrity, and thus believed to be important in the prevention of DNA damage and cancer. In zinc deficient rat glioma C6 cells, the DNA binding activities of p53, NF-κB, and activator protein 1 (AP-1) binding to their consensus DNA sequences were decreased (Ho and Ames 2002; Ho et al. 2001) whereas zinc deficiency in C6 cells showed increased oxidative stress and also induced DNA repair protein expression, compared to zinc sufficient condition (Ho and Ames 2002). Following exposure to TNF-α, zinc deficient porcine pulmonary artery-derived endothelial cells showed an increased oxidative stress, increased activation of NF-κB and AP-1 and increased production of IL-6 in comparison to zinc sufficient cells (Hennig et al. 1999). In zinc deficient rats, increased concentration of thiobarbituric acid-reactive substance (TBARS), known as a lipid peroxidation biomarker, was detected in the multiple tissues such as liver, brain and testes (Yousef et al. 2002).

One clinical trial of 30 mg zinc supplementation on oxidative stress was conducted in 56 patients with Type-2 diabetes mellitus (Roussel et al. 2003). Following 6 months of zinc supplementation, plasma zinc increased and plasma TBARS significantly decreased, whereas the placebo group showed no such changes (Roussel et al. 2003). Increased plasma lipid peroxidation by-products and decreased erythrocyte superoxide dismutase (SOD) were reported to be associated with decreased zinc status in children with chronic giardiasis (Demirci et al. 2003). The effects of vitamin C and zinc supplementation on osmotic fragility and lipid peroxidation of erythrocytes were studied in 34 zinc deficient hemodialysis patients (Candan et al. 2002). Patients were randomized to receive vitamin C (250 mg daily), zinc (20 mg daily) or a placebo for 3 months. The results revealed that supplementation with vitamin C and zinc improved osmotic fragility and decreased the level of the plasma lipid peroxidation by-product, malonyl dialdehyde (MDA).

Another recent human study by supplementation with multiple anti-oxidants have demonstrated that the combination of zinc and other anti-oxidant nutrients significantly decreased inflammatory cytokines and oxidative stress bio-markers in patients with colorectal adenoma, especially in smoking patients, compared to placebo control group (Hopkins et al. 2010). Our earlier studies have clearly demonstrated that following zinc supplementation, oxidative stress as assessed by the generation of lipid peroxidation and DNA oxidation by-products, inflammatory cytokines, and *ex vivo* TNF-α induced activation of NF-κB in isolated PMNC, were significantly decreased compared to placebo supplemented normal human subjects (Prasad et al. 2004). Our recent studies in elderly subjects and SCD patients confirmed that zinc supplementation significantly increased plasma zinc level and decreased plasma oxidative stress bio-markers, and inflammatory cytokines (Bao et al. 2008). These data strongly suggest that zinc certainly function as an anti-oxidant agent, which could play a protective role in the development and progression of cancers; however, further definitive clinical trial in human cancer patients or in population with high-risk for the development of cancer are warranted.

Molecular Link Between NF-κB, A20, Zinc and Cancer

NF-κB is one of the major immune response mediator transcription factors, and alteration of NF-κB activation is known to play critical roles in the development of chronic diseases including cancer. This transcription factor is activated by many environmental stimuli including inflammatory cytokines (IL-1β, TNF-α, and IL-6), LPS, protein kinase C activators (phorbol esters, platelet-activating factor), ROS, ultraviolet light and ionizing radiation, and other cellular stresses (Barnes 1997; Perkins 1997). NF-κB activation regulates the expression of numerous genes such as inflammatory cytokines (IL-1β, TNF-α, granulocyte macrophage colony stimulating factor, TNF superfamily member 4 and 7, and IL-2), chemokines (IL-8 and MCP-1), enzymes (iNOS and inducible cyclooxygenase), transforming growth factor 2, adhesion molecules (ICAM-1, VCAM-1, and E-selectin), receptors (IL-2 receptor-α), and other immune mediators, thereby controlling several immune responses including innate and adaptive immune response, stress response, and cell survival and proliferation. TNF-α and IL-1β not only activate NF-κB but are themselves induced by NF-κB activation (Barnes 1997; Perkins 1997). This may lead to positive feedback-loop amplification, with chronic activation of NF-κB in many cells including cancer cells. NF-κB, rather than acting alone, co-operates with other transcription factors, such as AP-1 and C/EBP (NF-κB-bZip interactions), to amplify gene expression. This may explain the wide range of genes expressed in different types of cells (Baldwin 1996).

NF-κB is normally present in the cytoplasm in an inactive form by binding to an inhibitory protein of NF-κB (IκB), which has several subunits such as IκB-α, IκB-β, and IκB-γ (Barnes 1997; Perkins 1997; Baldwin 1996). The activation state of NF-κB is determined by binding to IκB. Cytosolic NF-κB becomes active and translocates to the nucleus only when IκB is dissociated from the NF-κB heterodimer p50/p65. Many stimuli activate NF-κB via phosphorylation of IκB proteins through the action of specific kinases such as IκB kinase (IKK). Phosphorylation of IκB results in the attachment of ubiquitin residues and subsequent degradation by the multifunctional proteolytic enzyme proteasome complex (Barnes 1997; Perkins 1997; Baldwin 1996). Dissociation of IκB from NF-κB results in their rapid translocation to the nucleus for activation of NF-κB target genes. Loss of regulation of the normally latent NF-κB contributes the deregulated growth, resistance to apoptosis, and propensity to metastasize as observed in many human cancers, and thus targeting NF-κB activation has been recognized as a promising strategy for the prevention and/or treatment of human cancers.

Accumulating evidence suggests that zinc may play an important role in the regulation of NF-κB activation; however, the regulation of NF-κB activation by zinc appears to be cell type specific. Evidence show that zinc is required for NF-κB DNA binding activity either by purified proteins, recombinant NF-κB p50, or Th_0 cell lines-derived nuclear protein extracts (Otsuka et al. 1995; Prasad et al. 2001; Zabel et al. 1991). However, a number of *in vitro* studies show that zinc inhibits LPS-, ROS-, or TNF-α-induced NF-κB activation in endothelial cells, pancreatic cells, cancer cells, and PMNC (Prasad et al. 2004, 2011; Bao et al. 2008, 2010; Ho and Ames 2002; Ho et al. 2001, 2003; Connell et al. 1997), consistent with decreased expression of inflammatory cytokines, oxidative stress, anti-apoptotic protein C-1AP2, and activated C-Jun NH_2-terminal kinases, which promotes apoptotic pathways (Uzzo et al. 2002, 2006). Thus, over-expression of anti-apoptotic proteins controlled by NF-κB family members has been implicated as a key element of drug resistance in a wide variety of tumors (Uzzo et al. 2002, 2006), suggesting that inhibitors of NF-κB would an useful strategy for the treatment of human malignancies. Therefore, there are inhibitors of NF-κB activation that are different from IκB protein. One such endogenous inhibitor of NF-κB activation is A20 (also known as TNF-α induced protein 3, TNFAIP3), a cytoplasmic zinc finger-transactivating factor that plays a key role in the negative regulation of inflammation via inhibition of IL-1β- and TNF-α-induced NF-κB activation (Heyninck and Beyaert 1999; Jaattela et al. 1996; Song et al. 1996).

A20 is expressed through regulation of NF-κB activation in various types of cells in response to a number of stimuli such as TNF-α, IL-1β, LPS, PMA, ROS as well as other stimuli (Song et al. 1996). A20 was originally reported to protect cells from TNF-α-induced cytotoxicity by inhibiting the activation of NF-κB, which leads to decreased IL-1β and TNF-α signaling as demonstrated in endothelial cells and other cells (Song et al. 1996). A20 deficient ($A20^{-/-}$) mice developed severe inflammation and cachexia, and were hypersensitive to both LPS and TNF and died prematurely (Lee et al. 2000). A20 deficient cells failed to terminate TNF-induced NF-κB responses. The evidence shows that A20 inhibits NF-κB signaling by TNF-α and IL-1β via TNF-receptor associated factor (TRAF) pathways in endothelial cells (Heyninck and Beyaert 1999; Jaattela et al. 1996; Beyaert et al. 2000). Recently, A20 has also been found to contain two ubiquitin-editing domains for de-ubiquitinating proteins to inhibit NF-κB activation (Hymowitz and Wertz 2010; Malynn and Ma 2009).

Emerging evidence also suggest that A20 may play a key role in the development and progression of tumors, and its role in tumorigenesis has been shown cell-specific. For example, A20 has been identified as a tumor suppressor in the development and progression of several B-cell lymphomas (Hymowitz and Wertz 2010; Malynn and Ma 2009; Verstrepen et al. 2010; Honma et al. 2009; Schmitz et al. 2009). However, A20 is highly expressed in certain transformed cells and poorly differentiated cancer cells, although its role is not clear (Hymowitz and Wertz 2010; Malynn and Ma 2009; Verstrepen et al. 2010). Recently, one study revealed that over-expression of A20 in human salivary adenoid cystic carcinoma cells inhibits tumor cell invasion and cell growth, and NF-κB activation (Zhang et al. 2007), suggesting that A20 may function as anti-tumor agent not only in B-cell lymphomoid malignant cells, but in other cancer cells as well.

The inhibitory role of zinc in NF-κB-mediated inflammation has been considered to be associated with A20 in non-T cells. Our recent studies have shown that zinc increases A20 and A20-TRAF1 complex, and decreases the production of inflammatory cytokines and oxidative stress in HL-60, TPH-1, and HUVEC cells, compared to zinc sufficient cells (Prasad et al. 2004, 2011; Bao et al. 2010).

Silencing of A20 by its anti-sense mRNA increased TNF-alpha and IL-1 beta production in zinc-sufficient cells (Prasad et al. 2011), suggesting that zinc down-regulates the production of inflammatory cytokines via A20 pathway, which is due to deregulation of NF-κB activity.

The Role of Zinc in the Regulation of p53 and Cancer

Zinc finger protein p53, a key tumor suppressor, plays a critical role in the repression of tumorigenesis by triggering cell cycle arrest, cellular senescence, or cell death by apoptosis in response to a range of cellular stresses; for example, DNA damage and activated oncogenes. These wide ranges of biological processes generate an efficient anti-tumor barrier that eliminates incipient tumor cells (Bartkova et al. 2005; Gorgoulis et al. 2005; Vilborg et al. 2010). Normally, p53 is expressed at a low level due to its rapid protein turnover. Cellular stresses induce the stabilization of p53 protein through phosphorylation and other post-translational modifications such as acetylation. Stress-induced p53 activates the transcription of target downstream genes such as p21, GADD45, Bax, Puma, and Noxa, leading to a p53-dependent biological response including cell cycle arrest and apoptosis (Vogelstein et al. 2000), ultimately contributing to tumor suppression (Vilborg et al. 2010). The turnover of p53 is regulated by the p53 target gene encoding murine double minute 2 (MDM2), a p53 negative regulator responsible for p53 nuclear export and proteasomal degradation (Wellinghausen and Rink 1998). MDM2 is an E3 ubiquitin ligase that continuously conjugates ubiquitin molecules to lysine residues of p53, thereby targeting p53 for proteasomal degradation, and thus maintaining low constitutive p53 levels in the cells (Kruse and Gu 2009). Induction of DNA damage causes activation of protein kinases such as ATM, ATR, Chk1, Chk2, and DNA-dependent protein kinase, which phosphorylates serine residues in the N-terminal domain of p53. These phosphorylation events abolish the p53/MDM2 interaction and ubiquitination-dependent degradation of p53, with a consequent increase in the protein level of p53, and its translocation to the nucleus where it triggers the transcription of p53 target genes (Wickremasinghe et al. 2011). Inactivation of p53 function by mutation, deletion or depressed expression of its gene increases susceptibility to tumorigenesis (Kruse and Gu 2009; Pietsch et al. 2008). The mutation of p53 is the most frequently mutated gene in cancer that occurs in approximately 50% of all human tumors (Soussi and Wiman 2007).

A large number of evidence suggest that zinc may play a crucial role in the biology of p53 in which p53 protein binds to DNA through a structural complex domain stabilized by zinc. Several studies have shown that (Han et al. 2009) zinc deficiency decreases nuclear translocation of p53 and increases p53 mutation, leading to the inactivation of p53 function in several cell lines including human normal prostate cells and prostate cancer cells in comparison to the physiological zinc condition (Yan et al. 2008; Han et al. 2009). Although increased expression of p53 mRNA has been observed in zinc deficient cells (Yan et al. 2008;

Han et al. 2009), the mechanism has not been fully elucidated. Decreased cellular zinc level by its specific chelator also results in the disruption of p53-DNA inter-reaction, leading to p53 inactivation (Fong et al. 1997, 2003a, 2011). Several *in vivo* studies have demonstrated that dietary zinc deficiency results in increased esophageal cell proliferation, increased expression and mutations of p53, and the Ha-*ras* oncogene as well as increased tumor development in rats. However, these adverse effects were corrected with zinc replenishment (Fong et al. 1978, 1997, 2011). These data support the essential role of zinc in p53-mediated DNA damage response/repair mechanisms and protection against cancer development.

Our recent study have shown that zinc can reactivate p53 activity through inhibition of MDM2, resulting in the inhibition of cell growth and induction of apoptosis in colon and breast cancer cells. Chelation of cellular zinc by TPEN, a specific zinc chelator, suppressed reactivation of the p53 and its downstream target genes such as p21(WAF1) and Bax (Azmi et al. 2011). An additional new study revealed that zinc can rescue wild type and mutant p53 activity consistent with increased chemo-sensitivity in breast cancer SKBR3 (R175H mutation positive) and glioblastoma U373MG (R273H mutation positive) cells (Puca et al. 2011). The administration of zinc to U373MG-induced tumor xenografts increased drug-induced tumor regression *in vivo*, which correlated with increased wild-type p53 protein conformation. These results suggest that the use of zinc might restore drug sensitivity and inhibit tumor growth by reactivation of p53 function (Puca et al. 2011). Therefore, the essentiality of zinc in the regulation of p53 activity through stabilization of DNA-protein integrity may contribute to its protective role against the development and progression of tumors.

The Role of Zinc in the Regulation of p21 in Cancer

Zinc finger protein p21$^{WAF1/Cip1}$ is a member of the Cip/Kip family of cyclin kinase inhibitors (CKIs) (el-Deiry et al. 1993; Xiong et al. 1993), and plays an important role in the regulation of cell cycle progression through the inhibition of cyclin/cyclin depend kinase (CDK) complexes, resulting in cell cycle arrest and apoptosis. p21 is one of the p53-mediated downstream target gene products responsive to cellular stresses such as DNA damage, and thus p21 has been considered as a tumor suppressor. Cellular stresses such as DNA damage induces the expression of p21, which leads to cell growth arrest at the G1 and G2 phases or S phase (Niculescu et al. 1998). Cellular p21 level is mediated by various mechanisms such as transcriptional regulation, epigenetic silencing, and mRNA stability, as well as ubiquitin-dependent and -independent protein degradation. p21 is a short-lived protein, and proteasome inhibition leads to an increase in p21 protein levels by increasing its half-life (Sheaff et al. 2000).

Emerging evidence suggests that zinc might be involved in the regulation of p21 activity in tumorigenesis (Wong et al. 2007). The studies reported in the literature showed that zinc deficiency significantly decreased the levels of nuclear p21 protein and its mRNA abundance as well as its promoter activity in human hepatoblastoma (HepG2) cells, compared to the physiological zinc condition (Wong et al. 2007; Cui et al. 2002; Fraker and Telford 1997). This alteration in p21 caused by zinc deficiency is consistent with the depression of G1/S cell cycle progression and the promotion of apoptosis in HepG2 cells (Wong et al. 2007; Cui et al. 2002). The effect of zinc in the regulation of p21 is not unusual because we have already discussed the role of zinc in the regulation of p53, which is upstream regulator of p21.

Another recent study has shown that zinc deficiency increased p-Akt (active form), and decreased nuclear p21 and p53, consistent with induction of cell cycle at G0/G1 in human prostate cancer, LNCaP cells, compared to the physiological zinc condition (Han et al. 2009). Another recent report confirmed that zinc could suppress cell proliferation and induce G0/G1 cell cycle arrest and apoptosis through the deregulation of several apoptosis-associated genes of such as Bax, $p21^{WAF1}$, and cyclin D1 in human esophageal squamous cell carcinoma (ESCC) (Guo et al. 2011). These data suggest that zinc plays a protective role in the development and progression of esophageal squamous cell carcinoma, potentially through the regulation of zinc-dependent regulation of p21. Therefore, zinc may exhibit an anti-tumor effect through the regulation of p21 function during the development and progression of cancers, suggesting that zinc supplementation studies in clinical settings are warranted.

The Role of Zinc in the Regulation of MicroRNAs (miRNAs) in Cancer

MicroRNAs (miRNAs) are small, non-protein-coding RNA molecules (around 21–24 nucleotides) that act as post-transcriptional gene regulators by specific binding to the 3′ untranslated region (3′UTR) of target mRNAs to control protein synthesis or degradation of the mRNA. They are currently recognized as regulator of expression of most genes, and consequently play critical roles in a wide array of biological processes, including cell differentiation, proliferation, death, metabolism and energy homeostasis (DeSano and Xu 2009; Perera and Ray 2007). A large number of miRNAs have been reported to be associated with chronic diseases including cancers, and are suspected to be mechanistically associated with these chronic diseases. However, the exact role of these miRNAs in the pathogenesis of cancer with respect to the effects of zinc action has not been elucidated.

Although the role of zinc in the regulation of tumor-associated miRNAs has not been reported yet, emerging evidence suggest the existence of the interaction between zinc finger proteins and tumor-associated miRNAs. For example, miR-125 is highly expressed in cancers such as prostate cancer and pancreatic cancer, and has been considered a potent oncogenic molecule. The evidence shows that miR-125 inhibits the mRNA expression of p53, a zinc-finger transcription factor, in cancer cells (Vilborg et al. 2010), suggesting that miR-125a/b might play a role in the regulation of p53 mRNA during tumorigenesis. miRNA-181a, a tumor-associated miRNA, has been reported to decrease the expression of a large number of zinc finger genes (ZNFs) (Huang et al. 2010). These limited results suggest that miRNAs may be involved in the regulation of zinc finger proteins during tumorigenesis.

A number of zinc finger proteins have also been reported to be involved in the regulation of tumor-associated miRNAs. For example, the promyelocytic leukemia zinc finger (PLZF), a zinc-dependent transcription factor for tumor suppression, has been identified as a repressor of miR-221/miR-222, tumor-associated miRNAs, by direct binding to their putative regulatory region. Silencing of PLZF by its siRNA in melanomas unblocks miR-221 and miR-222, which in turn promotes the progression of the neoplasia through down-modulation of p27Kip1/CDKN1B and c-KIT receptor, leading to enhanced proliferation and differentiation blockade of the melanoma cells, respectively (Felicetti et al. 2008). Another zinc finger protein, zinc ribbon domain-containing 1 (ZNRD1), has been shown to inhibit cell growth, reduce tumor microvessel densities and inhibit the VEGF (vascular endothelial growth factor) production, consistent with the up-regulation of the expression of miR-214 and down-regulation of the expression of miR-296 in leukemia cell line K562 (Hong et al. 2011). These evidences suggest that anti-oncogenic zinc finger proteins may exhibit anti-tumor effect through regulation of tumor-associated miRNAs. Therefore, zinc may be involved in the inter-reaction between zinc finger proteins and miRNAs during tumorigenesis. However, in-deep mechanistic studies are warranted for elucidating the possible protective role of zinc in the development and progression of tumors through the regulation of tumor-associated miRNAs.

Anti-tumor Effect *in vitro and in vivo* of Zinc

Anti-tumor Effect of Zinc in vitro

A large number of *in vitro* studies have demonstrated that the physiological zinc level could exhibit anti-tumor effect by inhibiting cell cycle, cell growth and proliferation, cancer cell invasion, by regulating oncogenic signaling pathways such as NF-κB, AP-1, Notch-1, and PI3K/Akt. Moreover, zinc is also known for induction of mitochondria-mediated apoptosis, cytotoxicity, up-regulation of zinc-dependent activities of tumor suppressors (such as p21, p53, and A20) and stabilization of protein-DNA binding integrity in many different normal and cancer cell lines (such as pancreatic cancer cells, prostate cancer cells, and liver cancer cells) (Feng et al. 2000, 2002, 2008; Costello and Franklin 2011; Liang et al. 1999; Ishii et al. 2001a, b). The loss of zinc could be responsible for the development and progression of human malignancies, and thus suggesting that retention of the normal levels of cellular zinc might exhibit cytotoxic effects on the malignant cells. Exposure of the human pancreatic cancer Panc1 cells to a physiological concentration of 2.5–10 μM zinc has been reported to increase the cellular level of zinc, which resulted in 60–80% inhibition of cell proliferation, compared to the zinc deficient condition. This cytotoxic effect indicates that incorporation of zinc into malignant pancreatic cells could exhibit anti-tumor effects (Costello et al. 2011).

Moreover, one recent study demonstrates that short time (1–4 h) exposure to high concentration of zinc (200 μM) decreased Notch-1 binding activity through a PI3K/Akt-dependent, cytoplasmic retention of intracellular Notch domain (ICN) of Notch-1 and RBP-Jk, leading to inactivation of Notch-1 signaling in human embryonic kidney HEK 293 cells (Baek et al. 2007). Notch signaling plays a pivotal role in cell proliferation and apoptosis, which are involved in the development and functioning of a wide variety of organisms and cell types (Wang et al. 2008, 2010). Up-regulation of Notch-1 signaling has been observed in many tumors. Thus, the inactivation of Notch signaling network by zinc may contribute to the inhibition of cell growth and proliferation (Baek et al. 2007); however, more oncogenic pathways by which zinc may mediate its anti-tumor effect during the development and progression of tumors require future in-depth investigations.

Anti-tumor Effect of Zinc in vivo

Zinc and prostate cancer: Several early studies have demonstrated that the exposure of human malignant prostate LNCaP and PC-3 cells to physiological levels of zinc results in the induction of apoptosis via mitochondrial cytochrome c-mediated apoptogenesis and inhibition of cell growth while having no effect on HPR-1 cells derived from human normal prostatic epithelial cells (Feng et al. 2002; Costello and Franklin 1998; Costello et al. 2005). The zinc accumulation in PC-3 and BPH was higher than that in HPR-1 cells, consistent with the evidence that prostate tumor tissues or cells have significantly lower levels of zinc compared to normal prostate tissues or cells, suggesting that the zinc-induced apoptosis could be associated with the status of cellular zinc (Feng et al. 2002; Costello and Franklin 1998; Costello et al. 2005). Further studies have shown that *in vivo* treatment (28 days of treatment) with zinc increased zinc accumulation and citrate production in human malignant prostate cells PC-3-induced tumor tissues and inhibited tumor growth in nude mice (Feng et al. 2003). This inhibitory effect of zinc appears to result from zinc-induced apoptosis by regulation of mitochondrial membrane permeability related Bax/Bcl 2 proteins (Feng et al. 2003).

Recently, the protective role of dietary zinc in prostate cancer has been investigated in TRAMP (transgenic adenocarcinoma of the mouse prostate) mouse model (Prasad et al. 2010). The results showed that tumor weights were significantly higher when the dietary zinc intake was either deficient or high in comparison to normal zinc intake level, suggesting that an optimal dietary zinc intake may play a protective role against prostate cancer. Furthermore, normal zinc-supplemented animals show a decreased plasma insulin-like growth factor (IGF)-1 and a low ratio of IGF-1/IGF binding protein-3, a sensitive tumor biomarker, suggesting that zinc may modulate IGF-1 metabolism in relation to carcinogenesis. These data indicate that optimal prostate zinc concentration has a protective role against prostate cancer.

Zinc and esophageal tumor: A number of early *in vivo* studies have demonstrated that dietary zinc deficiency increases tumor cell proliferation and carcinogen-induced esophageal tumor incidences in both mice and rats, compared to the zinc sufficient condition (Fong et al. 1978, 1982, 1984a, b, 1987, 2003b; Fong and Newberne 1978; Fong and Magee 1999). More recent studies have confirmed that zinc supplementation to carcinogen-treated animals could prevent oral and stomach tumor development, consistent with decreased expression of cyclin D1 and COX-2, and induction of apoptosis in zinc-deficient carcinogen-treated rats (Fong et al. 2011; Wan et al. 2010). Zn supplementation also significantly reduced cell proliferation in non-lesional tongue squamous epithelia, thereby suppressing tumor development. These *in vivo* data suggest that zinc supplementation may be efficacious in the chemoprevention of human esophageal cancer.

Zinc and stomach tumor: Emerging evidence also suggests that zinc deficiency is associated with high incidences of esophageal and other cancers in humans and experimental animals (Ng et al. 1984; Joint Iran-International Agency for Research on Cancer Study Group 1977; Yang 1980), and this led to a highly proliferative hyperplastic condition in the upper gastrointestinal tract in the laboratory animals (Ng et al. 1984) whereas Zn replenishment reduced the incidence of lingual, esophageal, and forestomach tumors in Zn-deficient rats and mice. Recent study showed that zinc supplementation reduces the incidence of carcinogen-induced forestomach tumor and the severity of preneoplastic and neoplastic lesions in zinc sufficient mice of tumor-suppressor-deficient mouse strain (Ng et al. 1984; Sun et al. 2010), suggesting that zinc may play a protective role in the development and progression of stomach tumor in humans. The exact mechanism(s) by which zinc may protect against the development of stomach cancer is not clear, and thus further studies are required for fully elucidating the protective role of zinc against stomach cancer.

Zinc and colon tumor: The protective role of zinc against the development and progression of colon tumors has been investigated in animal models. The evidence revealed that decreased tissue level of zinc was associated with increased incidence of carcinogen-induced colon tumor, which is consistent with increased level of oxidative stress (Dani et al. 2007). Administration of zinc to carcinogen-treated rats significantly increased tissue concentrations of zinc in the colon following carcinogen (DMH) treatment and decreased the colon tumor incidence, tumor size and aberrant crypt foci number along with decreased production of oxidative stress. These results suggest that zinc could have a positive beneficial effect against carcinogen-induced colonic preneoplastic progression in rat model (Dani et al. 2007; Chadha and Dhawan 2010a, b; Chadha et al. 2010). Therefore, these *in vitro* and *in vivo* studies strongly suggest that zinc may play a key protective role against the development and progression of colon tumors.

Human Zinc Deficiency and Cancer

Human zinc deficiency decreases T lymphocyte function, especially T cell-mediated immune function, and increases the production of inflammatory cytokines and oxidative stress, and impairs DNA-protein structure and function. A large number of clinical and epidemiological studies have indicated that zinc deficiency could be associated with the development and progression of many tumors such as prostate cancer, esophageal cancer, head and neck cancer, and lung cancer (Costello and Franklin 2011; Joint Iran-International Agency for Research on Cancer Study Group 1977; Yang 1980; Schrauzer et al. 1977; Schrauzer and White 1978; Kristal et al. 1999; Ogunlewe and Osegbe 1989; Feustel et al. 1989; Lekili et al. 1991; Whelan et al. 1983; Allen et al. 1985).

One early clinical observation showed that blood zinc level was significantly decreased in 26 patients with prostate cancer compared to 15 patients with benign prostatic hyperplasia (BPH) (62.81 vs 93.53 μg zinc/mL) (Lekili et al. 1991), consistent with evidence from other studies (Lekili et al. 1991; Whelan et al. 1983; Chirulescu et al. 1987). The clinical *in situ* studies demonstrate that malignant prostate tissue has remarkably decreased zinc content (Ogunlewe and Osegbe 1989; Dhar et al. 1973; Feustel et al. 1982), consistent with altered expression of zinc transporter proteins such as Zip1, compared to normal or BPH prostate tissue (Ogunlewe and Osegbe 1989; Dhar et al. 1973; Feustel et al. 1982; Franklin et al. 2003). These results strongly suggest that zinc may play a key role in the development and progression of prostate cancer.

One early case-control study conducted in lung cancer patients (Allen et al. 1985) showed that mean serum zinc concentration in 75 patients with lung cancer was 67.4 vs 96.0 μg zinc/dL for normal subjects (equal to or greater than 90 μg zinc/dL considered as normal). Patients with low serum zinc levels (less than 70 μg/dl) had significantly higher urine zinc excretion, consistent with depressed T cell response function, compared to patients with normal serum zinc levels. These data indicate that these patients have a mild chronic zinc deficient state. After 6 months of high level of oral zinc therapy (220 mg, three times daily for 6 weeks), lung cancer patients with zinc deficiency had normalization of T cell response function, whereas the placebo patients with zinc deficiency demonstrated continued T cell dysfunction (Allen et al. 1985).

Another case-control study was conducted to examine the effect of zinc status on clinical morbidities in 47 patients with newly diagnosed head and neck cancer with metastatic disease having severe co-morbid conditions (Prasad et al. 1997, 1998; Doerr et al. 1997, 1998). The results showed that at baseline approximately 50% of subjects were zinc-deficient based on cellular zinc criteria and had decreased production of Th1 cytokines but not Th2 cytokines, decreased NK cell lytic activity and decreased proportion of CD^{4+} CD^{45RA+} cells in the peripheral blood. The tumor size and overall stage of the disease was correlated with baseline zinc status, but not with prognostic nutritional index (PNI), alcohol intake, or smoking. Zinc deficiency was also associated with increased unplanned hospitalizations. The disease-free interval was highest for the group which had both zinc sufficient and sufficient nutrition status. Zinc deficiency and cell mediated immune dysfunctions were frequently present in patients with head and neck cancer when seen initially. Zinc deficiency resulted in an imbalance of Th1 and Th2 functions. Therefore, zinc deficiency was associated with increased tumor size, overall stage of the cancer and increased unplanned hospitalizations (Prasad et al. 1997, 1998; Doerr et al. 1997, 1998). These results suggest that zinc deficiency may play an important role in the development and progression of head and neck cancer as indicated above.

Recent studies have also demonstrated that zinc deficiency was found in children with Down's syndrome, a 50 times higher risk of leukemia (Blair et al. 2008), and malignant lymphoma (Cavdar et al. 2009). Additional new *in situ* study revealed that cellular or tissue zinc levels are markedly decreased in pancreatic cancer, with concurrent down-regulation of ZIP3 zinc uptake transporter and ras responsive element binding protein-1 (RREB-1), a transcription factor for zinc transporter proteins, as compared with normal pancreatic ductal/acinar epithelium (Costello et al. 2011). These changes occur in early stage malignancy and persisted during the progression of malignancy. These data suggest that low cellular zinc status may be associated with the development and progression of pancreatic cancer, providing new insight into important factors and events in pancreatic carcinogenesis, which can lead to the development of early biomarkers and new efficacious therapeutic agents including zinc supplementation.

Dietary Zinc or Zinc Supplementation and Cancer

Since zinc deficiency appears to contribute to the development and progression of tumors, the high dietary zinc intake or zinc supplementation could be an attractive approach to increase the tissue or cellular zinc level, which would likely play a protective role against the development and progression of cancers.

Prostate cancer: As indicated previously that zinc deficiency is associated with prostate cancer, which is supported by a large number of experimental and clinical studies. However, the data from a large number of early epidemiological studies are not consistent. Modest to moderate inverse association between zinc and prostate cancer were observed in the case-control study for dietary zinc intake (Key et al. 1997) or zinc supplementation (Kristal et al. 1999). For example, one large population case-control study (n = 697 vs 666) showed that zinc supplementation to patients with prostate cancer has some protective role against the development and progression of prostate cancer (Kristal et al. 1999) whereas other case-control studies have not observed such a protective association for dietary (West et al. 1991; Andersson et al. 1996) or combined dietary and supplemental zinc intake (Kolonel et al. 1988; Vlajinac et al. 1997). Moreover, one study with the supplementation of more than 100 mg zinc daily has shown an opposite effect on the risk of advanced prostate cancer (Leitzmann et al. 2003). Differences in findings among these studies may be due to small number of positive case patients, very high dose of zinc supplementation, different ranges of dietary zinc intake among the human subjects, other dietary confounder such as high calcium intake and cadmium contamination, and misclassification of zinc intake by assessing post-diagnosis diet rather than diet in an etiologically relevant period. Another possible source of misclassification is in the assessment of zinc using food frequency questionnaires or dietary records (Platz and Helzlsouer 2001; Costello et al. 2004; Krone and Harms 2003).

One recent population-based cohort study including 525 men aged <80 year demonstrates that with a median follow-up of 6.4 year, 218 (42%) men died of prostate cancer and 257 (49%) died of other causes. High dietary zinc intake was associated with reduced risk of prostate cancer-specific mortality in this population-based study. The association was stronger in men with localized tumors and zinc intake was not associated with mortality from other causes (Epstein et al. 2011). These results suggest that high dietary intake of zinc could be associated with lower prostate cancer-specific mortality after diagnosis, particularly in men with localized disease.

Head and neck cancer: Several recent clinical studies have shown the beneficial effect of zinc supplementation in patients diagnosed with head and neck cancer (Lin et al. 2006, 2008, 2009, 2010). The results demonstrate that zinc supplementation used in conjunction with radiotherapy and or chemotherapy could decrease the development of severe mucositis and dermatitis, increases 3–5 year overall local-free and disease-free survival rate, compared to the patients in the placebo group. These data suggest that zinc supplementation in conjunction with chemo-radiotherapy attenuate local tumor recurrence and improve the overall survival of patients with advanced nasopharyngeal carcinoma.

Lung and other cancers: The beneficial effect of zinc supplementation in patients diagnosed with other tumors has also been reported (Lee and Jacobs 2005). In a 16 year follow-up study with 34,708 postmenopausal women (aged 55–69 years), the results showed that high dietary heme iron intake may increase the risk of lung cancer, whereas high dietary zinc may decrease the risk of lung cancer among women who consume high-dose vitamin C supplements. Another large population case-control study also demonstrated that normal zinc intake exhibit a weak protective effect in the development and progression of meningioma, compared to the subjects with low zinc intake (Dimitropoulou et al. 2008). These data indicate that high dietary zinc intake or oral zinc supplementation may have a protective role in the development and progression of these tumors. However, larger well-controlled populations must be included in the clinical trial design with oral zinc supplementation for assessing the protective role of zinc against the development and progression of human malignancies in the future.

Conclusions and Perspectives

We attempted to summarize the "state-of-our-knowledge" on the role of zinc in human health and disease as succinctly as possible and during such attempt we could cite all the published results, and thus we sincerely apologize to those authors whose work was not cited. In summary, evidences are compelling in favor of the beneficial role of dietary zinc in maintaining normal physiological conditions, and that supplementation of zinc could be useful for the prevention and/or treatment of human diseases including cancer. However, further mechanistic and well-designed clinical trials are needed in order to fully appreciate the health benefit of zinc for cancer and other chronic diseases.

Acknowledgements We thank Ms. Amanda C. Sehmer and Ms. Ginny W. Bao for editing the manuscript.

References

Allen JI, Bell E, Boosalis MG, Oken MM, McClain CJ, Levine AS, Morley JE (1985) Association between urinary zinc excretion and lymphocyte dysfunction in patients with lung cancer. Am J Med 79(2):209–215

Andersson SO, Wolk A, Bergstrom R, Giovannucci E, Lindgren C, Baron J, Adami HO (1996) Energy, nutrient intake and prostate cancer risk: a population-based case-control study in Sweden. Int J Cancer 68(6):716–722

Antoniou LD, Shalhoub RJ, Schechter GP (1981) The effect of zinc on cellular immunity in chronic uremia. Am J Clin Nutr 34(9):1912–1917

Azmi AS, Philip PA, Beck FW, Wang Z, Banerjee S, Wang S, Yang D, Sarkar FH, Mohammad RM (2011) MI-219-zinc combination: a new paradigm in MDM2 inhibitor-based therapy. Oncogene 30(1):117–126

Baek SH, Kim MY, Mo JS, Ann EJ, Lee KS, Park JH, Kim JY, Seo MS, Choi EJ, Park HS (2007) Zinc-induced downregulation of Notch signaling is associated with cytoplasmic retention of Notch1-IC and RBP-Jk via PI3k-Akt signaling pathway. Cancer Lett 255(1):117–126

Baldwin AS Jr (1996) The NF-kappa B and I kappa B proteins: new discoveries and insights. Annu Rev Immunol 14:649–683

Bao B, Prasad AS, Beck FW, Godmere M (2003) Zinc modulates mRNA levels of cytokines. Am J Physiol Endocrinol Metab 285(5):E1095–E1102

Bao B, Prasad AS, Beck FW, Snell D, Suneja A, Sarkar FH, Doshi N, Fitzgerald JT, Swerdlow P (2008) Zinc supplementation decreases oxidative stress, incidence of infection, and generation of inflammatory cytokines in sickle cell disease patients. Transl Res 152(2):67–80

Bao B, Prasad AS, Beck FW, Fitzgerald JT, Snell D, Bao GW, Singh T, Cardozo LJ (2010) Zinc decreases C-reactive protein, lipid peroxidation, and inflammatory cytokines in elderly subjects: a potential implication of zinc as an atheroprotective agent. Am J Clin Nutr 91(6):1634–1641

Bao B, Prasad AS, Beck FW, Bao GW, Singh T, Ali S, Sarkar FH (2011) Intracellular free zinc up-regulates IFN-gamma and T-bet essential for Th1 differentiation in Con-A stimulated HUT-78 cells. Biochem Biophys Res Commun 407(4):703–707

Barnes PJ (1997) Nuclear factor-kappa B. Int J Biochem Cell Biol 29(6):867–870

Bartkova J, Horejsi Z, Koed K, Kramer A, Tort F, Zieger K, Guldberg P, Sehested M, Nesland JM, Lukas C, Orntoft T, Lukas J, Bartek J (2005) DNA damage response as a candidate anti-cancer barrier in early human tumorigenesis. Nature 434(7035):864–870

Bettger WJ (1993) Zinc and selenium, site-specific versus general antioxidation. Can J Physiol Pharmacol 71(9):721–724

Beyaert R, Heyninck K, Van HS (2000) A20 and A20-binding proteins as cellular inhibitors of nuclear factor-kappa B-dependent gene expression and apoptosis. Biochem Pharmacol 60(8):1143–1151

Blair CK, Roesler M, Xie Y, Gamis AS, Olshan AF, Heerema NA, Robison LL, Ross JA (2008) Vitamin supplement use among children with Down's syndrome and risk of leukaemia: a Children's Oncology Group (COG) study. Paediatr Perinat Epidemiol 22(3):288–295

Candan F, Gultekin F, Candan F (2002) Effect of vitamin C and zinc on osmotic fragility and lipid peroxidation in zinc-deficient haemodialysis patients. Cell Biochem Funct 20(2):95–98

Castro L, Freeman BA (2001) Reactive oxygen species in human health and disease. Nutrition 17(2):161, 163–161, 165

Castro L, Alvarez MN, Radi R (1996) Modulatory role of nitric oxide on superoxide-dependent luminol chemiluminescence. Arch Biochem Biophys 333(1):179–188

Cavdar AO, Gozdasoglu S, Babacan E, Mengubas K, Unal E, Yavuz G, Tacyildiz N (2009) Zinc and selenium status in pediatric malignant lymphomas. Nutr Cancer 61(6):888–890

Chadha VD, Dhawan D (2010a) (65)Zn kinetics as a biomarker of DMH induced colon carcinogenesis. Hell J Nucl Med 13(3):257–260

Chadha VD, Dhawan DK (2010b) Ultrastructural changes in rat colon following 1,2-dimethylhydrazine-induced colon carcinogenesis: protection by zinc. Oncol Res 19(1):1–11

Chadha VD, Garg ML, Dhawan D (2010) Influence of extraneous supplementation of zinc on trace elemental profile leading to prevention of dimethylhydrazine-induced colon carcinogenesis. Toxicol Mech Methods 20(8):493–497

Chirulescu Z, Chiriloiu C, Suciu A, Pirvulescu R (1987) Variations of zinc, calcium and magnesium in normal subjects and in patients with neoplasias. Med Interne 25(4):257–261

Connell P, Young VM, Toborek M, Cohen DA, Barve S, McClain CJ, Hennig B (1997) Zinc attenuates tumor necrosis factor-mediated activation of transcription factors in endothelial cells. J Am Coll Nutr 16(5):411–417

Costello LC, Franklin RB (1998) Novel role of zinc in the regulation of prostate citrate metabolism and its implications in prostate cancer. Prostate 35(4):285–296

Costello LC, Franklin RB (2011) Zinc is decreased in prostate cancer: an established relationship of prostate cancer! J Biol Inorg Chem 16(1):3–8

Costello LC, Franklin RB, Feng P, Tan M (2004) Re: Zinc supplement use and risk of prostate cancer. J Natl Cancer Inst 96(3):239–240

Costello LC, Franklin RB, Feng P (2005) Mitochondrial function, zinc, and intermediary metabolism relationships in normal prostate and prostate cancer. Mitochondrion 5(3):143–153

Costello LC, Bernard AL, Desouki MM, Zou J, Zou J, Bagasra O, Johnson LA, Hanna N, Franklin RB (2011) Decreased zinc and down regulation of ZIP3 zinc uptake transporter in the development of pancreatic adenocarcinoma. Cancer Biol Ther 12(4)

Cui L, Schoene NW, Zhu L, Fanzo JC, Alshatwi A, Lei KY (2002) Zinc depletion reduced Egr-1 and HNF-3beta expression and apolipoprotein A-I promoter activity in Hep G2 cells. Am J Physiol Cell Physiol 283(2):C623–C630

Dani V, Goel A, Vaiphei K, Dhawan DK (2007) Chemopreventive potential of zinc in experimentally induced colon carcinogenesis. Toxicol Lett 171(1–2):10–18

De Marzo AM, Platz EA, Sutcliffe S, Xu J, Gronberg H, Drake CG, Nakai Y, Isaacs WB, Nelson WG (2007) Inflammation in prostate carcinogenesis. Nat Rev Cancer 7(4):256–269

DeCoursey TE, Morgan D, Cherny VV (2003) The voltage dependence of NADPH oxidase reveals why phagocytes need proton channels. Nature 422(6931):531–534

Demirci M, Delibas N, Altuntas I, Oktem F, Yonden Z (2003) Serum iron, zinc and copper levels and lipid peroxidation in children with chronic giardiasis. J Health Popul Nutr 21(1):72–75

DeSano JT, Xu L (2009) MicroRNA regulation of cancer stem cells and therapeutic implications. AAPS J 11(4):682–692

Dhar NK, Goel TC, Dube PC, Chowdhury AR, Kar AB (1973) Distribution and concentration of zinc in the subcellular fractions of benign hyperplastic and malignant neoplastic human prostate. Exp Mol Pathol 19(2):139–142

Dimitropoulou P, Nayee S, Liu JF, Demetriou L, van Tongeren M, Hepworth SJ, Muir KR (2008) Dietary zinc intake and brain cancer in adults: a case-control study. Br J Nutr 99(3):667–673

Dimitrova AA, Strashimirov DS, Russeva AL, Andreeva-Gateva PA, Lakova ET, Tzachev KN (2005) Effect of zinc on the activity of Cu/Zn superoxide dismutase and lipid profile in Wistar rats. Folia Med (Plovdiv) 47(1):42–46

Doerr TD, Prasad AS, Marks SC, Beck FW, Shamsa FH, Penny HS, Mathog RH (1997) Zinc deficiency in head and neck cancer patients. J Am Coll Nutr 16(5):418–422

Doerr TD, Marks SC, Shamsa FH, Mathog RH, Prasad AS (1998) Effects of zinc and nutritional status on clinical outcomes in head and neck cancer. Nutrition 14(6):489–495

el-Deiry WS, Tokino T, Velculescu VE, Levy DB, Parsons R, Trent JM, Lin D, Mercer WE, Kinzler KW, Vogelstein B (1993) WAF1, a potential mediator of p53 tumor suppression. Cell 75(4):817–825

Epstein MM, Kasperzyk JL, Andren O, Giovannucci EL, Wolk A, Hakansson N, Andersson SO, Johansson JE, Fall K, Mucci LA (2011) Dietary zinc and prostate cancer survival in a Swedish cohort. Am J Clin Nutr 93(3):586–593

Ertekin MV, Uslu H, Karslioglu I, Ozbek E, Ozbek A (2003) Effect of oral zinc supplementation on agents of oropharyngeal infection in patients receiving radiotherapy for head and neck cancer. J Int Med Res 31(4):253–266

Ertekin MV, Koc M, Karslioglu I, Sezen O (2004) Zinc sulfate in the prevention of radiation-induced oropharyngeal mucositis: a prospective, placebo-controlled, randomized study. Int J Radiat Oncol Biol Phys 58(1):167–174

Falchuk KH (1998) The molecular basis for the role of zinc in developmental biology. Mol Cell Biochem 188(1–2):41–48

Felicetti F, Errico MC, Bottero L, Segnalini P, Stoppacciaro A, Biffoni M, Felli N, Mattia G, Petrini M, Colombo MP, Peschle C, Care A (2008) The promyelocytic leukemia zinc finger-microRNA-221/-222 pathway controls melanoma progression through multiple oncogenic mechanisms. Cancer Res 68(8):2745–2754

Feng P, Liang JY, Li TL, Guan ZX, Zou J, Franklin R, Costello LC (2000) Zinc induces mitochondria apoptogenesis in prostate cells. Mol Urol 4(1):31–36

Feng P, Li TL, Guan ZX, Franklin RB, Costello LC (2002) Direct effect of zinc on mitochondrial apoptogenesis in prostate cells. Prostate 52(4):311–318

Feng P, Li TL, Guan ZX, Franklin RB, Costello LC (2003) Effect of zinc on prostatic tumorigenicity in nude mice. Ann N Y Acad Sci 1010:316–320

Feng P, Li T, Guan Z, Franklin RB, Costello LC (2008) The involvement of Bax in zinc-induced mitochondrial apoptogenesis in malignant prostate cells. Mol Cancer 7:25

Feustel A, Wennrich R, Steiniger D, Klauss P (1982) Zinc and cadmium concentration in prostatic carcinoma of different histological grading in comparison to normal prostate tissue and adenofibromyomatosis (BPH). Urol Res 10(6):301–303

Feustel A, Wennrich R, Schmidt B (1989) Serum-Zn-levels in prostatic cancer. Urol Res 17(1):41–42

Fleshner NE, Klotz LH (1998) Diet, androgens, oxidative stress and prostate cancer susceptibility. Cancer Metastasis Rev 17(4):325–330

Fong LY, Magee PN (1999) Dietary zinc deficiency enhances esophageal cell proliferation and N-nitrosomethylbenzylamine (NMBA)-induced esophageal tumor incidence in C57BL/6 mouse. Cancer Lett 143(1):63–69

Fong LY, Newberne PM (1978) Nitrosobenzylmethylamine, zinc deficiency and oesophageal cancer. IARC Sci Publ 19:503–513

Fong LY, Sivak A, Newberne PM (1978) Zinc deficiency and methylbenzylnitrosamine-induced esophageal cancer in rats. J Natl Cancer Inst 61(1):145–150

Fong LY, Lee JS, Chan WC, Newberne PM (1982) Zinc deficiency and the induction of oesophageal tumors in rats by benzylmethylamine and sodium nitrite. IARC Sci Publ 41:679–683

Fong LY, Lee JS, Chan WC, Newberne PM (1984a) Zinc deficiency and the development of esophageal and forestomach tumors in Sprague–Dawley rats fed precursors of N-nitroso-N-benzylmethylamine. J Natl Cancer Inst 72(2):419–425

Fong LY, Ng WL, Newberne PM (1984b) N-nitrosodimethylamine-induced forestomach tumours in male Sprague–Dawley rats fed a zinc-deficient diet. IARC Sci Publ 57:543–546

Fong LY, Lui CP, Ma-Tung L, Ng WL (1987) Zinc-deficiency and the development of malignant lymphoma in rats given a single intragastric dose of N-methyl-N-nitrosourea. IARC Sci Publ 84:261–263

Fong LY, Lau KM, Huebner K, Magee PN (1997) Induction of esophageal tumors in zinc-deficient rats by single low doses of N-nitrosomethylbenzylamine (NMBA): analysis of cell proliferation, and mutations in H-ras and p53 genes. Carcinogenesis 18(8):1477–1484

Fong LY, Mancini R, Nakagawa H, Rustgi AK, Huebner K (2003a) Combined cyclin D1 overexpression and zinc deficiency disrupts cell cycle and accelerates mouse forestomach carcinogenesis. Cancer Res 63(14):4244–4252

Fong LY, Ishii H, Nguyen VT, Vecchione A, Farber JL, Croce CM, Huebner K (2003b) p53 deficiency accelerates induction and progression of esophageal and forestomach tumors in zinc-deficient mice. Cancer Res 63(1):186–195

Fong LY, Jiang Y, Rawahneh ML, Smalley KJ, Croce CM, Farber JL, Huebner K (2011) Zinc supplementation suppresses 4-nitroquinoline 1-oxide-induced rat oral carcinogenesis. Carcinogenesis 32(4):554–560

Forman HJ, Torres M (2002) Reactive oxygen species and cell signaling: respiratory burst in macrophage signaling. Am J Respir Crit Care Med 166(12 Pt 2):S4–S8

Fraker PJ, Telford WG (1997) A reappraisal of the role of zinc in life and death decisions of cells. Proc Soc Exp Biol Med 215(3):229–236

Fraker PJ, Gershwin ME, Good RA, Prasad A (1986) Interrelationships between zinc and immune function. Fed Proc 45(5):1474–1479

Franklin RB, Ma J, Zou J, Guan Z, Kukoyi BI, Feng P, Costello LC (2003) Human ZIP1 is a major zinc uptake transporter for the accumulation of zinc in prostate cells. J Inorg Biochem 96(2–3):435–442

Fridovich I (1997) Superoxide anion radical (O2-.), superoxide dismutases, and related matters. J Biol Chem 272(30):18515–18517

Goel A, Dani V, Dhawan DK (2005) Protective effects of zinc on lipid peroxidation, antioxidant enzymes and hepatic histoarchitecture in chlorpyrifos-induced toxicity. Chem Biol Interact 156(2–3):131–140

Gorgoulis VG, Pratsinis H, Zacharatos P, Demoliou C, Sigala F, Asimacopoulos PJ, Papavassiliou AG, Kletsas D (2005) p53-dependent ICAM-1 overexpression in senescent human cells identified in atherosclerotic lesions. Lab Invest 85(4):502–511

Guo W, Zou YB, Jiang YG, Wang RW, Zhao YP, Ma Z (2011) Zinc induces cell cycle arrest and apoptosis by upregulation of WIG-1 in esophageal squamous cancer cell line EC109. Tumour Biol 32(4):801–808

Han D, Antunes F, Canali R, Rettori D, Cadenas E (2003) Voltage-dependent anion channels control the release of the superoxide anion from mitochondria to cytosol. J Biol Chem 278(8):5557–5563

Han CT, Schoene NW, Lei KY (2009) Influence of zinc deficiency on Akt-Mdm2-p53 and Akt-p21 signaling axes in normal and malignant human prostate cells. Am J Physiol Cell Physiol 297(5):C1188–C1199

Hennig B, Meerarani P, Toborek M, McClain CJ (1999) Antioxidant-like properties of zinc in activated endothelial cells. J Am Coll Nutr 18(2):152–158

Heyninck K, Beyaert R (1999) The cytokine-inducible zinc finger protein A20 inhibits IL-1-induced NF-kappaB activation at the level of TRAF6. FEBS Lett 442(2–3):147–150

Ho E, Ames BN (2002) Low intracellular zinc induces oxidative DNA damage, disrupts p53, NFkappa B, and AP1 DNA binding, and affects DNA repair in a rat glioma cell line. Proc Natl Acad Sci U S A 99(26):16770–16775

Ho E, Quan N, Tsai YH, Lai W, Bray TM (2001) Dietary zinc supplementation inhibits NFkappaB activation and protects against chemically induced diabetes in CD1 mice. Exp Biol Med (Maywood) 226(2):103–111

Ho E, Courtemanche C, Ames BN (2003) Zinc deficiency induces oxidative DNA damage and increases p53 expression in human lung fibroblasts. J Nutr 133(8):2543–2548

Hong L, Han Y, Li S, Yang J, Gong T, Li J, Zheng J, Zhang H, Zhao Q, Wu K, Fan D (2011) Role of ZNRD1 (zinc ribbon domain-containing 1) in angiogenesis of leukaemia cells. Cell Biol Int 35(4):321–324

Honma K, Tsuzuki S, Nakagawa M, Tagawa H, Nakamura S, Morishima Y, Seto M (2009) TNFAIP3/A20 functions as a novel tumor suppressor gene in several subtypes of non-Hodgkin lymphomas. Blood 114(12):2467–2475

Hopkins MH, Fedirko V, Jones DP, Terry PD, Bostick RM (2010) Antioxidant micronutrients and biomarkers of oxidative stress and inflammation in colorectal adenoma patients: results from a randomized, controlled clinical trial. Cancer Epidemiol Biomarkers Prev 19(3):850–858

Huang S, Wu S, Ding J, Lin J, Wei L, Gu J, He X (2010) MicroRNA-181a modulates gene expression of zinc finger family members by directly targeting their coding regions. Nucleic Acids Res 38(20):7211–7218

Hymowitz SG, Wertz IE (2010) A20: from ubiquitin editing to tumour suppression. Nat Rev Cancer 10(5):332–341

Ishii K, Usui S, Sugimura Y, Yoshida S, Hioki T, Tatematsu M, Yamamoto H, Hirano K (2001a) Aminopeptidase N regulated by zinc in human prostate participates in tumor cell invasion. Int J Cancer 92(1):49–54

Ishii K, Usui S, Sugimura Y, Yamamoto H, Yoshikawa K, Hirano K (2001b) Inhibition of aminopeptidase N (AP-N) and urokinase-type plasminogen activator (uPA) by zinc suppresses the invasion activity in human urological cancer cells. Biol Pharm Bull 24(3):226–230

Jaattela M, Mouritzen H, Elling F, Bastholm L (1996) A20 zinc finger protein inhibits TNF and IL-1 signaling. J Immunol 156(3):1166–1173

Joint Iran-International Agency for Research on Cancer Study Group (1977) Esophageal cancer studies in the Caspian littoral of Iran: results of population studies–a prodrome. J Natl Cancer Inst 59(4):1127–1138

Kagi JH, Schaffer A (1988) Biochemistry of metallothionein. Biochemistry 27(23):8509–8515

Key TJ, Silcocks PB, Davey GK, Appleby PN, Bishop DT (1997) A case-control study of diet and prostate cancer. Br J Cancer 76(5):678–687

Khandrika L, Kumar B, Koul S, Maroni P, Koul HK (2009) Oxidative stress in prostate cancer. Cancer Lett 282(2):125–136

Kocyigit A, Gur S, Erel O, Gurel MS (2002) Associations among plasma selenium, zinc, copper, and iron concentrations and immunoregulatory cytokine levels in patients with cutaneous leishmaniasis. Biol Trace Elem Res 90(1–3):47–55

Kolonel LN, Yoshizawa CN, Hankin JH (1988) Diet and prostatic cancer: a case-control study in Hawaii. Am J Epidemiol 127(5):999–1012

Kristal AR, Stanford JL, Cohen JH, Wicklund K, Patterson RE (1999) Vitamin and mineral supplement use is associated with reduced risk of prostate cancer. Cancer Epidemiol Biomarkers Prev 8(10):887–892

Krone CA, Harms LC (2003) Re: Zinc supplement use and risk of prostate cancer. J Natl Cancer Inst 95(20):1556–1557

Kruse JP, Gu W (2009) Modes of p53 regulation. Cell 137(4):609–622

Lachance PA, Nakat Z, Jeong WS (2001) Antioxidants: an integrative approach. Nutrition 17(10):835–838

Landmesser U, Harrison DG (2001) Oxidative stress and vascular damage in hypertension. Coron Artery Dis 12(6):455–461

Lee DH, Jacobs DR Jr (2005) Interaction among heme iron, zinc, and supplemental vitamin C intake on the risk of lung cancer: Iowa Women's Health Study. Nutr Cancer 52(2):130–137

Lee EG, Boone DL, Chai S, Libby SL, Chien M, Lodolce JP, Ma A (2000) Failure to regulate TNF-induced NF-kappaB and cell death responses in A20-deficient mice. Science 289(5488):2350–2354

Leitzmann MF, Stampfer MJ, Wu K, Colditz GA, Willett WC, Giovannucci EL (2003) Zinc supplement use and risk of prostate cancer. J Natl Cancer Inst 95(13):1004–1007

Lekili M, Ergen A, Celebi I (1991) Zinc plasma levels in prostatic carcinoma and BPH. Int Urol Nephrol 23(2):151–154

Liang JY, Liu YY, Zou J, Franklin RB, Costello LC, Feng P (1999) Inhibitory effect of zinc on human prostatic carcinoma cell growth. Prostate 40(3):200–207

Lin LC, Que J, Lin LK, Lin FC (2006) Zinc supplementation to improve mucositis and dermatitis in patients after radiotherapy for head-and-neck cancers: a double-blind, randomized study. Int J Radiat Oncol Biol Phys 65(3):745–750

Lin LC, Que J, Lin KL, Leung HW, Lu CL, Chang CH (2008) Effects of zinc supplementation on clinical outcomes in patients receiving radiotherapy for head and neck cancers: a double-blinded randomized study. Int J Radiat Oncol Biol Phys 70(2):368–373

Lin YS, Lin LC, Lin SW (2009) Effects of zinc supplementation on the survival of patients who received concomitant chemotherapy and radiotherapy for advanced nasopharyngeal carcinoma: follow-up of a double-blind randomized study with subgroup analysis. Laryngoscope 119(7):1348–1352

Lin YS, Lin LC, Lin SW, Chang CP (2010) Discrepancy of the effects of zinc supplementation on the prevention of radiotherapy-induced mucositis between patients with nasopharyngeal carcinoma and those with oral cancers: subgroup analysis of a double-blind, randomized study. Nutr Cancer 62(5):682–691

Malynn BA, Ma A (2009) A20 takes on tumors: tumor suppression by an ubiquitin-editing enzyme. J Exp Med 206(5):977–980

Minelli A, Bellezza I, Conte C, Culig Z (2009) Oxidative stress-related aging: a role for prostate cancer? Biochim Biophys Acta 1795(2):83–91

Ng WL, Fong LY, Newberne PM (1984) Forestomach squamous papillomas in the rat: effect of dietary zinc deficiency on induction. Cancer Lett 22(3):329–332

Niculescu AB III, Chen X, Smeets M, Hengst L, Prives C, Reed SI (1998) Effects of p21(Cip1/Waf1) at both the G1/S and the G2/M cell cycle transitions: pRb is a critical determinant in blocking DNA replication and in preventing endoreduplication. Mol Cell Biol 18(1):629–643

Ogunlewe JO, Osegbe DN (1989) Zinc and cadmium concentrations in indigenous blacks with normal, hypertrophic, and malignant prostate. Cancer 63(7):1388–1392

Otsuka M, Fujita M, Aoki T, Ishii S, Sugiura Y, Yamamoto T, Inoue J (1995) Novel zinc chelators with dual activity in the inhibition of the kappa B site-binding proteins HIV-EP1 and NF-kappa B. J Med Chem 38(17):3264–3270

Perera RJ, Ray A (2007) MicroRNAs in the search for understanding human diseases. BioDrugs 21(2):97–104

Perkins ND (1997) Achieving transcriptional specificity with NF-kappa B. Int J Biochem Cell Biol 29(12):1433–1448

Pietsch EC, Sykes SM, McMahon SB, Murphy ME (2008) The p53 family and programmed cell death. Oncogene 27(50):6507–6521

Platz EA, Helzlsouer KJ (2001) Selenium, zinc, and prostate cancer. Epidemiol Rev 23(1):93–101

Prasad AS (1979) Clinical, biochemical, and pharmacological role of zinc. Annu Rev Pharmacol Toxicol 19:393–426

Prasad AS (1988) Zinc in growth and development and spectrum of human zinc deficiency. J Am Coll Nutr 7(5):377–384

Prasad AS (1995) Zinc: an overview. Nutrition 11(1 Suppl):93–99

Prasad AS (1998) Zinc and immunity. Mol Cell Biochem 188(1–2):63–69

Prasad AS (2003) Zinc deficiency. BMJ 326(7386):409–410

Prasad AS (2007) Zinc: mechanisms of host defense. J Nutr 137(5):1345–1349

Prasad AS (2008) Clinical, immunological, anti-inflammatory and antioxidant roles of zinc. Exp Gerontol 43(5):370–377

Prasad AS (2009) Zinc: role in immunity, oxidative stress and chronic inflammation. Curr Opin Clin Nutr Metab Care 12(6):646–652

Prasad AS, Miale A Jr, Farid Z, Sandstead HH, Schulert AR (1963) Zinc metabolism in patients with the syndrome of iron deficiency anemia, hepatosplenomegaly, dwarfism, and hypognadism. J Lab Clin Med 61:537–549

Prasad AS, Dardenne M, Abdallah J, Meftah S, Brewer GJ, Bach JF (1987) Serum thymulin and zinc deficiency in humans. Trans Assoc Am Physicians 100:222–231

Prasad AS, Meftah S, Abdallah J, Kaplan J, Brewer GJ, Bach JF, Dardenne M (1988) Serum thymulin in human zinc deficiency. J Clin Invest 82(4):1202–1210

Prasad AS, Kaplan J, Brewer GJ, Dardenne M (1989) Immunological effects of zinc deficiency in sickle cell anemia (SCA). Prog Clin Biol Res 319:629–647

Prasad AS, Fitzgerald JT, Hess JW, Kaplan J, Pelen F, Dardenne M (1993) Zinc deficiency in elderly patients. Nutrition 9(3):218–224

Prasad AS, Beck FW, Grabowski SM, Kaplan J, Mathog RH (1997) Zinc deficiency: changes in cytokine production and T-cell subpopulations in patients with head and neck cancer and in noncancer subjects. Proc Assoc Am Physicians 109(1):68–77

Prasad AS, Beck FW, Doerr TD, Shamsa FH, Penny HS, Marks SC, Kaplan J, Kucuk O, Mathog RH (1998) Nutritional and zinc status of head and neck cancer patients: an interpretive review. J Am Coll Nutr 17(5):409–418

Prasad AS, Bao B, Beck FW, Sarkar FH (2001) Zinc activates NF-kappaB in HUT-78 cells. J Lab Clin Med 138(4):250–256

Prasad AS, Bao B, Beck FW, Kucuk O, Sarkar FH (2004) Antioxidant effect of zinc in humans. Free Radic Biol Med 37(8):1182–1190

Prasad AS, Beck FW, Bao B, Fitzgerald JT, Snell DC, Steinberg JD, Cardozo LJ (2007) Zinc supplementation decreases incidence of infections in the elderly: effect of zinc on generation of cytokines and oxidative stress. Am J Clin Nutr 85(3):837–844

Prasad AS, Beck FW, Snell DC, Kucuk O (2009) Zinc in cancer prevention. Nutr Cancer 61(6):879–887

Prasad AS, Mukhtar H, Beck FW, Adhami VM, Siddiqui IA, Din M, Hafeez BB, Kucuk O (2010) Dietary zinc and prostate cancer in the TRAMP mouse model. J Med Food 13(1):70–76

Prasad AS, Bao B, Beck FW, Sarkar FH (2011) Zinc-suppressed inflammatory cytokines by induction of A20-mediated inhibition of nuclear factor-kappaB. Nutrition 27(7–8):816–823

Puca R, Nardinocchi L, Porru M, Simon AJ, Rechavi G, Leonetti C, Givol D, D'Orazi G (2011) Restoring p53 active conformation by zinc increases the response of mutant p53 tumor cells to anticancer drugs. Cell Cycle 10(10):1679–1689

Roussel AM, Kerkeni A, Zouari N, Mahjoub S, Matheau JM, Anderson RA (2003) Antioxidant effects of zinc supplementation in Tunisians with type 2 diabetes mellitus. J Am Coll Nutr 22(4):316–321

Schafer FQ, Buettner GR (2001) Redox environment of the cell as viewed through the redox state of the glutathione disulfide/glutathione couple. Free Radic Biol Med 30(11):1191–1212

Schmitz R, Hansmann ML, Bohle V, Martin-Subero JI, Hartmann S, Mechtersheimer G, Klapper W, Vater I, Giefing M, Gesk S, Stanelle J, Siebert R, Kuppers R (2009) TNFAIP3 (A20) is a tumor suppressor gene in Hodgkin lymphoma and primary mediastinal B cell lymphoma. J Exp Med 206(5):981–989

Schrauzer GN, White DA (1978) Selenium in human nutrition: dietary intakes and effects of supplementation. Bioinorg Chem 8(4):303–318

Schrauzer GN, White DA, Schneider CJ (1977) Cancer mortality correlation studies–IV: associations with dietary intakes and blood levels of certain trace elements, notably se-antagonists. Bioinorg Chem 7(1):35–56

Shankar AH, Prasad AS (1998) Zinc and immune function: the biological basis of altered resistance to infection. Am J Clin Nutr 68(2 Suppl):447S–463S

Sheaff RJ, Singer JD, Swanger J, Smitherman M, Roberts JM, Clurman BE (2000) Proteasomal turnover of p21Cip1 does not require p21Cip1 ubiquitination. Mol Cell 5(2):403–410

Song HY, Rothe M, Goeddel DV (1996) The tumor necrosis factor-inducible zinc finger protein A20 interacts with TRAF1/TRAF2 and inhibits NF-kappaB activation. Proc Natl Acad Sci U S A 93(13):6721–6725

Soussi T, Wiman KG (2007) Shaping genetic alterations in human cancer: the p53 mutation paradigm. Cancer Cell 12(4):303–312

Stadtman ER (1992) Protein oxidation and aging. Science 257(5074):1220–1224

Sun J, Liu J, Pan X, Quimby D, Zanesi N, Druck T, Pfeifer GP, Croce CM, Fong LY, Huebner K (2011) Effect of Zinc Supplementation on N-nitrosomethylbenzylamine-induced forestomach tumor development and progression in tumor suppressor-deficient mouse strains. Carcinogenesis 32(3):351–358

Sutcliffe S, Platz EA (2007) Inflammation in the etiology of prostate cancer: an epidemiologic perspective. Urol Oncol 25(3):242–249

Touyz RM (2004) Reactive oxygen species and angiotensin II signaling in vascular cells – implications in cardiovascular disease. Braz J Med Biol Res 37(8):1263–1273

Uzzo RG, Leavis P, Hatch W, Gabai VL, Dulin N, Zvartau N, Kolenko VM (2002) Zinc inhibits nuclear factor-kappa B activation and sensitizes prostate cancer cells to cytotoxic agents. Clin Cancer Res 8(11):3579–3583

Uzzo RG, Crispen PL, Golovine K, Makhov P, Horwitz EM, Kolenko VM (2006) Diverse effects of zinc on NF-kappaB and AP-1 transcription factors: implications for prostate cancer progression. Carcinogenesis 27(10):1980–1990

Verstrepen L, Verhelst K, van Loo G, Carpentier I, Ley SC, Beyaert R (2010) Expression, biological activities and mechanisms of action of A20 (TNFAIP3). Biochem Pharmacol 80(12):2009–2020

Vilborg A, Wilhelm MT, Wiman KG (2010) Regulation of tumor suppressor p53 at the RNA level. J Mol Med 88(7):645–652

Vlajinac HD, Marinkovic JM, Ilic MD, Kocev NI (1997) Diet and prostate cancer: a case-control study. Eur J Cancer 33(1):101–107

Vogelstein B, Lane D, Levine AJ (2000) Surfing the p53 network. Nature 408(6810):307–310

Wan SG, Taccioli C, Jiang Y, Chen H, Smalley KJ, Huang K, Liu XP, Farber JL, Croce CM, Fong LY (2010) Zinc deficiency activates S100A8 inflammation in the absence of COX-2 and promotes murine oral-esophageal tumor progression. Int J Cancer 129(2):331–345

Wang Z, Li Y, Banerjee S, Sarkar FH (2008) Exploitation of the Notch signaling pathway as a novel target for cancer therapy. Anticancer Res 28(6A):3621–3630

Wang Z, Li Y, Ahmad A, Azmi AS, Banerjee S, Kong D, Sarkar FH (2010) Targeting Notch signaling pathway to overcome drug resistance for cancer therapy. Biochim Biophys Acta 1806(2):258–267

Ward PA (1995) Cytokines, inflammation, and autoimmune diseases. Hosp Pract (Minneap) 30(5):35–41

Wellinghausen N, Rink L (1998) The significance of zinc for leukocyte biology. J Leukoc Biol 64(5):571–577

West DW, Slattery ML, Robison LM, French TK, Mahoney AW (1991) Adult dietary intake and prostate cancer risk in Utah: a case-control study with special emphasis on aggressive tumors. Cancer Causes Control 2(2):85–94

Whelan P, Walker BE, Kelleher J (1983) Zinc, vitamin A and prostatic cancer. Br J Urol 55(5):525–528

Wickremasinghe RG, Prentice AG, Steele AJ (2011) p53 and Notch signaling in chronic lymphocytic leukemia: clues to identifying novel therapeutic strategies. Leukemia 25(9):1400–1407

Wong SH, Zhao Y, Schoene NW, Han CT, Shih RS, Lei KY (2007) Zinc deficiency depresses p21 gene expression: inhibition of cell cycle progression is independent of the decrease in p21 protein level in HepG2 cells. Am J Physiol Cell Physiol 292(6):C2175–C2184

Xiong Y, Hannon GJ, Zhang H, Casso D, Kobayashi R, Beach D (1993) p21 is a universal inhibitor of cyclin kinases. Nature 366(6456):701–704

Yan M, Song Y, Wong CP, Hardin K, Ho E (2008) Zinc deficiency alters DNA damage response genes in normal human prostate epithelial cells. J Nutr 138(4):667–673

Yang CS (1980) Research on esophageal cancer in China: a review. Cancer Res 40(8 Pt 1):2633–2644

Yousef MI, El-Hendy HA, El-Demerdash FM, Elagamy EI (2002) Dietary zinc deficiency induced-changes in the activity of enzymes and the levels of free radicals, lipids and protein electrophoretic behavior in growing rats. Toxicology 175(1–3):223–234

Zabel U, Schreck R, Baeuerle PA (1991) DNA binding of purified transcription factor NF-kappa B. Affinity, specificity, Zn2+ dependence, and differential half-site recognition. J Biol Chem 266(1):252–260

Zalba G, San JG, Moreno MU, Fortuno MA, Fortuno A, Beaumont FJ, Diez J (2001) Oxidative stress in arterial hypertension: role of NAD(P)H oxidase. Hypertension 38(6):1395–1399

Zhang Z, Rigas B (2006) NF-kappaB, inflammation and pancreatic carcinogenesis: NF-kappaB as a chemoprevention target (review). Int J Oncol 29(1):185–192

Zhang B, Guan CC, Chen WT, Zhang P, Yan M, Shi JH, Qin CL, Yang Q (2007) A20 inhibits human salivary adenoid cystic carcinoma cells invasion via blocking nuclear factor-kappaB activation. Chin Med J (Engl) 120(20):1830–1835

Chapter 13
Diet-Induced Epigenetic Changes and Cancer Prevention: A Mantra for Healthy Living

Ajay Goel and Gaurav Chaturvedi

Contents

A. Goel (✉)
Gastrointestinal Cancer Research Laboratory, Division of Gastroenterology, Baylor Research Institute and Charles A Sammons Cancer Center, Baylor University Medical Center, 3500 Gaston Avenue, Suite H-250 Hoblitzllee, Dallas, TX 75246, USA
e-mail: ajay.goel@baylorhealth.edu

G. Chaturvedi
Department of Molecular and Integrative physiology, University of Kansas Medical Center, Kansas City, KS, USA
e-mail: gchaturv@yahoo.com

S. Shankar and R.K. Srivastava (eds.), *Nutrition, Diet and Cancer*,
DOI 10.1007/978-94-007-2923-0_13, © Springer Science+Business Media B.V. 2012

Abstract In today's world, survival is mostly about making smart choices. Keeping our body healthy and disease free too is about making smart lifestyle and dietary choices. There is a growing sense that diet becomes a part of 'who we are' and 'how we express ourselves' in the world. As a matter of fact one question that is often raised is "why is diet so important"? The answer is that diet is the vehicle for obtaining the nutrients our bodies require to function optimally. What we eat and how much we eat dramatically influences the nutrition our cells receive. Therefore, the health and vitality of our bodies, on a cellular level, is directly determined by the state of nutrition. As a result, diet has become one of the fundamental contributors to both health and disease. Recent scientific evidence suggests that in addition to the presence of other dietary nutrients, diets are also an important source of essential dietary phytochemicals, also referred to as 'polyphenols'. Growing body of literature indicates that some of these dietary compounds and their secondary metabolites can have a tremendous effect on the way our bodies respond to various challenges posed by various diseases and aging. Not only this, preclinical and clinical studies in the last decade have convincingly demonstrated that the health promoting effect of various dietary agents extend far beyond than what was initially perceived, and that some of these compounds also possess potent anti-cancer activities. In this regard, multiple lines of evidence have provided unprecedented clues that dietary and environmental factors not only regulate various cell-signaling and growth regulatory pathways within cancer cells, but also directly influence epigenetic mechanisms. Epigenetic changes subsequently permit re-expression of tumor suppressor genes that promote apoptosis and growth inhibition of the tumor cells- a novel and previously unrecognized molecular mechanism supporting the underlying chemopreventive potential of many dietary agents. The term 'epigenetics' refers to heritable changes that are not encoded in the DNA sequence itself, but plays an important role in the control of gene expression. In mammals, the three key epigenetic mechanisms include changes in DNA methylation, histone modifications and non-coding RNAs. Although epigenetic changes can be inherited in the somatic cells, unlike genetic alterations, these modifications are potentially reversible. This potentially reversible nature of epigenetic signatures within growth regulatory genes makes them attractive avenues for developing innovative and promising chemopreventive and therapeutic endeavors in the future. From a nutritional perspective, this is quite fascinating because people are becoming increasingly aware of the beneficial effects of various food sources that are rich in dietary polyphenols, also referred to as superfoods. Although at this point in time we may not appreciate the significance of the dietary changes we all are making, nonetheless, such a behavior sets the stage for generating more scientific and epidemiologic data that will further help in highlighting the concept of chemoprevention by dietary agents at an epigenetic level. Cancer chemoprevention through the use of diet-derived, safe and natural polyphenols certainly seems to be a promising and inexpensive way to alleviate the pressure that weighs down the healthcare system because of rapidly increasing number of cancer patients throughout the world.

Abbreviations

5-aza-CdR	5-aza-2-deoxycytidine
AM	allyl mercaptan
COPD	chronic obstructive pulmonary disease
DADS	diallyl disulfide
DIM	3,3′-diindolylmethane
DNMT	DNA methyltransferase
EGCG	epigallocatechin-3-gallate
EMT	epithelial-mesenchymal transition
HAT	histone acetyltransferase
HDAC	histone deacetylase
HMT	histone methyltransferase
LINE	Long Interspersed Nuclear Elements
miRNA	microRNA
PEITC	phenethyl isothiocyanate
PsA	psammaplin A
SAH	S-adenosyl-L-homocysteine
SAM	S-adenosyl methionine
SFN	sulforaphane
SGR	sanguinarine
TSA	Trichostatin A

Epigenetic Mechanisms and Cancer

Conrad H. Waddington, a developmental biologist was the first to use the term ‘epigenetics’ in 1942. “Epigenetics” refers to potentially reversible and heritable changes in gene expression that occur without a permanent alteration in the DNA

Disclosures None of the authors have any potential conflicts to disclose

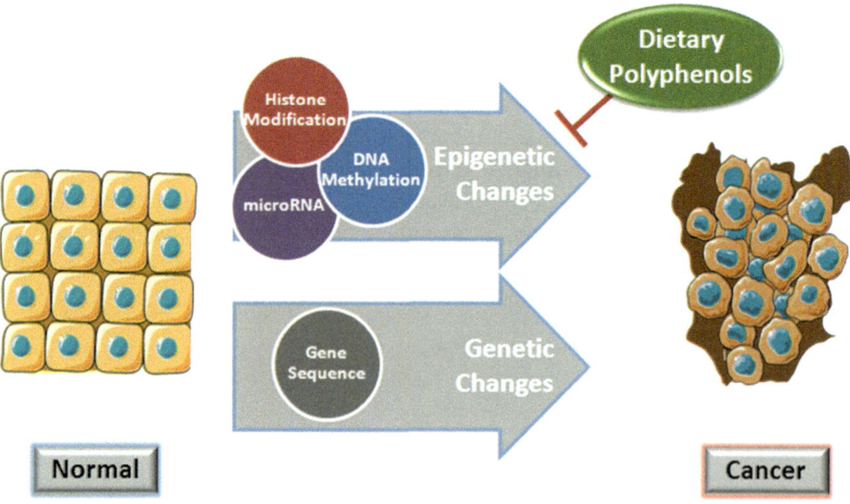

Fig. 13.1 Key epigenetic mechanisms involved in human cancers. Most human cancers evolve as a result of increased accumulation of both 'genetic' and 'epigenetic' alterations in the growth regulatory genes. However, genetic changes, such as gene mutations and deletions, are static and irreversible. In contrast, epigenetic changes, such as DNA methylation, histone modifications and microRNAs are easily influenced by dietary and environmental factors, and are hence reversible in nature. Based upon the data summarized in this article, there is a growing evidence to suggest that dietary polyphenols can potentially impact all three epigenetic modifications, which in turn contributes towards their chemopreventive potential

sequence. Although indirect, epigenetic alterations are sufficiently powerful to regulate the dynamics of gene expression in a manner analogous to genetic events such as mutations or deletions (Rodriguez-Paredes and Esteller 2011). DNA methylation changes, histone modifications, and post transcriptional gene regulation by non-coding microRNAs (miRNAs) are the best known and distinct mechanisms that fall under the umbrella of "epigenetics" (Fig. 13.1). These three epigenetic changes collectively are responsible for maintaining and influencing the "epigenome" within mammalian cells (Ducasse and Brown 2006). Epigenetic alterations affect complete nuclear organization of the genetic material including transcriptional stability, DNA folding, nucleosome positioning and chromatin compaction. These processes synergistically determine whether a gene is silenced or expressed and also regulate the timing and tissue-specificity of the expression of associated genes. Any kind of disruption of the epigenome potentially has an influence on disease development, including cancer. Therefore, disease susceptibility is clearly a manifestation of complex interplay between the genetic makeup and epigenetic marks imprinted within one's genome, a process that can be modulated by a variety of endogenous and exogenous influences, including environmental, lifestyle and dietary factors (Jaenisch and Bird 2003).

In recent years ample evidence has accumulated indicating that *'epigenetic'* alterations in cancer cells are one of the primary contributors towards tumor cell heterogeneity. Therefore, it is becoming increasingly clear that epigenetic plasticity together with the genetic lesions drives tumor progression (Rodriguez-Paredes and Esteller 2011). Even though some tumors are inherited, majority of cancers result from changes that accumulate throughout the life because of the exposure to various exogenous factors such as nutrients, infections, physical activity, social behavior and other environmental factors. Even when cancer initiation and progression is driven by acquired genetic alterations, epigenetic disruption of gene expression plays an equally important role in the disease development (Dolinoy et al. 2007b). Furthermore, diet and environment-mediated epigenetic perturbations arguably play a crucial role in the cancer progression in humans (Dolinoy et al. 2007a; Herceg 2007).

From a clinical standpoint, epigenetics offers a promising and attractive avenue waiting to be further explored from a therapeutic angle. Not surprisingly, epigenetic alterations thus have an edge over genetic changes (mutations, gene deletions and gene re-arrangements etc.), as these are potentially reversible. Consequently, epigenetically modified genes can be restored; methylation silenced genes can be demethylated, and histone complexes can be rendered transcriptionally active through the modification of acetylation and methylation of various histones via nutrients, drugs and other dietary interventions. This sets a stage for designing optimal chemopreventive and therapeutic strategies by exploiting the potential of epigenetic therapy. The following sections provide a summarized view of our current understanding of each of the three epigenetic mechanisms, and wherever possible, description has been provided on the interaction and crosstalk that exists between various epigenetic alterations to inactivate tumor suppressor gene expression in cancer cells.

DNA Methylation

DNA methylations and histone modifications are an essential component of the epigenetic machinery, and together these two processes cooperate in the regulation of gene expression and chromatin architecture (Deaton and Bird 2011). In mammalian cells, DNA methylation occurs at the 5′ position of the cytosine residues within CpG dinucleotides by the addition of a methyl group to form 5-methylcytosine as shown in Fig. 13.2 (Issa and Kantarjian 2009). CpG dinucleotides are often enriched in the promoter regions of genes, as well as regions of large repetitive sequences, such as centromeric repeats, LINE and ALU retrotransposon elements, that are distributed throughout the human genome (Bird 2002). Short CpG-rich regions are also called as "CpG islands", and these are present in more than 50% of human gene promoters (Taberlay and Jones 2011; Wang and Leung 2004). The majority of CpG islands usually remain unmethylated during

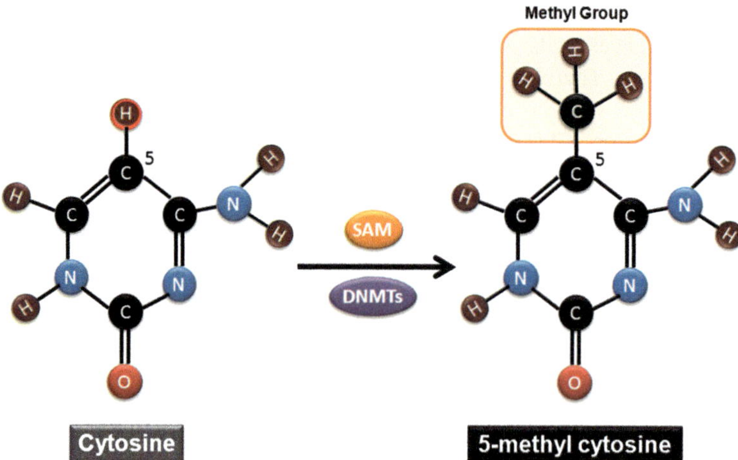

Fig. 13.2 A schematic for a DNA methylation reaction. A simple reaction that depicts the conversion of cytosine residues within the CpG dinucleotides into 5-methylctosine by DNA methyltransferases (DNMT). DNMTs catalyze the transfer of a methyl group (CH3) from S-adenosylmethionine (SAM) to the 5-carbon position of cytosine

development and in undifferentiated normal cells (Suzuki and Bird 2008). However, hyper-methylation of CpG islands within gene promoters can result in gene silencing, while promoters of transcriptionally active genes typically remain hypo-methylated (Suzuki and Bird 2008). DNA methylation can prevent (Prendergast and Ziff 1991) or promote (Jones et al. 1998) the recruitment of regulatory proteins to DNA and thus can lead to gene silencing. In other instances, it can provide binding sites for methyl-binding (sequestering) domain proteins, which can orchestrate gene repression through interaction with histone modifying enzymes.

DNA methyltransferases (DNMTs) are a class of enzymes that catalyze the addition of methyl groups at the 5-carbon position on the cytosine residues that occur in the context of CpG dinucleotide sequences. There are three main categories of DNMT enzymes; DNMT1, which is the major maintenance enzyme that preserves existing methylation patterns following DNA replication by adding methyl groups to the hemi/partially-methylated CpG sites (Plass and Soloway 2002); DNMT3a and DNMT3b on the other hand serve as *de novo* methyltransferases, which act independent of replication and have equal preference for both un-methylated and hemi-methylated DNA sequences (Berletch et al. 2007). It is now well-established that DNA methylation-induced transcriptional silencing of genes plays a major role in multiple human malignancies (Laird 2005). In fact, it is now believed that aberrant DNA methylation is perhaps the most frequent mechanism for the transcriptional inactivation (or silencing) of tumor suppressor genes in human cancers (Herman and Baylin 2003). Several detailed and informative reviews on the association between DNA methylation and cancer are available, but these are beyond the scope of this chapter (Dehan et al. 2009; McCabe et al. 2009; Ushijima and Asada 2010).

Histone Modifications

On a relatively macroscopic scale, chromatin structure is frequently influenced by diverse histone modifications, which also play an important role in gene regulation and pathogenesis of multiple human cancers (Esteller 2011). Chromatin proteins serve as scaffolds to package eukaryotic DNA into higher order of chromatin fibers. Each nucleosome encompasses ~146 bp of DNA wrapped around an octamer of histone proteins. These octamers consist of subunit dimers of H2A, H2B, H3 and H4 core histone proteins (Zhang et al. 1999). The histone proteins coordinate the changes between tightly packed DNA (or heterochromatin), which is inaccessible to transcription, and lightly packed DNA (or euchromatin), which is available for active transcription by permitting binding access to appropriate transcription factors (Lund and van Lohuizen 2004). These changes typically occur in the 'histone tails', which extend from the core octamer. The histone tails comprise of a globular C-terminal domain and an unstructured N-terminal tail (Luger et al. 1997). Most of the post-translational modifications including methylation, acetylation, phosphorylation, ribosylation, ubiquitination, sumoylation and biotinylation occur at the N-terminal histone tails (Kouzarides 2007). Lysine, arginine and serine residues within these histone tails are the major sites of such modifications (Kouzarides 2007). Unlike DNA methylation, histone modifications can lead to either activation or repression of the associated gene, depending upon which residues are involved and the type of modification introduced. For example, lysine acetylation always associates with transcriptional activation, while its methylation may lead to its transcriptional activation or repression depending upon which specific lysine residues are modified. For instance, tri-methylation of lysine 4 on histone H3 (H3K4me3) is enriched at transcriptionally active gene promoters (Liang et al. 2004), whereas tri-methylation of H3K9 (H3K9me3) and H3K27 (H3K27me3) is present at transcriptionally repressed gene promoters (Kouzarides 2007). Together, H3K9me3 and H3K27me3 histone modifications constitute the two key gene silencing mechanisms in human cancer cells.

As is the case with DNA methylation changes, various histone modifications are potentially reversible as well, and these processes are dynamically regulated by groups of enzymes that either add or remove covalent modifications from the histone proteins (Ellis et al. 2009; Iacobuzio-Donahue 2009). Histone acetyltransferases (HATs) and histone methyltransferases (HMTs) add acetyl and methyl groups, respectively, whereas histone deacetylases (HDACs) and histone demethylases (HDMs) remove acetyl and methyl groups, respectively, from the histone proteins (Haberland et al. 2009; Wang et al. 2008d). A number of histone-modifying enzymes including various HATs, HMTs, HDACs, and HDMs have been identified in the recent years, although the detailed molecular mechanisms underlying their enzymatic activity are still poorly understood.

microRNAs

Previously non-coding RNAs were recognized for their catalytic functions in facilitating RNA splicing. However, more recently, in addition to DNA methylation and histone modifications, microRNAs (miRNAs or miRs) have emerged as key mediators of epigenetic gene regulation in mammals. Although we have begun to appreciate the role of miRNAs in the post-transcriptional regulation of gene expression, this currently remains a fascinating and an active area of research investigation (Winter and Diederichs 2011; Winter et al. 2009).

miRNAs are single-stranded small RNA molecules of ~19–24 nucleotides in length. miRNAs regulate gene expression through a sequence-specific base pairing of 3′ untranslated regions of their target messenger RNA (mRNA, which results in the degradation of mRNA or translational inhibition of the affected target gene (He and Hannon 2004). Their tissue-specific expression and the fact that they control a wide spectrum of biological processes including cell proliferation, apoptosis and differentiation, makes them vital for normal cell physiology. Therefore any aberration in miRNA expression levels within normal cells can be catastrophic, and data have begun to emerge that aberrant expression of certain subsets of miRNAs is intimately linked to carcinogenesis. In fact, the unique tissue-specificity of miRNA in different tissues has permitted researchers to utilize miRNA expression profiles to classify human cancers and develop disease-specific biomarkers for the early detection of various human cancers (Calin et al. 2004; Peter 2009).

Interestingly miRNAs can themselves be regulated by other epigenetic mechanisms, such as DNA methylation (Balaguer et al. 2010; Saito and Jones 2006). This reciprocal influence of epigenetics and miRNA suggests that its deregulation during carcinogenesis has an important implication on global regulation of epigenetics and cancer. Several detailed and informative reviews on the associations between miRNA and cancer have been published elsewhere (Inui et al. 2010; Kai and Pasquinelli 2010; Paranjape et al. 2009).

Epigenetic Therapy

Epigenetic therapy is a fascinating new area in the field of drug development for cancer prevention and therapy. The concept of epigenetic therapy stems primarily because epigenetic defects, unlike genetic defects, are potentially reversible (Miyamoto and Ushijima 2005; Rodriguez-Paredes and Esteller 2011). Besides their therapeutic potential, epigenetic drugs also hold a great promise for the prevention of various diseases, including cancer (Gilbert et al. 2004). There is growing enthusiasm that epigenetic drugs alone, or in combination with conventional anticancer drugs may prove to be a significant advance over the currently available anticancer regimens, which are notoriously toxic by themselves (Gravina et al. 2010; Horrobin 2003). Considering that epigenetic alterations are associated with a broad range of human diseases, it is plausible that the scope of epigenetic therapy will be enormous and likely to expand beyond cancer therapeutics in the future.

Even though the current generation of epigenetic drugs primarily target and inhibit the activity and expression of DNMTs and HDACs, it is highly likely that additional epigenetic mechanisms that are involved in the regulation of gene expression might exist, but such targets remain unrecognized at this point in time. Current generation of epigenetic drugs that are presently under evaluation in various pre-clinical and clinical trials can be classified into two main groups, based on their ability to either inhibit DNMTs or HDACs. Among the DNMT inhibitors, nucleoside inhibitors, such as 5-azacytidine (5-Aza-CR, or commercially marketed as Vidaza) and 5-aza-2-deoxycytidine (5-Aza-CdR, available as Decitabine) are the most important and widely studied epigenetic drugs (Komashko and Farnham 2010). In addition to this, certain non-nucleoside inhibitors such as procainamide, procaine and EGCG have also shown a limited potential for inhibiting DNMT activity in various experimental and clinical studies (Berletch et al. 2008; Gao et al. 2009; Gu et al. 2009; Tada et al. 2007). With regards to HDAC inhibitors, trichostatin A (TSA), suberoylanilide hydroxamic acid (SAHA), valproic acid and phenyl butyrate have all shown some success and these compounds have been widely used in various studies (Jones et al. 2010; Kim et al. 2010). Several of these potentially useful epigenetic drugs are undergoing various stages of preclinical and clinical evaluation for the treatment of different types of solid tumors and hematological malignancies (Gilbert et al. 2004).

Despite possessing some encouraging proof for their efficacy, the current generation of epigenetic drugs has found limited clinical usefulness mostly due to the undesired toxicity associated with these compounds. Since the DNMTs and HDACs lack sufficient target specificity, it is not unimaginable that these molecules may inadvertently participate in the activation of certain oncogenes leading to accelerated tumor progression instead of growth inhibition of the neoplastic cells (Sato et al. 2003). Moreover, the therapy may not last long enough to have a biologically effective influence on the gene expression as post-therapy epigenetic states may revert back to their original state due to the reversible nature of DNA methylation patterns (Costello and Plass 2001). In light of the facts that there is lack of target specificity in addition to high levels of toxicity profiles associated with the synthetic epigenetic, there is a dire need for discovering and developing safer and more specific epigenetic chemopreventive and therapeutic drugs. Epidemiological and experimental data in recent years have clearly provided evidence that diet and diet-derived plant polyphenols have potent anti-cancer properties, and some of these effects are orchestrated via modulation of epigenetic machinery within cancer cells (Link et al. 2010).

Dietary Factors and Their Influence on Epigenetic Mechanisms

One of the most alluring facet of diet-induced epigenetic alterations is that unlike genetic changes, epigenetic changes are reversible and can be potentially modified by the environment, diet or other pharmacological interventions. The reversible nature of epigenetic modifications has been the main inspiration for developing therapeutic strategies by targeting the activity of various epigenetic factors, such as DNMTs and HDACs, in order to prevent or treat various diseases including human cancers (Teodoridis et al. 2004; Yoo and Jones 2006). In the following sections, we will briefly provide a historical perspective, followed by the current state of evidence for the interactions between the environment, nutrition and the epigenome – all of the characteristics that provide a compelling rationale for the use of dietary agents for the chemoprevention of human cancers. In this regard, we will briefly describe how epigenetic changes are vital for defining a wide spectrum of growth and developmental features in the plants, as well as animals and humans. We will finally review how dietary and environmental factors have such a profound relationship on epigenetic alterations in human cancers.

Vernalization in Plants

The effect of environment and epigenetic factors has long been studied in plants. One of the best examples of environmental influences on the plant physiology governed by their epigenetic status is the phenomenon of vernalization, a process in which the exposure of a plant to lower temperatures induces earlier flowering (Sheldon et al. 2000a). This process was best understood when a protein encoded by the *flowering locus C* (*FLC*) gene, which acts as a repressor of flowering in Arabidopsis was firstly identified (Sheldon et al. 2000b). Vernalization down-regulates *FLC* activity and induces premature flowering. The suppression of *FLC* activity was found to be associated with a reduction of histone H3 trimethyl-lysine 4 (H3K4) and acetylation of both histones H3 and H4 in the neighborhood of the promoter-translation start site of the *FLC* gene.

Agouti Mice, Nutrition and Epigenetics

One of the classical evidences to demonstrate that nutritional changes alone can modulate the epigenetic status of mammals comes from the studies done in mice. These experiments demonstrate the influence of mother's diet in shaping the epigenome of her offspring were done in mice carrying the agouti viable yellow (*Avy*) gene. The normal function of the *Avy* gene is to confer a wild-type brown coat color. However, dominant mutations at the *Avy* locus cause a pleiotropic syndrome, which confers excessive amounts of yellow pigment on the coat, in conjunction with other systemic defects including obesity, a non-insulin-dependent diabetic-like condition, and the vulnerability to develop various types of cancers (Yen et al. 1994). In these mice, the expression of the *Avy* allele is dependent on its methylation status. When methylated, the *Avy* gene behaves like a wild type allele and is expressed only in the hair follicle. In contrast, when unmethylated, the gene is expressed ubiquitously in different cell types and results in the full agouti syndrome. Intermediate levels of *Avy* methylation cause a mottled appearance, thereby providing a direct readout of the methylation status of the allele via the coat color and other aspects of the agouti phenotype. Wolff and colleagues showed that by feeding pregnant Avy dams diets that are rich in folic acid (which acts as a methyl donor), it was possible to modify the expression of the agouti gene in the offspring (Wolff et al. 1998). A higher proportion of offspring with wild type coat color were obtained from folic acid supplemented dams, which was consistent with the higher levels of DNA methylation of the agouti gene (Waterland 2003; Waterland and Jirtle 2003). Another remarkable feature of the *Avy* mouse model is that this provides an evidence that the epigenetic marks established by dietary supplementation with methyl donors can also be passed on to the successive generations via the female germline. Later on, it was realized that such effects were mediated by polycomb group of proteins (Blewitt et al. 2006). These results are of essence as these indicate that an individual's adult health is heavily influenced by early prenatal factors, and that our health is not only determined by what we eat, but also what our parents ate during our embryonic stages.

Epigenetic Changes Induced by Maternal Behavior and Diet

The direct effects of the environmental influences on the epigenetic status in mammals are somewhat poorly understood. One of the remarkable examples in this regard is the effect of maternal care behavior on the offspring of rodents. Studies have shown that higher level of pup-licking, grooming and "arched-back nursing" by rat mothers have a direct influence on the modification of DNA methylation levels at the glucocorticoid receptor (GR) gene promoter in the hippocampus of the offspring. These changes in DNA methylation lead to reduced histone acetylation and binding of a transcription factor (NGFI-A) to the GR promoter, which caused its transcriptional silencing (Weaver et al. 2004a). Remarkably, introduction of a histone deacetylase (HDAC) inhibitor abolished the differences in histone acetylation, DNA methylation, NGFI-A binding, expression of the GR and hypothalamic–pituitary–adrenal responses to stress (Weaver et al. 2004b). These researchers subsequently showed that differences in maternal care modify the expression of more than 900 genes in the offspring. The probable involvement of epigenetic reprogramming in these effects was strongly implied by the observation that some of these changes could be rather easily modified by treatment with an

HDAC inhibitor or by using the methyl donor, methionine (Weaver et al. 2006). Thus, these data illustrate how an epigenetic determinant of maternal behavior can be successfully transmitted across various generations. Likewise, maternal dietary proteins have also been shown to affect transcriptional regulation of myostatin gene in skeletal muscle of Meishan Pigs (Liu et al. 2011). It has been reported that maternal high-fat diet exposure *in-utero* can disrupt peripheral circadian gene expression in nonhuman primates (Suter et al. 2011). In addition, magnesium deficiency has also been shown to alter CpG methylation in hepatic hydroxysteroid dehydrogenase-2 promoter of the offspring in rats (Takaya et al. 2011).

Nutritional Deficiency and Human Cancers

There is an ever increasing awareness that nutritional deficiencies may be one of the most critical factors that associate with the development of many human cancers. For instance, nutrients such as folic acid, B vitamins and SAM (S-adenosyl methionine) are key components of the methyl-metabolism pathway, and methyl-donating nutrient-rich diet can rapidly alter gene expression, especially during early development when the epigenome is first being established. As a result, diets can rather easily influence the degree of methylation by affecting the availability of methyl donors, including folate, choline, and methionine, as well as DNMT activity (Davis and Ross 2007, 2008; Ross 2003). A classic example of the dietary influences in DNA methylation and cancer is the finding that dietary methyl deficiencies (of folate, choline, and methionine) in animals may alter hepatic DNA methylation patterns and induce liver cancer, even in the absence of a carcinogen (Poirier 1994). It has further been shown that that only early-stage re-feeding of a methyl-rich diet during methyl-deficiency-induced hepatocarcinoma can help mitigate aberrant DNA methylation defects. These studies highlight that the timing of the availability of methyl donors can be a critical factor in any interventional strategy that is established in a disease that is primarily driven by aberrant DNA methylation (Pogribny et al. 2006). Selenium is another nutrient that has been linked with DNA methylation, both in the cultured cell studies and the animal experiments. It has been shown that in rats fed with selenium-rich diets, both liver and colon DNA were significantly hypo-methylated, thus providing a rationale for potential chemopreventive efficacy of selenium rich diets (Davis and Ross 2007). Such effects of selenium were linked to its ability to inhibit both DNMT1 activity and its protein expression (Davis et al. 2000), and provide a mechanistic explanation for its chemopreventive potential in these animal tumors.

Other Nutritional Factors Influencing Epigenetics

Various environmental factors have the ability to affect epigenetic mechanisms, but nutrition perhaps remains the most important cause that influences epigenomic makeup most profoundly. A number of biologically active food constituents have been shown to affect the energy metabolism associated processes through changes in DNA methylation status of genes. In obese individuals, excess adipose tissue accumulates over time when the energy intake far exceeds the energy expenditure. Adipocytes being a rich source of endocrine factors and other pro-inflammatory cytokines (such as TNF-α and IL-6) cause increased inflammation that is strongly associated with carcinogenesis (Aggarwal et al. 2006). In fact, inflammatory bowel disease has been shown to be a driver of aberrant DNA methylation in the colon (Issa and Kantarjian 2009). One potential mechanism for this effect is through the activity of IL-6, which supports the aberrant methylation of the *p53* gene promoter via up-regulation of DNMT1 gene expression (Hodge et al. 2005).

Dietary Polyphenols, Chemoprevention and the Role of Epigenetics

Plant-derived polyphenols constitute one of the largest, natural, and ubiquitous groups of phytochemicals that are consumed as part of the diet and as health supplements. One of the primary functions of these plant-derived polyphenols is to protect plants from photosynthetic stress, reactive oxygen species, and consumption by herbivores. Polyphenols are also an essential part of the human diet, with flavonoids and phenolic acids being the most common ones present across a wide range of food classes. Not surprisingly, there is a growing realization that lower incidence of cancer in certain populations in the world, may probably be due to consumption of certain nutrients, especially polyphenol rich diets (Quideau et al. 2011). Consequently, a systematic dissection of the chemopreventive potential of polyphenolic compounds in the recent years has provided compelling scientific evidence that lends credence to the health benefits, including anti-cancer effects, that people have derived from these botanicals for centuries (Perez-Jimenez et al. 2011). Cancer chemoprevention and chemotherapy, which utilizes pharmacological or natural agents to impede, arrest or reverse carcinogenesis at its earliest stages' remains the most practical and promising approach for the management of cancer patients.

Based on the comprehensive body of literature that has been gathered from a large number of studies in cultured cells, animal models and human clinical trials, dietary polyphenols have begun to gain recognition as potential chemopreventive agents in different types of cancers (Cui et al. 2010; Singh et al. 2010). Polyphenols are abundantly present in several fruits, vegetables and nuts, and some examples of such botanicals and their active principles are depicted in Fig. 13.3. Some estimates suggest that more than 8,000 different dietary polyphenols exist, and these can be divided into ten different general classes based on their chemical structure (Bravo 1998). Phenolic acids, flavonoids, stilbenes and lignans are the most abundantly occurring polyphenols that are also an integral part of everyday nutrition worldwide. Some of the most studied and promising cancer chemopreventive polyphenols

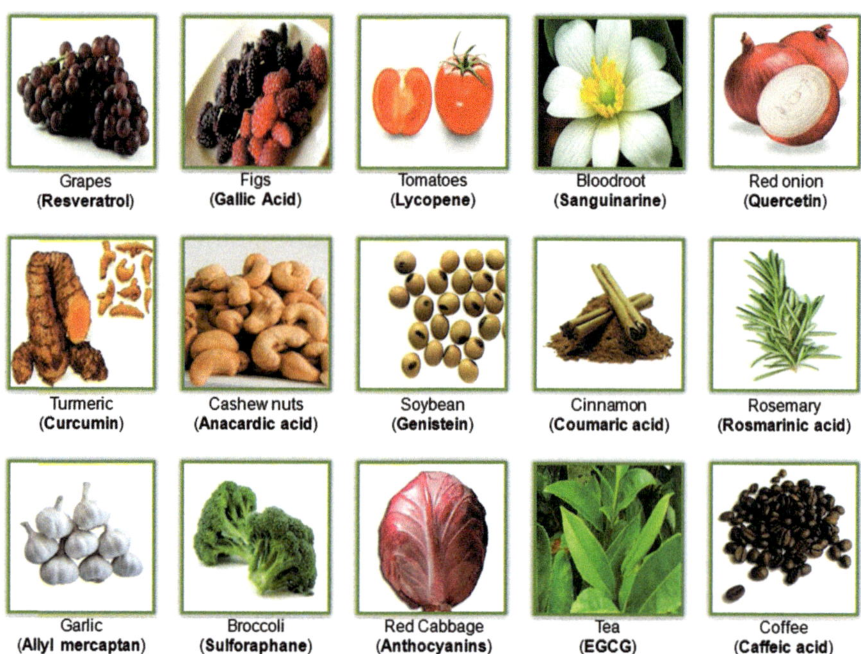
Grapes
(Resveratrol)
Figs
(Gallic Acid)
Tomatoes
(Lycopene)
Bloodroot
(Sanguinarine)
Red onion
(Quercetin)
Turmeric
(Curcumin)
Cashew nuts
(Anacardic acid)
Soybean
(Genistein)
Cinnamon
(Coumaric acid)
Rosemary
(Rosmarinic acid)
Garlic
(Allyl mercaptan)
Broccoli
(Sulforaphane)
Red Cabbage
(Anthocyanins)
Tea
(EGCG)
Coffee
(Caffeic acid)

Fig. 13.3 Partial illustration of dietary botanicals that influence epigenetic mechanisms in cancer cells. The figure illustrates photographs from some of the key botanicals that have the ability to modulate epigenetic mechanisms in cancer cells. The active principles present within each of the plants are shown within *parenthesis*

include EGCG (from green tea), curcumin (from curry) and resveratrol (from grapes and berries). Significant gains of knowledge have been made in understanding the molecular mechanisms underpinning the chemopreventive effects of polyphenols, and consequently, a wide range of mechanisms and gene targets have been identified for individual compounds. Various mechanistic explanations for their chemopreventive efficacy include their ability to interrupt or reverse the carcinogenesis process by acting on intracellular signaling network molecules involved in the initiation and/or promotion of cancer, or their potential to arrest or reverse the progression stage of cancer (Surh 2003). Polyphenolic compounds may also trigger apoptosis in cancer cells through the modulation of a number of key elements in cell signal transduction pathways linked to apoptosis, such as caspases and *bcl-2* genes (Surh 2003). Several elegant reviews have described in detail specific genetic and signaling mechanisms that are targeted by different polyphenols, and this is beyond the scope of this article (Aggarwal and Shishodia 2006; Shishodia et al. 2007). Recent research has suggested that some of the chemopreventive potential of dietary polyphenols may in part be due to their ability to modulate epigenetic alterations in cancer cells. This is of interest, as epigenetic modifications occur early and are potentially reversible, making dietary polyphenol-induced chemoprevention of various human cancers an attractive possibility from a clinical standpoint. This article provides a comprehensive review of the chemopreventive effects of various dietary polyphenols in regulating specific epigenetic alterations in human cancers. In the following sections of this chapter, we will summarize the existing data on the role of a large number of dietary agents on various epigenetic modifications in human cancers.

DNA Methylation Changes Induced by Dietary Polyphenols in Human Cancers

As described earlier, hyper-methylation induced transcriptional silencing of tumor suppressor genes constitutes a frequent epigenetic defect in majority of human cancers. Therefore, reversal of gene hypermethylation, which may in part be achieved by inhibiting DNMT activity in cancer cells, is a plausible and promising avenue for developing epigenetic drugs. In spite of the promising effects DNMT inhibitors have thus far shown in the clinical studies, their usefulness has been limited due to their lack of specificity and undesirable toxicity. In contrast to synthetic DNMT inhibitory drugs, several dietary polyphenols have now been discovered that have potent DNMT inhibitory activity and ability to reverse methylation-induced silencing. Although there is yet a poor understanding of how these dietary polyphenols achieve DNMT inhibition, nonetheless, these are found to be safe and non-toxic- a feature that clearly distinguishes them from the synthetic DNMT inhibitors. In the sections below and Table 13.1, we will summarize data gathered from various experimental studies that have demonstrated the promising efficacy of various dietary polyphenols on DNA methylation-related epigenetic changes in a variety of human cancer models.

Genistein

Genistein, which is one of the many phytoestrogens contained in soybeans, has been extensively studied for its ability to act as a DNA demethylating agent. Stronger than other soy isoflavones (Biochanin A or diadzein), genistein has been shown to induce a dose-dependent inhibition of the DNMT activity (Fang et al. 2005a; Li et al. 2009a). The treatment of KYSE510 esophageal squamous cell carcinoma (ESCC) cells with genistein partially reversed DNA hypermethylation and reactivated *p16*, *RARβ* and *MGMT* genes (Fang et al. 2005a). Reversal of DNA hypermethylation and reactivation of *RAR*β expression was also observed in KYSE150 cells and multiple prostate cancer cell lines. In addition, genistein in combination with other DNMT or HDAC inhibitors (such as TSA), demonstrated a synergistic effect and demonstrated an enhanced efficacy for the reactivation of

Table 13.1 DNA methylation changes induced by dietary polyphenols in human cancers

Cancer	Dietary agent	Plant source	Molecular mechanism	Concentration	References
Breast	Lycopene	Tomatoes	Unknown	2 μM	King-Batoon et al. (2008)
Breast	Baicalein	Indian trumpet	DNMT inhibitor	20–40 μM	Paluszczak et al. (2010)
Breast	Betanin	Beetroot red	DNMT inhibitor	20–40 μM	Paluszczak et al. (2010)
Breast	Ellagic acids	Berries	DNMT inhibitor	20–40 μM	Paluszczak et al. (2010)
Breast	Caffeic acid	Coffea	DNMT inhibitor	1–50 μM	Lee and Zhu (2006)
Breast	Catechin	Green tea	DNMT inhibitor	5–50 μM	Lee et al. (2005)
Breast	Chlorogenic acid	Coffea	DNMT inhibitor	1–50 μM	Lee and Zhu (2006)
Breast	Galangin	Galangal root, propolis	DNMT inhibitor	20 μM	Paluszczak et al. (2010)
Breast	Cyanidin	Berries, grapes	DNMT inhibitor	20–40 μM	Paluszczak et al. (2010)
Breast	Phloretin	Apples	DNMT inhibitor	20–40 μM	Paluszczak et al. (2010)
Breast	Piceatannol (resveratrol metabolite)	Grapes, blueberries	DNMT inhibitor	20–40 μM	Paluszczak et al. (2010)
Breast	Protocatechuric acid	Olives	DNMT inhibitor	20–40 μM	Paluszczak et al. (2010)
Breast	Rosmarinic acid /Rosmarinic	Rosemary	DNMT inhibitor	20–40 μM	Paluszczak et al. (2010)
Breast	Sinapic acid	Sinapis (mustard)	DNMT inhibitor	20–40 μM	Paluszczak et al. (2010)
Breast	Resveratrol	Grapes, wines, eucalyptus	DNMT inhibitor	20–40 μM	Stefanska et al. (2010)
Esophageal	Naringenin	Citrus	DNMT inhibitor	20–50 μM	Fang et al. (2007)
Esophageal	Apigenin	Parsley, celery	DNMT inhibitor	20–50 μM	Fang et al. (2007)
Esophageal	Garcinol	Garcinia	DNMT inhibitor	20–50 μM	Fang et al. (2007))
Esophageal	Epicatechin gallate	Green tea	DNMT inhibitor	20–50 μM	Fang et al. (2003)
Esophageal	Epigallocatechin	Green tea	DNMT inhibitor	20–50 μM	Fang et al. (2003)
Esophageal	Myricetin	Berries	DNMT inhibitor	5–25 μM	Paluszczak et al. (2010)
Esophageal	Fisetin	Poison ivy	DNMT inhibitor	5–20 μM	Lee et al. (2005)
Esophageal	Epicatechin	Green tea	DNMT inhibitor	50 μM	Lee et al. (2005)
Prostate	Isothiocyanates	Broccoli, broccoli sprouts	Unknown	2.5 μM	Wang et al. (2007)
Prostate	Genistein	Soy	DNMT inhibitor	3.75–100 μM	Fang et al. (2005b)
Prostate	Biochanin A	Soy	DNMT inhibitor	20–100 μM	Fang et al. (2007)
Colon	Quercetin	Citrus	DNMT inhibitor	5–20 μM	Lee et al. (2005)
Colon	Sulforaphane	Broccoli	↓ DNMTs expression	50 μM	Traka et al. (2005)
Oral	Epigalocatechin-3-gallate	Green tea	DNMT inhibitor	20–100 μM	Kato et al. (2008, 236)

methylation-silenced genes (Fang et al. 2005a). Similarly, in another study, low, nontoxic concentration of genistein demethylated the promoter of the *GSTP1* tumor suppressor gene in MDA-MB-468 breast cancer cells (King-Batoon et al. 2008). This observation was further corroborated, when the treatment of renal and prostate cancer cells with genistein lead to the reversal of hypermethylation and reactivation of B-cell translocation gene 3 (*BTG3*), a known tumor suppressor gene in some malignancies (Majid et al. 2009, 2010b).

Curiously, in contrast to cell culture studies that reported genistein to induce demethylation of tumor suppressor genes via DNMT inhibition, a few animal studies have observed an opposite phenomenon for the increased DNA methylation following similar treatments. In one such study, male mice were treated with either genistein or with control diets for 2–4 weeks, and methylation changes were analyzed in different tissues using differential methylation hybridization arrays (Day et al. 2002). It was observed that prostate cancer tissues in these animals demonstrated a net overall increase in DNA methylation compared to untreated control animals. Similarly, another study determined whether maternal feeding of genistein would affect the DNA methylation in the offspring by altering their epigenome *in utero* (Dolinoy et al. 2006). The study end-points included the assessment for coat/fur color, DNA methylation levels, and the body weight changes in genetically identical heterozygous yellow agouti (*Avy/a*) offspring. Expression of the transcriptionally active *Avy* allele usually leads to yellow fur, obesity and formation of multiple tumors in these mice. On the other hand, CpG methylation of an intracisternal A particle retrotransposon upstream of the *Agouti* gene correlates inversely with ectopic *Agouti* expression. The results from this study revealed that genistein induced CpG hypermethylation of six CpG sites within this critical gene region, which not only caused a shift in the animal coat-color more toward a pseudoagouti characteristic (more brown fur), but also associated with a decreased incidence of adult-onset obesity in the *Avy/a* offspring. Guerrero-Bosagna et al. evaluated the sexual maturity, morphometric parameters and DNA methylation status in mice treated with genistein and daidzein (Guerrero-Bosagna et al. 2008). In this instance, soy-isoflavin rich diet resulted in an advancement of sexual maturation in female pups as a result of hypermethylation-induced inactivation of *Acta1* gene, a phenomenon that was exclusively observed in the female pups (Guerrero-Bosagna et al. 2008). In contrast, Tang et al. reported that treatment of neonatal mice with genistein prevented the hypermethylation of *nucleosomal binding protein* 1 (*Nsbp*1) in the uterus throughout life, which lead to the induction of uterine adenocarcinoma in aging animals (Tang et al. 2008).

More recently, the effect of genistein treatment on DNA methylation in humans has also been evaluated. A double-blind, randomized trial was conducted in 34 healthy premenopausal women who received 40 or 140 mg isoflavones daily (including genistein, daidzein, and glycitein) through one menstrual cycle (Qin et al. 2009). After the completion of the study, methylation status of five breast cancer-related genes that are also frequent targets aberrant methylation (*p16, RASSF1A, RARβ2, ER,* and *CCND2*) was performed in the intraductal tissue specimens. As was the case in a couple of animal studies, it was noted that genistein treatment associated with the hypermethylation of the *RARβ2* and *CCND2* genes. On the other hand, recent experiences with the human cervical (Jha et al. 2010), prostate (Vardi et al. 2010), and colon cancer (Wang and Chen 2010) cell lines have clearly demonstrated that genistein is a potent DNA demethylating agent, due to its ability to demethylate multiple tumor suppressor genes in these cells. Despite some inconsistencies in the data in different cancer models, these studies clearly suggest that genistein has potent ability to modulate DNMT activities and the methylation status of tumor suppressor genes in various human cancers.

Epigallocatechin-3-Gallate (EGCG)

EGCG is a major polyphenol that is present in green tea. EGCG is methylated by catechol-O-methyltransferase (COMT), the enzyme which is responsible for the inactivation of catechol molecules, including dietary polyphenols. The methyl group during this process is donated by S-adenosyl methionine (SAM), and subsequent demethylation of SAM results in the formation of S-adenosyl-L-homocysteine (SAH). Since SAH is a potent inhibitor of DNMT, its generation has been hypothesized as one of the key mechanism for the demethylating property of this compound. In addition, EGCG can form hydrogen bonds with various residues in the catalytic pocket of DNMT, and hence can act as its direct inhibitor (Fang et al. 2003; Lee et al. 2005). EGCG has also been shown to be an efficient inhibitor of human dihydrofolate reductase (DHFR). Similar to other anti-folate compounds, EGCG acts by modulating folic acid metabolism, inhibiting DNA and RNA synthesis and by altering DNA methylation in the cancer cells (Navarro-Peran et al. 2007).

DNA demethylating potential of EGCG was first demonstrated in a study, in which human esophageal cancer cells upon treatment with EGCG resulted in a concentration- and time-dependent reversal of hypermethylation of several known tumor suppressor genes including *p16*, *RAR*, *MGMT*, and *MLH1* genes (Fang et al. 2007). In another independent study, treatment of oral cancer cells with EGCG partially reversed the hypermethylation status of the *RECK* gene and significantly enhanced the expression level of *RECK* transcripts (Kato et al. 2008). In a human prostate cancer cell line, exposure to green tea polyphenols caused the re-expression of the *GSTP1* gene (Pandey et al. 2010). Likewise, treatment of MCF-7 breast cancer cells with EGCG resulted in decrease of *hTERT* promoter methylation (Berletch et al. 2008; Guilleret and Benhattar 2004; Quante et al. 2005).

In contrast to all these reports favoring EGCG's ability to demethylate transcriptionally silenced genes, others failed to observe similar epigenetic activity for this polyphenol. Chuang et al. examined the methylation status and expression status of six different genes/repetitive elements (*p16, RARβ, MAGE-A1, MAGE-B2* and *Alu*) in three independent cell lines (T24, HT29, and PC3) (Chuang et al. 2005). Treatment with EGCG did not cause either DNA demethylation or re-expression of any of the analyzed genes. Stresemann et al. also performed a comparative analysis of a variety of compounds that had previously been reported to inhibit

DNMT activity in cancer cell lines, including EGCG (Stresemann et al. 2006). Total cytosine methylation levels and the methylation status of *TIMP3* were analyzed in different cell lines. The authors discovered that EGCG did not inhibit DNA methylation or there was any change in total methylated cytosine content in any of these cell lines.

The ability of EGCG to reverse DNA hypermethylation and reactivate methylation-silenced genes *in vivo* is still somewhat debatable. Topical treatment of EGCG inhibits UVB induced global DNA hypomethylation pattern in chronically UVB-exposed mice (Mittal et al. 2003). Kinney et al. recently tested whether oral consumption of green tea polyphenols (GTP) could affect normal or cancer-specific DNA methylation *in vivo*, using a mice model (Morey Kinney et al. 2009). Wild-type and transgenic adenocarcinoma of mouse prostate (TRAMP) mice were orally fed with green tea polyphenols in drinking water. To monitor DNA methylation, 5-methyl-deoxycytidine (5mdC) levels, methylation of the B1 repetitive element, and methylation of the *Mage-a8* gene were quantitatively measured. GTP treatment did not inhibit tumor progression in TRAMP mice and no dose-dependent alterations in DNA methylation status were observed. Similarly, Yuasa et al. performed a retrospective analysis examining the methylation status of several genes in primary gastric carcinomas in relation to past lifestyle of the patients, including dietary habits (Yuasa et al. 2005, 2009). Methylation of *CDX2* and *BMP-2* in this study correlated with the decreased intake of green tea and cruciferous vegetables. Of interest, in a phase II randomized, placebo-controlled trial of green tea extract (GTE) in patients with high-risk oral premalignant lesions, the clinical response rate was significantly higher in all GTE arms at different doses versus placebo (Tsao et al. 2009). Although most of the evidence related to the epigenetic properties of natural tea compounds has focused on EGCG, other catechins such as catechin, epicatechin, epicatechin gallate and apigallocatechin have also been found to share similar features, though with somewhat less prominent DNMT inhibitory activity compared to EGCG (Fang et al. 2003, 2007; Lee et al. 2005). Collectively, all the above reports do suggest the potential of green tea polyphenols in mediating DNA methylation in various cancer cells, which may in part be the mechanism underlying their chemopreventive potential.

Curcumin

Curcumin, the major component of turmeric, has long been known for its potent anti-inflammatory, anti-angiogenic and antioxidant, wound healing and anticancer effects in various diseases. From an epigenetic standpoint, recently it was shown that curcumin and one of its major metabolites, tetrahydrocurcumin can inhibit the activity of *M.SssI*, an DNMT1 analog. However, curcumin-induced inhibition of this enzymatic activity was lower than the other compounds, such as EGCG, that were compared in this study (Fang et al. 2007; Kuck et al. 2010; Liu et al. 2009).

More interestingly, curcumin exposure to genomic DNA of MV4-11 leukemia cell line induced a decrease in global DNA methylation comparable to decitabine (Liu et al. 2009).

Resveratrol and Rosmarinic Acid

Resveratrol, a phytoalexin made naturally by several plants, is being envisioned as a promising dietary polyphenol to impact a variety of human diseases, including cancer. Such a promise is primarily because of its potential anti-cancer, anti-inflammatory, blood-sugar-lowering and other beneficial cardiovascular characteristics. There is limited evidence about the potential demethylating activity of this compound. Both resveratrol and rosmarinic acid have been shown to be a weak DNMT inhibitors in nuclear extracts from MCF7 cells, and both of these compounds were unable to reverse the methylation of several tumor suppressor genes (Paluszczak et al. 2010). Nonetheless, although no significant effect on its own, resveratrol improved the action of adenosine analogues to inhibit methylation and increased the expression of RARβ2 in MCF-7 breast cancer cells (Stefanska et al. 2010).

Rosmarinic acid is a natural polyphenol antioxidant carboxylic acid found in many *Lamiaceae* herbs used commonly as culinary herbs such as lemon balm, rosemary, oregano, sage, thyme and peppermint. Rosmarinic acid has been recently shown to be a potent inhibitor of DNMT1 activity in nuclear extracts from MCF7 breast cancer cells and decrease the protein levels of DNMT1. However, this compound was unable to demethylate and reactivate known hypermethylated genes such as *RASSF1A*, *GSTP1* and *HIN-1* in this cell line (Paluszczak et al. 2010).

Lycopene, Sulforaphane, Coffee Polyphenols and Isothiocyanates

Lycopene is a bright red carotene and carotenoid pigment found in tomatoes and other red fruits and vegetables. Lycopene can modulate the expression of numerous genes relevant to cell cycle control, DNA repair, and apoptosis in breast cancer cells as evidenced from several gene microarray studies (Chalabi et al. 2006, 2007). In addition, treatment of MDA-MB-468 breast cancer cells with a single dose of lycopene partially demethylated the promoter of the *GSTP1* tumor suppressor gene, with a concomitant increase in expression (King-Batoon et al. 2008).

Sulforaphane, a dietary phytochemical obtained from broccoli, has been implicated in several physiological processes, which is consistent with its anti-carcinogenic activity. Although the effects of sulforaphane as a demethylating agent have not been specifically studied, this compound was found to downregulate DNMT1 in CaCo-2 colon cancer cells (Traka et al. 2005).

Caffeic acid and chlorogenic acid are catechol-containing coffee polyphenols, which in a manner analogous to the tea polyphenols, have been proposed to have demethylating potential. Lee et al. studied the effects of these two compounds on the *in vitro* methylation of synthetic DNA substrates and also on the methylation status of the promoter region of *RARβ* in two human breast cancer cells lines (Lee and Zhu 2006). The presence of caffeic acid or chlorogenic acid inhibited in a concentration-dependent manner the DNA methylation catalyzed by DNMT1, predominantly through a non-competitive mechanism. This inhibition, similar to other dietary polyphenols, was largely due to the increased formation of SAH. Treatment of MCF-7 and MAD-MB-231 human breast cancer cells with these two compounds partially inhibited the methylation of the promoter region of *RARβ*.

Isothiocyanates comprise of another class of dietary compounds that are known to affect the epigenome. Isothiocyanates are metabolites of glucosynolates present in a wide variety of cruciferous vegetables and are known to possess anti-cancer properties. Treatment of prostate cancer cells with 2-phenethyl isothiocyanate, a metabolite of gluconasturtin from watercress, was shown to demethylate and help restore the expression of *GSTP1* (Wang et al. 2007). Similarly, treatment with unrelated isothiocyanates prevented the esophageal tumorigenesis induced by the methylating agent *N*-nitrosomethylbenzylamine (NMBA) in male rats (Wilkinson et al. 1995). In addition to various dietary polyphenols described above, further compounds exist for which the evidence to modulate DNA methylation is less robust. Several of these additional compounds are not described here, but are listed in the Table 13.1.

Histone Modifications Induced by Diet-Related Polyphenols

Not only DNA methylation alterations, evidence gathered in the recent decade indicates that dietary polyphenols can also regulate gene expression through changes in histone modifications (Fig. 13.4). Several polyphenols are known to possess potent histone deacetylation (HDAC) and histone acetyl transferase (HAT) regulatory activities. The data in the following sections together with the reports listed in the Table 13.2 summarize the current understanding on the effects of dietary polyphenols on histone modifications that might play a significant role in the chemopreventive potential of these botanicals.

Curcumin

Data from both *in vitro* and *in vivo* experiments suggests that curcumin has potent histone modifying characteristics, and that it may act as a powerful HAT inhibitor. Using computational screening algorithms, curcumin has been shown to bind to HAT enzymes in a covalent manner (Marcu et al. 2006; Singh and Misra 2009).

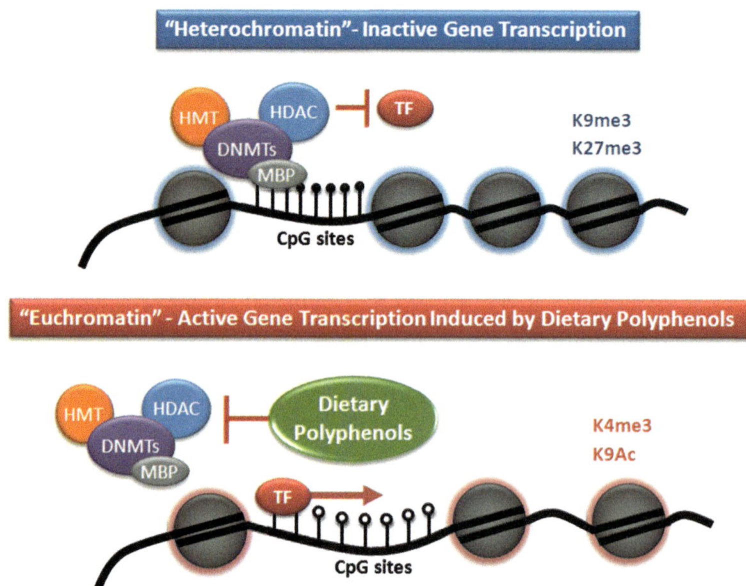

Fig. 13.4 Schematic figure of epigenetic regulation mechanism and the effect of dietary polyphenols in cancer cells. *Upper panel*; this figure illustrates how the packaging of DNA around the histone cores (shown as *large gray circles*). In cancers, tumor suppressor genes become frequently "inactivated" (shown in the *upper panel*) due to aberrant hypermethylation of the CpG islands (shown as *black lollipops*) within gene promoters. Hypermethylation of genes very complex, and requires the participation of several key enzymes during this process. DNA methyltransferases (DNMTs) are responsible for transfer of methyl group to 5′-cytosine. Methyl binding proteins (MBPs) work in concert with DNMTs to facilitate the process of methylation of CpG residues. In addition, histone methyltransferases (HMT) and histone deacetylases (HDAC) are responsible for the methylation and de-acetylation of lysine residues within histone tails, respectively. A combination of methylation and histone modifications causes conformational changes in chromatin structure that lead to changes in DNA accessibility for transcription factors (TF). Such an inactive state of gene transcription is also referred to as "heterochromatin". *Lower panel*; Dietary polyphenols have the ability to block all these enzymes in specific ways, allow the active binding of transcription factors to the unmethylated DNA (shown as *empty lollipops*) and restore the chromatin to the "euchromatin" form. K4me3 and K9Ac are both activating histone marks, while *K9me3* and *K27me3* represent repressive histone marks within cancer cells

Moreover, curcumin effectively prevents histone hyper-acetylation induced by the histone deacetylase (HDAC) inhibitor MS-275 in both PC3-M and HeLa cell lines, as well as peripheral blood lymphocytes (Kutluay et al. 2008; Singh and Misra 2009). Curcumin strongly inhibits p300/CBP activity in cell extracts from multiple cancers including cervix, hepatoma and leukemia (Kang et al. 2005; Mai et al. 2006; Sbardella et al. 2008). Using prostate PC3-M cells and peripheral blood lymphocytes, curcumin was shown to selectively promote proteasome-dependent degradation of p300/CBP without affecting other HATs such as PCAF or GCN5 (Marcu et al. 2006). Inhibition of p300/CBP caused repression of histones H3/H4

Table 13.2 Histone modifications induced by diet-related polyphenols in human cancers

Cancer	Dietary agent	Plant source	Molecular mechanism	Concentration	References
Alveolar macrophages	Theophylline	Black and green tea	HDAC activator	10 μM	Cosio et al. (2009)
Breast	6-methoxy-2E,9E-humuladien-8-one	Ginger	HDAC inhibitor	1.25 μM	Chung et al. (2008)
Cervix	Butein	Varnish Tree	SIRT1 induction	100 μM	Howitz et al. (2003)
Cervix	Caffeic acid	Coffea	HDAC inhibitor	1–2.54 mM	Waldecker et al. (2008)
Cervix	Curcumin	Turmeric	HAT/HDAC inhibitor	6.25–135 μM	Bora-Tatar et al. (2009)
Cervix	Isoliquiritigenin	Liquorice	SIRT1 activator	100 μM	Howitz et al. (2003)
Cervix	Chlorogenic acid	Coffea	HDAC inhibitor	0.375 mM	Bora-Tatar et al. (2009)
Colon	Cinnamic acid	Cinnamon	HDAC inhibitor	1–2 mM	Waldecker et al. (2008)
Colon	Coumaric acid	Cinnamon	HDAC inhibitor	1–2 mM	Waldecker et al. (2008)
Colon	3,3-diindolylmethane	Broccoli	HDAC inhibitor	10–60 μM	Bhatnagar et al. (2009)
Erythroleukemia	Diallyl disulfide	Garlic	HDAC inhibitor	20–200 μM	Lea and Randolph (2001)
Erythroleukemia	S-allylmercaptocysteine	Garlic	HDAC inhibitor	20–250 μM	Lea et al. (2002)
Esophageal	Biochanin A	Soy	HDAC inhibitor	20–100 μM	Fang et al. (2005a)
Esophageal	Sulforaphane	Broccoli	HDAC inhibitor	15–25 μM	Fang et al. (2005a)
Esophageal	Daidzein	Soy	HDAC inhibitor	12.8–100 μM	Fang et al. 2005a)
Hepatoma	Silibinin	Milk thistle	↑ histone acetylation	120–240 μM	Lah et al. (2007)
Leukemia	Garcinol	Garcinia	HAT inhibitor	5–100 μM	Arif et al. (2007)
Leukemia	Anacardic acid	Cashew nuts	HAT inhibitor	3–200 μM	Souto et al. (2008)
Leukemia	Ursolic Acid	Basil	HDAC inhibitor	5–20 μM	Chen et al. (2009)
Lymphocytes	Epicatechin	Green tea	HAT inhibitor	100 μM	Choi et al. (2009)
Lymphocytes	Epicatechin gallate	Green tea	HAT inhibitor	100 μM	Choi et al. (2009)
Lymphocytes	Epigallocatechin	Green tea	HAT inhibitor	100 μM	Choi et al. (2009)
Lymphocytes	Epigalocatechin-3-gallate	Green tea	HAT/HMT inhibitor	5–100 μM	Choi et al. (2009)
Liver; cervix	Sanguinarine	Opium poppy	HAT/HMTinhibitor	5–75 μM	Selvi et al. (2009)
Myeloid leukemia	Flavone	Feijoa	HDAC inhibitor	170–340 μM	Bontempo et al. (2007)
Prostate	Isothiocyanates	Broccoli, wasabi	HDAC inhibitor	20–100 μM	Wang et al. (2008a)

and non-histone proteins such as p53, HIV-Tat protein, as well as HAT-dependent chromatin transcription (Balasubramanyam et al. 2004).

Curcumin has further been shown to modulate the immunologic memory of CD8+ T-lymphocytes, in part, through deacetylation of H3K9 at the promoter region of several key transcription factors such as *Eomesodermin* and its targets *perforin* and *granzyme B* (Araki et al. 2008). Besides human cells, curcumin treatment has also been linked to strong inhibition of the *Plasmodium falciparum* HAT's nuclear activity which induced hypoacetylation of H3K9 and -K14 (Cui and Miao 2007). The same group further demonstrated that curcumin-related H3K9 hypoacetylation at the promoter region of certain genes was associated with the transcriptional silencing of the genes (Cui et al. 2007). Several independent studies have subsequently corroborated the HAT inhibitory effect of curcumin in animal models. In addition, data has revealed the beneficial effects of curcumin on the progression of streptozotocin-induced diabetes-related nephropathy in male Sprague-Dawley rats. In this animal model, curcumin treatment was associated with inhibition of p300, NF-*k*B, H3S10 phosphorylation and H3 hyperacetylation (Chiu et al. 2009; Tikoo et al. 2008). Furthermore, two independent groups have further provided data that suggests that curcumin acts as a protective agent against cardiac hypertrophy, inflammation and fibrosis in animal models by suppressing HAT activity (p300) and by downregulating *GATA4*, *NF-κF* and *TGFβ/Smad* signaling pathways (Li et al. 2008; Morimoto et al. 2008). In these studies, curcumin abrogated H3/H4 acetylation, *GATA4* acetylation levels and the relative levels of p300/GATA4 complex, which is otherwise markedly increased in the hypertensive hearts of these rats (Li et al. 2008; Morimoto et al. 2008). Finally, in addition to HAT-inhibitory effects of curcumin, recent studies have inconclusively suggested that curcumin may also possess HDAC-inhibitory activity (Kang et al. 2005). Using Burkitt-lymphoma Raji cells, curcumin treatment was associated with down-regulation of HDAC1, HDAC3 and HDAC8 proteins, whereas H4 protein expression was up-regulated (Chen et al. 2007; Liu et al. 2005). Although these results certainly require further experimental confirmation, another recent study has supported the HDAC–inhibitory effects of curcumin (Bora-Tatar et al. 2009).

EGCG and Other Green Tea Polyphenols

EGCG is one of the key epigenetic modulators in the cancer cells, even though in this context much of its efficacy has been related to its ability to demethylate genes by inhibiting DNMT activity. However, recent data suggests that EGCG may also act as a histone modifier. Among all the catechins present in green tea, EGCG was found to be the most promising and potent modulators of histone marks in cancer cells (Choi et al. 2009). Additionally, EGCG treatment inhibited the acetylation of p65 and the expression of NF-κB target genes in response to diverse stimuli (Choi et al. 2009). The activity of EGCG toward other histone modifying enzymes such as HDACs, SIRTs and HMTs remains controversial. While two previous studies failed to notice any appreciable changes in activity of these enzymes (Choi et al. 2009; Nair et al. 2008), Pandey et al. demonstrated that green tea polyphenols showed both inhibition of HDAC activity and reduction in mRNA expression of various HDACs (HDAC 1, 2 and 3) in prostate cancer cells. These changes were subsequently associated with time-dependent increases in the acetylation of H3 and H4 (Pandey et al. 2010). Besides its effect on HAT and HDAC activities, EGCG has also been shown to affect polycomb group (PcG) of protein complexes PRC2 (EED) and PRC1 (BMI-1) in immortalized keratinocytes and skin cancer cells (Balasubramanian et al. 2010). Both PRC1 and PRC2 actively participate in epigenetic regulation of gene expression by increasing histone methylation and by reducing acetylation, which causes chromatin compaction and transcriptional silencing of various genes in the cancer cells (Balasubramanian et al. 2010). Treatment of skin cancer cells with EGCG reduced the expression of BMI-1 and EZH2, which was associated with reduction in survival and global reduction in histone H3K27me3 (Balasubramanian et al. 2010).

Other than EGCG, there is very limited data on the regulation of epigenetic activity by other polyphenols present in green tea. In this context, although there are no studies on the epigenetic properties of polyphenon B (black tea polyphenol) in cultured cancer cells, in a single study on DAB-induced liver cancer animal model, polyphenon B was shown to induce significant decrease in HDAC1 expression in male Sprague-Dawley rats (Murugan et al. 2009). Theophylline, which shows structural similarity to caffeine, is also present at low concentrations in tea. Cosio et al. evaluated the HDAC modulatory effect of theophylline in smokers and patients with chronic obstructive pulmonary disease (COPD), a disease that is known to be linked with decreased HDAC activity (Cosio et al. 2004). Of interest, theophylline treatment was associated with down-regulation of the inflammatory response through modulation of HAT, HDAC activity, and NF-κB activation. In addition, low-doses of theophylline increased HDAC activity in epithelial cells and macrophages, and further reduced IL-8 and TNFα (Cosio et al. 2009; Ito et al. 2002). This effect was observed at therapeutic concentrations and occurred independently of phosphodiesterase inhibition (Ito et al. 2002).

Resveratrol

Resveratrol, presumed to play a significant role in the reduction of cardio-vascular events (Artaud-Wild et al. 1993), is also being considered as a potent anti-cancer agent. Multiple studies have shown that resveratrol is associated with activation of NAD^+ dependent histone deacetylase sirtuin 1 (SIRT1) and p300 in multiple *in vitro* and *in vivo* models (Gracia-Sancho et al. 2010; Wang et al. 2008b). Although it is still controversial whether resveratrol's chemopreventive effects are by virtue of its ability to directly induce SIRT1 (Beher et al. 2009; Kaeberlein et al. 2005; Malik et al. 2010), recent animal studies have demonstrated that cancer preventive effects of resveratrol are in fact significantly dependent on SIRT expression in APCmin/+

mice. These data highlight the importance of SIRT1 activation as a key factor in resveratrol-induced chemoprevention in human cancers (Boily et al. 2009). It has also been demonstrated that SIRT1 negatively regulates the expression of surviving by through H3K9 deacetylation within its promoter region (Wang et al. 2008c). In addition, SIRT1 mediates BRCA1 signaling in breast cancer cells by inhibiting tumor growth through transcriptional repression of various oncogenes (Wang et al. 2008b). Recently, it was demonstrated that resveratrol treatment also enhanced p53 acetylation and apoptosis in prostate cancer cells by inhibiting MTA1/NuRD complex (Kai et al. 2010).

Allyl-Derivatives

Different allyl-derivatives from garlic were among one of the first compounds that were described to have an effect on histone acetylation. These reports suggest that these compounds may inhibit HDAC enzyme activity in mouse and human leukemia cells (Lea and Randolph 2001; Lea et al. 1999. Various allyl-derivates such as allyl mercaptan (AM), diallyl disulfide (DADS), S-allylcysteine(SAC), S-allylmercaptocysteine (SAMC) and allicin induce increased histone acetylation (H3/H4) in cultured cancer cells and in rat livers (Lea et al. 2001 #297 Lea et al. 2002). Among various allyl-derivatives and precursors, AM is perhaps the most potent HDAC inhibitor in colorectal cancer and leukemic cells (Druesne et al. 2004; Nian et al. 2008). Similar to other HDAC-inhibitors, AM increases histone H3 acetylation on the *CDKN1A* gene, with an associated increase in the binding of transcription factor Sp3 and p53 to its promoter region (Nian et al. 2008). Although less significant, several studies have shown that DADS treatment in cultured colorectal cancer cells also produced increased acetylation of H3 and H4, and a simultaneous up-regulation of *CDKN1A* (Arunkumar et al. 2007; Druesne-Pecollo et al. 2006, 2007; Zhao et al. 2006). Both SAMC and DADS treatments have been shown to associate with increased *E-cadherin* expression, which happens as a consequence of HDAC inhibition (Druesne-Pecollo et al. 2007). Similarly, animal studies with allyl-derivatives clearly indicated that AM and/or DADS treatment increased acetylation of histones and caused up-regulation of p21 expression in normal liver and hepatoma cells, as well as in rat colonocytes (Druesne-Pecollo et al. 2007; Zhao et al. 2006). Although these findings are very encouraging, there is concern about the high concentrations of allyl-derivatives used in animal studies, which are unlikely to be physiologically achievable in humans if such compounds are considered for clinical intervention. Considering this, it was proposed that SAMC may be a safer and more effective choice, as it was shown to induce growth arrest in mouse erythroleukemia cells at relatively low concentrations (Lea et al. 2002). However, SAMC is inherently a weaker HDAC inhibitor that AM or DADS, as evidenced by its effect in prostate cancer cell lines (Chu et al. 2006).

Sulforaphane and Other Isothiocyanate Derivatives

Sulforaphane (SFN) and other isothiocyanates such as phenethyl isothiocyanate (PEITC) are the main constituents that are present at high levels in broccoli. Several studies have confirmed the potent HDAC inhibitory activity of isothiocyanates. Using human kidney cells and colorectal cancer cells, it was demonstrated that one of the SFN metabolites (SFN-Cys) acts as a HDAC inhibitor (Myzak et al. 2004). In a similar manner, HDAC inhibition in cell lines and animals was associated with increased histone H3/H4 acetylation. Such effects of SFN were associated with increased H4 acetylation in the *p21* and *Bax* promoters, which resulted in the significant up-regulation of both gene and protein expression in prostate cancer cells (Myzak et al. 2007; Pledgie-Tracy et al. 2007). In a mice model, it was demonstrated that SFN-containing diet is optimal for achieving biologically relevant SFN tissue concentrations (Hu et al. 2006). SFN-enriched diets in these animals were shown to suppress tumor development in APC min/+ mice via increase in overall H3/H4 histone acetylation, and a concomitant up-regulation of p21 expression (Myzak et al. 2006). Additionally, in a pilot study in human volunteers, consumption of broccoli sprouts resulted in a significant inhibition of blood HDAC activity (Myzak et al. 2007). SFN treatment induced changes in the gene expression of numerous genes in human colon cancer cell lines, although it is unclear whether these changes are a consequence of modifications in their corresponding histone marks (Schwab et al. 2008). In support of this, squamous esophageal cells treated with SFN showed a marked increase in the RARβ expression in a similar manner as Trichostatin A (TSA) and 5-aza-CdR, the two potent HDAC and DNMT inhibitors, respectively (Fang et al. 2005b).

Allyl-isothiocyanate (AITC), one of the first compounds isolated from broccoli, was shown to increase acetylation of histones, independent of its HAT activity, in mouse erythroleukemia cells (Lea et al. 2001). These findings have subsequently been confirmed in other studies in which isothiocyanates have been shown to inhibit HDAC activity which associated with an up-regulation of p21/Bax expression in various cancer cell lines (Beklemisheva et al. 2006; Ma et al. 2006; Wang et al. 2007, 2008d).

Anacardic Acid and Garcinol

Anacardic acid (AA) is the most active principle present in cashew nuts, and has been shown to be a potent and specific HAT inhibitor. HAT inhibitory activity of AA associates with the down-regulation of p300, PCAF and Tip60 HAT factors (Balasubramanyam et al. 2003; Sun et al. 2006). AA exerts its effect by inhibiting HAT-dependent transcription, which strongly correlates with simultaneous histone H3 and/or H4 hypoacetylation in HeLa and MCF7 cancer cells (Balasubramanyam et al. 2003; Eliseeva et al. 2007). In fact knowledge gained from the HAT inhibitory activity of AA has paved path for the development of new synthetic HAT inhibitors and activators (Chandregowda et al. 2009; Sbardella et al. 2008; Souto et al. 2008). Only very few studies have evaluated the molecular biological relevance of AA-related HAT inhibitory activity. Sung et al. showed that AA inhibits both inducible and constitutive NF-κB activation, and suppresses activation of IκBα kinase which leads to abrogation of its phosphorylation and eventual degradation in multiple cancer cells (Sung et al. 2008). In addition, using human dermal fibroblasts it was demonstrated that AA effectively inhibits UV-induced cancer formation and premature skin aging by reducing UV-enhanced levels of *c-H2AX*, *p53*, and acetylation of H3 (Kim et al. 2009).

Garcinol is a cytotoxic poly-isoprenylated benzophenone derivative from garcinia fruit rinds. Similar to anacardic acid, garcinol is a potent inhibitor of different HATs, such as, p300 and PCAF (Balasubramanyam et al. 2004; Chandregowda et al. 2009; Mai et al. 2006). A recent mechanistic work using fluorescence, docking and mutational studies, has revealed that garcinol induces alteration in the secondary structure of the HAT proteins (Arif et al. 2007). Analogous to curcumin and AA, garcinol also possesses significant histone H3 and H4 deacetylating activities (Arif et al. 2007). In addition, garcinol also has the ability to inhibit auto-acetylation of p300, which is one of the key regulatory mechanisms for its catalytic activity in HeLa core histones (Arif et al. 2007). Although none of the studies have specifically evaluated the effects of garcinol on gene-specific histone modifications, existing data indicates that garcinol and/or its synthetic derivate LTK14, down-regulates the expression of multiple genes in cervical cancer cells and T-lymphocytes (Mantelingu et al. 2007).

3,3′-Diindolylmethane, Isoflavones and Soy Peptides

The brassica family of vegetables, such as broccoli or cauliflower contain indole-3-carbinol which upon digestion turns into an active compound 3,3′-Diindolylmethane (DIM). Bhatnagar et al. found that this compound significantly inhibited the expression of HDAC1, HDAC2 and HDAC3 in colon cancer cells, and was also associated with strong inhibition of anti-apoptotic protein survivin, both in colon cancer cells and APC min/+ mice (Bhatnagar et al. 2009). An insight into the mechanism responsible for HDAC1 inhibition using colon cancer cell lines has recently revealed that DIM selectively induces proteasome-mediated degradation of class I histone deacetylases (HDAC1-3 and HDAC 8), which in turn results in increased p21 and p27 expression (Li et al. 2010a). In another study, treatment of MCF-7 breast cancer cells with DIM prevented histone H4 acetylation at the *COX-2* gene promoter, thus inhibiting over-expression of this gene (Degner et al. 2009).

Genistein is the major isoflavone present in soybeans. Recent evidence indicates that genistein possesses the highest histone modifying activities in comparison to the other isoflavones, biochanin A and diadzein. In the few available studies, genistein has been shown to increase histone acetylation in esophageal squamous and prostate cancer cells (Fang et al. 2005a; Hong et al. 2004; Majid et al. 2009). In further support of this, several studies have revealed an increased activation of HAT following genistein treatment in renal and prostate cancers. In such instances HAT activation lead to the increased mRNA expression of *CREBBP, HAT1, PCAF* and *EP300* (Majid et al. 2008, 2010b). In addition, there is evidence suggesting that genistein inhibits the expression of SIRT1, one of the NAD$^+$ dependent histone deacetylases (Kikuno et al. 2008).

Quercetin, Sanguinarine and Dihydrocoumarin

Quercetin, which is primarily present in citrus fruits and buckwheat, is a potent anti-tumor dietary polyphenol. Quercetin activated NAD$^+$ dependent histone deacetylase SIRT1 in yeast, but this effect was less pronounced compared to resveratrol (Howitz et al. 2003). Ruiz et al. evaluated the effect of quercetin on the TNFα mediated expression of interferon-g-inducible protein 10 (*IP-10*) and macrophage inflammatory protein 2 (*MIP-2*) genes in murine intestinal epithelial cells (Ruiz et al. 2007). Treatment with quercetin was associated with the inhibition of the HAT activity on the promoter region of these genes, which resulted in reduced gene expression (Ruiz et al. 2007).

Sanguinarine (SGR) is commonly extracted from several plants such as bloodroot (*Sanguinaria canadensis*) or from the root, stem and leaves of the opium poppy. SGR has been shown to induce conformational changes by interacting with chromatin (Selvi et al. 2009). This compound potently inhibited HAT activity in rat liver and cervix cancer cell lines, which was associated with dose-dependent decrease in H3/H4 acetylation. In addition, binding of SGR to chromatin inhibited H3K4 and H3R17 methylation, an epigenetic mark that is associated with transcriptional activation more efficiently than H3K9 methylation.

Dihydrocoumarin (DHC) is an active compound found in sweet clover that is widely used in food and cosmetic industries. DHC has recently been identified as an inhibitor of the HDAC family of sirtuins, which have an established role in the ageing process (Olaharski et al. 2005). DHC disrupted heterochromatin silencing and inhibited yeast Sir2p and human SIRT1/2 deacetylase activity, which caused p53 acetylation and increase in apoptosis *in vitro* (Olaharski et al. 2005). In addition to the well-described effects of various dietary polyphenols on histone modifications described above, there are several other such compounds for which limited evidence exists for their ability to modulate histone modifications. Several such additional compounds are not mentioned here, but are listed in the Table 13.2.

Polyphenols Induced Changes in miRNA Expression

Among various epigenetic modifiers, microRNAs are the most recently discovered regulators of gene expression. In spite of the limited evidence, sufficient data exists to indicate that several dietary polyphenols can also modulate gene expression by targeting various oncogenic or tumor suppressive miRNAs. In the section, we will summarize the current evidence supporting the effect of dietary polyphenols on specific target miRNAs (Table 13.3 and Fig. 13.5).

EGCG

EGCG has been recently found to modulate the miRNA expression in human hepatocellular carcinoma HepG2 cells. Tsang et al. performed microarray analysis in this cell line after EGCG treatment and discovered that this compound modified the expression of a subset of 61 miRNAs (Tsang and Kwok 2010). miR-16, one of the miRNAs up-regulated by EGCG, is known to regulate the anti-apoptotic protein Bcl-2. Interestingly, EGCG treatment in this study also induced apoptosis and down-regulated Bcl-2 in HepG2 cells.

Curcumin

The anti-cancer effects of curcumin have recently been linked to changes in miRNA expression. Treatment of BxPC-3 pancreatic cancer cell lines with curcumin, followed by microRNA expression profiling, revealed significant changes in the expression levels of 29 miRNAs (Sun et al. 2008). In this study, up-regulation of miR-22 was one of the most significant curcumin-induced changes. Functional studies showed that up-regulation of miRNA-22 expression by curcumin or by transfection with miRNA-22 mimetics in the PxBC-3 pancreatic cancer cell line suppressed expression of two of its known target genes, *SP1* and *ESR1*. In other recently published study, Ali et al. have further analyzed potential of curcumin in treatment of pancreatic cancer in combination with Gemcitabine, a standard agent used for the care of pancreatic cancer patients (Ali et al. 2010). In this study, the researchers demonstrated that treatment with either curcumin or curcumin-analogues potentiated apoptotic effects of gemcitabine, which resulted in induction of miR-200b/c and inhibition of miR-21 expression. In addition, increased PTEN expression correlated with increased miR-21 expression in this study (Ali et al. 2010). More recently, it was demonstrated that curcumin promoted increased apoptosis in lung adenocarcinoma cells by inducing miR-186 cell signaling pathway (Zhang et al. 2010). Similarly, another recent report indicated that curcumin regulated the expression of miR-21 which in turn regulated metastasis and invasion in colorectal cancer cells (Mudduluru et al. 2011).

Table 13.3 microRNA expression changes induced by the dietary polyphenols

Cancer	Dietary agent	Plant source	microRNAs	Target genes	Concentration	References
Colon	Curcumin	Turmeric	miR-21	*PDCD4*	10 μM	Mudduluru et al. (2011)
Liver	EGCG	Green tea	miR-16	*BCLl2*	100 μM	Tsang and Kwok (2010)
Lung	Curcumin	Turmeric	miR-186	*Caspase-10*	–	Zhang et al. (2010))
Pancreas	3,3-diindolylmethane	Broccoli	miR-200 (a-c), let-7 (a-f), miR-146a	*ZEB1, EGFR*	25 μM	Li et al. (2009b, 2010b)
Pancreas	Genistein	Soy	miR-200 (a-c), let-7 (a-f), mir-27b, miR-146a	*ZEB1, ZBTB10, EGFR*	25 μM	Li et al. (2009b, 2010b), Parker et al. (2009), Sun et al. (2009)
Prostate	Genistein	Soy	miR-1296	*MCM2*	25–50 μM	Majid et al. (2010a)
Prostate	Genistein	Soy	miR-221/222	*ARHI*	–	Chen et al. (2011))

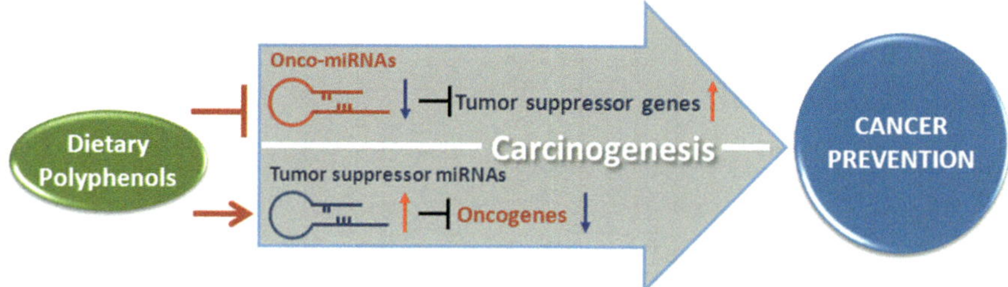

Fig. 13.5 Effects of dietary polyphenols on microRNA (miRNA) expression. Dependent on various factors, miRNA can have either an oncogenic role (called onco-miRNAs) if the target mRNA is a tumor suppressor gene, or a tumor suppressive role (tumor-suppressor miRNAs) if the target molecule is an oncogene. Dietary polyphenols have the ability to impact expression level of miRNAs and allow up-regulation of the tumor suppressor gene expression (*red arrows*) as well as down-regulation of oncogenes in order to achieve their chemopreventative potential

Genistein and 3,3′-Diindolylmethane (DIM)

Isoflavones, genistein and DIM have been found to regulate the miRNA expression in pancreatic cancer cells. Li et al. recently compared the expression of miRNAs between gemcitabine-sensitive and gemcitabine-resistant pancreatic cancer cells and investigated whether the treatment of cells with these two dietary compounds could affect the expression of several miRNAs (Li et al. 2009b). The expression of the miR-200 and let-7 family was significantly down-regulated in gemcitabine-resistant cells, which showed epithelial-mesenchymal transition (EMT) characteristics. Interestingly, restoration of miR-200 expression or the treatment of gemcitabine-resistant cells with DIM or isoflavones (a combination of genistein, diadzin, and glycitein) resulted in the reversal of the EMT features, leading to epithelial morphology. In another study, these investigators have further shown that treatment with these compounds up-regulates miR-146a in pancreatic cancer cell, and this was associated with reduction in cell invasion and metastasis (Li et al. 2010b). This effect was associated with down-regulation of EGFR and NF-κB regulatory kinase interleukin-1 receptor associated kinase. Re-expression of miR-146a inhibited the invasive capacity of pancreatic cancer cells with concomitant down-regulation of EGFR and interleukin 1 receptor–associated kinase 1 (IRAK-1) further pointing the significance of polyphenol mediated anticancer effect (Li et al. 2010b). Another study demonstrated that genistein inhibits cell growth and modulates the expression of miR-27a and one of its targets (gene zinc finger and BTB domain containing 10 or *ZBTB10*) in human uveal melanoma cell lines (Sun et al. 2009). Lastly, in an observational study, Parker et al. observed that genistein is able to induce changes in miRNA expression in ovarian cancer cell lines (Parker et al. 2009). In another study, it was shown that miR-1296 and genistein regulate mini chromosome maintenance (MCM) in prostate cancer cells (Majid et al. 2010a). More recently, Chen and colleagues showed evidence for mir-221/miR-222 and genistein-induced regulation of ARHI gene in prostate cancer cells (Chen et al. 2011).

Indole-3-Carbinol and Phenethyl Isothiocyanate

A recently published study focused on the potential of natural compounds as chemopreventive agents after environmental cigarette smoke (ECS) exposure in animals (Izzotti et al. 2010). In this study, microarray miRNA expression analysis was performed in the lungs of either ECS-free or ECS-exposed rats treated with the orally administered chemopreventive agents including indole-3-carbinol and phenethyl isothiocyanate (both found in cruciferous vegetables). Interestingly, none of the above chemopreventive agents appreciably affected the baseline microRNA expression in non-exposed lungs, indicating potential safety. However, all of them attenuated ECS-induced alterations to a variable extent and with different patterns, indicating potential preventive efficacy.

Summary

The take home message from the data presented in this chapter is that dietary polyphenols which were once considered as mere health supplements are now earning more attention and respect as essential ingredients for living and maintaining a healthier lifestyle. While the anecdotal epidemiological evidence has historically supported the idea of different diet and good health, experimental evidence accumulated in the recent years from various pre-clinical and clinical studies clearly support the idea that dietary polyphenols have potentially beneficial effects on multitude of health conditions, including cancer. This chapter provides a novel perspective on the potential chemoprevention by diet and dietary agents, as the extensive data summarized here suggest that beneficial effects of different dietary polyphenols may in part be attributable to their epigenetic properties, including changes in the DNA methylation pattern, regulation of histone modifications and changes in the expression of specific miRNAs. Although the health effects of dietary polyphenols in humans are generally considered promising, there are definite challenges and limitations of the current data in better understanding the molecular mechanisms responsible for these effects. Consequently, until sufficient preclinical and clinical data has been gathered on the epigenetic changes, one should interpret and extrapolate these results with a grain of salt. In addition, clinical studies are required in the immediate future to further examine the safety profile of various dietary polyphenols. It is really exciting to witness that we have at least shun our reluctance to accept the idea of "complementary and alternate system of medicine" and have begun to cautiously embrace the "goodness" of certain diets and diet-related factors that has been in existence for centuries. The fact that currently there is an unprecedented interest in further exploration and enthusiasm to explore the efficacy of various dietary polyphenols from an epigenomic perspective clearly mandates the trust we have begun to pose in the mantra of healthier living through the use of certain diets and dietary supplements rich in health-promoting polyphenols. Needless to mention that although the current evidence on the topic is very superficial, but in light of burgeoning scientific and domestic inquisitiveness on the potential usefulness of dietary polyphenols, it is not unrealistic to picture that these compounds may play a central role in the care of cancer patients in the near future.

Acknowledgement The present work was supported in part by grant R01 CA129286 from the National Cancer Institute, National Institutes of Health.

References

Aggarwal BB, Shishodia S (2006) Molecular targets of dietary agents for prevention and therapy of cancer. Biochem Pharmacol 71:1397–1421

Aggarwal BB, Shishodia S, Sandur SK, Pandey MK, Sethi G (2006) Inflammation and cancer: how hot is the link? Biochem Pharmacol 72:1605–1621

Ali S, Ahmad A, Banerjee S, Padhye S, Dominiak K, Schaffert JM, Wang Z, Philip PA, Sarkar FH (2010) Gemcitabine sensitivity can be induced in pancreatic cancer cells through modulation of miR-200 and miR-21 expression by curcumin or its analogue CDF. Cancer Res 70:3606–3617

Araki Y, Fann M, Wersto R, Weng NP (2008) Histone acetylation facilitates rapid and robust memory CD8 T cell response through differential expression of effector molecules (eomesodermin and its targets: perforin and granzyme b). J Immunol 180:8102–8108

Arif M, Kumar GV, Narayana C, Kundu TK (2007) Autoacetylation induced specific structural changes in histone acetyltransferase domain of P300: probed by surface enhanced Raman spectroscopy. J Phys Chem B 111:11877–11879

Artaud-Wild SM, Connor SL, Sexton G, Connor WE (1993) Differences in coronary mortality can be explained by differences in cholesterol and saturated fat intakes in 40 countries but not in France and Finland. A paradox. Circulation 88:2771–2779

Arunkumar A, Vijayababu MR, Gunadharini N, Krishnamoorthy G, Arunakaran J (2007) Induction of apoptosis and histone hyperacetylation by diallyl disulfide in prostate cancer cell line PC-3. Cancer Lett 251:59–67

Balaguer F, Link A, Lozano JJ, Cuatrecasas M, Nagasaka T, Boland CR, Goel A (2010) Epigenetic silencing of miR-137 is an early event in colorectal carcinogenesis. Cancer Res 70:6609–6618

Balasubramanian S, Adhikary G, Eckert RL (2010) The Bmi-1 polycomb protein antagonizes the (-)-epigallocatechin-3-gallate-dependent suppression of skin cancer cell survival. Carcinogenesis 31:496–503

Balasubramanyam K, Swaminathan V, Ranganathan A, Kundu TK (2003) Small molecule modulators of histone acetyltransferase P300. J Biol Chem 278:19134–19140

Balasubramanyam K, Altaf M, Varier RA, Swaminathan V, Ravindran A, Sadhale PP, Kundu TK (2004) Polyisoprenylated benzophenone, garcinol, a natural histone acetyltransferase inhibitor, represses chromatin transcription and alters global gene expression. J Biol Chem 279:33716–33726

Beher D, Wu J, Cumine S, Kim KW, Lu SC, Atangan L, Wang M (2009) Resveratrol is not a direct activator of SIRT1 enzyme activity. Chem Biol Drug Des 74:619–624

Beklemisheva AA, Fang Y, Feng J, Ma X, Dai W, Chiao JW (2006) Epigenetic mechanism of growth inhibition induced by phenylhexyl isothiocyanate in prostate cancer cells. Anticancer Res 26:1225–1230

Berletch JB, Andrews LG, Tollefsbol TO (2007) A method to detect DNA methyltransferase I gene transcription in vitro in aging systems. Methods Mol Biol 371:73–80

Berletch JB, Liu C, Love WK, Andrews LG, Katiyar SK, Tollefsbol TO (2008) Epigenetic and genetic mechanisms contribute to telomerase inhibition by EGCG. J Cell Biochem 103:509–519

Bhatnagar N, Li X, Chen Y, Zhou X, Garrett SH, Guo B (2009) 3,3′-diindolylmethane enhances the efficacy of butyrate in colon cancer prevention through down-regulation of survivin. Cancer Prev Res (Phila) 2:581–589

Bird A (2002) DNA methylation patterns and epigenetic memory. Genes Dev 16:6–21

Blewitt ME, Vickaryous NK, Paldi A, Koseki H, Whitelaw E (2006) Dynamic reprogramming of DNA methylation at an epigenetically sensitive allele in mice. PLoS Genet 2:E49

Boily G, He XH, Pearce B, Jardine K, McBurney MW (2009) SirT1-null mice develop tumors at normal rates but are poorly protected by resveratrol. Oncogene 28:2882–2893

Bontempo P, Mita L, Miceli M, Doto A, Nebbioso A, de Bellis F, Conte M, Minichiello A, Manzo F, Carafa V, Basile A, Rigano D, Sorbo S, Castaldo Cobianchi R, Schiavone EM, Ferrara F, De Simone M, Vietri M, Cioffi M, Sica V, Bresciani F, de Lera AR, Altucci L, Molinari AM (2007) Feijoa sellowiana derived natural flavone exerts anti-cancer action displaying HDAC inhibitory activities. Int J Biochem Cell Biol 39:1902–1914

Bora-Tatar G, Dayangac-Erden D, Demir AS, Dalkara S, Yelekci K, Erdem-Yurter H (2009) Molecular modifications on carboxylic acid derivatives as potent histone deacetylase inhibitors: activity and docking studies. Bioorg Med Chem 17:5219–5228

Bravo L (1998) Polyphenols: chemistry, dietary sources, metabolism, and nutritional significance. Nutr Rev 56:317–333

Calin GA, Sevignani C, Dumitru CD, Hyslop T, Noch E, Yendamuri S, Shimizu M, Rattan S, Bullrich F, Negrini M, Croce CM (2004) Human microRNA genes are frequently located at fragile sites and genomic regions involved in cancers. Proc Natl Acad Sci U S A 101:2999–3004

Chalabi N, Delort L, le Corre L, Satih S, Bignon YJ, Bernard-Gallon D (2006) Gene signature of breast cancer cell lines treated with lycopene. Pharmacogenomics 7:663–672

Chalabi N, Satih S, Delort L, Bignon YJ, Bernard-Gallon DJ (2007) Expression profiling by whole-genome microarray hybridization reveals differential gene expression in breast cancer cell lines after lycopene exposure. Biochim Biophys Acta 1769:124–130

Chandregowda V, Kush A, Reddy GC (2009) Synthesis of benzamide derivatives of anacardic acid and their cytotoxic activity. Eur J Med Chem 44:2711–2719

Chen Y, Shu W, Chen W, Wu Q, Liu H, Cui G (2007) Curcumin, both histone deacetylase and p300/CBP-specific inhibitor, represses the activity of nuclear factor kappa B and Notch 1 in Raji cells. Basic Clin Pharmacol Toxicol 101:427–433

Chen IH, Lu MC, Du YC, Yen MH, Wu CC, Chen YH, Hung CS, Chen SL, Chang FR, Wu YC (2009) Cytotoxic triterpenoids from the stems of Microtropis japonica. J Nat Prod 72:1231–1236

Chen Y, Zaman MS, Deng G, Majid S, Saini S, Liu J, Tanaka Y, Dahiya R (2011) MicroRNAs 221/222 and genistein-mediated regulation of ARHI tumor suppressor gene in prostate cancer. Cancer Prev Res (Phila) 4:76–86

Chiu J, Khan ZA, Farhangkhoee H, Chakrabarti S (2009) Curcumin prevents diabetes-associated abnormalities in the kidneys by inhibiting p300 and nuclear factor-kappab. Nutrition 25:964–972

Choi KC, Jung MG, Lee YH, Yoon JC, Kwon SH, Kang HB, Kim MJ, Cha JH, Kim YJ, Jun WJ, Lee JM, Yoon HG (2009) Epigallocatechin-3-gallate, a histone acetyltransferase inhibitor, inhibits EBV-induced B lymphocyte transformation via suppression of RelA acetylation. Cancer Res 69:583–592

Chu Q, Ling MT, Feng H, Cheung HW, Tsao SW, Wang X, Wong YC (2006) A novel anticancer effect of garlic derivatives: inhibition of cancer cell invasion through restoration of E-cadherin expression. Carcinogenesis 27:2180–2189

Chuang JC, Yoo CB, Kwan JM, Li TW, Liang G, Yang AS, Jones PA (2005) Comparison of biological effects of non-nucleoside DNA methylation inhibitors versus 5-aza-2′-deoxycytidine. Mol Cancer Ther 4:1515–1520

Chung IM, Kim MY, Park WH, Moon HI (2008) Histone deacetylase inhibitors from the rhizomes of Zingiber zerumbet. Pharmazie 63:774–776

Cosio BG, Mann B, Ito K, Jazrawi E, Barnes PJ, Chung KF, Adcock IM (2004) Histone acetylase and deacetylase activity in alveolar macrophages and blood monocytes in asthma. Am J Respir Crit Care Med 170:141–147

Cosio BG, Iglesias A, Rios A, Noguera A, Sala E, Ito K, Barnes PJ, Agusti A (2009) Low-dose theophylline enhances the anti-inflammatory effects of steroids during exacerbations of COPD. Thorax 64:424–429

Costello JF, Plass C (2001) Methylation matters. J Med Genet 38:285–303

Cui L, Miao J (2007) Cytotoxic effect of curcumin on malaria parasite Plasmodium falciparum: inhibition of histone acetylation and generation of reactive oxygen species. Antimicrob Agents Chemother 51:488–494

Cui L, Miao J, Furuya T, Li X, Su XZ (2007) PfGCN5-mediated histone H3 acetylation plays a key role in gene expression in Plasmodium falciparum. Eukaryot Cell 6:1219–1227

Cui X, Jin Y, Hofseth AB, Pena E, Habiger J, Chumanevich A, Poudyal D, Nagarkatti M, Nagarkatti PS, Singh UP, Hofseth LJ (2010) Resveratrol suppresses colitis and colon cancer associated with colitis. Cancer Prev Res (Phila) 3:549–559

Davis CD, Ross SA (2007) Dietary components impact histone modifications and cancer risk. Nutr Rev 65:88–94

Davis CD, Ross SA (2008) Evidence for dietary regulation of microRNA expression in cancer cells. Nutr Rev 66:477–482

Davis CD, Uthus EO, Finley JW (2000) Dietary selenium and arsenic affect DNA methylation in vitro in caco-2 cells and in vivo in rat liver and colon. J Nutr 130:2903–2909

Day JK, Bauer AM, Desbordes C, Zhuang Y, Kim BE, Newton LG, Nehra V, Forsee KM, Macdonald RS, Besch-Williford C, Huang TH, Lubahn DB (2002) Genistein alters methylation patterns in mice. J Nutr 132:2419S–2423S

Deaton AM, Bird A (2011) CpG islands and the regulation of transcription. Genes Dev 25:1010–1022

Degner SC, Papoutsis AJ, Selmin O, Romagnolo DF (2009) Targeting of aryl hydrocarbon receptor-mediated activation of cyclooxygenase-2 expression by the indole-3-carbinol metabolite 3,3′-diindolylmethane in breast cancer cells. J Nutr 139:26–32

Dehan P, Kustermans G, Guenin S, Horion J, Boniver J, Delvenne P (2009) DNA methylation and cancer diagnosis: new methods and applications. Expert Rev Mol Diagn 9:651–657

Dolinoy DC, Weidman JR, Waterland RA, Jirtle RL (2006) Maternal genistein alters coat color and protects Avy mouse offspring from obesity by modifying the fetal epigenome. Environ Health Perspect 114:567–572

Dolinoy DC, Huang D, Jirtle RL (2007a) Maternal nutrient supplementation counteracts bisphenol A-induced DNA hypomethylation in early development. Proc Natl Acad Sci U S A 104:13056–13061

Dolinoy DC, Weidman JR, Jirtle RL (2007b) Epigenetic gene regulation: linking early developmental environment to adult disease. Reprod Toxicol 23:297–307

Druesne N, Pagniez A, Mayeur C, Thomas M, Cherbuy C, Duee PH, Martel P, Chaumontet C (2004) Diallyl disulfide (DADS) increases histone acetylation and p21(waf1/cip1) expression in human colon tumor cell lines. Carcinogenesis 25:1227–1236

Druesne-Pecollo N, Pagniez A, Thomas M, Cherbuy C, Duee PH, Martel P, Chaumontet C (2006) Diallyl disulfide increases CDKN1A promoter-associated histone acetylation in human colon tumor cell lines. J Agric Food Chem 54:7503–7507

Druesne-Pecollo N, Chaumontet C, Pagniez A, Vaugelade P, Bruneau A, Thomas M, Cherbuy C, Duee PH, Martel P (2007) In vivo treatment by diallyl disulfide increases histone acetylation in rat colonocytes. Biochem Biophys Res Commun 354:140–147

Ducasse M, Brown MA (2006) Epigenetic aberrations and cancer. Mol Cancer 5:60

Eliseeva ED, Valkov V, Jung M, Jung MO (2007) Characterization of novel inhibitors of histone acetyltransferases. Mol Cancer Ther 6:2391–2398

Ellis L, Atadja PW, Johnstone RW (2009) Epigenetics in cancer: targeting chromatin modifications. Mol Cancer Ther 8:1409–1420

Esteller M (2011) Epigenetic changes in cancer. F1000 Biol Rep 3:9

Fang MZ, Wang Y, Ai N, Hou Z, Sun Y, Lu H, Welsh W, Yang CS (2003) Tea polyphenol (-)-epigallocatechin-3-gallate inhibits DNA methyltransferase and reactivates methylation-silenced genes in cancer cell lines. Cancer Res 63:7563–7570

Fang MZ, Chen D, Sun Y, Jin Z, Christman JK, Yang CS (2005a) Reversal of hypermethylation and reactivation of p16INK4a, RARbeta, and MGMT genes by genistein and other isoflavones from soy. Clin Cancer Res 11:7033–7041

Fang MZ, Jin Z, Wang Y, Liao J, Yang GY, Wang LD, Yang CS (2005b) Promoter hypermethylation and inactivation of O(6)-methylguanine-DNA methyltransferase in esophageal squamous cell carcinomas and its reactivation in cell lines. Int J Oncol 26:615–622

Fang M, Chen D, Yang CS (2007) Dietary polyphenols may affect DNA methylation. J Nutr 137:223S–228S

Gao Z, Xu Z, Hung MS, Lin YC, Wang T, Gong M, Zhi X, Jablon DM, You L (2009) Promoter demethylation of WIF-1 by epigallocatechin-3-gallate in lung cancer cells. Anticancer Res 29:2025–2030

Gilbert J, Gore SD, Herman JG, Carducci MA (2004) The clinical application of targeting cancer through histone acetylation and hypomethylation. Clin Cancer Res 10:4589–4596

Gracia-Sancho J, Villarreal G Jr, Zhang Y, Garcia-Cardena G (2010) Activation of SIRT1 by resveratrol induces KLF2 expression conferring an endothelial vasoprotective phenotype. Cardiovasc Res 85:514–519

Gravina GL, Festuccia C, Marampon F, Popov VM, Pestell RG, Zani BM, Tombolini V (2010) Biological rationale for the use of DNA methyltransferase inhibitors as new strategy for modulation of tumor response to chemotherapy and radiation. Mol Cancer 9:305

Gu B, Ding Q, Xia G, Fang Z (2009) EGCG inhibits growth and induces apoptosis in renal cell carcinoma through TFPI-2 overexpression. Oncol Rep 21:635–640

Guerrero-Bosagna CM, Sabat P, Valdovinos FS, Valladares LE, Clark SJ (2008) Epigenetic and phenotypic changes result from a continuous pre and post natal dietary exposure to phytoestrogens in an experimental population of mice. BMC Physiol 8:17

Guilleret I, Benhattar J (2004) Unusual distribution of DNA methylation within the hTERT CpG island in tissues and cell lines. Biochem Biophys Res Commun 325:1037–1043

Haberland M, Montgomery RL, Olson EN (2009) The many roles of histone deacetylases in development and physiology: implications for disease and therapy. Nat Rev Genet 10:32–42

He L, Hannon GJ (2004) MicroRNAs: small RNAs with a big role in gene regulation. Nat Rev Genet 5:522–531

Herceg Z (2007) Epigenetics and cancer: towards an evaluation of the impact of environmental and dietary factors. Mutagenesis 22:91–103

Herman JG, Baylin SB (2003) Gene silencing in cancer in association with promoter hypermethylation. N Engl J Med 349:2042–2054

Hodge DR, Peng B, Cherry JC, Hurt EM, Fox SD, Kelley JA, Munroe DJ, Farrar WL (2005) Interleukin 6 supports the maintenance of p53 tumor suppressor gene promoter methylation. Cancer Res 65:4673–4682

Hong T, Nakagawa T, Pan W, Kim MY, Kraus WL, Ikehara T, Yasui K, Aihara H, Takebe M, Muramatsu M, Ito T (2004) Isoflavones stimulate estrogen receptor-mediated core histone acetylation. Biochem Biophys Res Commun 317:259–264

Horrobin DF (2003) Are large clinical trials in rapidly lethal diseases usually unethical? Lancet 361:695–697

Howitz KT, Bitterman KJ, Cohen HY, Lamming DW, Lavu S, Wood JG, Zipkin RE, Chung P, Kisielewski A, Zhang LL, Scherer B, Sinclair DA (2003) Small molecule activators of sirtuins extend Saccharomyces cerevisiae lifespan. Nature 425:191–196

Hu R, Khor TO, Shen G, Jeong WS, Hebbar V, Chen C, Xu C, Reddy B, Chada K, Kong AN (2006) Cancer chemoprevention of intestinal polyposis in ApcMin/+ mice by sulforaphane, a natural product derived from cruciferous vegetable. Carcinogenesis 27:2038–2046

Iacobuzio-Donahue CA (2009) Epigenetic changes in cancer. Annu Rev Pathol 4:229–249
Inui M, Martello G, Piccolo S (2010) MicroRNA control of signal transduction. Nat Rev Mol Cell Biol 11:252–263
Issa JP, Kantarjian HM (2009) Targeting DNA methylation. Clin Cancer Res 15:3938–3946
Ito K, Lim S, Caramori G, Cosio B, Chung KF, Adcock IM, Barnes PJ (2002) A molecular mechanism of action of theophylline: induction of histone deacetylase activity to decrease inflammatory gene expression. Proc Natl Acad Sci U S A 99:8921–8926
Izzotti A, Calin GA, Steele VE, Cartiglia C, Longobardi M, Croce CM, de Flora S (2010) Chemoprevention of cigarette smoke-induced alterations of microRNA expression in rat lungs. Cancer Prev Res (Phila) 3:62–72
Jaenisch R, Bird A (2003) Epigenetic regulation of gene expression: how the genome integrates intrinsic and environmental signals. Nat Genet 33(SUPPL):245–254
Jha AK, Nikbakht M, Parashar G, Shrivastava A, Capalash N, Kaur J (2010) Reversal of hypermethylation and reactivation of the RARbeta2 gene by natural compounds in cervical cancer cell lines. Folia Biol (Praha) 56:195–200
Jones PL, Veenstra GJ, Wade PA, Vermaak D, Kass SU, Landsberger N, Strouboulis J, Wolffe AP (1998) Methylated DNA and MeCP2 recruit histone deacetylase to repress transcription. Nat Genet 19:187–191
Jones K, Nourse J, Corbett G, Gandhi MK (2010) Sodium valproate in combination with ganciclovir induces lysis of EBV-infected lymphoma cells without impairing EBV-specific T-cell immunity. Int J Lab Hematol 32:E169–E174
Kaeberlein M, McDonagh T, Heltweg B, Hixon J, Westman EA, Caldwell SD, Napper A, Curtis R, Distefano PS, Fields S, Bedalov A, Kennedy BK (2005) Substrate-specific activation of sirtuins by resveratrol. J Biol Chem 280:17038–17045
Kai ZS, Pasquinelli AE (2010) Microrna assassins: factors that regulate the disappearance of miRNAs. Nat Struct Mol Biol 17:5–10
Kai L, Samuel SK, Levenson AS (2010) Resveratrol enhances p53 acetylation and apoptosis in prostate cancer by inhibiting MTA1/NuRD complex. Int J Cancer 126:1538–1548
Kang J, Chen J, Shi Y, Jia J, Zhang Y (2005) Curcumin-induced histone hypoacetylation: the role of reactive oxygen species. Biochem Pharmacol 69:1205–1213
Kato K, Long NK, Makita H, Toida M, Yamashita T, Hatakeyama D, Hara A, Mori H, Shibata T (2008) Effects of green tea polyphenol on methylation status of RECK gene and cancer cell invasion in oral squamous cell carcinoma cells. Br J Cancer 99:647–654
Kikuno N, Shiina H, Urakami S, Kawamoto K, Hirata H, Tanaka Y, Majid S, Igawa M, Dahiya R (2008) Genistein mediated histone acetylation and demethylation activates tumor suppressor genes in prostate cancer cells. Int J Cancer 123:552–560
Kim MK, Shin JM, Eun HC, Chung JH (2009) The role of p300 histone acetyltransferase in UV-induced histone modifications and MMP-1 gene transcription. PLoS One 4:E4864
Kim SH, Kang HJ, Na H, Lee MO (2010) Trichostatin a enhances acetylation as well as protein stability of ERalpha through induction of p300 protein. Breast Cancer Res 12:R22
King-Batoon A, Leszczynska JM, Klein CB (2008) Modulation of gene methylation by genistein or lycopene in breast cancer cells. Environ Mol Mutagen 49:36–45
Komashko VM, Farnham PJ (2010) 5-Azacytidine treatment reorganizes genomic histone modification patterns. Epigenetics 5:229–240
Kouzarides T (2007) Chromatin modifications and their function. Cell 128:693–705
Kuck D, Singh N, Lyko F, Medina-Franco JL (2010) Novel and selective DNA methyltransferase inhibitors: docking-based virtual screening and experimental evaluation. Bioorg Med Chem 18:822–829
Kutluay SB, Doroghazi J, Roemer ME, Triezenberg SJ (2008) Curcumin inhibits herpes simplex virus immediate-early gene expression by a mechanism independent of p300/CBP histone acetyltransferase activity. Virology 373:239–247
Lah JJ, Cui W, Hu KQ (2007) Effects and mechanisms of silibinin on human hepatoma cell lines. World J Gastroenterol 13:5299–5305
Laird P (2005) Cancer epigenetics. Hum Mol Genet 14:R65–R76

Lea MA, Randolph VM (2001) Induction of histone acetylation in rat liver and hepatoma by organosulfur compounds including diallyl disulfide. Anticancer Res 21:2841–2845

Lea MA, Randolph VM, Patel M (1999) Increased acetylation of histones induced by diallyl disulfide and structurally related molecules. Int J Oncol 15:347–352

Lea MA, Randolph VM, Lee JE, Desbordes C (2001) Induction of histone acetylation in mouse erythroleukemia cells by some organosulfur compounds including allyl isothiocyanate. Int J Cancer 92:784–789

Lea MA, Rasheed M, Randolph VM, Khan F, Shareef A, Desbordes C (2002) Induction of histone acetylation and inhibition of growth of mouse erythroleukemia cells by S-allylmercaptocysteine. Nutr Cancer 43:90–102

Lee WJ, Zhu BT (2006) Inhibition of DNA methylation by caffeic acid and chlorogenic acid, two common catechol-containing coffee polyphenols. Carcinogenesis 27:269–277

Lee WJ, Shim JY, Zhu BT (2005) Mechanisms for the inhibition of DNA methyltransferases by tea catechins and bioflavonoids. Mol Pharmacol 68:1018–1030

Li HL, Liu C, de Couto G, Ouzounian M, Sun M, Wang AB, Huang Y, He CW, Shi Y, Chen X, Nghiem MP, Liu Y, Chen M, Dawood F, Fukuoka M, Maekawa Y, Zhang L, Leask A, Ghosh AK, Kirshenbaum LA, Liu PP (2008) Curcumin prevents and reverses murine cardiac hypertrophy. J Clin Invest 118:879–893

Li Y, Liu L, Andrews LG, Tollefsbol TO (2009a) Genistein depletes telomerase activity through cross-talk between genetic and epigenetic mechanisms. Int J Cancer 125:286–296

Li Y, Vandenboom TG 2nd, Kong D, Wang Z, Ali S, Philip PA, Sarkar FH (2009b) Up-regulation of miR-200 and let-7 by natural agents leads to the reversal of epithelial-to-mesenchymal transition in gemcitabine-resistant pancreatic cancer cells. Cancer Res 69:6704–6712

Li Y, Li X, Guo B (2010a) Chemopreventive agent 3,3′-diindolylmethane selectively induces proteasomal degradation of class I histone deacetylases. Cancer Res 70:646–654

Li Y, Vandenboom TG, Wang Z, Ali S, Philip PA, Sarkar FH (2010b) miR-146a suppresses invasion of pancreatic cancer cells. Cancer Res 70:1486–1495

Liang G, Lin JC, Wei V, Yoo C, Cheng JC, Nguyen CT, Weisenberger DJ, Egger G, Takai D, Gonzales FA, Jones PA (2004) Distinct localization of histone H3 acetylation and H3-K4 methylation to the transcription start sites in the human genome. Proc Natl Acad Sci U S A 101:7357–7362

Link A, Balaguer F, Goel A (2010) Cancer chemoprevention by dietary polyphenols: promising role for epigenetics. Biochem Pharmacol 80:1771–1792

Liu HL, Chen Y, Cui GH, Zhou JF (2005) Curcumin, a potent anti-tumor reagent, is a novel histone deacetylase inhibitor regulating B-NHL cell line Raji proliferation. Acta Pharmacol Sin 26:603–609

Liu Z, Xie Z, Jones W, Pavlovicz RE, Liu S, Yu J, Li PK, Lin J, Fuchs JR, Marcucci G, Li C, Chan KK (2009) Curcumin is a potent DNA hypomethylation agent. Bioorg Med Chem Lett 19:706–709

Liu X, Wang J, Li R, Yang X, Sun Q, Albrecht E, Zhao R (2011) Maternal dietary protein affects transcriptional regulation of myostatin gene distinctively at weaning and finishing stages in skeletal muscle of Meishan pigs. Epigenetics 6:899–907

Luger K, Mader AW, Richmond RK, Sargent DF, Richmond TJ (1997) Crystal structure of the nucleosome core particle at 2.8 A resolution. Nature 389:251–260

Lund AH, van Lohuizen M (2004) Epigenetics and cancer. Genes Dev 18:2315–2335

Ma X, Fang Y, Beklemisheva A, Dai W, Feng J, Ahmed T, Liu D, Chiao JW (2006) Phenylhexyl isothiocyanate inhibits histone deacetylases and remodels chromatins to induce growth arrest in human leukemia cells. Int J Oncol 28:1287–1293

Mai A, Rotili D, Tarantino D, Ornaghi P, Tosi F, Vicidomini C, Sbardella G, Nebbioso A, Miceli M, Altucci L, Filetici P (2006) Small-molecule inhibitors of histone acetyltransferase activity: identification and biological properties. J Med Chem 49:6897–6907

Majid S, Kikuno N, Nelles J, Noonan E, Tanaka Y, Kawamoto K, Hirata H, Li LC, Zhao H, Okino ST, Place RF, Pookot D, Dahiya R (2008) Genistein induces the p21WAF1/CIP1 and p16iNK4a tumor suppressor genes in prostate cancer cells by epigenetic mechanisms involving active chromatin modification. Cancer Res 68:2736–2744

Majid S, Dar AA, Ahmad AE, Hirata H, Kawakami K, Shahryari V, Saini S, Tanaka Y, Dahiya AV, Khatri G, Dahiya R (2009) BTG3 tumor suppressor gene promoter demethylation, histone modification and cell cycle arrest by genistein in renal cancer. Carcinogenesis 30:662–670

Majid S, Dar AA, Saini S, Chen Y, Shahryari V, Liu J, Zaman MS, Hirata H, Yamamura S, Ueno K, Tanaka Y, Dahiya R (2010a) Regulation of minichromosome maintenance gene family by microRNA-1296 and genistein in prostate cancer. Cancer Res 70:2809–2818

Majid S, Dar AA, Shahryari V, Hirata H, Ahmad A, Saini S, Tanaka Y, Dahiya AV, Dahiya R (2010b) Genistein reverses hypermethylation and induces active histone modifications in tumor suppressor gene B-cell translocation gene 3 in prostate cancer. Cancer 116:66–76

Malik R, Kashyap A, Bansal K, Sharma P, Rayasam GV, Davis JA, Bora RS, Ray A, Saini KS (2010) Comparative deacetylase activity of wild type and mutants of SIRT1. Biochem Biophys Res Commun 391:739–743

Mantelingu K, Reddy BA, Swaminathan V, Kishore AH, Siddappa NB, Kumar GV, Nagashankar G, Natesh N, Roy S, Sadhale PP, Ranga U, Narayana C, Kundu TK (2007) Specific inhibition of p300-HAT alters global gene expression and represses HIV replication. Chem Biol 14:645–657

Marcu MG, Jung YJ, Lee S, Chung EJ, Lee MJ, Trepel J, Neckers L (2006) Curcumin is an inhibitor of p300 histone acetylatransferase. Med Chem 2:169–174

McCabe MT, Brandes JC, Vertino PM (2009) Cancer DNA methylation: molecular mechanisms and clinical implications. Clin Cancer Res 15:3927–3937

Mittal A, Piyathilake C, Hara Y, Katiyar SK (2003) Exceptionally high protection of photocarcinogenesis by topical application of (–)-epigallocatechin-3-gallate in hydrophilic cream in SKH-1 hairless mouse model: relationship to inhibition of UVB-induced global DNA hypomethylation. Neoplasia 5:555–565

Miyamoto K, Ushijima T (2005) Diagnostic and therapeutic applications of epigenetics. Jpn J Clin Oncol 35:293–301

Morey Kinney SR, Zhang W, Pascual M, Greally JM, Gillard BM, Karasik E, Foster BA, Karpf AR (2009) Lack of evidence for green tea polyphenols as DNA methylation inhibitors in murine prostate. Cancer Prev Res (Phila) 2:1065–1075

Morimoto T, Sunagawa Y, Kawamura T, Takaya T, Wada H, Nagasawa A, Komeda M, Fujita M, Shimatsu A, Kita T, Hasegawa K (2008) The dietary compound curcumin inhibits p300 histone acetyltransferase activity and prevents heart failure in rats. J Clin Invest 118:868–878

Mudduluru G, George-William JN, Muppala S, Asangani IA, Regalla K, Nelson LD, Allgayer H (2011) Curcumin regulates miR-21 expression and inhibits invasion and metastasis in colorectal cancer. Biosci Rep 31(3):185–197

Murugan RS, Vinothini G, Hara Y, Nagini S (2009) Black tea polyphenols target matrix metalloproteinases, reck, proangiogenic molecules and histone deacetylase in a rat hepatocarcinogenesis model. Anticancer Res 29:2301–2305

Myzak MC, Karplus PA, Chung FL, Dashwood RH (2004) A novel mechanism of chemoprotection by sulforaphane: inhibition of histone deacetylase. Cancer Res 64:5767–5774

Myzak MC, Dashwood WM, Orner GA, Ho E, Dashwood RH (2006) Sulforaphane inhibits histone deacetylase in vivo and suppresses tumorigenesis in Apc-minus mice. FASEB J 20:506–508

Myzak MC, Tong P, Dashwood WM, Dashwood RH, Ho E (2007) Sulforaphane retards the growth of human PC-3 xenografts and inhibits HDAC activity in human subjects. Exp Biol Med (Maywood) 232:227–234

Nair S, Hebbar V, Shen G, Gopalakrishnan A, Khor TO, Yu S, Xu C, Kong AN (2008) Synergistic effects of a combination of dietary factors sulforaphane and (-) epigallocatechin-3-gallate in HT-29 AP-1 human colon carcinoma cells. Pharm Res 25:387–399

Navarro-Peran E, Cabezas-Herrera J, Campo LS, Rodriguez-Lopez JN (2007) Effects of folate cycle disruption by the green tea polyphenol epigallocatechin-3-gallate. Int J Biochem Cell Biol 39:2215–2225

Nian H, Delage B, Pinto JT, Dashwood RH (2008) Allyl mercaptan, a garlic-derived organosulfur compound, inhibits histone deacetylase and enhances Sp3 binding on the P21WAF1 promoter. Carcinogenesis 29:1816–1824

Olaharski AJ, Rine J, Marshall BL, Babiarz J, Zhang L, Verdin E, Smith MT (2005) The flavoring agent dihydrocoumarin reverses epigenetic silencing and inhibits sirtuin deacetylases. PLoS Genet 1:E77

Paluszczak J, Krajka-Kuzniak V, Baer-Dubowska W (2010) The effect of dietary polyphenols on the epigenetic regulation of gene expression in MCF7 breast cancer cells. Toxicol Lett 192:119–125

Pandey M, Shukla S, Gupta S (2010) Promoter demethylation and chromatin remodeling by green tea polyphenols leads to re-expression of GSTP1 in human prostate cancer cells. Int J Cancer 126:2520–2533

Paranjape T, Slack FJ, Weidhaas JB (2009) MicroRNAs: tools for cancer diagnostics. Gut 58:1546–1554

Parker LP, Taylor DD, Kesterson J, Metzinger DS, Gercel-Taylor C (2009) Modulation of microRNA associated with ovarian cancer cells by genistein. Eur J Gynaecol Oncol 30:616–621

Perez-Jimenez J, Fezeu L, Touvier M, Arnault N, Manach C, Hercberg S, Galan P, Scalbert A (2011) Dietary intake of 337 polyphenols in French adults. Am J Clin Nutr 93:1220–1228

Peter ME (2009) Let-7 and miR-200 microRNAs: guardians against pluripotency and cancer progression. Cell Cycle 8:843–852

Plass C, Soloway PD (2002) DNA methylation, imprinting and cancer. Eur J Hum Genet 10:6–16

Pledgie-Tracy A, Sobolewski MD, Davidson NE (2007) Sulforaphane induces cell type-specific apoptosis in human breast cancer cell lines. Mol Cancer Ther 6:1013–1021

Pogribny IP, Ross SA, Wise C, Pogribna M, Jones EA, Tryndyak VP, James SJ, Dragan YP, Poirier LA (2006) Irreversible global DNA hypomethylation as a key step in hepatocarcinogenesis induced by dietary methyl deficiency. Mutat Res 593:80–87

Poirier LA (1994) Methyl group deficiency in hepatocarcinogenesis. Drug Metab Rev 26:185–199

Prendergast GC, Ziff EB (1991) Methylation-sensitive sequence-specific DNA binding by the c-Myc basic region. Science 251:186–189

Qin W, Zhu W, Shi H, Hewett JE, Ruhlen RL, Macdonald RS, Rottinghaus GE, Chen YC, Sauter ER (2009) Soy isoflavones have an antiestrogenic effect and alter mammary promoter hypermethylation in healthy premenopausal women. Nutr Cancer 61:238–244

Quante M, Heeg S, von Werder A, Goessel G, Fulda C, Doebele M, Nakagawa H, Beijersbergen R, Blum HE, Opitz OG (2005) Differential transcriptional regulation of human telomerase in a cellular model representing important genetic alterations in esophageal squamous carcinogenesis. Carcinogenesis 26:1879–1889

Quideau S, Deffieux D, Douat-Casassus C, Pouységu L (2011) Plant polyphenols: chemical properties, biological activities, and synthesis. Angew Chem Int Ed 50:586–621

Rodriguez-Paredes M, Esteller M (2011) Cancer epigenetics reaches mainstream oncology. Nat Med 17:330–339

Ross SA (2003) Diet and DNA methylation interactions in cancer prevention. Ann N Y Acad Sci 983:197–207

Ruiz PA, Braune A, Holzlwimmer G, Quintanilla-Fend L, Haller D (2007) Quercetin inhibits TNF-induced NF-kappaB transcription factor recruitment to proinflammatory gene promoters in murine intestinal epithelial cells. J Nutr 137:1208–1215

Saito Y, Jones PA (2006) Epigenetic activation of tumor suppressor microRNAs in human cancer cells. Cell Cycle 5:2220–2222

Sato N, Maitra A, Fukushima N, van Heek NT, Matsubayashi H, Iacobuzio-Donahue CA, Rosty C, Goggins M (2003) Frequent hypomethylation of multiple genes overexpressed in pancreatic ductal adenocarcinoma. Cancer Res 63:4158–4166

Sbardella G, Castellano S, Vicidomini C, Rotili D, Nebbioso A, Miceli M, Altucci L, Mai A (2008) Identification of long chain alkylidenemalonates as novel small molecule modulators of histone acetyltransferases. Bioorg Med Chem Lett 18:2788–2792

Schwab M, Reynders V, Loitsch S, Steinhilber D, Schroder O, Stein J (2008) The dietary histone deacetylase inhibitor sulforaphane induces human beta-defensin-2 in intestinal epithelial cells. Immunology 125:241–251

Selvi BR, Pradhan SK, Shandilya J, Das C, Sailaja BS, Shankar GN, Gadad SS, Reddy A, Dasgupta D, Kundu TK (2009) Sanguinarine interacts with chromatin, modulates epigenetic modifications, and transcription in the context of chromatin. Chem Biol 16:203–216

Sheldon CC, Finnegan EJ, Rouse DT, Tadege M, Bagnall DJ, Helliwell CA, Peacock WJ, Dennis ES (2000a) The control of flowering by vernalization. Curr Opin Plant Biol 3:418–422

Sheldon CC, Rouse DT, Finnegan EJ, Peacock WJ, Dennis ES (2000b) The molecular basis of vernalization: the central role of Flowering Locus C (FLC). Proc Natl Acad Sci U S A 97:3753–3758

Shishodia S, Chaturvedi MM, Aggarwal BB (2007) Role of curcumin in cancer therapy. Curr Probl Cancer 31:243–305

Singh N, Misra K (2009) Computational screening of molecular targets in Plasmodium for novel non resistant anti-malarial drugs. Bioinformation 3:255–262

Singh UP, Singh NP, Singh B, Hofseth LJ, Price RL, Nagarkatti M, Nagarkatti PS (2010) Resveratrol (trans-3,5,4′-trihydroxystilbene) induces silent mating type information regulation-1 and down-regulates nuclear transcription factor-kappaB activation to abrogate dextran sulfate sodium-induced colitis. J Pharmacol Exp Ther 332:829–839

Souto JA, Conte M, Alvarez R, Nebbioso A, Carafa V, Altucci L, de Lera AR (2008) Synthesis of benzamides related to anacardic acid and their histone acetyltransferase (HAT) inhibitory activities. ChemMedChem 3:1435–1442

Stefanska B, Rudnicka K, Bednarek A, Fabianowska-Majewska K (2010) Hypomethylation and induction of retinoic acid receptor beta 2 by concurrent action of adenosine analogues and natural compounds in breast cancer cells. Eur J Pharmacol 638:47–53

Stresemann C, Brueckner B, Musch T, Stopper H, Lyko F (2006) Functional diversity of DNA methyltransferase inhibitors in human cancer cell lines. Cancer Res 66:2794–2800

Sun Y, Jiang X, Chen S, Price BD (2006) Inhibition of histone acetyltransferase activity by anacardic acid sensitizes tumor cells to ionizing radiation. FEBS Lett 580:4353–4356

Sun M, Estrov Z, Ji Y, Coombes KR, Harris DH, Kurzrock R (2008) Curcumin (diferuloylmethane) alters the expression profiles of microRNAs in human pancreatic cancer cells. Mol Cancer Ther 7:464–473

Sun Q, Cong R, Yan H, Gu H, Zeng Y, Liu N, Chen J, Wang B (2009) Genistein inhibits growth of human uveal melanoma cells and affects microRNA-27a and target gene expression. Oncol Rep 22:563–567

Sung B, Pandey MK, Ahn KS, Yi T, Chaturvedi MM, Liu M, Aggarwal BB (2008) Anacardic acid (6-nonadecyl salicylic acid), an inhibitor of histone acetyltransferase, suppresses expression of nuclear factor-kappaB-regulated gene products involved in cell survival, proliferation, invasion, and inflammation through inhibition of the inhibitory subunit of nuclear factor-kappaBalpha kinase, leading to potentiation of apoptosis. Blood 111:4880–4891

Surh YJ (2003) Cancer chemoprevention with dietary phytochemicals. Nat Rev Cancer 3:768–780

Suter M, Bocock P, Showalter L, Hu M, Shope C, McKnight R, Grove K, Lane R, Aagaard-Tillery K (2011) Epigenomics: maternal high-fat diet exposure in utero disrupts peripheral circadian gene expression in nonhuman primates. FASEB J 25:714–726

Suzuki MM, Bird A (2008) DNA methylation landscapes: provocative insights from epigenomics. Nat Rev Genet 9:465–476

Taberlay PC, Jones PA (2011) DNA methylation and cancer. Prog Drug Res 67:1–23

Tada M, Imazeki F, Fukai K, Sakamoto A, Arai M, Mikata R, Tokuhisa T, Yokosuka O (2007) Procaine inhibits the proliferation and DNA methylation in human hepatoma cells. Hepatol Int 1:355–364

Takaya J, Iharada A, Okihana H, Kaneko K (2011) Magnesium deficiency in pregnant rats alters methylation of specific cytosines in the hepatic hydroxysteroid dehydrogenase-2 promoter of the offspring. Epigenetics 6:573–578

Tang WY, Newbold R, Mardilovich K, Jefferson W, Cheng RY, Medvedovic M, Ho SM (2008) Persistent hypomethylation in the promoter of nucleosomal binding protein 1 (Nsbp1) correlates with overexpression of Nsbp1 in mouse uteri neonatally exposed to diethylstilbestrol or genistein. Endocrinology 149:5922–5931

Teodoridis JM, Strathdee G, Brown R (2004) Epigenetic silencing mediated by CpG island methylation: potential as a therapeutic target and as a biomarker. Drug Resist Updat 7:267–278

Tikoo K, Meena RL, Kabra DG, Gaikwad AB (2008) Change in post-translational modifications of histone H3, heat-shock protein-27 and map kinase p38 expression by curcumin in Streptozotocin-induced type I diabetic nephropathy. Br J Pharmacol 153:1225–1231

Traka M, Gasper AV, Smith JA, Hawkey CJ, Bao Y, Mithen RF (2005) Transcriptome analysis of human colon caco-2 cells exposed to sulforaphane. J Nutr 135:1865–1872

Tsang WP, Kwok TT (2010) Epigallocatechin gallate up-regulation of miR-16 and induction of apoptosis in human cancer cells. J Nutr Biochem 21:140–146

Tsao AS, Liu D, Martin J, Tang XM, Lee JJ, El-Naggar AK, Wistuba I, Culotta KS, Mao L, Gillenwater A, Sagesaka YM, Hong WK, Papadimitrakopoulou V (2009) Phase ii randomized, placebo-controlled trial of green tea extract in patients with high-risk oral premalignant lesions. Cancer Prev Res (Phila) 2:931–941

Ushijima T, Asada K (2010) Aberrant DNA methylation in contrast with mutations. Cancer Sci 101:300–305

Vardi A, Bosviel R, Rabiau N, Adjakly M, Satih S, Dechelotte P, Boiteux JP, Fontana L, Bignon YJ, Guy L, Bernard-Gallon DJ (2010) Soy phytoestrogens modify DNA methylation of GSTP1, RASSF1A, EPH2 and BRCA1 promoter in prostate cancer cells. In Vivo 24:393–400

Waldecker M, Kautenburger T, Daumann H, Busch C, Schrenk D (2008) Inhibition of histone-deacetylase activity by short-chain fatty acids and some polyphenol metabolites formed in the colon. J Nutr Biochem 19:587–593

Wang Z, Chen H (2010) Genistein increases gene expression by demethylation of WNT5a promoter in colon cancer cell line SW1116. Anticancer Res 30:4537–4545

Wang Y, Leung FC (2004) An evaluation of new criteria for CpG islands in the human genome as gene markers. Bioinformatics 20:1170–1177

Wang LG, Beklemisheva A, Liu XM, Ferrari AC, Feng J, Chiao JW (2007) Dual action on promoter demethylation and chromatin by an isothiocyanate restored GSTP1 silenced in prostate cancer. Mol Carcinog 46:24–31

Wang LG, Liu XM, Fang Y, Dai W, Chiao FB, Puccio GM, Feng J, Liu D, Chiao JW (2008a) De-repression of the p21 promoter in prostate cancer cells by an isothiocyanate via inhibition of HDACS and c-Myc. Int J Oncol 33:375–380

Wang RH, Sengupta K, Li C, Kim HS, Cao L, Xiao C, Kim S, Xu X, Zheng Y, Chilton B, Jia R, Zheng ZM, Appella E, Wang XW, Ried T, Deng CX (2008b) Impaired DNA damage response, genome instability, and tumorigenesis in SIRT1 mutant mice. Cancer Cell 14:312–323

Wang RH, Zheng Y, Kim HS, Xu X, Cao L, Luhasen T, Lee MH, Xiao C, Vassilopoulos A, Chen W, Gardner K, Man YG, Hung MC, Finkel T, Deng CX (2008c) Interplay among BRCA1, SIRT1, and survivin during BRCA1-associated tumorigenesis. Mol Cell 32:11–20

Wang Z, Zang C, Rosenfeld JA, Schones DE, Barski A, Cuddapah S, Cui K, Roh TY, Peng W, Zhang MQ, Zhao K (2008d) Combinatorial patterns of histone acetylations and methylations in the human genome. Nat Genet 40:897–903

Waterland RA (2003) Do maternal methyl supplements in mice affect DNA methylation of offspring? J Nutr 133:238, Author reply 239

Waterland RA, Jirtle RL (2003) Transposable elements: targets for early nutritional effects on epigenetic gene regulation. Mol Cell Biol 23:5293–5300

Weaver IC, Cervoni N, Champagne FA, D'Alessio AC, Sharma S, Seckl JR, Dymov S, Szyf M, Meaney MJ (2004a) Epigenetic programming by maternal behavior. Nat Neurosci 7:847–854

Weaver IC, Diorio J, Seckl JR, Szyf M, Meaney MJ (2004b) Early environmental regulation of hippocampal glucocorticoid receptor gene expression: characterization of intracellular mediators and potential genomic target sites. Ann N Y Acad Sci 1024:182–212

Weaver IC, Meaney MJ, Szyf M (2006) Maternal care effects on the hippocampal transcriptome and anxiety-mediated behaviors in the offspring that are reversible in adulthood. Proc Natl Acad Sci U S A 103:3480–3485

Wilkinson JT, Morse MA, Kresty LA, Stoner GD (1995) Effect of alkyl chain length on inhibition of N-nitrosomethylbenzylamine-induced esophageal tumorigenesis and DNA methylation by isothiocyanates. Carcinogenesis 16:1011–1015

Winter J, Diederichs S (2011) MicroRNA biogenesis and cancer. Method Mol Biol 676:3–22

Winter J, Jung S, Keller S, Gregory RI, Diederichs S (2009) Many roads to maturity: microRNA biogenesis pathways and their regulation. Nat Cell Biol 11:228–234

Wolff GL, Kodell RL, Moore SR, Cooney CA (1998) Maternal epigenetics and methyl supplements affect agouti gene expression in Avy/a mice. FASEB J 12:949–957

Yen TT, Gill AM, Frigeri LG, Barsh GS, Wolff GL (1994) Obesity, diabetes, and neoplasia in yellow A(vy)/- mice: ectopic expression of the agouti gene. FASEB J 8:479–488

Yoo CB, Jones PA (2006) Epigenetic therapy of cancer: past, present and future. Nat Rev Drug Discov 5:37–50

Yuasa Y, Nagasaki H, Akiyama Y, Sakai H, Nakajima T, Ohkura Y, Takizawa T, Koike M, Tani M, Iwai T, Sugihara K, Imai K, Nakachi K (2005) Relationship between CDX2 gene methylation and dietary factors in gastric cancer patients. Carcinogenesis 26:193–200

Yuasa Y, Nagasaki H, Akiyama Y, Hashimoto Y, Takizawa T, Kojima K, Kawano T, Sugihara K, Imai K, Nakachi K (2009) DNA methylation status is inversely correlated with green tea intake and physical activity in gastric cancer patients. Int J Cancer 124:2677–2682

Zhang Y, Ng HH, Erdjument-Bromage H, Tempst P, Bird A, Reinberg D (1999) Analysis of the NuRD subunits reveals a histone deacetylase core complex and a connection with DNA methylation. Genes Dev 13:1924–1935

Zhang J, Du Y, Wu C, Ren X, Ti X, Shi J, Zhao F, Yin H (2010) Curcumin promotes apoptosis in human lung adenocarcinoma cells through miR-186* signaling pathway. Oncol Rep 24:1217–1223

Zhao J, Huang WG, He J, Tan H, Liao QJ, Su Q (2006) Diallyl disulfide suppresses growth of HL-60 cell through increasing histone acetylation and p21WAF1 expression in vivo and in vitro. Acta Pharmacol Sin 27:1459–1466

Chapter 14
Western Diet-Induced Pancreatic Cancer

M. Mura Assifi and Guido Eibl

Contents

Abstract Major changes in our dietary patterns since the introduction of agriculture and more recently after the industrial revolution may underlie the development of many chronic diseases that plague human societies today. A lifestyle of increased energy consumption together with decreased energy expenditure is undoubtly the basis of the high prevalence of obesity in the Western Civilization. Diet-induced obesity is strongly associated with cardiovascular complications, type 2 diabetes, and cancer, including pancreatic cancer. The underlying mechanisms may include insulin-resistance with elevated circulating levels of insulin and other growth factors, e.g. insulin-like growth factor-1, and inflammation with increased levels of inflammatory cytokines and eicosanoids. Studies that unravel the mechanisms mediating and driving the tumor promoting effects of diet-induced obesity are clearly needed to halt the deleterious consequences of obesity on the development of pancreatic and other types of human cancers.

M.M. Assifi • G. Eibl (✉)
Department of Surgery, UCLA David Geffen School of Medicine, UCLA Center for Excellence in Pancreatic Diseases, Hirschberg Laboratory for Pancreatic Cancer Research, 675 Charles E. Young Drive South, MRL 2535, Los Angeles, CA 90095-7330, USA
e-mail: muraassifi@gmail.com; GEibl@mednet.ucla.edu

S. Shankar and R.K. Srivastava (eds.), *Nutrition, Diet and Cancer*,
DOI 10.1007/978-94-007-2923-0_14,

Evolution of the Human Diet: From Paleolithic Times to Present

In the Western world chronic disease plays a significant part in morbidity and mortality. These chronic illnesses are believed to be largely due to a loss of balance between genetic susceptibility and lifestyle factors such as nutrition, exercise, and exposure to toxic agents. Industrial era foods, including refined carbohydrates, saturated fats, and cereals have become the mainstay of diets in several developed nations. Such trends, once considered a luxury of the wealthy, are now being observed in all classes of society, along with the associated affect on human health.

The genome of hominoids has evolved over the past several million years. Compared with late Paleolithic hunter-gatherers, who lived approximately 35,000 years ago, our gene pool has undergone little change (Eaton et al. 1988), while our culture and environment have changed beyond recognition. The conflict between our late Paleolithic genome and current lifestyle factors is considered to form the basis for much of the human pathology observed today (Klein 1999; Wilson 1998). The similarities in our genome make the differences between late Paleolithic and modern diet increasingly relevant. In the late Paleolithic era, seasonal and climate effects contributed to regional variation in diet, and periods of abundance and shortage. Overall, the hunter-gatherer diet from centuries ago was high in protein and low in fat. Fruits, roots, and legumes accounted for 65–70% of the Paleolithic diet. The daily protein intake for hunter-gatherers from this century was 34%, with intake from the late Paleolithic era possibly even higher (Eaton and Konner 1985; Foley 1982). A significant benefit of their diet was the decreased fat content associated with game meat. The fat consumed was largely polyunsaturated, in contrast to the large saturated fat burden found in the Western diet. The amount of carbohydrate intake varied with the proportion of meat ingested but like the Western diet, accounted for 45–50% of their total energy intake (Colditz et al. 1995). However, vegetables and fruits contributed to most of the carbohydrate consumption two centuries ago, whereas current carbohydrate intake is mainly from refined sugars and cereal grains. Another notable feature in the pre-agricultural diet was the high fiber intake. Compared with the current daily energy intake in Western diets, fiber consumption was increased fivefold in the Paleolithic diet (Popkin et al. 2006).

With the introduction of agriculture and animal husbandry about 10,000 years ago, the lifestyle of late Paleolithic hunter-gatherers underwent significant change and advancement. There was no longer a need to expend great amounts of energy to procure nourishment, diminishing the inherent connection between food acquisition and physical activity (Eaton and Easton 2003). Furthermore, with the development of improved food preservation and storage, food became more readily available and the time span between meals was considerably shortened. Moreover, the agricultural and technological advancement in the last two centuries changed the quantity and types of foods available. The advent of food processing centers created new combinations of nutrients, producing high caloric, energy-dense foods that were not available to our Paleolithic ancestors (Cordain et al. 2005). Examples of these types of food include cereals, bagels, pizza, baked goods, soft drinks, and candy. Therefore, not only did the quantity of food increase in the post-agricultural diet, but there was a change in nutrient quality as well.

In contrast to the late Paleolithic diet, contemporary Westernized humans consume a diet low in protein, high in fat and carbohydrates, and low in fiber. In the standard American diet, only 12% of total dietary energy is from protein and 42% is from fat, double the amount found in the pre-agricultural diet (Popkin et al. 2006). Current recommendations call for 20–35% of total daily energy contribution from fat (Food and Nutrition Board 2002). Furthermore, 7–10% of the average American's daily energy intake comes from alcohol.

Today, dairy products, cereals, refined sugars, refined vegetable oils, and alcohol make up 72.1% of the total daily energy consumed in the United States population (Peto 2001). Ingestion of high caloric, energy-dense food may begin during infancy with the increased popularity of formula feeding (Malik et al. 2006). In addition, the use of high-fructose corn syrup as sweetener in soft drinks is growing as a new worldwide trend. Caloric sweetener consumption in beverages has been associated with increased weight gain in several studies (Josefson 2001). In the United States, caloric sweeteners account for greater than one third of all carbohydrates consumed (Popkin and Nielsen 2003).

The cultural changes that rapidly progressed after the Industrial Revolution had a profound impact on civilization in positive and negative ways. Efforts to improve housing, sanitation, and medical care resulted in a drop in infant mortality and increased life expectancy. Further developments in technology and health care led to extraordinary advances within society and were integral to the success of our species and quality of life. However, such extensive progress came with a price, and was accompanied by many chronic degenerative conditions, referred to as the "diseases of civilization" (Popkin et al. 2006).

Obesity Epidemiology and Implications

Since the Industrial Revolution $\sim$200 years ago, human consumption of protein has decreased while ingestion of fat has substantially increased. Concurrent advances in technology have afforded much of the population with a more sedentary lifestyle. As a result of these changes and other influences, there has been a dramatic increase in obesity over the last 20 years. In the United States, the prevalence of obesity increased from 15% to 33% among adults between 1980 and 2004 (Flegal et al. 2002; Ogden et al. 2006). According to the CDC in 2009, 33 states had an obesity prevalence greater than or equal to 25%, with nine of these states having a prevalence of greater or equal to 30% (Centers for Disease Control and Prevention 2010).

Body mass index (BMI), calculated as weight in kilograms divided by height in meters squared, is frequently used to define obesity. Healthy adults are classified as having a BMI of 18.5–24.9. Overweight individuals have a BMI of 25.0–29.9, and obese persons are defined as having a BMI equal to or greater than 30 (World Health Organization Expert Committee and World Health Organization 1995). BMI is frequently utilized in clinical situations to estimate body fat, even though it fails to distinguish between fat mass and lean mass. Despite this limitation, BMI is widely used and is a common reference point for comparison between studies. Other methods to define obesity include waist circumference, skinfold thickness, and bioimpedance, each with their own limitations to consider (Kopelman 2000).

Analysis of height and weight measurements from the National Health and Nutrition Examination Survey (NHANES), a national representation of the United States population, demonstrate an increase in prevalence of adult obesity since 1980. After a relatively stable period from 1960 to 1980, the prevalence of obesity was noted to increase 8% points between 1988 and 1994 (Flegal et al. 1998; Kuczmarski et al. 1994). Further analysis of data from 1999 to 2000 demonstrated a continued increase in obesity in both men and women (Eaton et al. 1988). The most recent analysis examining data from 1999–2000 to 2008–2009 showed an increase of 4.7% points (95% CI 0.5–9.0) in men and an increase of 2.1% points (95% CI −2.1 to 6.3) for women (Flegal et al. 2010). Although the prevalence of obesity remains high at 33.8% (95% CI 31.6–36%) overall, the increase in obesity does not appear to be continuing at the same rate as observed in the past.

Several factors have contributed to the rise of overweight and obesity. Predisposition for weight gain is influenced by genes, although the extent is unclear. For instance, the activity level of the satiety center found in the hypothalamus is genetically predetermined (Swaab et al. 1995), as are the relative amounts of hormones, like ghrelin, that are known to stimulate appetite (Moran et al. 2004). Furthermore, leptin, a hormone associated with body weight and food intake, is produced by adipocytes in various quantities, but its complex role in fat metabolism is being further investigated (Maffei et al. 1995). Rather than genes alone, the interactions between genes and environment are more likely to promote the development of obesity. The observation that overweight and obesity run in families can be better attributed to learned lifestyle behaviors and environmental factors instead of pure genetics.

Excessive weight gain is largely influenced by energy intake and energy expenditure. Current trends in the diet of the developing world are shifting to high caloric, energy dense foods and high energy beverages (Popkin 2006; Popkin et al. 2006). These diets consist of foods containing high saturated fats, usually in the form of edible oil, with lower protein and fiber and refined carbohydrates. Changes like these taken together with decreased physical activity provide a ready environment for the development of obesity. Physical activity accounts for 20–50% of all energy expenditure, and has been inversely associated with obesity in several developed countries. In fact, children in the United States have an approximate fivefold increased relative risk of obesity if they watch greater than 5 h of television daily compared with those children who watch less than 2 h per day (Gortmaker et al. 1996).

Overweight and obesity affect physiological function in several ways, facilitating the development of many medical problems. Excess body fat, especially when concentrated in the truncal region, is associated with insulin resistance, type 2 diabetes mellitus, and cardiovascular mortality (Foley 1982; American Diabetes Association 1994). The Nurses Cohort Study found that when compared to women with a BMI of less than 21, the risk of diabetes increased fivefold for women with a BMI of 25, and 93-fold in women with a BMI of 35 or greater (Colditz et al. 1995). Furthermore, the Framingham Heart Study found that obesity was an independent risk factor for congestive heart failure (Hubert et al. 1983; Hubert 1986). In the same study, the risk of death was increased by 1% for each pound gained between age 30 and 42 years of age, and further increased up to 2% in those ages 50–62 years.

Aside from a few known high-risk cancer causing foods, like alcohol consumption and aflatoxin, there is no single dietary factor that has clearly been identified as a carcinogen (Peto 2001). However, several studies have recently drawn attention to the link between cancer and obesity (Josefson 2001). In 2002, the International Agency for Research on Cancer (IARC) reported that the percentages of cancer attributed to obesity were 11% for colon cancer, 9% for postmenopausal breast cancer, 39% for endometrial cancer, and 37% for esophageal cancer (Vainio and Bianchini 2002). In addition, a landmark study by Calle et al. concluded that approximately 10% of all cancer deaths among non-smokers in the United States were secondary to being overweight (Calle et al. 2003).

In summary, there has been a striking increase in obesity over the past 20 years in the United States, and approximately one-third of the world's population is currently considered to be overweight or obese. Obesity is a complex disease process influenced by diet, genes, and environmental factors, and is linked to several diet-related diseases, including cancer. There are several proposed mechanisms to explain the relationship between diet and carcinogenesis, but much is still unknown. The greatest challenge lies in using the established data to implement broader strategies for the prevention of diet-related disease.

Pancreatic Cancer: Incidence and Risk Factors

In 2010, 43,140 individuals were diagnosed with pancreatic cancer in the United States, with an estimated 36,800 deaths (Jemal et al. 2010), making pancreatic cancer the fourth leading cause of cancer death nationally. Pancreatic cancer accounts for roughly 2.5% of all cancers diagnosed globally (Ferlay et al. 2010), and is the eighth or ninth most frequent cause of cancer mortality worldwide (Maisonneuve and Lowenfels 2010).

The global distribution of pancreatic cancer seems to vary with latitude. In both men and women, rates are increased threefold in northern countries when compared to those that are closer to the equator (Ferlay et al. 2008). In the United States, approximately 80% of cases occur in patients 60–80 years of age, with a median age at diagnosis of 72 years (Raimondi et al. 2007). Pancreatic cancer occurs more frequently in men than women and is more common in black populations when compared to white populations.

Several risk factors have been identified that increase the incidence and development of pancreatic cancer. Except for nitrosamines, no definitive link has been demonstrated between diet and pancreatic cancer (Zheng and Lee 2009). However, several studies have found high caloric intake and obesity to be strong risk factors (Michaud et al. 2001; Reeves et al. 2007; Berrington de Gonzalez et al. 2003). In a pooled analysis from 13 prospective cohort studies from the PANSCAN consortium, obesity was associated with a 20% increased risk of pancreatic cancer development (Arslan et al. 2010). Furthermore, studies found that a larger waist-to-hip ratio and waist circumference were both significantly related to pancreatic cancer incidence (Arslan et al. 2010; Larsson et al. 2005).

Exposure to noxious substances has also been shown to increase the risk for pancreatic neoplasms. The risk from cigarette smoking is as high as 70–100% for pancreatic cancer, and does not return to baseline until at least 10 years after cessation (Iodice et al. 2008). Alcohol, a known risk factor for liver and esophageal malignancies, has also been linked to pancreatic tumors. A recent meta-analysis identified heavy alcohol consumption (three or more drinks per day) to be associated with a 22% increased risk of pancreatic cancer development (Tramacere et al. 2010).

Pancreatic cancer risk has been related to several benign medical conditions as well, most notably seen in chronic pancreatitis and diabetes mellitus. Patients with chronic pancreatitis in a large retrospective cohort study were found to have a 14-fold increased risk of pancreatic cancer (Lowenfels et al. 1993). This association is dramatically strengthened in patients with autosomal dominant hereditary pancreatitis, a rare condition arising during childhood. In this patient population, the risk is roughly 70% greater, with a lifetime risk of 40–55% (Malka et al. 2002).

Diabetes mellitus has been linked to pancreatic cancer in several studies, but it is unclear if diabetes is a risk factor for cancer development or a manifestation of cancer pathology. Both type 1 and 2 diabetes pose an elevated risk for pancreatic cancer. But patients with chronic ($\geq$10 years) type 2 diabetes have up to a 50% increased risk (Everhart and Wright 1995; Huxley et al. 2005). Furthermore, unexpected diabetes onset has been reported as an early symptom of pancreatic cancer in approximately one-third of all patients (Chari et al. 2008).

Pancreatic cancer has historically been associated with poor outcomes. Ductal adenocarcinoma and its variants comprise 80–90% of all pancreatic neoplasms, and are associated with an overall survival of less than 5%. Approximately 70% of ductal cancers arise within the pancreatic head or uncinate process. At the time of diagnosis, ductal cancers measure roughly 3 cm in diameter and are frequently associated with lymph node and vessel involvement. About 40% of people have metastatic disease when first diagnosed (Bradley 2008).

Surgical resection remains the mainstay of treatment for pancreatic cancer, and holds the only possibility for cure. Preoperative staging with CT scans or MRI is a widely used method to determine tumor resectability. Circumferential encasement, invasion or occlusion of the portal vein, superior mesenteric vein, or superior mesenteric artery are ominous signs and are generally considered to be associated with unresectable lesions. Management of patients with metastatic disease or unresectable tumors is limited to treatment with chemotherapy. Patients with resectable disease, however, undergo surgical resection. For lesions in the head of the pancreas and uncinate process, pancreaticoduodenectomy, commonly known as a Whipple procedure, is performed. For tumors in the body and tail of the pancreas a distal pancreatectomy, with or without splenectomy, is done.

Median survival for patients with advanced disease ranges from 8 to 12 months. In contrast, patients undergoing pancreaticoduodenectomy have a 5-year survival of 25–35% (Yeo et al. 1995; Kazanjian et al. 2008). Despite the vast technical progress made in the surgical management of pancreatic cancer over the past 60 years, the overall survival of the disease remains low.

The aggressive nature attributed to pancreatic cancer is associated with genetic mutations in oncogenes, tumor suppressor genes, and excessive expression of growth factors and their receptors (McCormick and Lemoine 1998). Mutations of the K-*ras* oncogene are found in most pancreatic cancers and precursor lesions. K-*ras* plays a key role in regulating growth, resulting in permanent activation and continuous cell growth when mutated. *p53*, a tumor suppressor gene, is mutated in approximately 75% of all pancreatic neoplasms, interfering with DNA synthesis and repair, cell proliferation, and apoptosis (Michaud et al. 2001). The epidermal growth factor receptor (EGFR) family has been found to be upregulated in pancreatic cancer, which correlates with tumor angiogenesis, invasiveness, and poorer prognosis.

In addition, pancreatic ductal cancer is now thought to progress in a stepwise fashion, similar to colon cancer. Progression from histologically normal ductal epithelium to low and high-grade pancreatic intraepithelial neoplasia (PanIN) lesions are associated with specific genetic mutations. K-*ras* mutations and *HER2*/neu overexpression are the earliest changes observed, with inactivation of *p53* and *DPC4* occurring in the later stages of disease progression (Wilentz et al. 2000).

Western Diet and Pancreatic Cancer

There is growing evidence linking the rise of obesity worldwide to cancer development. In the United States, more than 85,000 new cancer cases annually are related to obesity (Engquist and Chang 2011). In fact, recent study demonstrated that as BMI increases by 5 kg/m^2, cancer mortality rises by 10% (Prospective Studies Collaboration 2009). Calle et al. showed that among a cohort of 900,000 adults in the United States between 1982 and 1998, there was a stepwise progression of risk between obesity and all cancers (Popkin 2006). Compared to women with a BMI less than 25, the risk of cancer development was 8% higher in women with a BMI 25–29.9, 18% increased for BMI 30–34.9, 32% higher for BMI 35–39.9, and 62% higher for BMI greater or equal to 40. Men with a BMI $\geq$35 had a 2.61 relative risk of death from pancreatic cancer when compared to men with a BMI 18.5–24.9. Women with a BMI $\geq$40 had a 2.76 relative risk of death from pancreatic cancer (Popkin 2006).

Although the correlation between obesity and cancer initiation and promotion is well accepted, the underlying mechanisms are still debated and need to be explored in more detail. Obesity in general is considered to induce a systemic, sub-clinical inflammatory state with an increase in circulating and tissue levels of pro-inflammatory mediators. Several mechanisms have been proposed and tested to explain the relationship between obesity and cancer, including pancreatic cancer. Currently, extensive research has focused on the potential link between adipokines and cancer risk (van Kruijsdijk et al. 2009). Adipokines, hormones produced by adipose tissue, include leptin, adiponectin, resistin, and visfatin. In the non-obese state, leptin acts on the hypothalamus to decrease appetite and increase energy expenditure. In obesity, high levels of circulating leptin have been identified, suggesting leptin resistance (Hursting et al. 2003). Colon, prostate, and breast cancers have been associated with increased serum leptin levels (Birmingham et al. 2009), while adiponectin has been found to be negatively associated with endometrial, breast, colon, and prostate cancers (Hursting and Berger 2010). In addition, adiponectin has been shown to inhibit tumor growth and angiogenesis in animal models (Brakenhielm et al. 2004). The relationship of resistin and visfatin with cancer development are less defined at this time. A recent study investigating fatless A-Zip/F-1 mice, which have no circulating levels of adipokines, found these mice to demonstrate accelerated tumor formation, suggesting that adipokines were not necessary for tumorigenesis (Nunez et al. 2006). Although these mice lack white adipose tissue, the A-Zip/F-1 mice are diabetic with high serum levels of insulin, insulin-like growth factor (IGF-1), and pro-inflammatory cytokines. It has been suggested that these pro-inflammatory agents and the associated carcinogenesis-linked signaling pathways may play a larger role in the development of cancer, even in the absence of adipose tissue.

There is great interest in studying the role of IGF-1 in diet-induced cancer development. Obesity is a known risk factor for type II diabetes which is characterized by insulin resistance and increased levels of insulin and IGF-1. IGF-1 acts directly on cells through the IGF-1 receptor, which is highly expressed in several tumors (Hursting et al. 2003). Elevated levels of IGF-1 have been associated with increased risk of breast and prostate cancer (Rowlands et al. 2009; The Endogenous Hormones and Breast Cancer Collaborative Group 2010). In a recent study, men greater than 50 years of age had a significantly increased risk of cancer death associated with elevated IGF-1 levels after adjusting for age, adiposity, exercise, and smoking status (Major et al. 2010). However, a reduction in IGF-1 levels has been shown to contribute to the anti-proliferative, pro-apoptotic effects of calorie restriction (Hursting et al. 2003). Insulin and IGF-1 signal downstream mainly through the phosphatidylinositol 3-kinase (PI3K)/Akt pathway regulating cell proliferation and metabolism by integrating the extracellular signals with the intracellular environment (Luo et al. 2003). Constitutive activation of the PI3K/Akt pathway has been shown to occur in pancreatic cancers despite the lack of common genetic mutations in the upstream elements of this pathway. Activation of the PI3K/Akt pathway in pancreatic cancer is increasingly believed to be maintained by high levels of insulin and IGF-1 within the pancreatic micro-environment.

Obesity and cancer development have also been linked to chronic inflammation. Calorie restriction or physical activity has been shown to decrease the circulating levels of some pro-inflammatory cytokines and decrease cancer risk (Mai et al. 2003). In addition, the nuclear factor-kappa B (NF-kappaB) pathway, which increases cytokine production and promotes inflammation, has been shown to contribute to tumorigenesis in colon cancer in an in vivo study but has not been thoroughly investigated (Greten et al. 2004).

Conclusions and Recommendations

It is beyond doubt that the human diet changed significantly and profoundly since the dawn of agriculture and more recently after the industrial revolution. New food processing technologies, availability of new and calorie-denser food items, together with definite lifestyle changes are believed to be the root of many chronic diseases that plague the Western Civilization. Obesity imposes an incredible health and socioeconomic burden on our society. Strong evidence today exists that links obesity to cancer development, including pancreatic cancer, although the exact operative pathways and processes are still poorly understood and are just beginning to be explored in sufficient detail. The central role of the exocrine and endocrine pancreas within the digestive system, collecting numerous inputs and processing them to regulate various mechanisms, makes it – at least putatively – very sensitive to various changes in food intake and composition. To dissect the mechanisms that underlie diet-driven cancer development in the pancreas – and other organs – and to formulate, test, and ultimately implement efficacious preventive interventions are a challenge for years to come. However, we as the scientific community must face these challenges to understand the impact of the altered dietary environment we live in and to divert the path that otherwise lies ahead of us.

References

American Diabetes Association (1994) Nutrition recommendations and principles for people with diabetes mellitus. Diabetes Care 17(5):519–522

Arslan AA, Helzlsouer KJ, Kooperberg C, Shu XO et al (2010) Pancreatic cancer cohort consortium (PanScan): anthropometric measures, body mass, index, and pancreatic cancer: a pooled analysis from the pancreatic cancer cohort consortium (PanScan). Arch Intern Med 170(9):791–802

Berrington de Gonzalez A, Sweetland S, Spencer E (2003) A meta-analysis of obesity and the risk of pancreatic cancer. Br J Cancer 89(3):519–523

Birmingham JM, Busik JV, Hansen-Smith FM, Fenton JI (2009) Novel mechanism for obesity-induced colon cancer progression. Carcinogenesis 30(4):690–697

Bradley EL (2008) Long-term survival after pancreatoduodenectomy for ductal adenocarcinoma: the emperor has no clothes? Pancreas 37(4):349–351

Brakenhielm E, Veitonmaki N, Cao R, Kihara S et al (2004) Adiponectin-induced antiangiogenesis and antitumor activity involve caspase-mediated endothelial cell apoptosis. Proc Natl Acad Sci U S A 101(8):2476–2481

Calle EE, Rodriguez C, Walker-Thurmond K, Thun MJ (2003) Overweight, obesity, and mortality from cancer in a prospectively studied cohort of U.S. adults. N Engl J Med 348(17):1625–1638

Centers for Disease Control and Prevention (2010) Overweight and obesity, U.S. obesity trends 1985–2009. http://www.cdc.gov/obesity/data/trends.html

Chari ST, Leibson CL, Rabe KG, Timmons LJ et al (2008) Pancreatic cancer-associated diabetes mellitus: prevalence and temporal association with diagnosis of cancer. Gastroenterology 134(1):95–101

Colditz GA, Willet WC, Rotnisky A, Manson JE (1995) Weight gain as a risk factor for clinical diabetes in women. Arch Int Med 122(7):481–486

Cordain L, Eaton SB, Sebastian A, Mann N et al (2005) Origins and evolution of the Western diet: health implications for the 21st century. Am J Clin Nutr 81(2):341–354

Eaton SB, Easton SB (2003) An evolutionary perspective on human physical activity: implications for health. Comp Biochem Physiol A Mol Integr Physiol 136(1):153–159

Eaton SB, Konner MJ (1985) Paleolithic nutrition. A consideration of its nature and current implications. N Eng J Med 312(3):283–289

Eaton SB, Konner M, Shostak M (1988) Stone agers in the fast lane: chronic degenerative diseases in evolutionary perspective. Am J Med 84(4):739–749

Engquist KB, Chang M (2011) Obesity and cancer risk: recent review and evidence. Curr Oncol Rep 13(1):71–76

Everhart J, Wright D (1995) Diabetes mellitus as a risk factor for pancreatic cancer. A meta-analysis. JAMA 273(20):1605–1609

Ferlay J, Shin HR, Bray F, Forman D et al (2008) GLOBOCAN 2008, Cancer incidence and mortality worldwide: IARC Cancer Base No 10. Lyon, International Agency for Research on Cancer, 2010. http://globocan.iarc.fr

Ferlay J, Shin HR, Bray F, Forman D et al (2010) Estimates of worldwide burden of cancer in 2008: GLOBOCAN 2008. Int J Cancer 127(12):2893–2917

Flegal KM, Carroll MD, Kuczmarski RJ, Johnson CL (1998) Overweight and obesity in the United States: prevalence and trends, 1960–1994. Int J Obes Relat Metab Disord 22(1):339–347

Flegal KM, Carroll MD, Cl O, Johnson CL (2002) Prevalence and trends in obesity among US adults, 1999–2000. JAMA 288(14):1723–1727

Flegal KM, Carroll MD, Ogden CL, Curtin LR (2010) Prevalence and trends in obesity among US adults, 1999–2008. JAMA 303(3):235–241

Foley R (1982) A reconsideration of the role of predation on large mammals in tropical hunter-gatherer adaptation. Man 17(3):393–402

Food and Nutrition Board (2002) Dietary reference intakes for energy, carbohydrate, fiber, fat, fatty acids, cholesterol, protein, and amino acids (macronutrients). National Academic Press, Washington, DC

Gortmaker SL, Must A, Sobal AM, Peterson K et al (1996) Television viewing as a cause of increasing obesity among children in the United States, 1986–1990. Arch Pediatr Adolesc Med 150(4):356–362

Greten FR, Eckmann L, Greten TF, Park JM et al (2004) IKK [beta] links inflammation and tumorigenesis in a mouse model of colitis-associated cancer. Cell 118(3):285–296

Hubert HB (1986) The importance of obesity in the development of coronary risk factors and disease: the epidemiological evidence. Annu Rev Public Health 7:493–502

Hubert HB, Feinleib M, McNamara PM, Castelli WP (1983) Obesity as an independent risk factor for cardiovascular disease: a 26-year follow-up of participants in the Framingham Heart Study. Circulation 67(5):968–977

Hursting SD, Berger NA (2010) Energy balance, host-related factors, and cancer progression. J Clin Oncol 28(26):4058–4065

Hursting SD, Lavigne JA, Berrigan D, Perkins SN et al (2003) Calorie restriction, aging, and cancer prevention: mechanisms of action and applicability to humans. Annu Rev Med 54:131–152

Huxley R, Ansary-Moghaddam A, Berrington de Gonzalez A, Barzi F et al (2005) Type II diabetes and pancreatic cancer: a meta-analysis of 36 studies. Br J Cancer 92(11):2076–2083

Iodice S, Gandini S, Maisonneuve P, Lowenfels AB (2008) Tobacco and the risk of pancreatic cancer: a review and meta-analysis. Arch Surg 393(4):535–545

Jemal A, Siegel R, Xu J, Ward E (2010) Cancer statistics, 2010. CA Cancer J Clin 60(5):277–300

Josefson D (2001) Obesity and inactivity fuel global cancer epidemic. Br Med J 322(7292):945

Kazanjian KK, Hines OJ, Duffy JP, Yoon DY et al (2008) Improved survival following pancreaticoduodenectomy to treat adenocarcinoma of the pancreas: the influence of operative blood loss. Arch Surg 143(12):116–171

Klein RG (1999) The human career. Human biological and cultural origins. University of Chicago Press, Chicago. ISBN 0-226-43963-I

Kopelman PG (2000) Obesity as a medical problem. Nature 404(6778):635–643

Kuczmarski RJ, Flegal KM, Campbell SM, Johnson CL (1994) Increasing prevalence of overweight among US adults: the National Health and Nutrition Examination Surveys, 1960 to 1991. JAMA 272(3):205–211

Larsson SC, Permert J, Hakansson N, Naslund I et al (2005) Overall obesity, abdominal adiposity, diabetes and cigarette smoking in relation to the risk of pancreatic cancer in two Swedish population-based cohorts. Br J Cancer 93(11):1310–1315

Lowenfels AB, Maisonneuve P, Cavallini G, Ammann RW et al (1993) Pancreatitis and the risk of pancreatic cancer. International Pancreatitis Study Group. N Engl J Med 328(20):1433–1437

Luo J, Manningn BD, Cantley LC (2003) Targeting the PI3K-Akt pathway in human cancer: rationale and promise. Cancer Cell 4(4):257–262

Maffei M, Halaas J, Ravussin E, Pratley RE (1995) Leptin levels in human and rodent: measurement of plasma leptin and ob RNA in obese and weight-reduced subjects. Nat Med 1(11):1155–1161

Mai V, Colbert L, Berrigan D, Perkins SN et al (2003) Calorie restriction and diet composition modulate spontaneous intestinal tumorigenesis in Apc-min mice through different mechanisms. Cancer Res 63(8):1752–1755

Maisonneuve P, Lowenfels AB (2010) Epidemiology of pancreatic cancer: an update. Dig Dis 28(4–5):645–656

Major JM, Stolzenberg-Solomon RZ, Pollak MN, Snyder K et al (2010) Insulin-like growth factors and liver cancer risk in male smokers. Br J Cancer 103(7):1089–1092

Malik VS, Schulze MB, Hu FB (2006) Intake of sugar-sweetened beverages and weight gain: a systematic review. Am J Clin Nutr 84(2):274–288

Malka D, Hammel P, Maire F, Rufat P et al (2002) Risk of pancreatic adenocarcinoma in chronic pancreatitis. Gut 51(6):849–852

McCormick CSF, Lemoine NR (1998) Molecular biological events in the development of pancreatic cancer. In: Beger HG, Warshaw AL, Buchler MW et al (eds) The pancreas. Blackwell Science, Oxford, pp 907–921

Michaud DS, Giovannucci E, Willett WC, Colditz GA et al (2001) Physical activity, obesity, height, and the risk of pancreatic cancer. JAMA 286(8):921–929

Moran LF, Noakes M, Clifton PM, Wittert GA et al (2004) Ghrelin and measures of satiety are altered in polycystic ovary syndrome but not differentially affected by diet composition. J Clin Endocrinol Metab 89(7):3337–3344

Nunez NP, Oh WJ, Rozenberg J, Perella C et al (2006) Accelerated tumor formation in a fatless mouse with type 2 diabetes and inflammation. Cancer Res 66(10):5469–5476

Ogden CL, Carroll MD, Curtin LR, McDowell MA et al (2006) Prevalence of overweight and obesity in the United States, 1999–2004. JAMA 295(13):1549–1555

Peto J (2001) Cancer epidemiology in the last century and the next decade. Nature 411(6835):390–395

Popkin BM (2006) Global nutrition dynamics: the world is shifting rapidly toward a diet linked with noncommunicable diseases. Am J Clin Nutr 84(2):289–298

Popkin BM, Nielsen SJ (2003) The sweetening of the world's diet. Obes Res 11(11):1325–1332

Popkin BM, Kim S, Rusev ER, Du S et al (2006) Measuring the full economic costs of diet, physical activity and obesity-related chronic diseases. Obes Rev 7(3):271–293
Prospective Studies Collaboration (2009) Body-mass index and cause-specific mortality in 900,000 adults: a collaborative analysis of 57 prospective studies. Lancet 373(9669):1083–1096
Raimondi S, Maisonneuve P, Lohr JM, Lowenfels AB (2007) Early onset pancreatic cancer: evidence of a major role for smoking and genetic factors. Cancer Epidemiol Biomarkers Prev 16(9):1894–1897
Reeves GK, Pirie K, Beral V, Green J et al (2007) Cancer incidence and mortality in relation to body mass index in the million women study: cohort study. BMJ 335(7630):1134
Rowlands MA, Gunnell D, Harris R, Vatten LJ et al (2009) Circulating insulin-like growth factor peptides and prostate cancer risk: a systemic review and meta-analysis. Int J Cancer 124(10):2416–2429
Swaab DF, Purba JS, Hofman MA (1995) Alterations in the hypothalamic paraventricular nucleus and its oxytocin neurons (putative satiety cells) in Prader-Willi syndrome: a study of five cases. J Clin Endocrinol Metab 80(2):573–579
The Endogenous Hormones and Breast Cancer Collaborative Group (2010) Insulin-like growth factor 1 (IGF1), IGF binding protein 3 (IGFBP3), and breast cancer risk: pooled individual data analysis of 17 prospective studies. Lancet Oncol 11(6):530–542
Tramacere I, Scotti L, Jenab M, Bagnardi V et al (2010) Alcohol drinking and pancreatic cancer risk: a meta-analysis of the dose-relation risk. Int J Cancer 126(6):1474–1486
Vainio H, Bianchini F (2002) IARC handbooks of cancer prevention – weight control and physical activity. Oxford University Press, New York. ISBN 92-832-3006-X
van Kruijsdijk RC, van der Wall E, Visseren FL (2009) Obesity and cancer: the role of dysfunctional adipose tissue. Cancer Epidemiol Biomarkers Prev 18(10):2569–2578
Wilentz RE, Iacobuzio-Donahue CA, Argani P, McCarthy DM et al (2000) Loss of expression of DPC4 in pancreatic intraepithelial neoplasia: evidence that DPC4 inactivation occurs late in neoplastic progression. Cancer Res 60(7):2002–2006
Wilson EO (1998) Consilience. The unity of science. Knopf, New York. ISBN 0-679-45077-7
World Health Organization Expert Committee, World Health Organization, Geneva (1995) Physical status: the use and interpretation of anthropometry. WHO technical report series no. 854.
Yeo CJ, Cameron JL, Lillemoe KD, Sitzmann JV et al (1995) Pancreaticoduodenectomy for cancer of the head of the pancreas: 201 patients. Ann Surg 221(6):721–733
Zheng W, Lee SA (2009) Well-done meat intake, heterocyclic amine exposure, and cancer risk. Nutr Cancer 61(4):437–446

Chapter 15
Intracellular Signaling Network as a Prime Chemotherapy Target of Green Tea Catechin, (–)-Epigallocatechin-3-gallate

Brahma N. Singh, Sharmila Shankar, and Rakesh K. Srivastava

Contents

Abstract Chemoprevention is an attempt to use either naturally occurring or synthetic substances or their mixtures to intervene in the progress of carcinogenesis. Recently, it has been shown that green tea phytochemicals alter gene

B.N. Singh • R.K. Srivastava (✉)
Department of Pharmacology, Toxicology and Therapeutics, and Medicine,
The University of Kansas Cancer Center, The University of Kansas Medical Center,
3901 Rainbow Boulevard, Kansas City, KS 66160, USA
e-mail: bsingh@kumc.edu; rsrivastava@kumc.edu

S. Shankar
Department of Pathology and Laboratory Medicine, The University of Kansas Cancer Center, The University of Kansas Medical Center, 3901 Rainbow Boulevard, Kansas City, KS 66160, USA
e-mail: sshankar@kumc.edu

S. Shankar and R.K. Srivastava (eds.), *Nutrition, Diet and Cancer*,
DOI 10.1007/978-94-007-2923-0_15,

expression, directly or indirectly, thereby regulating the carcinogenic processes. Epigallocatechin-3-gallate (EGCG), the major antioxidant polyphenolic compound present in green tea, is a promising chemopreventive agent. EGCG has been shown to exert growth-inhibitory potential of various cancer cells in culture and antitumor activity *in vivo* models. EGCG could interact with various molecules like proteins, transcription factors, and enzymes, which block multiple stages of carcinogenesis. Moreover, much of the cancer chemopreventive effects of EGCG that regulates cell proliferation and apoptosis effects by altering the expression of cell cycle regulatory proteins, activating killer caspases, induction of phase II enzymes, mediation of anti-oxidative, anti-inflammation responses, and suppressing oncogenic transcription factors and pluripotency maintain factors. *In vitro* and *in vivo* studies have demonstrated that EGCG blocks carcinogenesis by affecting a wide array of signal transduction pathways involved in cell proliferation, transformation, inflammation, apoptosis, metastasis and invasion. EGCG stimulates telomere fragmentation through inhibiting telomerase activity. Recent reports demonstrated that EGCG inhibits DNA methyltransferases, proteases, and dihydrofolate reductase activities, which would affect transcription of tumor suppressor genes and protein synthesis. To develop EGCG as an anticarcinogenic agent, more clear understanding of the cell signaling pathways and the molecular targets responsible for chemopreventive and chemotherapeutic effects are needed. This review summarizes recent preclinical and clinical research on the EGCG-induced cellular signal transduction events which implicate in prevention and therapy of cancer.

Abbreviations

α-TNF	Alpha-tumor necrosis factor
AMPK	Adenosine monophosphate-activated protein kinase
AP1	Activator protein 1
AREs	Antioxidant responsive elements
Bcl-2	B-cell lymphoma-2
CAT	Catalase
CDKN2A	Cyclin dependent kinase 2A
Cdks	Cyclin-dependent kinases
c-IAP1	Cellular inhibitor of apoptosis protein1
COX-2	Cyclooxygenase-2
CpG	Cytosine-phosphate-guanine
CSCs	Cancer stem cells
CYP	Cytochrome P450
DHFR	Dihydrofolate reductase
DIABLO	Direct inhibitor of apoptosis-binding protein with low pI
DNMTs	DNA methyltransferases
EGCG	(-)-Epigallocatechin-3-gallate
EGFR	Epidermal growth factor receptor

EpRE	Electrophile-responsive element
ERK	Extracellular signal-regulated kinase
FAK	Focal adhesion kinase
FKHR	Forkhead homolog of rhabdosarcoma
GFRs	Growth factor receptors
GPx	Glutathione peroxidase
GR	Glutathione reductase
GST	Glutathione *S*-transferase
H_2O_2	Hydrogen peroxide
HATs	Histone acetyl transferases
HDACs	Histone deacetylases
HER	Human epidermal receptor
HIF	Hypoxia inducible factor
hTERT	human telomerase reverse transcriptase
HUVEC	Human vascular endothelial cell
IKK	I kappa B kinase
IL-1	Interleukin 1
JNK	Jun NH_2-terminal kinase
LPs	Lipopolysaccharides
MAP	Mitogen-activated protein
MBD	Methyl-CpG binding domain
Mcl-1	Myeloid cell leukemia 1
mdm2	mouse double minute 2
MEKK1	Mitogen-activated protein/ERK kinase 1
MLH1	MutL homologue 1
MMPs	Matrix metalloproteinases
MRLC	Myosin regulatory light chain
MT1-MMP	Membrane Type 1-matrix metalloproteinase
NFκB	Nuclear factor kappaB
NQO	NADPH quinone oxidoreductase
Nrf	NF-E2 p45-related factor
$O_2^{\bullet -}$	Superoxide anion radical
$^{\bullet}OH$	Hydroxyl radical
p90RSK	90 kDa ribosomal S6 kinase
PCNA	Proliferating cell nuclear antigen
PDGF	Platelet-derived growth factor
PGE2	Prostaglandins E2
PI3K	Phosphatidylinositol- 3-kinase
PKA	Protein kinase A
PPAR	Peroxisome proliferator-activated receptor
pRb	Retinoblastoma protein
PUMA	P53 upregulated modulator of apoptosis
RAR	Retinoic acid receptor
RECK	Reversion-inducing cysteine-rich protein with Kazal motifs
RTK	Receptor tyrosine kinase

RXRα	Retinoid X receptor alpha
SAM	*S*-adenosyl-methionine
siRNA	Small-interfering RNA
Smac	Second mitochondria-derived activator of caspase
SOD	Superoxide dismutase
STAT	Signal transducers and activators of transcription
TERT	Telomerase reverse transcriptase
TIMP	Tissue inhibitor of metalloproteinase
TRAIL	Tumor necrosis factor-related apoptosis-inducing ligand
TRAMP	Transgenic adenocarcinoma of the mouse prostate
TSGs	Tumor suppressor genes
uPA	Urokinase plasminogen activator
VEGF	Vascular endothelial growth factor
XIAP	X-linked inhibitor of apoptosis protein

Introduction

Green tea, black tea, and oolong tea are all derived from the dried leaves of the plant *Camellia sinensis* and contain an assortment of compounds, the most significant components of which are phytochemicals. Among all teas consumed in the world, green tea is best studied for its health benefits. (Masuda et al. 2011; Singh et al. 2011; Tang et al. 2010b, 2011; Tu et al. 2011; Yang et al. 2009). In recent years, green tea, has shown remarkable effects in inhibiting cancer cell growth both in cell culture system and in *in vivo* tumor models (Bettuzzi et al. 2006). It has been demonstrated that tea constituents exhibit various biological and pharmacological properties such anti-carcinogenic, anti-oxidative, anti-allergic, anti-virus, anti-hypertensive, anti-atherosclerosis, anti-cardiovascular disease and anti-hypercholesterolemic activities (Higdon and Frei 2003; Lambert and Yang 2003; Shankar et al. 2008a). Principles for these activities were shown to be a group of polyphenols, catechin. The major green tea catechins are (−)-epigallocatechin-3-gallate (EGCG), (−)-epigallocatechin (EGC), (−)-epicatechin-3-gallate (ECG) and (−)-epicatechin (Fig. 15.1). EGCG is the major catechin in green tea and accounts for 5–80% representing 200–300 mg/brewed cup of green tea (Khan et al. 2006).Tea catechins are characterized by the dihydroxyl or trihydroxyl substitutions on the B ring and the m-5,7-dihydroxyl substitutions on the A ring. The B ring seems to be the principal site of antioxidant reactions and the antioxidant activity is further increased by the trihydroxyl structure in the D ring (gallate) in EGCG (Singh et al. 2011).

The cancer-preventive effects of EGCG are widely supported by results from epidemiological, cell culture, animal and clinical studies. EGCG is known antioxidant compound and it is proposed that this flavonoid suppresses the inflammatory processes that lead to transformation, hyperproliferation, and initiation of carcinogenesis (Lopez-Lazaro et al. 2011; Thawonsuwan et al. 2010). EGCG inhibits cell proliferation and cell growth (Sanchez-Huerta et al. 2011). Polyphenols,

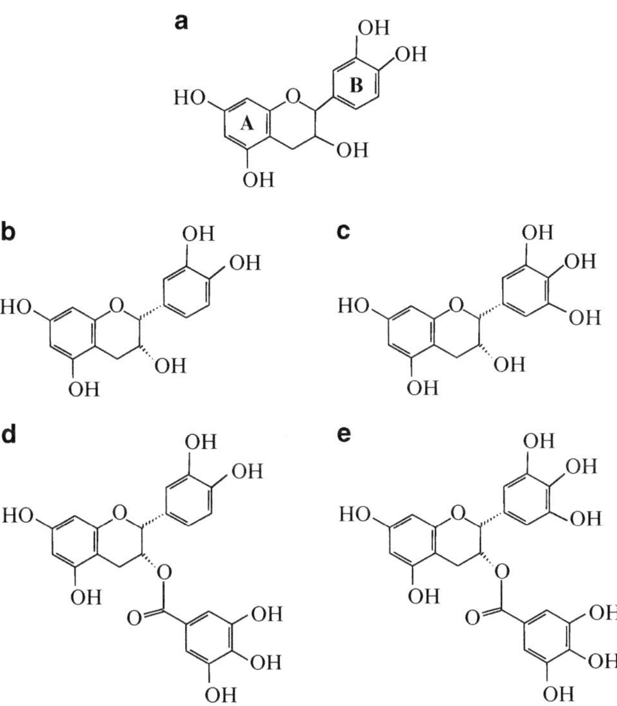

Fig. 15.1 Structures of green tea catechins. Figures are depicted (**a**) Catechin backbone, (**b**) (-)-Epicatechin, (**c**) (-)-Epicatechin-3-gallate, (**d**) (-)-Epigallocatechin and (**e**) (-)-Epigallocatechin-3-gallate

specifically, EGCG, have been shown to increase antioxidant activity in a variety of mouse organs and thus, enhancing the overall chemo-preventative effect of antioxidants in those cells and tissues (Higdon and Frei 2003; Hu et al. 2009). The experimental studies suggest an effect of this catechin which may block the promotion of tumor growth by sealing receptors in the affected cells (Sigler and Ruch 1993). Another possible mechanism indicates that this compound may facilitate direct binding to certain carcinogens (Sigler and Ruch 1993). Its inhibitory influences may ultimately suppress the final steps of carcinogenesis as well, namely angiogenesis and metastasis (Mukhtar and Ahmad 2000). Various animal studies have revealed that treatment with EGCG inhibits tumor incidence and multiplicity in different organ sites such as skin (UV radiation and chemically induced), lung, liver, breast, prostate, stomach, mammary gland and colon based on preclinical, observational, and clinical trial data (Mukhtar and Ahmad 2000; Yang et al. 2002).

Tumorigenesis is a multistep process that can be activated by any of various environmental carcinogens (cigarette smoke, industrial emissions, gasoline vapors), tumor promoters (phorbol esters and okadaic acid), and inflammatory agents (TNF-α and H_2O_2). These carcinogens are known to modulate the transcription machinery

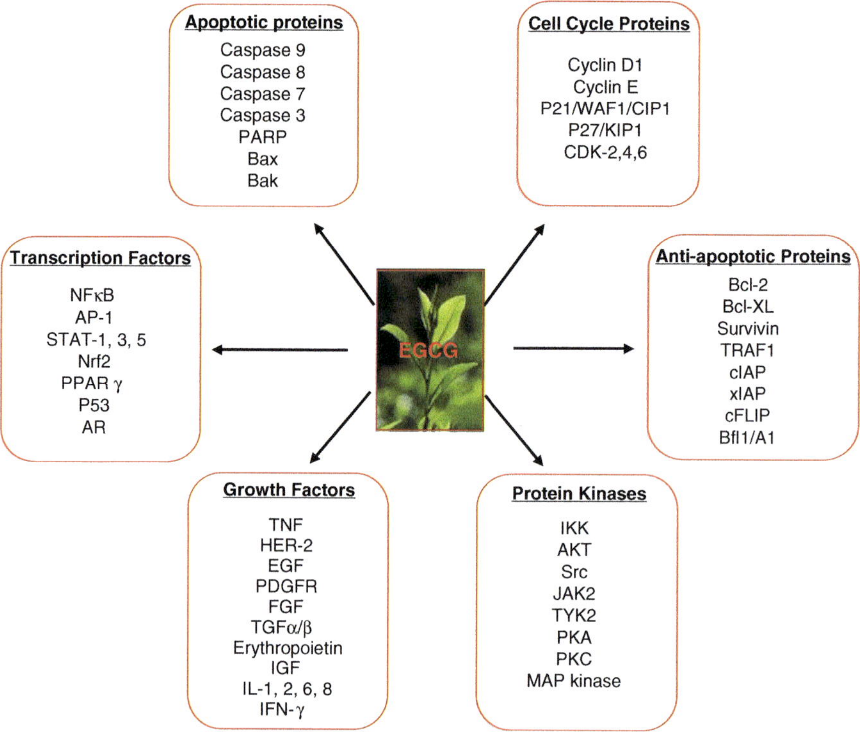

Fig. 15.2 Mechanism of actions of EGCG. The cancer chemopreventive effects of EGCG that regulates cell proliferation and cell growth by altering the expression of apoptotic, cell cycle, anti-apoptotic proteins, transcription, growth factors and different types of protein kinases

factors (e.g., NFκB, AP-1, STAT3), anti-apoptotic proteins (e.g., Akt, Bcl-2, Bcl-XL), proapoptotic proteins (e.g., caspases, PARP), protein kinases (e.g., IKK, JNK, MAP kinase), cell cycle proteins (e.g., cyclins, cyclin-dependent kinases), cell adhesion molecules, cyclooxygenase (COX)-2, and growth factor signaling pathways (Aggarwal and Shishodia 2006). Recently, tremendous progress has been made in elucidating the molecular mechanisms of cancer chemoprevention by EGCG (Yang et al. 2007). The suppression of various tumor biomarkers including growth factor receptor tyrosine kinases, cytokine receptor kinases, PI3K, phosphatases, ras, raf, MAP kinase, IKK, PKA, PKB, PKC, c-jun, c-fos, c-myc, cdks, cyclins, and related transducing proteins by tea polyphenols have been studied in our laboratory and others (Fig. 15.2). The IKK activity in LPs-activated murine macrophages (RAW 264.7 cells) was found to be inhibited by EGCG (Lin 2002; Singh et al. 2010c; Yuan et al. 2007). Besides, it regulates and promotes IL-23 dependent DNA repair and stimulates cytotoxic T cells activities in a tumor microenvironment. It also blocks carcinogenesis by modulating the signal transduction pathways involved in cancer development (Ahmed et al. 2004). EGCG was also shown to affect several biological pathways, including growth factor-mediated pathway, the mitogen activated protein (MAP) kinase-dependent pathway, and ubiquitin/proteasome degradation pathways (Khan et al. 2006; Yang et al. 2007).

A major challenge of cancer chemoprevention is to integrate new molecular findings into clinical practice. This review summarizes recent research on EGCG induced cellular signal transduction events that seems to have implications in the inhibition of cell proliferation and transformation, induction of apoptosis of preneoplastic and neoplastic cells as well as inhibition of angiogenesis, tumor invasion, and metastasis. This justifies the need for a systematic review on this topic.

Cellular Signaling in Cancer

Center to the cancer biology is disrupted intracellular signaling cascades, which transmit aberrant signals resulting in abnormal cellular functions. Consistent with this notion, targeting deregulated intracellular signaling cascades is considered to be a rational approach in achieving chemoprevention. Recent studies have shown that EGCG cancer chemopreventive agent exerts its effect by modulating one or more cell signaling pathways in a manner that interrupts the carcinogenic process (Shankar et al. 2007; Singh et al. 2011). Moreover, tea polyphenols display a vast array of cellular effects, they can affect all stages of cancer development by up- or down-regulating multiple key cellular proteins involved in diverse cellular signal transduction pathways: proliferation, differentiation, apoptosis, angiogenesis or metastasis, resulting in a potential beneficial effect (Khan et al. 2006; Shankar et al. 2007). The potential chemopreventive effect of EGCG seems to be quite specific, and cancer cell lines appear to be more sensitive than normal cells, since EGCG has shown higher cytotoxicity in cancer cells than in their normal counterparts. The inhibition of lung tumor in A/J mice by EGCG was associated with decreased cell proliferation, induced apoptosis, and decreased angiogenesis as well as with lower levels of phospho-c-jun and phospho-ERK1/2 in lung adenomas and carcinomas (Milligan et al. 2009).

Inhibition of oxidative stress constitutes the first line of defense system against carcinogenic insults and can be considered as most effective way for preventing cancer. It can be achieved by scavenging the reactive oxygen species (i.e. $^{\bullet}OH$ and $O_2^{\bullet-}$) or by inducing their detoxification through induction of phase-II conjugating enzymes (GST, glucuronidases and sulphotransferases) (Singh et al. 2009d, 2010a). Antioxidant enzymes (CAT, SOD, GPx and GR) are important components of the cellular stress response whereby a diverse array of electrophilic and oxidative toxicants can be removed from the cell before they are able to damage target cell DNA (Prakash et al. 2007; Singh et al. 2009a). In the tumor promotion step, mechanisms that stop or slow down cell division could be potentially beneficial (induction of cell cycle arrest, and apoptosis) in order to restore the lost balance between cell proliferation and apoptosis (Ahmad et al. 1997; Shankar et al. 2008a, b). At the latest phase of carcinogenesis (progression), the interruption of angiogenesis or the prevention of malignant cells to escape from original location and invade other tissues could also be potentially useful. During all the stages of cancer development many key proteins related to cellular antioxidant defences, cellular proliferation and survival transduction pathways (e.g. AKT, PI3K, MAP kinases, and NFκB) are upregulated, and anti-apoptotic members of Bcl-2 family genes (e.g. Bax and Bak), and tumor suppressor genes (p53, BRAC1 and BRAC2) are downregulated (Manson 2003; Surh 2003).

Anticarcinogenic Activity

Epigenetic modifications in particular, DNA hypermethylation and aberrant acetylation of non-histone proteins associated with inappropriate gene silencing contribute significantly to the initiation and progression of human cancer. The clinical studies suggest an effect of EGCG, which may block the promotion of tumor growth by blocking receptors in the affected cells. EGCG inhibits cancer-associated stages and exert an inhibitory effect on DNA methylation via blocking performance of DNMTs, antioxidant activity (Fang et al. 2003, 2007; Huang et al. 2007; Lee et al. 2005). Another possible mechanism indicates that EGCG may facilitate direct binding to certain cancer developing carcinogens (Fang et al. 2003). It has also been suggested that EGCG inhibits tumorigenesis in a variety of organs.

Recently, EGCG inhibited PDGF-induced apoptosis and cell cycle regulating pathways of vascular smooth muscle cells, resulting in inhibition of tumor growth, metastasis, and angiogenesis *in vivo* (Shankar et al. 2008a, b). Moreover, green tea polyphenols and EGCG have been shown to induce apoptosis, antioxidant and detoxifying protein levels in human lymphoid leukaemia cells and human prostate cancer cells (Hibasami et al. 1996). EGCG affected the proliferation and apoptosis of HCT-8 and HT29 (Zhang et al. 2011). EGCG caused G(2)/M phase arrest and M phase transition in HCT-8 cell line, and S phase arrest and G2 phase transition in HT29 cell line. EGCG down-regulated HES1 gene expression in both cell lines. EGCG upregulated JAG1 gene expression in both cell lines, however only the difference in HCT-8 was statistically significant (Zhang et al. 2011).

EGCG inhibited lipopolysaccharide-induced nitric oxide production and inducible nitric oxide synthase gene expression in isolated peritoneal macrophages by decreasing the activation of NFκB (Lin and Lin 1997). Many animal studies indicate that EGCG can inhibit the growth of malignant cells and induce apoptosis even in cancerous cell lines resistant to CD95-mediated apoptosis. Some results suggest that EGCG induce apoptosis due to their pro-oxidant effect. In a study where EGCG has been tested on oral cancer cell lines along with curcumin, EGCG blocked cell division in G1, whereas curcumin blocked cell division in S/G2M. EGCG has antiproliferative activities on tumor cells through the blockage of growth factor binding to the receptor and the suppression of mitogenic signal transduction (Khafif et al. 1998). Volatiles in tea have been found to be moderately cytotoxic against human carcinoma cells, with β-ionone and nerolidol exhibiting the strongest activity

(Babich et al. 2007). Procarcinogens such as *N*-nitrosodiethylamine and aflatoxins that are activated by cytochrome P450 enzymes are able to modify DNA and induce tumorigenesis (Singh et al. 2010b). Tea flavonoids can directly neutralise the procarcinogens by their strong antiradical activity, before cell membrane injury occur (Singh et al. 2010a). EGCG exhibits the highest protection against DNA scissions, mutations, and in non-enzymatic interception of superoxide anions. EGCG blocks urokinase, an enzyme which is essential for cancer growth and metastasis formation, by interfering with the enzyme's ability to recognize its substrates (Jankun et al. 1997). EGCG can also kill specifically transformed cells by adenovirus (Katiyar and Mukhtar 1996). EGCG inhibits DNA synthesis of rat hepatoma cells, leukemia cells and lung carcinoma cells (Sergediene et al. 1999). EGCG, in a transgenic mice model for skin cancer, has exhibited a preventive effect and/or improvement of the situation (Meeran et al. 2006). Sazuka et al. (1996) reported that the adhesion of lung carcinoma cells to fibronectin, a plasma protein, can be inhibited by EGCG, hindering cancer progression.

Chemopreventive Effects

Chemoprevention of cancer through the use of naturally occurring dietary agents recently has received an increasing interest, and dietary polyphenols have become not only important potential chemopreventive, but also therapeutic, natural agents. Chemoprevention, by definition, is a means of the therapy of precancerous lesions, which are called preinvasive neoplasia, dysplasia, or intraepithelial neoplasia, depending on the organ system. One misconception about chemoprevention is the thinking for complete prevention of cancer, an unachievable goal. Since the mechanism of cancer development is carcinogenesis, we believe that our key aim should be to prevent carcinogenesis process, which in turn will lead to lower cancer burden. We, therefore, define chemoprevention as *slowing the process of carcinogenesis*, a goal that can be met (Siddiqui et al. 2010). Polyphenols have been demonstrated to act on multiple key elements in intracellular signal transduction pathways related to cell proliferation, differentiation, apoptosis, inflammation, angiogenesis and metastasis; however, these molecular mechanisms of action are not completely characterized and many features remain to be elucidated (Aggarwal and Shishodia 2006).

The cancer chemopreventive effects of EGCG may be the result of decreased cell transformation and proliferation or increased cell cycle arrest and apoptosis (Babu et al. 2006; Chacko et al. 2010; Shankar et al. 2008b). *In vitro*, EGCG has been shown to cause growth inhibition and apoptosis in a number of human cancer cell lines including leukemia, melanoma, breast cancer, lung, and colon (Shankar et al. 2008a, b; Yang et al. 2006b, c). EGCG has been shown to possess chemopreventive effects against broad spectrum of carcinogens by inhibiting *N*-methylbenzylnitrosamine-induced esophagus (Yamane et al. 1995), azoxymethane- and *N*-methylnitrosourea-induced colon (Narisawa and Fukaura 1993), diethylnitrosamine-induced liver (Tamura et al. 1997), 7,12-dimethylbenz(*a*)anthraceneinduced mammary (Tamura et al. 1997), *N*-methyl-*N*'-nitro-*N*-nitrosoguanidine-induced glandular stomach, *N*-ethyl-*N*'-nitro-*N*-nitrosoguanidine-induced duodenum (Fujita et al. 1989), 4-(methylnitrosamimo)-1-(3-pyridyl)-1-butanone-induced pulmonary (Wang et al. 1992), diethylnitrosamine- and benzo(*a*)pyrene-induced lung and forestomach (Katiyar et al. 1993), *N*-nitrosobis(2-oxopropyl)amine-induced pancreatic (Majima et al. 1998) and UV-induced skin (Lu et al. 2001) carcinogenesis in the animal model. These effects have been extensively studied *in vitro* to try to elucidate the potential mechanism(s) of action of EGCG. Moreover, these chemopreventive effects have been observed *in vivo* in certain animal models; no clear and fully understandable mechanism(s) has been reported for EGCG. Currently, the molecular evidence to prove chemopreventive efficacy by animal studies is at its initial stage. However, an ever-growing number of studies are demonstrating that EGCG can prevent carcinogenesis.

Inhibition of Tumorigenesis and Possible Mechanism: Molecular Targets

Many mechanisms have been proposed for the biological activities of EGCG. This includes antioxidant activities, cell cycle arrest, induction of apoptosis, induction or inhibition of drug metabolism enzymes, modulation of cell signaling, inhibition of DNA methylation, effect on miRNA expression, DHFR, proteases, and telomerase (Fig. 15.2). With the availability of many reagents for signal transduction research, EGCG has been found to affect different signal transduction pathways, such as the inhibition of many protein kinases; suppression of the activation of transcription factors (e.g. AP-1 and NFκB) and blocking growth receptor mediated pathways. However, it is not clear which of these mechanisms occur *in vivo* and are relevant to the cancer-preventive activities of tea.

Antioxidative Effect

Tea polyphenols are characterized by the di- or tri-hydroxyl groups on the B-ring and the meta-5,7-dihydroxyl groups on the A ring (Fig. 15.1). The antioxidant activities of EGCG are due to the presence of phenolic groups that are sensitive to oxidation and can generate quinone. The antioxidative effect is further increased by the presence of the trihydroxyl structure in the D ring in EGCG (Wiseman et al. 1997). EGCG is powerful radical scavengers; protected neurons from the oxidative damage induced by a commonly used pro-oxidant such as *tert*-butylhydroperoxide (Sonee et al. 2004). Murakami et al. (2002) reported that EGCG can reduced the cytotoxicity evoked by H_2O_2 and increased the levels of the enzymes related to the oxidative stress, resulting in an enhanced cellular GSH content in a HepG2 (Table 15.1). EGCG from green tea induced H_2O_2 formation in human lung adenocarcinoma (H661) and in Ha-ras gene-transformed human bronchial (21BES) cells, but exogenously added catalase (CAT) prevented EGCG-induced cell apoptosis, which suggested that H_2O_2 is involved in the apoptotic process provoked by EGCG (Lee et al. 2000; Yang and Koo 2000). Moreover, in a clinical investigation, when HUVEC were incubated with EGCG or in pro-oxidant conditions, its restored cell viability and inhibited apoptosis, showing that phenolic compound differ in their antiapoptotic efficacy (Choi et al. 2003). Treatment of C57bl/6 J mice with this catechin has been reported to increase gene expression of c-GST, glutamate cysteine ligase, and hemeoxygenase-1 in an Nrf2-ARE-dependent manner (Rietveld and Wiseman 2003). Similar results have been reported in the tumor cells of colon cancer xenograft-bearing nude mice treated with dietary EGCG (Liu et al. 2003). These effects have been re-capitulated *in vitro* (Yuan et al. 2007). Increased expression of hemeoxygenase-1 and SOD was recorded when human mammary epithelial cells were treated with EGCG (Lambert and Elias 2010). This effect was reduced by siRNA-mediated disruption of Nrf2, suggesting a role for this pathway in the EGCG-mediated induction of these endogenous antioxidant systems.

Treatment of 24 month-old rats with EGCG (100 mg/kg, i.g.) decreased 50% hepatic levels of lipid peroxides and 39% protein carbonyls formation (Kumaran et al. 2008). EGCG treatment also increased the levels of antioxidant and antioxidant enzymes of hepatic compared to control one. These effects were not observed in young rats, suggesting that EGCG offered no improvement in antioxidant status in the absence of pre-existing oxidative stress (Senthil Kumaran et al. 2008; Srividhya et al. 2008). This may explain why other studies have failed to observe an effect of tea polyphenolics treatment. Treatment of Hepa1c1c7 human hepatoma cells with EGCG resulted in dose-dependent increases in NADPH:quinone reductase-1 and glutathione genes expression through the EpRE. LC–MS analysis of the cell culture medium revealed the presence of EGCG-20-glutathione further supporting this conclusion (Muzolf-Panek et al. 2008). EGCG induced apoptosis in 21BES cells. EGCG-mediated apoptosis was reduced by approximately 50% by inclusion of exogenous catalase (Yang et al. 2000). This result suggested that EGCG can induce apoptosis by an ROS dependent mechanism.

Induction of Apoptosis and Cell Cycle Arrest

Apoptosis is a highly ordered protective mechanism by which unwanted or damaged cells are eliminated before malignancy manifests. It is essential for normal development, turnover, and replacement of cells in the living system (Ahmad et al. 1997; Chen et al. 2010b). Cell apoptosis is characterized by typical morphological and biochemical hallmarks including chromatin condensation, membrane blebbing, cell shrinkage, nuclear DNA fragmentation and the formation of apoptotic bodies (Adhami et al. 2004). The cell subsequently breaks up into membrane-enclosed

Table 15.1 Regulation of cellular signaling by EGCG

S. No.	Molecular mechanisms	Molecular targets	References
1.	Induction of cell cycle arrest	↓ cyclin D; ↓ cyclin E; ↓ CDK1; ↓ CDK2; ↓ CDK4; ↓ CDK6; ↓ PCNA; ↑ 16; ↑ p18; ↑ p21; ↑ p27; ↑ pRb; ↑ p53; ↑ mdm2	Shankar et al. (2007, 2008a, b), Lin et al. (2010), and Lim and Cha (2011)
2.	Antioxidant(s)	↓ H_2O_2-induced apoptosis; ↑ H_2O_2 production; ↑ ROS; ↑ GSH; ↓ Nrf-2-mediated HO-1 activation	Wiseman et al. (1997), Sonee et al. (2004), and Kumaran et al. (2008)
	Phase I and II enzyme(s)	↓ CYP1A1 ↓ CYP2E	Chandra and De Mejia (2004), Syed et al. 2007
3.	Induction of apoptosis	↑ ↓ROS; ↑ caspase-3; ↑ caspase-8; ↑ caspase-9; ↑ cytochrome c; ↑ Smac/DIABLO; ↓↑ Bax; Bak; ↑ cleaved PPAR; ↓↑ Bcl-2; ↓ Bcl-xL; ↓ Bid; ↓ c-myc; = c-IAP1; ↓ c-IAP2; ↓ Mcl-1; ↓ survivin; ↓ XIAP	Ahmad et al. (1997), Chen et al. (2010b), Singh et al. (2011), and Tang et al. (2010a, 2011)
4.	Inhibition of proliferation and inflammation	↓ PI3K; ↓↑ AKT; ↓↑ ERK; ↓ p90RSK; ↓ FKHR; ↓ PDGF; ↓ PDGFRα; ↓ EGFR; ↓↑ c-fos; ↓ egr-1; ↓ AP-1; ↓ NF-kB; ↓ IKK; ↓ COX-2; ↑ JNK; ↑ Ras; ↑ MEKK1; ↑ MEK3; ↓↑ p38; ↑ IjB; ↑ AMPK; ↑ PGE2; ↑ TNF-α	Roy et al. (2010), Yang et al. (2006a), Masuda et al. (2001), Dong et al. (1997), Afaq et al. (2003b), and Singh et al. (2011)
5.	Angiogenesis	↓ HIF-1α; ↓ VEGF; ↓ VEGFR1; ↓VEGFR2 ↓ ErbB2; ↓ErbB3 ↑FOXO	Bartholome et al. (2010), Anton et al. (2007), and Masuda et al. (2003)

6.	Metastasis	↓ MMP-2; ↓ MMP-9; ↓ FAK; proMMP-2; ↓ MRLC; ↓ vimentin; ↓ laminin; ↓ integrina2b1; ↓ uPA; ↓ HuR; ↑ proMMP-7; ↑ TIMP-2; ↑ MT1-MMP		Berger et al. (2001), Givant-Horwitz et al. (2004), and Jankun et al. (1997)
7.	Epigenetic modifier(s)	↓ DNMTs; ↓ HAT ↓ acetylation of H3/H4		Fang et al. (2003), Nandakumar et al. (2011), and Chuang et al. (2005)
8.	Validate gene target(s)	RARb, MGMT, MLH1, CDKN2A, RECK, TERT, RXRa, CDX2, GSTP1, WIF1		Nandakumar et al. (2011) and Sanchez-Huerta et al. (2011)
9.	Proteasomal activity	↓ 20S/26S proteasome complex		Nam et al. (2001) and Khan et al. (2010)
10.	Inhibition of cancer(s)	***In vitro* model:** Esophageal; oral; prostate; breast; urinary; lung; colon; leukemia; lymphoma	***In vivo* model:** Skin, prostrate, colon and uterine cancer; human gastric, pancreatic and oral cancers	Fang et al. (2003), Nandakumar et al. (2011), Shankar et al. (2007, 2008b), Katiyar et al. (1993), Masuda et al. (2002), and Singh et al. (2011)

fragments, termed apoptosis bodies, which are rapidly recognized and engulfed by neighboring cells or macrophages (Aggarwal et al. 2004; Guo et al. 2005). Markedable, biochemical modifications occurs within the apoptosis bodies by phagocytosis. On the molecular basis, apoptosis can be induced by two major pathways: (i) at the plasma membrane upon ligation of the death receptor (extrinsic pathway) and (ii) at the mitochondria (intrinsic pathway).

The induction of different negative regulators of the cell cycle may be the consequence of this inhibition. Although EGCG has been shown to affect a number of factors associated with cell cycle progression, the direct inhibition of cyclin-dependent kinases is considered as the primary event (Khan et al. 2006). EGCG also induces the expression of p21 and p27 while decreasing the expression of cyclin D1 and the phosphorylation of retinoblastoma. However, EGCG inhibited LPs-induced phosphorylation of IKK, but failed to affect NFκB luciferase reporter gene activation in human colon cancer (HT-29) cells, suggesting that EGCG modulation of NFκB transcriptional activity is not necessarily dependent on IkBα degradation and subsequent release of NFκB proteins (Table 15.1; Kim et al. 2004b). EGCG-induced apoptosis was evidenced by nuclear condensation, increased protein levels of activated caspase-3, down-regulation of gelsolin and tropomyosin-4 (Tm-4), and up-regulation of tropomyosin-1(Tm-1) (Hsu and Liou 2011). By disrupting adherens junction formation, EGCG caused accumulation of extra-nuclear β-catenin aggregates in the cytosol and alterations of the protein content and mRNA expression of E-cadherin and β-catenin, but not N-cadherin, in MCF-7 cells. In human prostate carcinoma LNCaP cells, treatment with EGCG induced apoptosis and was associated with stabilization of p53 and also with a down-regulation of NFκB activity, resulting in a decreased expression of the anti-apoptotic protein Bcl-2 (Hastak et al. 2003). EGCG down-regulates the NFκB inducing kinase expression in human lung cancer cell PC-9 (Fujiki et al. 2001). Apoptosis induction by EGCG is more prominent in many cancer cells without affecting normal cells because NFκB is activated in the cancer cells (Table 15.1). Activation of NFκB promotes transcriptional up-regulation of Bcl-2 and Bcl-XL. Negative regulation of NFκB by EGCG decreases the expression of the proapoptotic protein Bcl-2 (Chen et al. 2001). EGCG (70% lethal dose) at the suprapharmacological concentration of 10 μg/ml increased the proportion of HNSCC cells in the G1 phase, decreased cyclin D1 protein expression and increased the levels of p21WAF1/CIP1 and p27KIP1 proteins (Masuda et al. 2001).

Many recent studies demonstrated that EGCG trigger cell growth arrest pathways at G1 stage of cell cycle through regulation of cyclin D1, cdk4, cdk6, p21/WAF1/CIP1 and p27/KIP1, and induced apoptosis through generation of ROS and caspase-3 and caspase-9 activation (Shankar et al. 2007). Treatment of MCF7 breast cancer cells with EGCG (30 μM) inhibited cell cycle arrest in G0/G1 phase. In prostate cancer cells, EGCG (10–80 μM) increased the expression of p16, p18, p21, p27 and p53, which are associated with negative regulation of cell cycle progression (Table 15.1). Overall, these findings suggest that green tea and its constituents induce growth arrest and apoptosis through multiple mechanisms and can be used for chemoprevention to target cancer cells. EGCG induces apoptosis by activating capase-3/7 and inhibiting the expression of Bcl-2, survivin and XIAP in prostate stem cancer cells. Furthermore, EGCG inhibits epithelial-mesenchymal transition by inhibiting the expression of vimentin, slug, snail and nuclear β-catenin, and the activity of LEF-1/TCF responsive reporter, and also retards CSC's migration and invasion, suggesting the blockade of signaling involved in early metastasis (Lin et al. 2010; Tang et al. 2010a). Interestingly, quercetin synergizes with EGCG in inducing apoptosis, and blocking CSC's migration and invasion. These data suggest that EGCG either alone or in combination with quercetin can eliminate CSC's-characteristics. EGCG inhibited expressions of Bcl-2 and Bcl-XL and induced expressions of Bax, Bak, Bcl-XS and PUMA. Furthermore, ras, raf-1 activities and ERK1/2 were down regulated, whereas the activities of MEKK1, JNK1/2 and p38 MAP kinases were upregulated (Shankar et al. 2007). Inhibition of craf-1 or ERK enhanced EGCG-induced apoptosis, whereas inhibition of JNK or p38 MAP kinase inhibited EGCG-induced apoptosis. EGCG promoted the activation of p90 ribosomal protein S6 kinase, and induced the activation of c-jun. Xenograft and TRAMP models have shown that green tea or EGCG can decrease the tumorigenic potential of prostate cancer (Shankar et al. 2007). EGCG treatment inhibited the growth of ARO cells in a dose-dependent manner. Furthermore, EGCG suppressed phosphorylation of EGFR, ERK1/2, JNK, and p38. These changes were associated with increased p21 and reduced cyclin B1/CDK1 expression. In addition, EGCG treatment increased the accumulation of sub-G1 cell, activated caspase-3 and cleaved PARP (Lim and Cha 2011).

Caspases, a ubiquitous family of cysteine proteases play key roles both as upstream initiators and downstream effectors in apoptosis (Shankar et al. 2011). This cascade leads to proteolytic cleavage of a variety of cytoplasmic and nuclear proteins, thereby favoring the prevalence of proapoptotic activities on antiapoptotic activities (Yang et al. 2006a, c). In an *in vivo* study, EGCG inhibited xenograft tumor size of TSGH-8301 cells in a nude mouse model. Based on an in vitro study, EGCG resulted in morphological changes and increased growth inhibition in a dose- and time-dependent manner in TSGH-8301 cells (Chen et al. 2011). Furthermore, sub-G1 populations were shown and caspase-9 and -3 activities were stimulated in EGCG-treated TSGH-8301 cells. Moreover, a caspase-9 inhibitor (Z-LEHD-FMK) and a caspase-3 inhibitor (Z-DEVD-FMK) were able to reduce EGCG-stimulated caspase-9 and -3 activities, respectively. Loss of mitochondrial membrane potential ($\Delta\Psi m$) resulted in an increase of protein levels of cytochrome c, Apaf-1, caspase-9 and -3 in TSGH-8301 cells following exposure to EGCG. Proteomic analysis revealed that EGCG affected the expression levels of various proteins, including HSP27, porin, tropomyosin 3 isoform 2, prohibitin and keratin 5, 14, 17 in TSGH-8301 cells. EGCG also suppressed AKT kinase activity and protein levels and also altered the expression levels of Bcl-2 family-related proteins such as Bcl-2, Bax, BAD and p-BAD. Treatment of human colorectal carcinoma HT-29 cells with EGCG resulted in nuclear condensation, DNA fragmentation, caspase activation, disruption of mitochondrial membrane potential and cytochrome c release, which all appeared to be mediated by the JNKs pathway (Chan et al. 2003). In addition, EGCG also invokes Bax oligomerization and depolarization of mitochondrial membranes to facilitate cytochrome c release into cytosol. Treatment of colon cancer cells with EGCG decreased cell proliferation index (based on Ki-67 expression), increased apoptotic index (cleaved caspase-3), decreased nuclear β-catenin levels, and decreased phospho-AKT levels (Roy et al. 2010; Yang et al. 2006a). EGCG abrogated the expression of anti-apoptotic Bcl-2 and Bcl-XL proteins and enhanced the levels of proapoptotic Bax proteins followed by caspase-3 activation (Smith et al. 2002). Moreover, EGCG–induced nuclear condensation, and poly(ADP)ribose polymerase cleavage (Lambert et al. 2005). EGCG also reduced the protein expression of cyclin D1, cyclin E, CDK2, CDK4, and CDK6. EGCG also inhibited the activity of CDK2 and CDK4, and caused Rb hypophosphorylation (Masuda et al. 2001). Head and neck squamous cell carcinoma cells were found to be more sensitive to the effects of EGCG; EGCG induced G0/G1 phase cell cycle arrest at concentrations lower than 20 μM (Masuda et al. 2001). The results suggest that EGCG exerts cancer preventive potential by inhibiting cell proliferation, promoting apoptosis, and modulating β-catenin and Akt signaling.

Effect on Phase I and II Enzymes

One of the most important mechanisms of chemoprevention by cruciferous plants extracts appears to be induction of phase II enzymes and inhibition of phase I enzymes (Smith et al. 2002). Procarcinogenic metabolism can be altered by EGCG by inhibiting phase-I drug-metabolizing enzymes CYPs, increasing the activity or modulating the gene expression of phase II conjugating-enzymes which can regulate several biological events such as acetylation, methylation, glucuronidation, sulphation and conjugation (Table 15.1; Schwarz et al. 2003). EGCG increased the activity of the phase II detoxifying enzymes GST and NQO in mouse liver, breast and prostate cancer cells. Similarly, drinks rich in tea phenols increased QR activity in the Hepa1c1c7 cells and in general, EGCG prevented glutathione depletion and ROS formation after an oxidative injury caused by different carcinogens which are formed reactive metabolites such as prooxidants (Chandra and De Mejia 2004). Consequently, tea also showed *in vitro* a protective effect on rat hepatic extracts, which was associated with a reduced level of CYP2E and an enhanced activity of phase II detoxifying enzyme UDPGT, suggesting that EGCG can regulate phase I and phase II drug metabolizing enzymes, although GST activity was unaffected (Maliakal et al. 2001). *In vitro* studies have demonstrated that EGCG possesses a strong inhibitory effect on CYP1A1 at the transcriptional level (Maliakal et al. 2001). Phenolic compounds can induce phase II conjugating enzymes, they can be considered as potential candidates for preventing tumor development (Maliakal et al. 2001). An ARE has been found in the promoters of antioxidant proteins (SOD, GPx, and CAT) and several drug-metabolizing enzymes (GST, and GR). Several signaling pathways have been involved in the activation of the ARE that binds transcription factor Nrf-2. In a study, it has been observed that in human hepatoma HepG2 cells, an EGCG rich green tea polyphenol extract induced the transcriptional potency of phase II detoxifying enzymes through ARE and decreased in Nrf-2-ARE binding in lung adenocarcinoma A549 cells (Syed et al. 2007).

Modulation of Intracellular Signaling Cascades

Inhibition of NFκB

NFκB is a family of closely related protein dimers or oxidative stress–sensitive transcription factor that bind to a common sequence motif in DNA called the κB site (Campbell et al. 2006). The identification of the p50 subunit of NFκB as a member of the REL family of viruses provided the first evidence that NFκB is linked to cancer. NFκB is sequestered in the cytoplasm in an inactive form through interaction with IκB. NFκB is activated by free radicals, inflammatory stimuli, cytokines, carcinogens, tumor promoters, endotoxins, γ-radiation, UV light, and X-rays. Upon activation, it is translocated to the nucleus, where it induces the expression of more than 200 genes that have been shown to suppress apoptosis and induce cellular transformation, proliferation, invasion, metastasis, chemo-resistance, radio-resistance, innate immunity and inflammation (Campbell et al. 2006).

Recent results also totally confirmed its pivotal roles in suppressing apoptosis in cancer cells (Aggarwal and Shishodia 2006; Ahmad et al. 1997). Phosphorylation and activation of IκB kinase is controlled by an NFκB-inducing kinase and there is crosstalk between activation of the MAP kinase/ERK pathway, and the NFκB - inducing kinase/I-κB kinase/ NFκB pathway (Shimizu et al. 2005). In the cytosol, NFκB is inactive when bound to I-κB (Fig. 15.3). The phosphorylation of I-κB by IKKs leads to proteasome dependent degradation of I-κB, resulting NFκB free (Hou et al. 2004). NFκB can activate the expression of a set of NFκB responsive genes when translocate into the nucleus. EGCG has been shown to inhibit the activation of NFκB in H891 head and neck cancer cells and MDA-MB-231 breast cancer cells (Masuda et al. 2002). Treatment of EGCG dose- and time-dependently increased I-κB level, and inhibited NFκB nuclear translocation in A431 epidermoid carcinoma cells (Gupta et al. 2003). EGCG has been shown to inhibit NFκB activity in human colon cancer cells (Shimizu and Weinstein 2005). EGCG suppresses the TNF-induced activation of IKK that leads to the inhibition of TNF-dependent phosphorylation and degradation of IκBα and translocation of the p65 subunit. Based on its ability to inhibit other kinases, emodin may act directly on the IKK complex to block phosphorylation of IκBα. Yang et al. (2007) found that EGCG suppresses NFκB activation by inhibiting IKK activity. Some act by suppressing Iκ-Bα degradation and p65 translocation or NFκB –DNA binding activity.

EGCG as well as TF inhibited activation of Akt and nuclear factor-kappaB (NF-kappaB) via blocking phosphorylation and subsequent degradation of inhibitor of kappaBalpha and kappaBbeta subunits, thereby downregulating cyclooxygenase-2. Treatment with EGCG in a dose- and time-dependent manner was found to inhibit

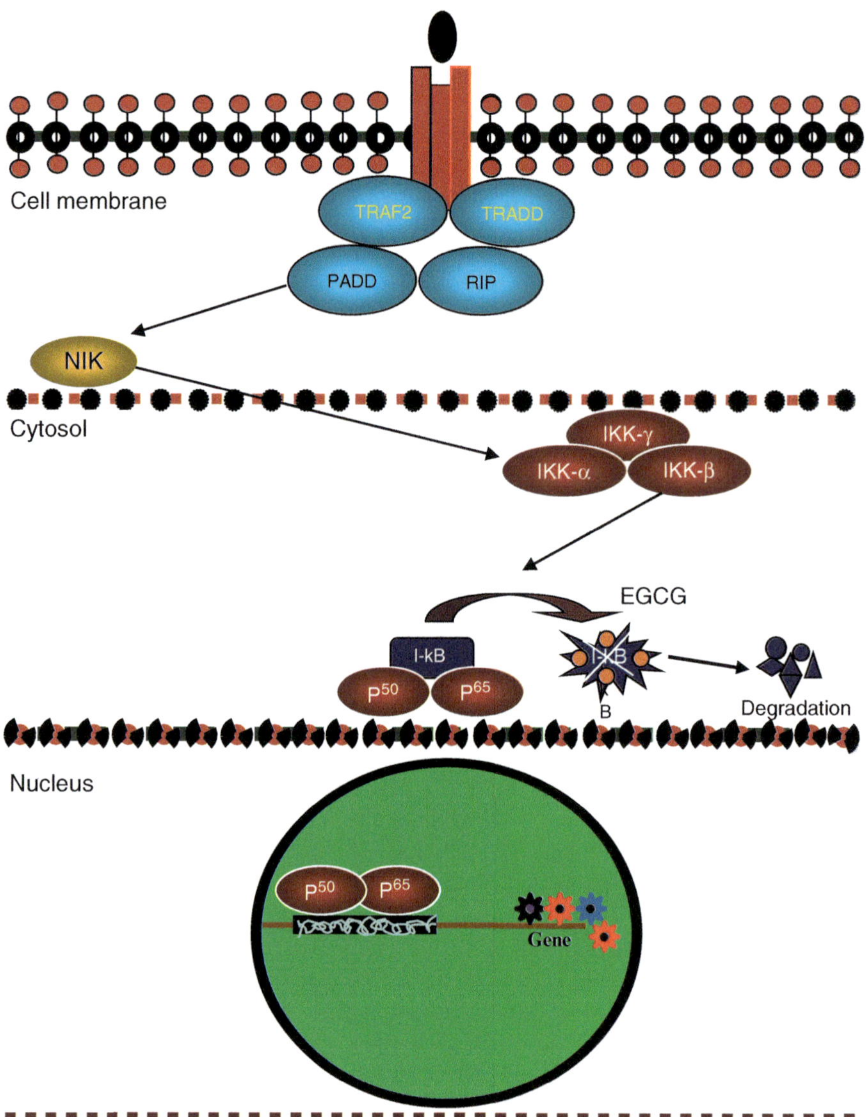

Fig. 15.3 Modulation of NF-κB pathway by EGCG. In the cytosol as a result of the binding of *p50* and *p65* to *I-κB*, *NF-κB* becomes inactive. When *I-κB* is phosphorylated by IKKs and degraded in a proteasome-dependent pathway, p50 and p65 are set free and are translocated into the nucleus to activate a specific set of genes. This pathway has been shown to be inhibited by EGCG both, possibly by inhibiting IKK-catalyzed phosphorylation of I-κB

UVB-mediated activation of NFκB in normal human epidermal keratinocytes (Afaq et al. 2003a). Gupta et al. (2004) identified NFκB/p65 component of the NFκB complex as a target for specific cleavage by caspases during EGCG-mediated apoptosis. Thus, one of the probable mechanisms by EGCG exercise their anti-tumor property is through the suppression of the NFκB signaling pathway. In normal human epidermal keratinocytes, UVB irradiation-induced NFκB activation was associated with increased I-kB phosphorylation and degradation and EGCG was shown to inhibit NFκB activation and nuclear translocation (Afaq et al. 2003a). Although, ROS have been suggested to be involved in the activation of the NFκB signaling system, and that its suppression by EGCG is due to its strong antioxidant and free radical quenching activities (Lee et al. 2004). It has been shown that the galloyl and phenolic groups at the 3' position on EGCG are responsible for its strong anti-inflammatory properties (Lin and Lin 1997).

Activation of FOXO Transcription Factors

FOXO transcription factors including FOXO1, FOXO3a, and FOXO4, exert critical biological functions in response to genotoxic stress. In mammals four FOXOs proteins are known (Roy et al. 2010; Shankar et al. 2008b, 2011). FOXOs induce cell cycle arrest, repair damaged DNA, or initiate apoptosis by modulating genes that control these processes. The importance of FOXO factors ascribes them under multiple levels of regulation including phosphorylation, acetylation/deacetylation, ubiquitination and protein-protein interactions (Srivastava et al. 2010). This function of FOXO is essential for the regulation of cancer cells and CSCs and progenitor cell pool in the hematopoietic system (Srivastava et al. 2010). The inhibition of PI3K/AKT and MEK/ERK pathways activated FOXO transcription factors. EGCG inhibited phosphorylation of AKT and ERK, and activated FOXO transcription factors, leading to cell cycle arrest and apoptosis and further enhanced FOXO activity and apoptosis (Shankar et al. 2008b). Recently, we have demonstrated that EGCG inhibited cell proliferation and colony formation, and induced apoptosis through caspase-3 activation in pancreatic cancer cells (Chen et al. 2010a; Roy et al. 2010; Shankar et al. 2008b).

Inhibition of AP-1 and MAP Kinases

AP-1 was originally identified by its binding to a DNA sequence in the SV40 enhancer. AP-1 transcription factor is a protein dimer composed of homo- or heterodimers members of the basic region leucine zipper protein superfamily, specifically, the Jun, Fos, and activating transcription factor proteins (Eferl and Wagner 2003). AP-1 has been implicated in regulation of genes involved in apoptosis and proliferation and may promote cell proliferation by activating the cyclin D1 gene, and repressing TSGs, such as p53, p21cip1/waf1 and p16 (Bakiri et al. 2000; Newton and Strasser 2000). Many stimuli, most notably serum, growth factors, and oncoproteins, are potent inducers of AP-1 activity; it is also induced by TNF and IL-1, as well as by a variety of environmental stresses, such as UV radiation. High AP-1 activity or activation of AP-1 has also been shown to be involved in the tumor promotion and progression of various types of cancers, such as lung, breast, and skin cancer (Eferl and Wagner 2003). The inhibition of AP-1 activity by EGCG was associated with inhibition of JNK activation but not ERK activation. Interestingly, in another study where EGCG blocked the UVB-induced c-Fos activation in a human keratinocyte cell line HaCaT, inhibition of p38 activation was suggested as the major mechanism underlying the effects of EGCG (Dong et al. 1997).

MAP kinases have been known to involve in variety of key physiologic processes, including cell apoptosis, differentiation, and death (Rose et al. 2010). In an animal study, it was shown that EGCG (5–20 μmol/L) in concentration dependent manner inhibited the MAP kinase pathway in JB6 mouse epidermal cell line (Dong et al. 1997). In NHEK cells, treatment with EGCG inhibited UVB-induced H_2O_2 production concomitant with block of UVB-induced phosphorylation of ERK1/2, JNK, and p38 proteins (Table 15.1; Afaq et al. 2003b). In mammalian cells, three major types of MAP kinases are presented; p38 MAP kinases, ERK, and c-JNK (Teng et al. 2005). Activated MAP kinases such as ERK, JNK, and p38 can activate ELK and c-Jun. The second messenger, phosphatidyl inositol-3,4,5-triphosphate synthesized by activate PI3K, which is necessary for phosphorylation of Akt, then Akt directly phosphorylates the proapoptotic protein Bad, thus enhancing the antiapoptotic function of Bcl-xL (Silverman and Maniatis 2001).

Recently, EGCG has been shown to inhibit MAP kinase pathway and activator protein-1 (AP-1) activity in human colon cancer cells. In a study, orally feeding of EGCG inhibits PI3K pathway in TRAMP model system (Adhami et al. 2004). The confirm involvement of MAP kinase pathways in the regulation of AP-1 activity by EGCG has been investigated. EGCG has been shown to inhibit c-Jun, ERK1/2 phosphorylation and the phosphorylation of ELK1 and MEK1/2 in Ha-ras-transformed human bronchial cells (Afaq et al. 2003b). In contrast to these reports, markedly increase AP-1 factor-associated responses through a MAP kinase signaling mechanism in normal human keratinocytes has been measured by EGCG, suggesting that the signaling mechanism of EGCG action could be markedly different in different cell types (Jeong et al. 2004; Shimizu and Weinstein 2005).

Inhibition of Epidermal Growth Factor Receptor (EGFR)–Mediated Signal Transduction Pathway

The EGFR (ErbB-1; HER1 in humans) is a cell surface glycoprotein receptor with an extracellular ligand-binding domain, a single transmembrane region, and an intracellular domain that exhibits intrinsic tyrosine kinase activity. The EGFR is a member of the ErbB family of receptors, a subfamily of four closely related receptor tyrosine kinases: EGFR (ErbB-1), HER2/neu (ErbB-2), HER3 (ErbB-3) and HER4 (ErbB-4) (Herbst 2004). Mutations that lead to EGFR overexpression (known as upregulation) or overexpression have been associated with a number of cancers, including lung cancer, anal cancers and glioblastoma multiforme (Zhang et al. 2007). A blockade of EGFR may lead the cancer cells to enter apoptosis (Zhang et al. 2010). Therefore, inhibition of EGFR abrogates the invasive potential of the cancer cells. Overexpression of HER-2/neu, an oncogene in the EGFR tyrosine kinase superfamily, is observed in breast, prostate, ovarian and lung cancers and it is recognized as a target for cancer therapy (Khan and Mukhtar 2010). Downstream events, the phosphorylation of ERK, STAT3, and Akt were subsequently blocked by the treatment with EGCG (Table 15.1; Adhami et al. 2004). Treatment with EGCG inhibited the constitutive ligand-mediated activation of the EGFR in both YCU-H891 head and neck squamous cell carcinoma and MDA-MB-231 breast carcinoma cell lines, indicating that it has the potential to break the autocrine loops that are established in several advanced cancers (Masuda et al. 2003). The results suggested that blocking the EGFR signaling by EGCG would potentially inhibit both cancer cell proliferation and angiogenesis. However, the cells were pre-incubated with EGCG before the addition of TGF-α, resulting the inhibition of EGFR-dependent STAT3 activation subsequently retarded VEGF synthesis in the cancer cells.

Recently, Ahmad observed that EGCG suppresses the expression of IL-6 and IL-8 *in vitro* (Ahmed 2010). EGCG blocks PDGF-induced proliferation and migration of rat pancreatic stellate cells (Masamune et al. 2005). EGCG binds to a specific metastasis associated 67 kDa laminin receptor that is expressed on a variety of tumor cells (Tachibana et al. 2004). When EGCG incorporated in plasma membrane directly interacts with Platelet-derived Growth Factor-BB (PDGF-BB), thereby preventing specific receptor binding leading to the inhibitory effects of EGCG on PDGF-induced cell signaling and mitogenesis. Moreover, Givant-Horwitz and associates (2004) reported that in human colon cancer cells, EGCG inhibits growth and activation of EGFR and human EGFR-2 signaling pathways. Based on these data, it was suggested that may be existence of EGCG receptor. EGCG has been shown to suppress the production of VEGF in swine granulosa cells and breast carcinoma cells (Chen et al. 2010a).

Inhibition of Overexpression of Cyclooxygenase-2 (COX-2)

COX is prostaglandin H synthase, the key regulatory enzyme for prostaglandin synthesis is transcribed from two distinct genes (COX-1 & COX-2). COX-1 is constitutively expressed in many tissues, but the expression of COX-2 is regulated by a variety of factors, such as mitogens, tumor promoters, cytokines, and growth factors (Plumb et al. 1999). Inappropriate COX-2 activity has been observed in practically every premalignant and malignant condition involving the colon, liver, pancreas, breast, lung, bladder, skin, stomach, head and neck, and esophagus (Subbaramaiah and Dannenberg 2003). Several transcription factors including AP-1, and NFκB can stimulate COX-2 transcription (Aggarwal and Shishodia 2006). Pretreatment with green tea extract enriched with EGCG inhibited COX-2 expression induced by TPA in mouse skin. EGCG can downregulate COX-2 in TPA-stimulated human mammary cells (MCF-10A) in culture (Kundu et al. 2003). Recent clinical research findings strongly suggest that development of chemopreventive compounds, which can inhibit COX-2 expression preferably without affecting COX-1, is a high priority for cancer research. EGCG inhibits mitogen-stimulated COX-2 expression in androgen-sensitive LNCaP and androgen-insensitive PC-3 human prostate carcinoma cells (Gerhauser et al. 2003; Hussain et al. 2005). It has been shown that EGCG reduces the activity of COX-2 following interleukin-1A stimulation of human chondrocytes (Ahmad et al. 2002). EGCG exhibited COX inhibition in LPs-induced macrophages (Table 15.1).

Inhibition of Proteasome Activity

The proteasome is a massive multicatalytic protease complex that is responsible for degrading most of the damage or misfold proteins. The proteasomal degradation pathway is essential for many cellular processes, including cell proliferation, down-regulation of cell death, development of drug resistance, regulation of gene expression and responses to oxidative stress, suggesting the use of proteasome inhibitors as potential novel anticancer drugs (Adams and Kauffman 2004; Ciechanover 1994). *In vitro* and *in vivo* studies shown that EGCG inhibits the chymotrypsin-like but not trypsin-like activity of the proteasome. Application of EGCG resulted in G0/G1 cell cycle arrest and accumulation of p27 and IκBα in LNCaP prostate cancer cells with both of which are targets for proteasomes (Nam et al. 2001). The difference of effective concentrations in cell-free systems (IC_{50} 0.09–0.2 mM) and in cell lines (IC_{50} 1–10 mM) suggests that EGCG may bind nonspecifically to proteins or other macromolecules in the cells, and therefore lower the effective concentration of EGCG at the active site of the protease and stability and cellular uptake of EGCG may also be an important factor. Inhibition of the chymotrypsin-like activity of the proteasome has been associated with induction of tumor cell apoptosis. The catalytic activities of the 20S/26S proteasome complex were inhibited by EGCG, resulting in intracellular accumulation of IκBα and subsequent inhibition of NFκB activation (Table 15.1; Khan et al. 2010).

Inhibition of Epigenetic Modifications

DNA methylation is a covalent biochemical modification, resulting in the addition of a methyl group to the fifth carbon position in the pyramidine ring of cytosine located in the CpG dinucleotides (Singh et al. 2010a). Hypermethylation often limits the accessibility of transcription factors to promoters, promote the methyl-CpG binding domain (MBD) binding, which results in recruitment of additional silencing-associated proteins, and ultimately, gene silencing (Volate et al. 2009). An estimated 60% of mammalian gene promoters contain CpG islands, many of these genes belongs to the house keeping category that are usually unmethylated and transcriptionally activate (Suzuki et al. 2008). It has been well known that CpG islands in certain genes, especially tumor suppressor genes, often become aberrantly hypermethylated during the development of cancer (Fig. 15.4a, b). Patterns of DNA

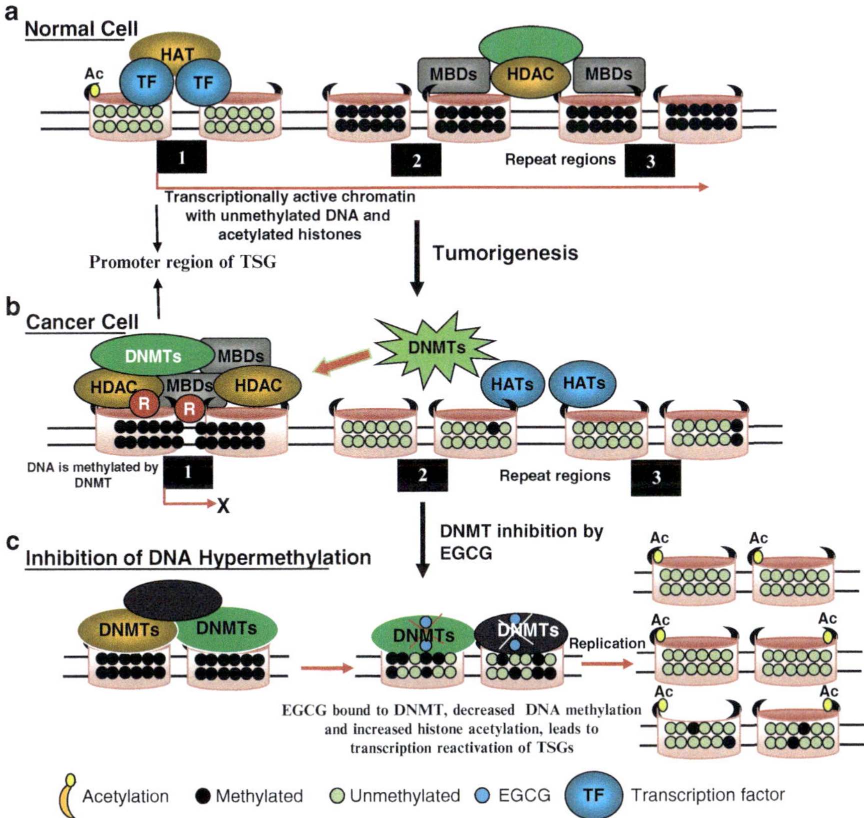

Fig. 15.4 Molecular modeling of the interaction between *EGCG* and *DNMT*. In normal cells (**a**), genes are generally unmethylated and packaged with acetylated histone proteins associated with *HAT* as well as basal transcription factor machinery. These epigenetic elements constitute an 'open' chromatin structure which favors transcription. In cancer cells, the same genes may become hypermethylated (**b**), and the methylated CpG sites are recognized by the methyl-binding proteins (*MBDs*), which are coupled with repressor (R) and histone deacetyltransferase (*HDAC*) proteins to remove the acetyl group from the histones, generating a tightly closed chromatin status to shut down gene expression. (**c**) DNMT activity is blocked by EGCG through forming hydrogen bonds with amino acids (Pro, Glu, Cys, Ser, and Arg) in the catalytic pocket of DNMT. Newly synthesized DNA strands are hemi-methylated after the first round of DNA replication and become progressively more demethylated after several rounds of replication due to the dilution effect. Using EGCG as a DNMT inhibitor, the silenced epigenetic modifications could be switched to an active status

methylation are established by the coordinated action of DNMTs and associated factors, such as the polycomb proteins, in the presence of S-adenosylmethionine (SAM) that serves as a methyl donor for methyl group. Demethylation of SAM results in the formation of *S*-adenosylhomocysteine (SAH), and evidences from clinical studies demonstrated that SAH is a potent inhibitor of DNMT (Plass and Soloway 2002).

EGCG can form hydrogen bonds with different residues in the catalytic pocket of DNMT, thus acting as a direct inhibitor of DNMT1 (Table 15.1; Fig. 15.4c). The inhibition of DNMT may prevent the methylation of the newly synthesized DNA strand, resulting in the reversal of the hypermethylation and the re-expression of the silenced genes (Fang et al. 2003). Finally, it has been shown that EGCG is also an efficient blocker of DHFR. Treatment of human colon cancers and prostate cancer cells with EGCG reactivated some methylation-silenced genes. Since then, several groups found similar *in vitro* results. Partial demethylation of hypermethylated RARb by EGCG was demonstrated in breast cancer cells such as MCF-7 and MDA-MB-231 (Nandakumar et al. 2011). EGCG partially reversed the hypermethylation status of the RECK gene and significantly enhanced the expression level of RECK mRNA in oral cancer cells. Repetitive elements such as p16, RARb, MAGE-A1, MAGE-B2 and Alu in T24, HT29, and PC3 cell lines for their DNA methylation levels and their mRNA expression levels using several demethylating agents. Recently, *in vivo* study showed that topical treatment of EGCG in hydrophilic cream inhibits UVB induced global DNA hypomethylation pattern in chronically UVB-exposed mice. Treatment with EGCG did induce neither induce DNA demethylation nor re-expression of the analyzed genes (Chuang et al. 2005). Treatment of MCF-7 breast cancer cells with EGCG resulted in activation of several genes and decrease in hTERT promoter methylation (Nandakumar et al. 2011; Sanchez-Huerta et al. 2011). EGCG acts through interaction with folic acid metabolism in cells, causing the inhibition of DNA synthesis and altering pattern of DNA methylation. EGCG was shown to affect various biologic pathways and inhibits DNMTs activity in human cancer cell lines (Fig. 15.4c). EGCG binds to DNMT1 and blocks the enzyme's active site. EGCG generates oxidizing agent H_2O_2 in a substantial amount, which is oxidized to DNMTs and other proteins might contribute to its inhibition of DNA methylation as well (Fang et al. 2003; Lee et al. 2005). The same action, however, may also cause oxidative damage and substantially increase its cytotoxicity. EGCG caused a concentration and time-dependent reversal of hypermethylation of TSGs such as p16, RAR, MGMT, and MLH1 genes in human esophageal cancer cells (Fang et al. 2007; Kato et al. 2008).

Inhibition of Dihydrofolate Reductase (DHFR) and Telomerase

DHFR, a methyl group shuttle required for the de novo synthesis of purines, thymidylic acid, and certain amino acids. Morrissette et al. (2010) reported that DHFR as a novel modulator of β-catenin and GSK3 signaling and raise several implications for clinical and can use for inflammatory disease and cancer. Recently, it was reported that EGCG acts as a potential inhibitor of DHFR (Lee et al. 2006). It exhibited kinetic characteristics of a slow tight binding inhibitor of 7, 8-dihydrofolate reduction with bovine liver DHFR (Ki 0.11 mM). The very low Ki value observed for bovine liver DHFR might be due to the fact that very low levels of the enzyme were used in the assay, and the inhibition was due to the strong binding activity of EGCG to the enzyme (a slow tight binding inhibitor, as reported), not necessarily by binding to the active site (Table 15.1; Navarro-Martinez et al. 2005). But EGCG acted as a classic reversible competitive inhibitor with chicken liver DHFR with a much larger Ki (10.3 mM). Folate depletion increased the sensitivity of these cell lines to the antifolate activities of EGCG.

Telomerase is important for maintaining the telomere nuclear protein endcaps of the chromosome and it has been shown to be overexpressed in many human cancers (Artandi 2002; Sharpless and DePinho 2004). In an animal study, treatment of mice bearing telomerase-positive colon cancer xenografts (HCT-L2) with 1.2 mg of EGCG per day for 80 days resulted in a 50% inhibition in tumor size (Naasani et al. 1998). Whereas mice bearing telomerase-negative tumors of the same parent cell line (HCT-S2R) were unresponsive to EGCG treatment. This interesting line of observation should be extended into other cell lines. Long-term treatment with EGCG (5–10 mM) was reported to inhibit telomerase and induce cell senescence (Naasani et al. 1998). At high nanomolar to low micromolar concentrations of EGCG inhibited telomerase activity in cell-free systems at neutral pH. The authors were concluded that EGCG decomposes by auto-oxidation to form a galloyl radical, which can covalently modify telomerase activity (Ju et al. 2005).

Inhibition of Angiogenesis

Angiogenesis is a complex event which requires endothelial cell sprouting, lumen formation, tubulogenesis and is regulated by the coordinated action of different transcription factors (Folkman 2002). Their interaction leads to endothelial cell differentiation and acquisition of arterial, venous and lymphatic properties. FOXO transcription factors play a crucial role in the regulation of tissue homeostasis in organs such as the pancreas and the ovaries and complex diseases such as diabetes and cancer (Nakae et al. 2002; Shankar et al. 2008a). We have recently shown that EGCG inhibits angiogenesis by enhancing FOXO transcriptional activity (Shankar et al. 2008a). Inhibition of AKT and MEK kinases synergistically induced FOXO transcriptional activity, which was further enhanced in the presence of EGCG. Phosphorylation deficient mutants of FOXO induced FOXO transcriptional activity, inhibited HUVEC cell migration and capillary tube formation. Inhibition of FOXO phosphorylation also enhanced antiangiogenic effects of EGCG through transcriptional activation of FOXO (Shankar et al. 2008a). Authors concluded that the activation of FOXO transcription factors through inhibition of these two pathways may have physiological significance in management of diabetic retinopathy, rheumatoid arthritis, psoriasis, cardiovascular diseases and cancer. Recently, Bartholome et al. (2010) reported that EGCG at 1 μM stimulated FOXO transcription factor nuclear accumulation and DNA binding activity. EGCG decreases ET-1 expression and secretion from endothelial cells, in part, via Akt- and AMPK-stimulated FOXO1 regulation of the ET-1 promoter. These findings may be relevant to beneficial cardiovascular actions of green tea (Reiter et al. 2010).

Moreover, EGCG exerts its insulin mimetic effects at least in part by phosphorylation of the FOXOs through a mechanism that is similar but not identical to insulin and IGF-1 induced FOXO phosphorylation (Anton et al. 2007).

Modulation of miRNA Expression

Small molecules known as MicroRNAs are a contemporary class of noncoding endogenous RNA molecules, generating great excitement in the clinical and scientific communities (Wang et al. 2010). miRNAs have been recently discovered as key regulators of gene expression by controlling the translation of a specific type of RNA called messenger RNA which relays the genetic instructions for making proteins (Croce and Calin 2005). Previous research has indicated that miRNAs are express in a tissue-specific manner and control a wide spectrum of biological processes including cell proliferation, apoptosis and differentiation. Although miRNA are vital to normal cell physiology, aberrant expression of these small non-coding RNAs has been linked to carcinogenesis (Croce 2009; Croce and Calin 2005). The recent discovery that miRNA expression is frequently dysregulated in cancer has uncovered an entirely new repertoire of molecular factors upstream of gene expression, which warrants extensive investigation to further elucidate their precise role in malignancy (Galluzzi et al. 2010; Kotani et al. 2009). The influence of miRNA on the epigenetic machinery and the reciprocal epigenetic regulation of miRNA expression suggest that its aberrant expression during carcinogenesis has an important implication for global regulation of cancer. Additionally, interaction among various components of the epigenetic machinery re-emphasizes the integrated nature of epigenetic mechanisms involved in the maintenance of global gene expression patterns in mammals. Treatment of human hepatocellular carcinoma HepG2 cells with EGCG has been recently found to inhibit the expression of oncogenic miRNA and induce level of tumor suppressive miRNAs (Fig. 15.5). Treatment of HepG2 with EGCG resulted in the expressions of 61 miRNAs. miR-16, one of the miRNAs up-regulated by EGCG, is known to regulate the anti-apoptotic protein Bcl-2, and interestingly EGCG treatment induced apoptosis and downregulated Bcl-2 in HepG2 cells (Tsang and Kwok 2010). Transfection with anti-miR-16 inhibitor suppressed miR-16 expression and counteracted the EGCG effects on Bcl-2 down-regulation and also induction of apoptosis in cells.

Miscellaneous Effects

EGCG was also shown to affect MMPs directly and indirectly. EGCG also inhibited the activation of MMPs by MT1-MMP (Oku et al. 2003). EGCG increased the expression of the tissue inhibitor of MMPs (TIMP1 and 2) at even lower concentrations (~1 μM), which provides an additional mechanism to suppress the

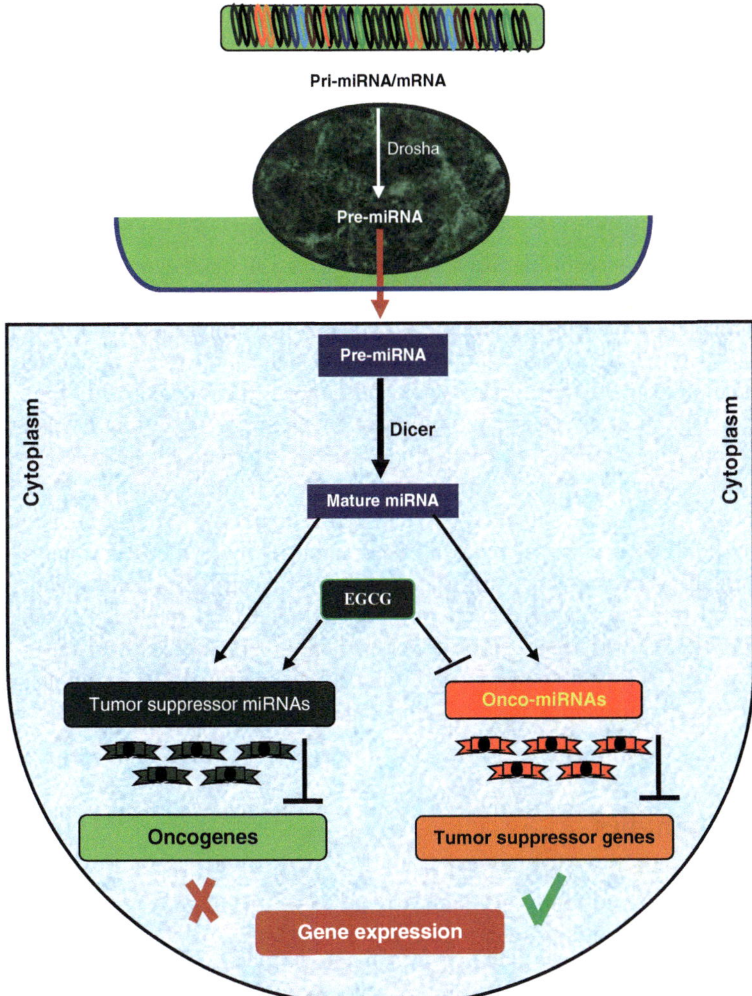

Fig. 15.5 Regulation of microRNA (miRNA) expression by EGCG. miRNA are transcribed in the nucleus into pri-miRNA (*primary miRNA*) which is further cleaved by Drosha into precursor miRNA (*pre-miRNA*). Pre-miRNA is exported from nucleus to the cytoplasm and further processed by Dicer into miRNA duplex. Single strand of miRNA duplex (also called mature miRNA) leads this complex to mRNA cleavage or translation repression, which is dependent on miRNA:mRNA complementarity. Dependent on various factors, miRNA can have either an oncogenic role (called *oncomiRNAs*) if the target mRNA is a tumor suppressor gene, or a tumor suppressive role (*tumor-suppressor miRNAs*) if the target molecule is an oncogene. EGCG can impact on expression level of miRNAs and participate in gene expression regulation

activity of MMPs. The activities of secreted MMP2 and MMP9 were inhibited by EGCG with IC_{50} values of 8–13 μM (Oku et al. 2003). These activities may contribute to the reported inhibition of metastasis and invasion following treatment of tumor-bearing mice with EGCG. Most recently, in several human colon carcinoma cell lines, EGCG was found to inhibit the activity of topoisomerase I at 3–17 μM concentration. By comparison, EGCG at concentrations up to 550 μM did not inhibit topoisomerase II activity (Berger et al. 2001). This is an interesting mechanism of action for EGCG given the relatively low concentrations necessary for inhibition and the correlation of topoisomerase I inhibition with phenomena, such as DNA damage, cell cycle arrest, and induction of apoptosis (Berger et al. 2001).

The uPA is a trypsin-like protease that converts the zymogen plasminogen into active plasmin. It is highly expressed in human cancer and has the ability to prevent apoptosis, stimulate angiogenesis, mitogenesis, cell migration, and to modulate cell adhesion (Barber et al. 2004). uPA, one of the hydrolases implicated in the degradation of the extracellular matrix and tumor invasion, is directly inhibited by EGCG (Jankun et al. 1997). Inhibition of uPA can decrease tumor size or even cause complete remission of cancers in mice. EGCG-induced suppression of uPA promoter activity as well as expression appears to be mediated by blocking ERK and p38 MAP kinase, but not JNK and AKT. Jankun et al. (1997) showed that EGCG binds to urokinase, blocking His^{57} and Ser^{195} of the uPA catalytic triad, and extending toward Arg^{35} from a positively charged loop of uPA. Thus, it was suggested that the cancer prevention action of EGCG is mediated by inhibition of uPA. EGCG was found to be a potent inhibitor of uPA expression in human fibrosarcoma HT 1,080 cells. In addition, EGCG inhibited uPA promoter activity and also destabilized uPA mRNA (Kim et al. 2004a).

Clinical Studies

Limited data are currently available from EGCG chemoprevention trials. EGCG offers several potential clinical advantages compared to other traditional cancer drugs. In contrast, EGCG is globally available as tea, is inexpensive to isolate, and can be administered orally (Sartippour et al. 2002). While traditional cancer drugs often destroy some healthy cells along with cancerous cells (Ahn et al. 2003a). EGCG appears to target biochemical and genetic functions unique to cancer cells (Hastak et al. 2003). Some of the anticarcinogenic agents currently in use have toxic adverse effects, but data from clinical trials reported to date suggest that EGCG has a very acceptable safety profile (Hastak et al. 2003). These benefits support further development of EGCG as a potentially useful anticarcinogenic agent. A prospective cohort study with over 8,000 individuals revealed that the daily consumption of green tea resulted in delayed cancer onset and a follow-up study of breast cancer patients found that stages I and II breast cancer patients experienced a lower recurrence rate and longer disease free period (Fujiki et al. 1999). Moreover, EGCG delivered in the form of capsule (200 mg p.o.) for 12 weeks has been reported to be effective in the patients with human papilloma virus–infected cervical lesions

(Ahn et al. 2003b). The positive results observed in phase II and phase III clinical trials along with exciting preclinical results indicate that ways and means to take EGCG "from bench to real-life situations" are on the horizon.

Summary, Conclusion and Future Prospects

Polyphenolic substances that are derived from the plants provide a new insight in prevention and therapy of cancer. The mechanisms of action of several dietary chemopreventive agents have gained considerable attention in cancer research. There is extensive research going on in elucidating the molecular mechanisms of cancer chemoprevention by green tea EGCG. Several mechanisms to explain the chemopreventive potentials of EGCG have been presented (Fig. 15.6), among which its effect to target specific cell signaling pathways have received considerable attention for regulating cellular proliferation and apoptosis. The diversified effects of EGCG may explain its broad pharmacologic activities in modulating cellular signaling pathways in cells. EGCG, in addition to other mechanisms, at human achievable dose, is known to activate cell death signals and induce apoptosis in precancerous or cancer cells, resulting in the inhibition of tumor development and/or progression (Fig. 15.6). In cancer cells, EGCG also causes inhibition of the activity of specific receptor tyrosine kinases and related downstream pathways of signal transduction.

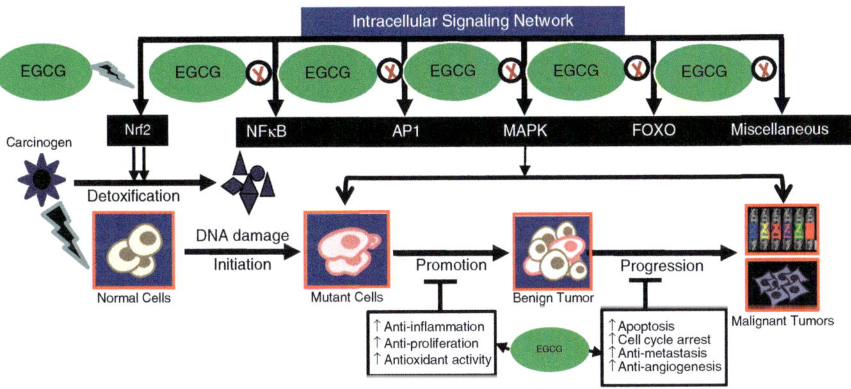

Fig. 15.6 Possible molecular targets for chemopreventive effects of EGCG on multi-stage carcinogenesis. Targeted suppression of inappropriately activated *NF-κB* or *AP-1* can ameliorate proinflammatory, proliferative, invasive, and metastastic signals. EGCG inhibits the activation of NF-κB, AP-1 and other proliferative signal mediators and activates *FOXO* transcription, which may account for its anti-proliferative, proapoptotic, antimetastatic and anti-angiogenic activities in cancer cells as well as anti-tumor promotional effects. In addition, EGCG stimulates the detoxification process via Nrf2-mediated de novo synthesis of antioxidant or phase-II enzymes while inhibiting metabolic activation of carcinogens, induces antioxidant defense networks, thereby interfering with the tumor initiation

Most modern medicines currently available for treating cancers are very expensive, toxic, and less effective in treating the disease. Thus, one must investigate further in detail the EGCG derived from green tea, described traditionally, for the prevention and treatment of cancer and other diseases. The understanding of the cell signaling pathways and the molecular events leading to carcinogenesis will provide more insight into the identification and development of potent chemopreventive/chemotherapeutic agents that specifically target these pathways. Future studies from *in vitro* systems should be integrated with studies *in vivo*, especially in ongoing clinical trials, to evaluate the applicability of these mechanisms in cancer prevention in humans. To fully elucidate the molecular mechanisms of action of EGCG with existing therapy in future studies, more in-depth *in vitro* and *in vivo* experiments are needed.

Acknowledgements We thank our lab members for critical reading of the manuscript. This work was supported in part by the grants from the National Institutes of Health (R01CA125262, RO1CA114469 and RO1CA125262-02S1) and Kansas Bioscience Authority.

References

Adams J, Kauffman M (2004) Development of the proteasome inhibitor Velcade (Bortezomib). Cancer Invest 22:304–311

Adhami VM, Siddiqui IA, Ahmad N, Gupta S, Mukhtar H (2004) Oral consumption of green tea polyphenols inhibits insulin-like growth factor-I-induced signaling in an autochthonous mouse model of prostate cancer. Cancer Res 64:8715–8722

Afaq F, Adhami VM, Ahmad N, Mukhtar H (2003a) Inhibition of ultraviolet B-mediated activation of nuclear factor kappaB in normal human epidermal keratinocytes by green tea Constituent (-)-epigallocatechin-3-gallate. Oncogene 22:1035–1044

Afaq F, Ahmad N, Mukhtar H (2003b) Suppression of UVB-induced phosphorylation of mitogen-activated protein kinases and nuclear factor kappa B by green tea polyphenol in SKH-1 hairless mice. Oncogene 22:9254–9264

Aggarwal BB, Shishodia S (2006) Molecular targets of dietary agents for prevention and therapy of cancer. Biochem Pharmacol 71:1397–1421

Aggarwal BB, Bhardwaj A, Aggarwal RS, Seeram NP, Shishodia S, Takada Y (2004) Role of resveratrol in prevention and therapy of cancer: preclinical and clinical studies. Anticancer Res 24:2783–2840

Ahmad N, Feyes DK, Nieminen AL, Agarwal R, Mukhtar H (1997) Green tea constituent epigallocatechin-3-gallate and induction of apoptosis and cell cycle arrest in human carcinoma cells. J Natl Cancer Inst 89:1881–1886

Ahmad N, Adhami VM, Gupta S, Cheng P, Mukhtar H (2002) Role of the retinoblastoma (pRb)-E2F/DP pathway in cancer chemopreventive effects of green tea polyphenol epigallocatechin-3-gallate. Arch Biochem Biophys 398:125–131

Ahmed S (2010) Green tea polyphenol epigallocatechin 3-gallate in arthritis: progress and promise. Arthritis Res Ther 12:208

Ahmed S, Wang N, Lalonde M, Goldberg VM, Haqqi TM (2004) Green tea polyphenol epigallocatechin-3-gallate (EGCG) differentially inhibits interleukin-1 beta-induced expression of matrix metalloproteinase-1 and -13 in human chondrocytes. J Pharmacol Exp Ther 308:767–773

Ahn WS, Huh SW, Bae SM, Lee IP, Lee JM, Namkoong SE, Kim CK, Sin JI (2003a) A major constituent of green tea, EGCG, inhibits the growth of a human cervical cancer cell line, CaSki cells, through apoptosis, G(1) arrest, and regulation of gene expression. DNA Cell Biol 22:217–224

Ahn WS, Yoo J, Huh SW, Kim CK, Lee JM, Namkoong SE, Bae SM, Lee IP (2003b) Protective effects of green tea extracts (polyphenon E and EGCG) on human cervical lesions. Eur J Cancer Prev 12:383–390

Anton S, Melville L, Rena G (2007) Epigallocatechin gallate (EGCG) mimics insulin action on the transcription factor FOXO1a and elicits cellular responses in the presence and absence of insulin. Cell Signal 19:378–383

Artandi SE (2002) Telomere shortening and cell fates in mouse models of neoplasia. Trends Mol Med 8:44–47

Babich H, Zuckerbraun HL, Weinerman SM (2007) In vitro cytotoxicity of (-)-catechin gallate, a minor polyphenol in green tea. Toxicol Lett 171:171–180

Babu PV, Sabitha KE, Shyamaladevi CS (2006) Therapeutic effect of green tea extract on oxidative stress in aorta and heart of streptozotocin diabetic rats. Chem Biol Interact 162:114–120

Bakiri L, Lallemand D, Bossy-Wetzel E, Yaniv M (2000) Cell cycle-dependent variations in c-Jun and JunB phosphorylation: a role in the control of cyclin D1 expression. EMBO J 19:2056–2068

Barber CG, Dickinson RP, Fish PV (2004) Selective urokinase-type plasminogen activator (uPA) inhibitors. Part 3: 1-isoquinolinylguanidines. Bioorg Med Chem Lett 14:3227–3230

Bartholome A, Kampkotter A, Tanner S, Sies H, Klotz LO (2010) Epigallocatechin gallate-induced modulation of FoxO signaling in mammalian cells and C. elegans: FoxO stimulation is masked via PI3K/Akt activation by hydrogen peroxide formed in cell culture. Arch Biochem Biophys 501:58–64

Berger SJ, Gupta S, Belfi CA, Gosky DM, Mukhtar H (2001) Green tea constituent (–)-epigallocatechin-3-gallate inhibits topoisomerase I activity in human colon carcinoma cells. Biochem Biophys Res Commun 288:101–105

Bettuzzi S, Brausi M, Rizzi F, Castagnetti G, Peracchia G, Corti A (2006) Chemoprevention of human prostate cancer by oral administration of green tea catechins in volunteers with high-grade prostate intraepithelial neoplasia: a preliminary report from a one-year proof-of-principle study. Cancer Res 66:1234–1240

Campbell KJ, O'Shea JM, Perkins ND (2006) Differential regulation of NF-kappaB activation and function by topoisomerase II inhibitors. BMC Cancer 6:101

Chacko SM, Thambi PT, Kuttan R, Nishigaki I (2010) Beneficial effects of green tea: a literature review. Chin Med 5:13

Chan HY, Wang H, Tsang DS, Chen ZY, Leung LK (2003) Screening of chemopreventive tea polyphenols against PAH genotoxicity in breast cancer cells by a XRE-luciferase reporter construct. Nutr Cancer 46:93–100

Chandra S, De Mejia GE (2004) Polyphenolic compounds, antioxidant capacity, and quinone reductase activity of an aqueous extract of Ardisia compressa in comparison to mate (Ilex paraguariensis) and green (Camellia sinensis) teas. J Agric Food Chem 52:3583–3589

Chen Z, Zhu QY, Tsang D, Huang Y (2001) Degradation of green tea catechins in tea drinks. J Agric Food Chem 49:477–482

Chen Q, Ganapathy S, Singh KP, Shankar S, Srivastava RK (2010a) Resveratrol induces growth arrest and apoptosis through activation of FOXO transcription factors in prostate cancer cells. PLoS One 5:e15288

Chen X, Lu W, Zheng Y, Gu K, Chen Z, Zheng W, Shu XO (2010b) Exercise, tea consumption, and depression among breast cancer survivors. J Clin Oncol 28:991–998

Chen NG, Lu CC, Lin YH, Shen WC, Lai CH, Ho YJ, Chung JG, Lin TH, Lin YC, Yang JS (2011) Proteomic approaches to study epigallocatechin gallate-provoked apoptosis of TSGH-8301 human urinary bladder carcinoma cells: roles of AKT and heat shock protein 27-modulated intrinsic apoptotic pathways. Oncol Rep 26:939–947

Choi JH, Rhee IK, Park KY, Kim JK, Rhee SJ (2003) Action of green tea catechin on bone metabolic disorder in chronic cadmium-poisoned rats. Life Sci 73:1479–1489

Chuang JC, Yoo CB, Kwan JM, Li TW, Liang G, Yang AS, Jones PA (2005) Comparison of biological effects of non-nucleoside DNA methylation inhibitors versus 5-aza-2′-deoxycytidine. Mol Cancer Ther 4:1515–1520

Ciechanover A (1994) The ubiquitin-proteasome proteolytic pathway. Cell 79:13–21

Croce CM (2009) Causes and consequences of microRNA dysregulation in cancer. Nat Rev Genet 10:704–714

Croce CM, Calin GA (2005) miRNAs, cancer, and stem cell division. Cell 122:6–7

Dong Z, Ma W, Huang C, Yang CS (1997) Inhibition of tumor promoter-induced activator protein 1 activation and cell transformation by tea polyphenols, (-)-epigallocatechin gallate, and theaflavins. Cancer Res 57:4414–4419

Eferl R, Wagner EF (2003) AP-1: a double-edged sword in tumorigenesis. Nat Rev Cancer 3:859–868

Fang MZ, Wang Y, Ai N, Hou Z, Sun Y, Lu H, Welsh W, Yang CS (2003) Tea polyphenol (-)-epigallocatechin-3-gallate inhibits DNA methyltransferase and reactivates methylation-silenced genes in cancer cell lines. Cancer Res 63:7563–7570

Fang JY, Tsai TH, Lin YY, Wong WW, Wang MN, Huang JF (2007) Transdermal delivery of tea catechins and theophylline enhanced by terpenes: a mechanistic study. Biol Pharm Bull 30:343–349

Folkman J (2002) Role of angiogenesis in tumor growth and metastasis. Semin Oncol 29:15–18

Fujiki H, Suganuma M, Okabe S, Sueoka E, Suga K, Imai K, Nakachi K, Kimura S (1999) Mechanistic findings of green tea as cancer preventive for humans. Proc Soc Exp Biol Med 220:225–228

Fujiki H, Suganuma M, Okabe S, Sueoka E, Sueoka N, Fujimoto N, Goto Y, Matsuyama S, Imai K, Nakachi K (2001) Cancer prevention with green tea and monitoring by a new biomarker, hnRNP B1. Mutat Res 480–481:299–304

Fujita Y, Yamane T, Tanaka M, Kuwata K, Okuzumi J, Takahashi T, Fujiki H, Okuda T (1989) Inhibitory effect of (-)-epigallocatechin gallate on carcinogenesis with N-ethyl-N′-nitro-N-nitrosoguanidine in mouse duodenum. Jpn J Cancer Res 80:503–505

Galluzzi L, Morselli E, Vitale I, Kepp O, Senovilla L, Criollo A, Servant N, Paccard C, Hupe P, Robert T, Ripoche H, Lazar V, Harel-Bellan A, Dessen P, Barillot E, Kroemer G (2010) miR-181a and miR-630 regulate cisplatin-induced cancer cell death. Cancer Res 70:1793–1803

Gerhauser C, Klimo K, Heiss E, Neumann I, Gamal-Eldeen A, Knauft J, Liu GY, Sitthimonchai S, Frank N (2003) Mechanism-based in vitro screening of potential cancer chemopreventive agents. Mutat Res 523–524:163–172

Givant-Horwitz V, Davidson B, Reich R (2004) Laminin-induced signaling in tumor cells: the role of the M(r) 67,000 laminin receptor. Cancer Res 64:3572–3579

Guo S, Yang S, Taylor C, Sonenshein GE (2005) Green tea polyphenol epigallocatechin-3 gallate (EGCG) affects gene expression of breast cancer cells transformed by the carcinogen 7,12-dimethylbenz[a]anthracene. J Nutr 135:2978S–2986S

Gupta S, Hussain T, Mukhtar H (2003) Molecular pathway for (-)-epigallocatechin-3-gallate-induced cell cycle arrest and apoptosis of human prostate carcinoma cells. Arch Biochem Biophys 410:177–185

Gupta S, Hastak K, Afaq F, Ahmad N, Mukhtar H (2004) Essential role of caspases in epigallocatechin-3-gallate-mediated inhibition of nuclear factor kappa B and induction of apoptosis. Oncogene 23:2507–2522

Hastak K, Gupta S, Ahmad N, Agarwal MK, Agarwal ML, Mukhtar H (2003) Role of p53 and NF-kappaB in epigallocatechin-3-gallate-induced apoptosis of LNCaP cells. Oncogene 22:4851–4859

Herbst RS (2004) Review of epidermal growth factor receptor biology. Int J Radiat Oncol Biol Phys 59:21–26

Hibasami H, Achiwa Y, Fujikawa T, Komiya T (1996) Induction of programmed cell death (apoptosis) in human lymphoid leukemia cells by catechin compounds. Anticancer Res 16:1943–1946

Higdon JV, Frei B (2003) Tea catechins and polyphenols: health effects, metabolism, and antioxidant functions. Crit Rev Food Sci Nutr 43:89–143

Hou Z, Lambert JD, Chin KV, Yang CS (2004) Effects of tea polyphenols on signal transduction pathways related to cancer chemoprevention. Mutat Res 555:3–19

Hsu YC, Liou YM (2011) The anti-cancer effects of (-)-epigalocathine-3-gallate on the signaling pathways associated with membrane receptors in MCF-7 cells. J Cell Physiol 226:2721–2730

Hu J, Zhou D, Chen Y (2009) Preparation and antioxidant activity of green tea extract enriched in epigallocatechin (EGC) and epigallocatechin gallate (EGCG). J Agric Food Chem 57:1349–1353

Huang CC, Wu WB, Fang JY, Chiang HS, Chen SK, Chen BH, Chen YT, Hung CF (2007) (-)-Epicatechin-3-gallate, a green tea polyphenol is a potent agent against UVB-induced damage in HaCaT keratinocytes. Molecules 12:1845–1858

Hussain T, Gupta S, Adhami VM, Mukhtar H (2005) Green tea constituent epigallocatechin-3-gallate selectively inhibits COX-2 without affecting COX-1 expression in human prostate carcinoma cells. Int J Cancer 113:660–669

Jankun J, Selman SH, Swiercz R, Skrzypczak-Jankun E (1997) Why drinking green tea could prevent cancer. Nature 387:561

Jeong WS, Kim IW, Hu R, Kong AN (2004) Modulatory properties of various natural chemopreventive agents on the activation of NF-kappaB signaling pathway. Pharm Res 21:661–670

Ju J, Hong J, Zhou JN, Pan Z, Bose M, Liao J, Yang GY, Liu YY, Hou Z, Lin Y, Ma J, Shih WJ, Carothers AM, Yang CS (2005) Inhibition of intestinal tumorigenesis in Apcmin/+ mice by (-)-epigallocatechin-3-gallate, the major catechin in green tea. Cancer Res 65:10623–10631

Katiyar SK, Mukhtar H (1996) Tea consumption and cancer. World Rev Nutr Diet 79:154–184

Katiyar SK, Agarwal R, Zaim MT, Mukhtar H (1993) Protection against N-nitrosodiethylamine and benzo[a]pyrene-induced forestomach and lung tumorigenesis in A/J mice by green tea. Carcinogenesis 14:849–855

Kato K, Long NK, Makita H, Toida M, Yamashita T, Hatakeyama D, Hara A, Mori H, Shibata T (2008) Effects of green tea polyphenol on methylation status of RECK gene and cancer cell invasion in oral squamous cell carcinoma cells. Br J Cancer 99:647–654

Khafif A, Schantz SP, Chou TC, Edelstein D, Sacks PG (1998) Quantitation of chemopreventive synergism between (-)-epigallocatechin-3-gallate and curcumin in normal, premalignant and malignant human oral epithelial cells. Carcinogenesis 19:419–424

Khan N, Mukhtar H (2010) Cancer and metastasis: prevention and treatment by green tea. Cancer Metastasis Rev 29:435–445

Khan N, Afaq F, Saleem M, Ahmad N, Mukhtar H (2006) Targeting multiple signaling pathways by green tea polyphenol (-)-epigallocatechin-3-gallate. Cancer Res 66:2500–2505

Khan N, Adhami VM, Mukhtar H (2010) Apoptosis by dietary agents for prevention and treatment of prostate cancer. Endocr Relat Cancer 17:R39–R52

Kim HJ, Yum KS, Sung JH, Rhie DJ, Kim MJ, Min DS, Hahn SJ, Kim MS, Jo YH, Yoon SH (2004a) Epigallocatechin-3-gallate increases intracellular [Ca2+] in U87 cells mainly by influx of extracellular Ca2+ and partly by release of intracellular stores. Naunyn Schmiedebergs Arch Pharmacol 369:260–267

Kim HS, Kim MH, Jeong M, Hwang YS, Lim SH, Shin BA, Ahn BW, Jung YD (2004b) EGCG blocks tumor promoter-induced MMP-9 expression via suppression of MAPK and AP-1 activation in human gastric AGS cells. Anticancer Res 24:747–753

Kotani A, Ha D, Hsieh J, Rao PK, Schotte D, den Boer ML, Armstrong SA, Lodish HF (2009) miR-128b is a potent glucocorticoid sensitizer in MLL-AF4 acute lymphocytic leukemia cells and exerts cooperative effects with miR-221. Blood 114:4169–4178

Kumaran G, Clamp AR, Jayson GC (2008) Angiogenesis as a therapeutic target in cancer. Clin Med 8:455–458

Kundu JK, Na HK, Chun KS, Kim YK, Lee SJ, Lee SS, Lee OS, Sim YC, Surh YJ (2003) Inhibition of phorbol ester-induced COX-2 expression by epigallocatechin gallate in mouse skin and cultured human mammary epithelial cells. J Nutr 133:3805S–3810S

Lambert JD, Elias RJ (2010) The antioxidant and pro-oxidant activities of green tea polyphenols: a role in cancer prevention. Arch Biochem Biophys 501:65–72

Lambert JD, Yang CS (2003) Mechanisms of cancer prevention by tea constituents. J Nutr 133:3262S–3267S

Lambert JD, Rice JE, Hong J, Hou Z, Yang CS (2005) Synthesis and biological activity of the tea catechin metabolites, M4 and M6 and their methoxy-derivatives. Bioorg Med Chem Lett 15:873–876

Lee MJ, Prabhu S, Meng X, Li C, Yang CS (2000) An improved method for the determination of green and black tea polyphenols in biomatrices by high-performance liquid chromatography with coulometric array detection. Anal Biochem 279:164–169

Lee KM, Yeo M, Choue JS, Jin JH, Park SJ, Cheong JY, Lee KJ, Kim JH, Hahm KB (2004) Protective mechanism of epigallocatechin-3-gallate against Helicobacter pylori-induced gastric epithelial cytotoxicity via the blockage of TLR-4 signaling. Helicobacter 9:632–642

Lee WJ, Shim JY, Zhu BT (2005) Mechanisms for the inhibition of DNA methyltransferases by tea catechins and bioflavonoids. Mol Pharmacol 68:1018–1030

Lee JH, Shim JS, Lee JS, Kim JK, Yang IS, Chung MS, Kim KH (2006) Inhibition of pathogenic bacterial adhesion by acidic polysaccharide from green tea (Camellia sinensis). J Agric Food Chem 54:8717–8723

Lim YC, Cha YY (2011) Epigallocatechin-3-gallate induces growth inhibition and apoptosis of human anaplastic thyroid carcinoma cells through suppression of EGFR/ERK pathway and cyclin B1/CDK1 complex. J Surg Oncol 104(7):776–780

Lin JK (2002) Cancer chemoprevention by tea polyphenols through modulating signal transduction pathways. Arch Pharm Res 25:561–571

Lin YL, Lin JK (1997) (-)-Epigallocatechin-3-gallate blocks the induction of nitric oxide synthase by down-regulating lipopolysaccharide-induced activity of transcription factor nuclear factor-kappaB. Mol Pharmacol 52:465–472

Lin SM, Wang SW, Ho SC, Tang YL (2010) Protective effect of green tea (-)-epigallocatechin-3-gallate against the monoamine oxidase B enzyme activity increase in adult rat brains. Nutrition 26:1195–1200

Liu TT, Liang NS, Li Y, Yang F, Lu Y, Meng ZQ, Zhang LS (2003) Effects of long-term tea polyphenols consumption on hepatic microsomal drug-metabolizing enzymes and liver function in Wistar rats. World J Gastroenterol 9:2742–2744

Lopez-Lazaro M, Calderon-Montano JM, Burgos-Moron E, Austin CA (2011) Green tea constituents (-)-epigallocatechin-3-gallate (EGCG) and gallic acid induce topoisomerase I- and topoisomerase II-DNA complexes in cells mediated by pyrogallol-induced hydrogen peroxide. Mutagenesis 26(4):489–498

Lu YP, Lou YR, Lin Y, Shih WJ, Huang MT, Yang CS, Conney AH (2001) Inhibitory effects of orally administered green tea, black tea, and caffeine on skin carcinogenesis in mice previously treated with ultraviolet B light (high-risk mice): relationship to decreased tissue fat. Cancer Res 61:5002–5009

Majima T, Tsutsumi M, Nishino H, Tsunoda T, Konishi Y (1998) Inhibitory effects of beta-carotene, palm carotene, and green tea polyphenols on pancreatic carcinogenesis initiated by N-nitorsobis(2-oxopropyl)amine in Syrian golden hamsters. Pancreas 16:13–18

Maliakal PP, Coville PF, Wanwimolruk S (2001) Tea consumption modulates hepatic drug metabolizing enzymes in Wistar rats. J Pharm Pharmacol 53:569–577

Manson MM (2003) Cancer prevention – the potential for diet to modulate molecular signalling. Trends Mol Med 9:11–18

Masamune A, Kikuta K, Satoh M, Suzuki N, Shimosegawa T (2005) Green tea polyphenol epigallocatechin-3-gallate blocks PDGF-induced proliferation and migration of rat pancreatic stellate cells. World J Gastroenterol 11:3368–3374

Masuda M, Suzui M, Weinstein IB (2001) Effects of epigallocatechin-3-gallate on growth, epidermal growth factor receptor signaling pathways, gene expression, and chemosensitivity in human head and neck squamous cell carcinoma cell lines. Clin Cancer Res 7:4220–4229

Masuda M, Suzui M, Lim JT, Deguchi A, Soh JW, Weinstein IB (2002) Epigallocatechin-3-gallate decreases VEGF production in head and neck and breast carcinoma cells by inhibiting EGFR-related pathways of signal transduction. J Exp Ther Oncol 2:350–359

Masuda M, Suzui M, Lim JT, Weinstein IB (2003) Epigallocatechin-3-gallate inhibits activation of HER-2/neu and downstream signaling pathways in human head and neck and breast carcinoma cells. Clin Cancer Res 9:3486–3491

Masuda M, Wakasaki T, Toh S, Shimizu M, Adachi S (2011) Chemoprevention of head and neck cancer by green tea extract: EGCG-the role of EGFR signaling and "Lipid Raft". J Oncol 2011:540148

Meeran SM, Mantena SK, Elmets CA, Katiyar SK (2006) (-)-Epigallocatechin-3-gallate prevents photocarcinogenesis in mice through interleukin-12-dependent DNA repair. Cancer Res 66:5512–5520

Milligan SA, Burke P, Coleman DT, Bigelow RL, Steffan JJ, Carroll JL, Williams BJ, Cardelli JA (2009) The green tea polyphenol EGCG potentiates the antiproliferative activity of c-Met and epidermal growth factor receptor inhibitors in non-small cell lung cancer cells. Clin Cancer Res 15:4885–4894

Morissette M, Samadi P, Hadj Tahar A, Belanger N, Di Paolo T (2010) Striatal Akt/GSK3 signaling pathway in the development of L-Dopa-induced dyskinesias in MPTP monkeys. Prog Neuropsychopharmacol Biol Psychiatry 34:446–454

Mukhtar H, Ahmad N (2000) Tea polyphenols: prevention of cancer and optimizing health. Am J Clin Nutr 71:1698S–1702S, discussion 1703S–1694S

Murakami C, Hirakawa Y, Inui H, Nakano Y, Yoshida H (2002) Effect of tea catechins on cellular lipid peroxidation and cytotoxicity in HepG2 cells. Biosci Biotechnol Biochem 66:1559–1562

Muzolf-Panek M, Gliszczynska-Swiglo A, de Haan L, Aarts JM, Szymusiak H, Vervoort JM, Tyrakowska B, Rietjens IM (2008) Role of catechin quinones in the induction of EpRE-mediated gene expression. Chem Res Toxicol 21:2352–2360

Naasani I, Seimiya H, Tsuruo T (1998) Telomerase inhibition, telomere shortening, and senescence of cancer cells by tea catechins. Biochem Biophys Res Commun 249:391–396

Nakae J, Biggs WH 3rd, Kitamura T, Cavenee WK, Wright CV, Arden KC, Accili D (2002) Regulation of insulin action and pancreatic beta-cell function by mutated alleles of the gene encoding forkhead transcription factor Foxo1. Nat Genet 32:245–253

Nam S, Smith DM, Dou QP (2001) Ester bond-containing tea polyphenols potently inhibit proteasome activity in vitro and in vivo. J Biol Chem 276:13322–13330

Nandakumar V, Vaid M, Katiyar SK (2011) (-)-Epigallocatechin-3-gallate reactivates silenced tumor suppressor genes, Cip1/p21 and p16INK4a, by reducing DNA methylation and increasing histones acetylation in human skin cancer cells. Carcinogenesis 32(4):537–544

Narisawa T, Fukaura Y (1993) A very low dose of green tea polyphenols in drinking water prevents N-methyl-N-nitrosourea-induced colon carcinogenesis in F344 rats. Jpn J Cancer Res 84:1007–1009

Navarro-Martinez MD, Navarro-Peran E, Cabezas-Herrera J, Ruiz-Gomez J, Garcia-Canovas F, Rodriguez-Lopez JN (2005) Antifolate activity of epigallocatechin gallate against Stenotrophomonas maltophilia. Antimicrob Agents Chemother 49:2914–2920

Newton K, Strasser A (2000) Ionizing radiation and chemotherapeutic drugs induce apoptosis in lymphocytes in the absence of Fas or FADD/MORT1 signaling. Implications for cancer therapy. J Exp Med 191:195–200

Oku N, Matsukawa M, Yamakawa S, Asai T, Yahara S, Hashimoto F, Akizawa T (2003) Inhibitory effect of green tea polyphenols on membrane-type 1 matrix metalloproteinase, MT1-MMP. Biol Pharm Bull 26:1235–1238

Plass C, Soloway PD (2002) DNA methylation, imprinting and cancer. Eur J Hum Genet 10:6–16

Plumb GW, Price KR, Williamson G (1999) Antioxidant properties of flavonol glycosides from tea. Redox Rep 4:13–16

Prakash D, Suri S, Upadhyay G, Singh BN (2007) Total phenol, antioxidant and free radical scavenging activities of some medicinal plants. Int J Food Sci Nutr 58:18–28

Reiter CE, Kim JA, Quon MJ (2010) Green tea polyphenol epigallocatechin gallate reduces endothelin-1 expression and secretion in vascular endothelial cells: roles for AMP-activated protein kinase, Akt, and FOXO1. Endocrinology 151:103–114

Rietveld A, Wiseman S (2003) Antioxidant effects of tea: evidence from human clinical trials. J Nutr 133:3285S–3292S

Rose BA, Force T, Wang Y (2010) Mitogen-activated protein kinase signaling in the heart: angels versus demons in a heart-breaking tale. Physiol Rev 90:1507–1546

Roy SK, Srivastava RK, Shankar S (2010) Inhibition of PI3K/AKT and MAPK/ERK pathways causes activation of FOXO transcription factor, leading to cell cycle arrest and apoptosis in pancreatic cancer. J Mol Signal 5:10

Sanchez-Huerta V, Gutierrez-Sanchez L, Flores-Estrada J (2011) (-)-Epigallocatechin 3-gallate (EGCG) at the ocular surface inhibits corneal neovascularization. Med Hypotheses 76:311–313

Sartippour MR, Shao ZM, Heber D, Beatty P, Zhang L, Liu C, Ellis L, Liu W, Go VL, Brooks MN (2002) Green tea inhibits vascular endothelial growth factor (VEGF) induction in human breast cancer cells. J Nutr 132:2307–2311

Sazuka M, Itoi T, Suzuki Y, Odani S, Koide T, Isemura M (1996) Evidence for the interaction between (-)-epigallocatechin gallate and human plasma proteins fibronectin, fibrinogen, and histidine-rich glycoprotein. Biosci Biotechnol Biochem 60:1317–1319

Schwarz RE, Donohue CA, Sadava D, Kane SE (2003) Pancreatic cancer in vitro toxicity mediated by Chinese herbs SPES and PC-SPES: implications for monotherapy and combination treatment. Cancer Lett 189:59–68

Senthil Kumaran V, Arulmathi K, Srividhya R, Kalaiselvi P (2008) Repletion of antioxidant status by EGCG and retardation of oxidative damage induced macromolecular anomalies in aged rats. Exp Gerontol 43:176–183

Sergediene E, Jonsson K, Szymusiak H, Tyrakowska B, Rietjens IM, Cenas N (1999) Prooxidant toxicity of polyphenolic antioxidants to HL-60 cells: description of quantitative structure-activity relationships. FEBS Lett 462:392–396

Shankar S, Suthakar G, Srivastava RK (2007) Epigallocatechin-3-gallate inhibits cell cycle and induces apoptosis in pancreatic cancer. Front Biosci 12:5039–5051

Shankar S, Chen Q, Srivastava RK (2008a) Inhibition of PI3K/AKT and MEK/ERK pathways act synergistically to enhance antiangiogenic effects of EGCG through activation of FOXO transcription factor. J Mol Signal 3:7

Shankar S, Ganapathy S, Hingorani SR, Srivastava RK (2008b) EGCG inhibits growth, invasion, angiogenesis and metastasis of pancreatic cancer. Front Biosci 13:440–452

Shankar S, Nall D, Tang SN, Meeker D, Passarini J, Sharma J, Srivastava RK (2011) Resveratrol inhibits pancreatic cancer stem cell characteristics in human and KrasG12D transgenic mice by inhibiting pluripotency maintaining factors and epithelial-mesenchymal transition. PLoS One 6:e16530

Sharpless NE, DePinho RA (2004) Telomeres, stem cells, senescence, and cancer. J Clin Invest 113:160–168

Shimizu M, Weinstein IB (2005) Modulation of signal transduction by tea catechins and related phytochemicals. Mutat Res 591:147–160

Shimizu M, Deguchi A, Lim JT, Moriwaki H, Kopelovich L, Weinstein IB (2005) (-)-Epigallocatechin gallate and polyphenon E inhibit growth and activation of the epidermal growth factor receptor and human epidermal growth factor receptor-2 signaling pathways in human colon cancer cells. Clin Cancer Res 11:2735–2746

Siddiqui IA, Asim M, Hafeez BB, Adhami VM, Tarapore RS, Mukhtar H (2010) Green tea polyphenol EGCG blunts androgen receptor function in prostate cancer. FASEB J 25(4):1098–1207

Sigler K, Ruch RJ (1993) Enhancement of gap junctional intercellular communication in tumor promoter-treated cells by components of green tea. Cancer Lett 69:15–19

Silverman N, Maniatis T (2001) NF-kappaB signaling pathways in mammalian and insect innate immunity. Genes Dev 15:2321–2342

Singh BN, Singh BR, Singh RL, Prakash D, Singh DP, Sarma BK, Upadhyay G, Singh HB (2009a) Polyphenolics from various extracts/fractions of red onion (Allium cepa) peel with potent antioxidant and antimutagenic activities. Food Chem Toxicol 47:1161–1167

Singh BN, Singh BR, Singh RL, Prakash D, Singh DP, Sarma BK, Upadhyay G, Singh HB (2009d) Polyphenolics from various extracts/fractions of red onion (Allium cepa) peel with potential antioxidant and antimutagenic activities. Food Chem Toxicol

Singh BN, Zhang G, Hwa YL, Li J, Dowdy SC, Jiang SW (2010a) Nonhistone protein acetylation as cancer therapy targets. Expert Rev Anticancer Ther 10:935–954

Singh HB, Singh BN, Singh SP, Nautiyal CS (2010b) Solid-state cultivation of Trichoderma harzianum NBRI-1055 for modulating natural antioxidants in soybean seed matrix. Bioresour Technol 101:6444–6453

Singh M, Tyagi S, Bhui K, Prasad S, Shukla Y (2010c) Regulation of cell growth through cell cycle arrest and apoptosis in HPV 16 positive human cervical cancer cells by tea polyphenols. Invest New Drugs 28:216–224

Singh BN, Shankar S, Srivastava RK (2011) Green tea catechin, epigallocatechin-3-gallate (EGCG): mechanisms, perspectives and clinical applications. Biochem Pharmacol 82(12):1807–1821

Smith DM, Wang Z, Kazi A, Li LH, Chan TH, Dou QP (2002) Synthetic analogs of green tea polyphenols as proteasome inhibitors. Mol Med 8:382–392

Sonee M, Sum T, Wang C, Mukherjee SK (2004) The soy isoflavone, genistein, protects human cortical neuronal cells from oxidative stress. Neurotoxicology 25:885–891

Srivastava RK, Unterman TG, Shankar S (2010) FOXO transcription factors and VEGF neutralizing antibody enhance antiangiogenic effects of resveratrol. Mol Cell Biochem 337:201–212

Srividhya R, Jyothilakshmi V, Arulmathi K, Senthilkumaran V, Kalaiselvi P (2008) Attenuation of senescence-induced oxidative exacerbations in aged rat brain by (-)-epigallocatechin-3-gallate. Int J Dev Neurosci 26:217–223

Subbaramaiah K, Dannenberg AJ (2003) Cyclooxygenase 2: a molecular target for cancer prevention and treatment. Trends Pharmacol Sci 24:96–102

Surh YJ (2003) Cancer chemoprevention with dietary phytochemicals. Nat Rev Cancer 3:768–780

Suzuki H, Tokino T, Shinomura Y, Imai K, Toyota M (2008) DNA methylation and cancer pathways in gastrointestinal tumors. Pharmacogenomics 9:1917–1928

Syed DN, Afaq F, Kweon MH, Hadi N, Bhatia N, Spiegelman VS, Mukhtar H (2007) Green tea polyphenol EGCG suppresses cigarette smoke condensate-induced NF-kappaB activation in normal human bronchial epithelial cells. Oncogene 26:673–682

Tachibana H, Fujimura Y, Yamada K (2004) Tea polyphenol epigallocatechin-3-gallate associates with plasma membrane lipid rafts: lipid rafts mediate anti-allergic action of the catechin. Biofactors 21:383–385

Tamura K, Nakae D, Horiguchi K, Akai H, Kobayashi Y, Satoh H, Tsujiuchi T, Denda A, Konishi Y (1997) Inhibition by green tea extract of diethylnitrosamine-initiated but not choline-deficient, L-amino acid-defined diet-associated development of putative preneoplastic, glutathione S-transferase placental form-positive lesions in rat liver. Jpn J Cancer Res 88:356–362

Tang GQ, Yan TQ, Guo W, Ren TT, Peng CL, Zhao H, Lu XC, Zhao FL, Han X (2010a) (-)-Epigallocatechin-3-gallate induces apoptosis and suppresses proliferation by inhibiting the human Indian Hedgehog pathway in human chondrosarcoma cells. J Cancer Res Clin Oncol 136:1179–1185

Tang SN, Singh C, Nall D, Meeker D, Shankar S, Srivastava RK (2010b) The dietary bioflavonoid quercetin synergizes with epigallocathechin gallate (EGCG) to inhibit prostate cancer stem cell characteristics, invasion, migration and epithelial-mesenchymal transition. J Mol Signal 5:14

Tang SN, Fu J, Nall D, Rodova M, Shankar S, Srivastava RK (2011) Inhibition of sonic hedgehog pathway and pluripotency maintaining factors regulate human pancreatic cancer stem cell characteristics. Int J Cancer

Teng B, Qin W, Ansari HR, Mustafa SJ (2005) Involvement of p38-mitogen-activated protein kinase in adenosine receptor-mediated relaxation of coronary artery. Am J Physiol Heart Circ Physiol 288:H2574–H2580

Thawonsuwan J, Kiron V, Satoh S, Panigrahi A, Verlhac V (2010) Epigallocatechin-3-gallate (EGCG) affects the antioxidant and immune defense of the rainbow trout, Oncorhynchus mykiss. Fish Physiol Biochem 36:687–697

Tsang WP, Kwok TT (2010) Epigallocatechin gallate up-regulation of miR-16 and induction of apoptosis in human cancer cells. J Nutr Biochem 21:140–146

Tu SH, Ku CY, Ho CT, Chen CS, Huang CS, Lee CH, Chen LC, Pan MH, Chang HW, Chang CH, Chang YJ, Wei PL, Wu CH, Ho YS (2011) Tea polyphenol (-)-epigallocatechin-3-gallate inhibits nicotine- and estrogen-induced alpha9-nicotinic acetylcholine receptor upregulation in human breast cancer cells. Mol Nutr Food Res 55:455–466

Volate SR, Muga SJ, Issa AY, Nitcheva D, Smith T, Wargovich MJ (2009) Epigenetic modulation of the retinoid X receptor alpha by green tea in the azoxymethane-Apc Min/+ mouse model of intestinal cancer. Mol Carcinog 48:920–933

Wang ZY, Hong JY, Huang MT, Reuhl KR, Conney AH, Yang CS (1992) Inhibition of N-nitrosodiethylamine- and 4-(methylnitrosamino)-1-(3-pyridyl)-1-butanone-induced tumorigenesis in A/J mice by green tea and black tea. Cancer Res 52:1943–1947

Wang Z, Li Y, Kong D, Ahmad A, Banerjee S, Sarkar FH (2010) Cross-talk between miRNA and Notch signaling pathways in tumor development and progression. Cancer Lett 292:141–148

Wiseman SA, Balentine DA, Frei B (1997) Antioxidants in tea. Crit Rev Food Sci Nutr 37:705–718

Yamane T, Takahashi T, Kuwata K, Oya K, Inagake M, Kitao Y, Suganuma M, Fujiki H (1995) Inhibition of N-methyl-N′-nitro-N-nitrosoguanidine-induced carcinogenesis by (-)-epigallocatechin gallate in the rat glandular stomach. Cancer Res 55:2081–2084

Yang TT, Koo MW (2000) Inhibitory effect of Chinese green tea on endothelial cell-induced LDL oxidation. Atherosclerosis 148:67–73

Yang CS, Chung JY, Yang G, Chhabra SK, Lee MJ (2000) Tea and tea polyphenols in cancer prevention. J Nutr 130:472S–478S

Yang CS, Maliakal P, Meng X (2002) Inhibition of carcinogenesis by tea. Annu Rev Pharmacol Toxicol 42:25–54

Yang CS, Lambert JD, Hou Z, Ju J, Lu G, Hao X (2006a) Molecular targets for the cancer preventive activity of tea polyphenols. Mol Carcinog 45:431–435

Yang CS, Sang S, Lambert JD, Hou Z, Ju J, Lu G (2006b) Possible mechanisms of the cancer-preventive activities of green tea. Mol Nutr Food Res 50:170–175

Yang SP, Wilson K, Kawa A, Raner GM (2006c) Effects of green tea extracts on gene expression in HepG2 and Cal-27 cells. Food Chem Toxicol 44:1075–1081

Yang CS, Lambert JD, Ju J, Lu G, Sang S (2007) Tea and cancer prevention: molecular mechanisms and human relevance. Toxicol Appl Pharmacol 224:265–273

Yang CS, Wang X, Lu G, Picinich SC (2009) Cancer prevention by tea: animal studies, molecular mechanisms and human relevance. Nat Rev Cancer 9:429–439

Yuan JM, Gao YT, Yang CS, Yu MC (2007) Urinary biomarkers of tea polyphenols and risk of colorectal cancer in the Shanghai Cohort Study. Int J Cancer 120:1344–1350

Zhang W, Weissfeld JL, Romkes M, Land SR, Grandis JR, Siegfried JM (2007) Association of the EGFR intron 1 CA repeat length with lung cancer risk. Mol Carcinog 46:372–380

Zhang Z, Stiegler AL, Boggon TJ, Kobayashi S, Halmos B (2010) EGFR-mutated lung cancer: a paradigm of molecular oncology. Oncotarget 1:497–514

Zhang CX, Wang SM, Jin HY (2011) Inhibitory effect and mechanism of (-)-epigallocatechin-3-gallate on HT29 and HCT-8 colorectal cancer cell lines and expression of HES1 and JAG1. Zhonghua Wei Chang Wai Ke Za Zhi 14:636–639

Chapter 16
Role of Dietary Antioxidants in Cancer

C.M. Ajila and S.K. Brar

Contents

Abstract Diets rich in fruits and vegetables are gaining increased importance due to their significant role in reducing the risk of degenerative disease such cancer, cardiovascular diseases and other chronic diseases. Many studies have shown that free radicals in the living organisms cause oxidative damage to different molecules, such as lipids, proteins, nucleic acids and these are involved in the interaction phases of many degenerative diseases. A diet is composed of food, which comprises a multitude of nutrients as well as non-nutritive components. Fruits and

C.M. Ajila • S.K. Brar (✉)
Institut national de la recherche scientifique, Centre Eau, Terre & Environnement/Centre for Water, Earth and Environment, Université du Québec, 490 de la Couronne, Québec (QC) G1K 9A9, Canada
e-mail: satinder.brar@ete.inrs.ca

S. Shankar and R.K. Srivastava (eds.), *Nutrition, Diet and Cancer*,
DOI 10.1007/978-94-007-2923-0_16,

vegetables contain many antioxidant compounds including phenolic compounds, carotenoids, anthocyanins and tocopherols. Antioxidants are substances that delay or prevent the oxidation of cellular oxidizable substrates. They exert their effect by scavenging reactive oxygen species (ROS) and reactive nitrogen species (RNS) or preventing the generation of ROS/RNS. The study of diet and cancer risk reduction is complicated not only by the multistage, multifactorial nature of the disease, but also because of the inherent complexities of any diet. This chapter discusses the chemopreventive role of dietary intake of fruits and vegetables in the development of cancers. It focuses on the role of different group of phytochemicals and its possible role in the chemoprevention of cancer.

Introduction

Cancer is one of the major leading causes of death in the world. According to World Cancer Report, cancer rates could further increase by 50% to 15 million new cases in the year 2020 (World Health Organization 2003). Malignant tumours were responsible for 12% cent of the nearly 56 million deaths worldwide from all causes in 2000. In many countries, more than a quarter of deaths are attributable to cancer. In 2000, 5.3 million men and 4.7 million women developed a malignant tumor and altogether 6.2 million died from the disease (World Health Organization 2003). Cancer has emerged as a major public health problem in developing countries, matching its effect in industrialized nations.

Generally, vegetables and fruits, dietary fiber, and certain micronutrients appear to be protective against cancer, whereas fat, excessive calories and alcohol seem to increase cancer risk. Foods are complex mixtures of nutrients and non-nutritive substances that are difficult to measure accurately, and the effects of individual constituents as well as the possible interactions among these constituents are difficult to unravel. Epidemiological evidences with data from animal and *in vitro* studies, strongly supports the relationships between dietary constituents and the risk of cancers. Diet plays a major role in cancer aetiology and prevention. Epidemiological studies proved the relation of antioxidant intake or low blood levels of antioxidants with increased cancer risk. Human epidemiological studies have revealed a protective effect of vegetable and fruit consumption for cancers of the stomach, esophagus, lung, oral cavity and pharynx, bladder, endometrium, pancreas, colon and rectum, breast, cervix, ovary and prostate (Block et al. 1992; Giovannucci 1999). Low dietary intake of fruits and vegetables doubles the risk of most types of cancers. Oxidants are capable of stimulating cell division, which is a critical factor in mutagenesis. When a cell with a damaged DNA strand divides, cell metabolism and duplication becomes irregular and causes mutation which in turn is an important factor in carcinogenesis. It is believed that antioxidants exert their protective effect by decreasing oxidative damage to DNA and by decreasing abnormal increases in cell division. Naturally occurring compounds in diet, particularly antioxidant compounds in plant products, have shown promise as potential chemo preventive agents. A variety of compounds found in these foods have known bioactive mechanisms and are suspected as anticancer agents; these include vitamins C and E, flavonoids, isothiocyanates, phytosterols, selenium, folic acid, dietary fiber, protease inhibitors, isoflavones, indoles, carotenoids and others (Papas 1998).

Free Radicals in Cancer

Oxygen is a highly reactive atom that is capable of becoming part of potentially damaging molecules commonly called "free radicals." Free radicals are capable of attacking the healthy cells of the body, causing them to lose their structure and function. Free radicals are electrically charged molecules, i.e., they have an unpaired electron, which causes them to seek out and capture electrons from other substances in order to neutralize themselves. The formation of free radical is chain reaction and until subsequent free radicals are deactivated, thousands of free radical reactions can occur within seconds of the initial reaction. Cells in humans and other organisms are constantly exposed to a variety of oxidizing agents and these may be present in air, food, and water, or they may be produced by metabolic activity within cells. The key factor is to maintain a balance between oxidants and antioxidants to sustain optimal physiological conditions. Overproduction of oxidants can cause an imbalance, leading to oxidative stress, especially in chronic bacterial, viral, and parasitic infections (Ames et al. 1993a, 1993b). Oxidative stress can cause oxidative damage to large biomolecules, such as lipids, proteins, and DNA, resulting in an increased risk for cancer and Cardiovascular diseases (Ames et al. 1993a).

Reactive oxygen species (ROS) is a term which encompasses all highly reactive, oxygen-containing molecules, including free radicals. Types of ROS include the hydroxyl radical, superoxide anion radical, hydrogen peroxide, singlet oxygen, nitric oxide radical, hypochlorite radical, and various lipid peroxides. Free radicals can react with membrane lipids, nucleic acids, proteins and enzymes, and other small molecules, resulting in cellular damage and finally leads to cancer (Fig. 16.1). ROS are generated by a number of pathways. Most of the oxidants produced by cells occur as:

1. A consequence of normal aerobic metabolism: approximately 90% of the oxygen utilized by the cell is consumed by the mitochondrial electron transport system.
2. Oxidative burst from phagocytes (white blood cells) as part of the mechanism by which bacteria and viruses are killed, and by which foreign proteins (antigens) are denatured.
3. Xenobiotic metabolism, i.e., detoxification of toxic substances

The term "oxidative stress" has been coined to represent a shift towards the pro-oxidants in the pro-oxidant/antioxidant balance that can occur as a result of an increase in oxidative metabolism. Increased oxidative stress at the cellular level

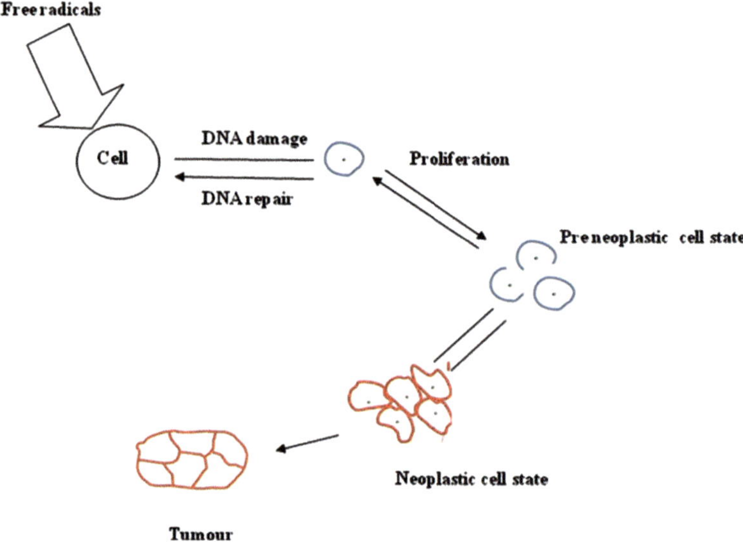

Fig. 16.1 Role of free radicals in cancer

is mainly due to factors such as exposure to alcohol, medications, trauma, cold, infections, poor diet, toxins, radiation, or strenuous physical activity etc. Oxidative damage to DNA, proteins, and other macromolecules has been implicated in the pathogenesis of a wide variety of diseases, such as heart disease and cancer (Halliwell 1994).

The reactive oxygen species (ROS) can damage the nucleic acids. The oxidative modification of the DNA constitutes the fundamental molecular event in carcinogenesis (Trueba et al. 2004). Oxidative DNA damage-induced mutagenesis is widely hypothesized to be a frequent event in the normal human cell. The enormous evidence suggests an important role of ROS in the expansion and progression of tumor clones, being considered a relevant class of carcinogens.

Antioxidants and Cancer Prevention

In higher eukaryotic aerobic organisms, including human beings, oxygen is the most important molecule for the existence of life. At the same time, oxygen represents a danger to their very existence due to its high reactivity. This fact has been termed the paradox of aerobic life. A number of reactive oxygen species are generated during normal aerobic metabolism, such as superoxide, hydrogen peroxide and the hydroxyl radical. In addition, singlet oxygen can be generated through photochemical events and lipid peroxidation can lead to peroxyl radical formation. These oxidants collectively contribute to aging and degenerative diseases such as cancer and atherosclerosis through oxidation of DNA, proteins and lipids (Ames et al. 1993b; Davies 1995). Carcinogenesis is a multistep process, and oxidative damage is linked to the formation of tumors through several mechanisms (Ames et al. 1993b). Oxidative stress induced by free radicals causes DNA damage which in turn leads to base mutation, single- and double-strand breaks, DNA cross-linking, and chromosomal breakage and rearrangement (Ames et al. 1993b).

Antioxidants are capable of stabilizing, or deactivating, free radicals before they attack cells. Antioxidants are absolutely critical for maintaining optimal cellular and systemic health and well-being. Antioxidant compounds can decrease mutagenesis, and thus carcinogenesis, both by decreasing oxidative damage to DNA and by decreasing oxidant-stimulated cell division (Ames et al. 1993a, b).The human body has an array of endogenous antioxidants such as catalase and superoxide dismutase; however, exogenous dietary antioxidants such as ascorbic acid (vitamin C), α-tocopherol (vitamin E) and carotenoids play important roles in reducing oxidative damage (Ames et al. 1993a).

Highly sophisticated and complex antioxidant protection system exist in human body to protect the cells and organ systems of the body against reactive oxygen species. It involves a variety of components, both endogenous and exogenous in origin that function interactively and synergistically to neutralize free radicals (Percival 1998).

These components include:

- Nutrient-derived antioxidants such as ascorbic acid (vitamin C), tocopherols and tocotrienols (vitamin E), carotenoids, and other low molecular weight compounds such as glutathione and lipoic acid.
- Antioxidant enzymes, e.g., superoxide dismutase, glutathione peroxidase, and glutathione reductase, which catalyze free radical quenching reactions.
- Metal binding proteins, such as ferritin, lactoferrin, albumin, and ceruloplasmin that sequester free iron and copper ions that are capable of catalyzing oxidative reactions.
- Numerous other antioxidant phytonutrients present in a wide variety of plant foods.

There are many evidences that dietary plant foods appear to be protective against different kinds of cancers (Krinsky and Johnson 2005). However, it is still not clear about the compounds involved in this effect and their mechanism of action. Among a number of mechanistic hypotheses, diet-derived antioxidants have been proposed to be protective against cancer mainly on the basis of their ability to reduce DNA damage caused by free radicals. Cancer cells are resistant to apoptosis and show a shift in energy production from mitochondrial oxidative phosphorylation to cytosolic glycolysis. Apoptosis resistance and metabolic reprogramming are linked in many cancer cells and both processes center on mitochondria. Different bioactive food components, separate or in support of pharmaceutical interventions, affecting various aspects of metabolism may, alone or in synergy, provide an important tool to reverse glycolytic to oxidative metabolism and enhance sensitivity to apoptosis (Keijer et al. 2011).

Table 16.1 Proposed mechanisms by which dietary phytochemicals may prevent cancer

Antioxidant activity
Scavenge free radicals and reduce oxidative stress
Inhibition of cell proliferation and oncogene expression
Induction of cell differentiation and tumor suppress gene expression
Induction of cell-cycle arrest and apoptosis
Inhibition of signal transduction pathways
Enzyme induction and enhancing detoxification
Phase II enzyme
Glutathione peroxidase
Catalase
Superoxide dismutase
Enzyme inhibition
Phase I enzyme (block activation of carcinogens)
Cyclooxygenase-2
Inducible nitric oxide synthase
Xanthine oxidase
Enhancement of immune functions and surveillance
Antiangiogenesis
Prevention of DNA binding
Regulation of steroid hormone metabolism
Regulation of estrogen metabolism
Antibacterial and antiviral effects

Antioxidant defenses of the body mainly consist of molecular and enzymatic factors; however, the composition of the network depends mainly in terms of concentration and components in different environments. Protection at the cellular level is mainly guaranteed by enzymes (superoxide dismutase, catalase, and glutathione peroxidase) and glutathione. At plasma level, non-enzymatic antioxidants play an important role. Antioxidant molecules are located in both the hydrophilic and hydrophobic compartments of plasma and try to decrease free radical concentration and to inactivate transition metal ions. Metal chelating antioxidants, such as transferrin, albumin, and ceruloplasmin avoid radical production by inhibiting the Fenton reaction catalyzed by copper or iron. Cancer-inducing oxidative damage might be prevented or limited by dietary antioxidants found in fruits and vegetables. Studies proved that phytochemicals in common fruits and vegetables can have complementary and overlapping mechanisms of action such as antioxidant activity and scavenging free radicals; regulation of gene expression in cell proliferation, cell differentiation, oncogenes, and tumor suppressor genes; induction of cell-cycle arrest and apoptosis; modulation of enzyme activities in detoxification, oxidation, and reduction; stimulation of the immune system; regulation of hormone metabolism; antibacterial and antiviral effects as shown in the Table 16.1 (Waladkhani and Clemens 1998; Sun et al. 2002; Chu et al. 2002).

Role of Phytochemicals in Cancer

It is widely accepted that a plant-based diet with high intake of fruits, vegetables, and other nutrient-rich plant foods may reduce the risk of oxidative stress-related diseases (World Cancer Research Fund/American Institute for Cancer Research 2007). Understanding the complex role of diet in such chronic diseases is challenging since a typical diet provides more than 25,000 bioactive food constituents, many of which may modify a multitude of processes that are related to these diseases. Because of the complexity of this relationship, it is likely that a comprehensive understanding of the role of these bioactive food components is needed to assess the role of dietary plants in human health and disease development. The "phyto-" of the word phytochemicals is derived from the Greek word phyto, which means plant. Phytochemicals are defined as bioactive non-nutrient plant compounds in fruits, vegetables, grains, and other plant foods that have been linked to reducing the risk of major chronic diseases. Phytochemicals can be classified as carotenoids, phenolics, alkaloids, and organosulfur compounds (Fig. 16.2). The most studied of the phytochemicals are phenolics and carotenoids.

Phenolic Compounds

Polyphenols are a large family of natural compounds which are secondary metabolites and are derivatives of the pentose phosphate, shikimate, and phenylpropanoid pathways in plants (Ryan et al. 1999). Phenolic compounds exhibit a wide range

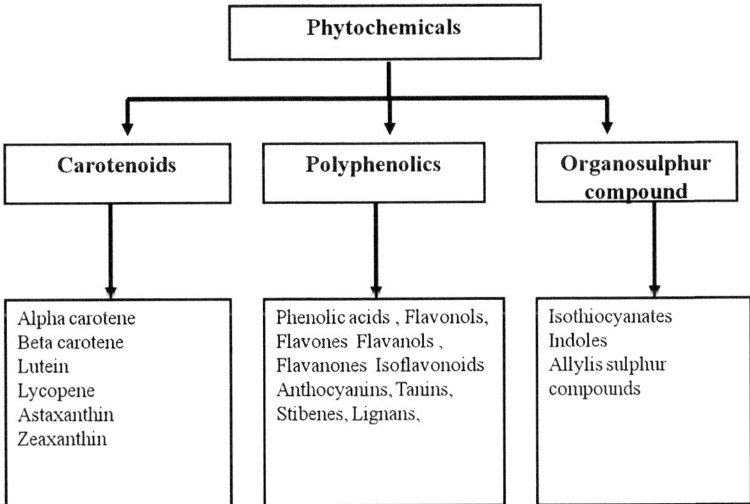

Fig. 16.2 Classification of phytochemical compounds present in fruits and vegetables

Table 16.2 Classes of phenolic compounds in plants

Class	Structure
Simple phenolics, benzoquinones	C_6
Hydroxybenzoic acids	C_6–C_1
Acetophenones, phenylacetic acids	C_6–C_2
Hydroxycinnamic acids, phenylpropanoids Napthoquinones	C_6–C_3
Xanthones	C_6–C_4
Stilbenes, anthroquinones	C_6–C_1–C_6
Flavonoids, isoflavanoids	C_6–C_2–C_6
Lignans, neolignanas	C_6–C_3–C_6
Bioflavoniods	$(C_6–C_3)_2$
Lignine	$(C_6–C_3–C_6)_2$
Condensed tannins	$(C_6–C_3)_n$
	$(C_6–C_3–C_6)_n$

of beneficial properties to health, such as: anti-allergenic, anti-inflammatory, antimicrobial, anti-oxidant, antithrombotic, cardio protective and vasodilatory effects (Singh et al. 2010). Several beneficial effects derived from phenolic compounds are mainly due to their antioxidant activity (Tagliazucchi et al. 2010). Many studies have reported the link between polyphenols and its health (Terao 2008; Del Rio et al. 2010). The antioxidant properties of phenolics are mainly due to their redox properties, which allow them to act as reducing agents, hydrogen donors and singlet oxygen quenchers. They also act as chelators of metal ions, preventing metal catalyzed formation of free radical species (Salah et al. 1995). Phenolic antioxidants interfere with the oxidation of lipid and other molecules by rapid donation of hydrogen atom to radicals. The phenoxy radical intermediates are relatively stable; therefore, a new chain reaction is not easily possible. The phenoxy radical intermediates also act as terminator of the propagation route by reacting with other free radical (Shahidi and Naczk 1995). Structurally, phenolic compounds comprise an aromatic ring, bearing one or more hydroxyl substituents, and range from simple phenolic molecules to highly polymerized compounds (Bravo 1998). Most naturally occurring phenolic compounds are present as conjugates with mono and polysaccharides, linked to one or more of the phenolic groups, and also may occur as functional derivatives, such as esters and methyl esters (Bravo 1998; Harborne et al. 1999). Phenolic compounds can be classified into several classes as shown in Table 16.2 (Adom and Liu 2002).

Phenolic Acids

The name phenolic acids describes phenols that posses one carboxylic acid functionality. Phenolic acids contain two distinguishing constitutive carbon frame works: the hydroxycinnamic and hydroxybenzoic structures. The numbers and position of the hydroxyl groups on the aromatic ring creates the variety. Hydroxybenzoic acids

Fig. 16.3 Structures of phenolic acids

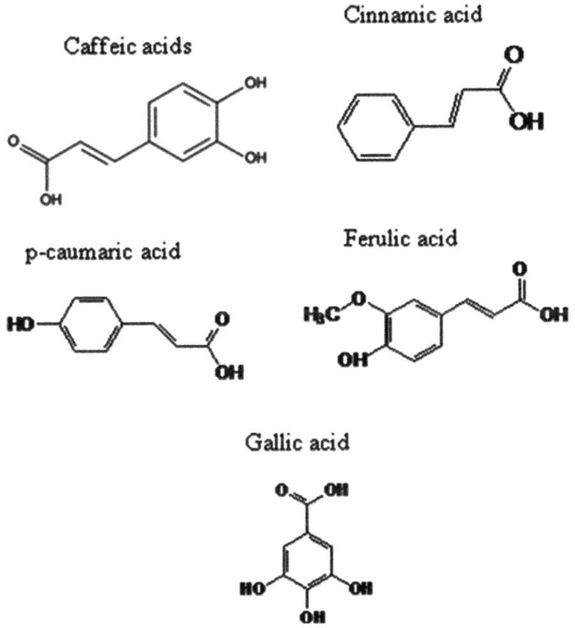

include gallic, p-hydroxybenzoic, protocatechuic, vanillic and syringic acids, which in common have the C6–C1 structure (Fig. 16.3). They are commonly present in the bound form and are typically a component of a complex structure, such as lignins and hydrolyzable tannins. They can also be found in the form of sugar derivatives and organic acids in plant foods. Hydroxycinnamic acids, on the other hand are aromatic compounds with a three carbon side chain (C6–C3) with caffeic, ferulic, p-caumaric and sinapic acids being the most common (Bravo 1998). They are mainly present in the bound form, linked to cell-wall structural components, such as cellulose, lignin, and proteins through ester bonds. Ferulic acids occur primarily in the seeds and leaves of plants, mainly covalently conjugated to mono- and disaccharides, plant-cell-wall polysaccharides, glycoproteins, polyamines, lignin, and insoluble carbohydrate biopolymers. Wheat bran is a good source of ferulic acids, which are esterified to hemicelluloses of the cell walls (Dewanto et al. 2002). Food processing, such as thermal processing, pasteurization, fermentation, and freezing, has a role in the release of these bound phenolic acids (Dewanto et al. 2002; Ajila et al. 2011). Caffeic, ferulic, p-coumaric, protocatechuic, and vanillic acids are present in almost all plants. Chlorogenic acids and curcumin are the major derivatives of hydroxycinnamic acids present in plants. Chlorogenic acids are the ester of caffeic acids and are the substrates for enzymatic oxidation leading to browning, particularly in apples and potatoes. Curcumin is made of two ferulic acids linked by a methylene in a diketone structure and is the major yellow pigment of mustard. Caffeic acid known to selectively block the biosynthesis of leukotrienes, components involved in immuno-regulation diseases, asthma and allergic reactions

(Koshihara et al. 1984). Caffeic acid and some of its esters might posses antitumour activity against colon carcinogenesis (Koshihara et al. 1984) and act as a selective inhibitors of human immunodeficiency virus type I integrase (King et al. 1999). Chlorogenic acid has been found to inhibit lipid peroxidation in rat liver induced by carbon tetrachloride, a potent liver carcinogen (Huang et al. 1997). Caffeic and ferulic acid found to detoxify carcinogen metabolites of polycyclic aromatic hydrocarbons (Huang et al. 1996). The interrelationship between antioxidative capacity and the vasodilatory activity of derivatives of hydroxybenzoic acid and hydroxycinnamic acid from wine has been well studied (Mudnic et al. 2010).

Flavonoids

Flavonoids are a group of phenolic compounds with antioxidant activity that have been identified in fruits, vegetables, and other plant foods and that have been linked to reducing the risk of major chronic diseases. More than 4,000 distinct flavonoids have been identified (Harborne et al. 1999). They commonly have a generic structure consisting of two aromatic rings (A and B rings) linked by three carbons that are usually in an oxygenated heterocycle ring, or C ring (Fig. 16.4). Flavonoids are low molecular weight compounds consisting of 15 carbon atoms, arranged in a C6–C3–C6 configuration. Essentially the structure consists of two aromatic rings A and B, joined by a 3-carbon bridge, usually in the form of a heterocyclic ring. Variations in substitution patterns to ring C result in the major flavonoids classes, i.e., flavonols, flavones, flavanones, flavanols (catechins), isoflavones, flavanols and anthocyanidins (Hollman and Katan 1999). Flavones and flavonols are the most widely occurring and structurally diverse compounds (Harborne et al. 1999). Substitutions to rings A and B give rise to different compounds of flavonoids and theses substitutions may include oxygenation, alkylation, glycosylation, acylation and sulfation (Hollman and Katan 1999; Pietta 2000). The epidemiological studies point out the possible role of flavonoids in preventing cardiovascular diseases and cancer (Chu et al. 2002; Wong et al. 2010) Flavonoids are wonderful molecules with vivid functional properties, such as anticancer, antiatherosclerotic, antimutagenic, antiviral, antineoplastic, antiallergic, antithrombotic and vasodilatory activity (Hollman and Katan 1999). Flavonoids are most frequently found in nature as conjugates in glycosylated or esterified forms but can occur as aglycones, especially as a result of the effects of food processing. Many different glycosides can be found in nature; approximately 80 different sugars have been discovered bound to flavonoids (Hollman and Arts 2000).

Quercetin is a strong antioxidant compounds and reported to have potential protective effects against degenerative disease such as cancer and heart disease. Quercetin has been found to down regulate expression of mutant p53 in breast cancer cells, arrest human leukemic T-cells in G1, inhibit tyrosine kinase, and inhibit heat shock proteins (Lamson and Brignall 2000). Quercetin has protected Caco-2

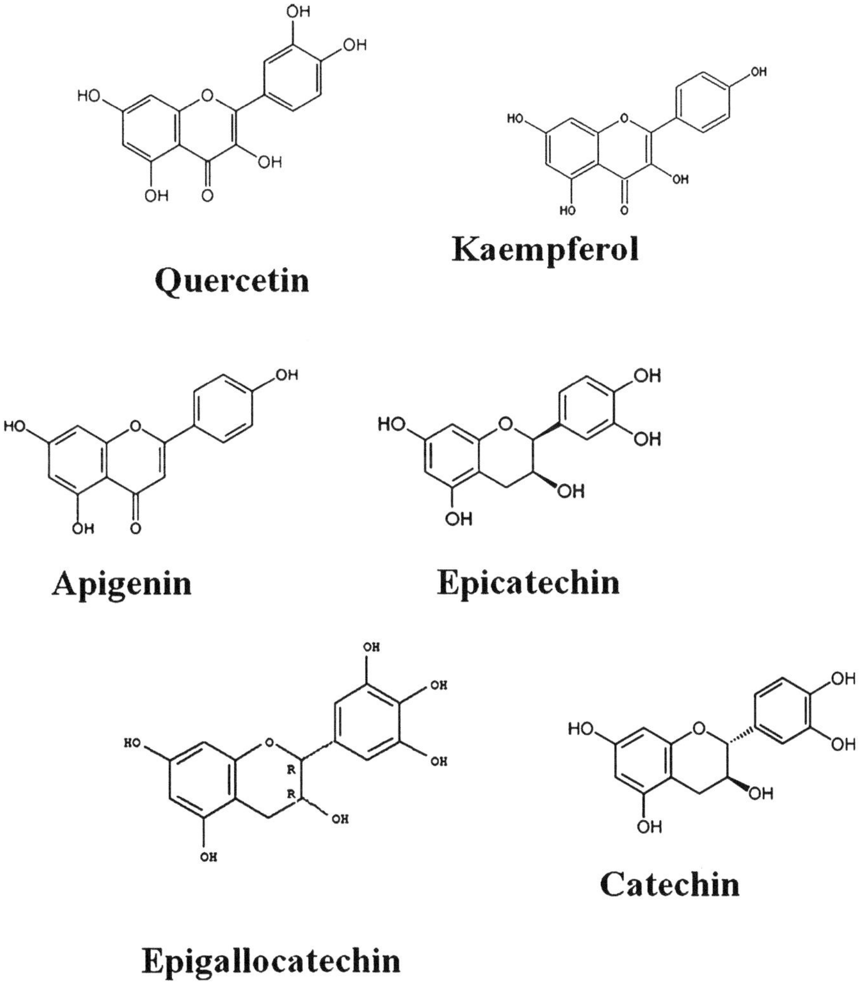

Quercetin

Kaempferol

Apigenin

Epicatechin

Epigallocatechin

Catechin

Fig. 16.4 Structures of flavonoids

cells from lipid peroxidation induced by hydrogen peroxide and Fe2+ (Peng and Kuo 2003). High doses of quercetin inhibited cell proliferation in colon carcinoma cell lines and in mammary adenocarcinoma cell lines (Woude et al. 2003). However, low doses of quercetin (10 μM) inhibited cell proliferation in Mol-4 Human Leukemia cells and also induced apoptosis (Mertens-Talcott et al. 2003). Quercetin inhibited intestinal tumor growth in mice, but not in rats. Quercetin decreased lipid oxidation and increased glutathione, protecting the liver from oxidative damage in mice liver treated with ethanol (Molina et al. 2003).

Antioxidant Vitamins

Free radicals which are one of the major reasons for cancer can cause lipid peroxidation in cell membranes and damage its function. Antioxidant vitamins can act as an effective scavenger of these radicals. This effect may protect against carcinogenesis. It was reported that Vitamin A administration can suppress mammary tumorigenesis in rats fed high dietary levels of PUFAs (Aylsworth et al. 1986) and also found that vitamin E deficiency can increase tumorigenesis in rats fed with high levels of PUFA (Ip 1982). Epidemiological studies have investigated the role of antioxidant vitamins such as retinol (vitamin A), alpha-tocopherol (vitamin E) and ascorbic acid (vitamin C) in protection effect against breast cancer. In the case of vitamin A, experimental evidence confirms its ability to block mammary carcinogenesis, but the epidemiological evidence is somewhat less convincing (Moon 1994). Vitamin A has both anti-initiating and antipromoting effects on mammary tumorigenesis and enhances cellular differentiation (Welsch 1987). Retinoids are also found to reduce the concentration of free radicals.

In the case of vitamin E, the antioxidant properties are more clearly established both in animals and in humans. Vitamin E administration reduces the incidence of carcinogen-induced rat mammary tumours (Kimmick et al. 1997). The presence of vitamin E deficiency increases tumour growth in animals fed high levels of PUFA compared to the standard diet without PUFA (Ip 1982).

A protective role for vitamin D in growth regulation and cell differentiation of cancer has been reported (Lipkin and Newmark 1999). Low vitamin levels have also been associated with increased colonic epithelial cell proliferation indices (Holt et al. 2002), increased adenoma risk (Peters et al. 2001) and colorectal cancer (Tangrea et al. 1997). One study reported a 29% reduction in the risk of breast cancer in women with a high dietary vitamin D/sun exposure index compared to a low index (John et al. 1999).

Epidemiologic studies have linked low folate intake with higher risk of several cancers, most notably colorectal (Giovannucci 2002) breast and uterine cervix cancer (Eichholzer et al. 2001). Long-term use of folate-containing multivitamin supplements has been associated with a 30–75% reduction in risk of colon cancer (Jacobs et al. 2001).

Use of vitamin C for cancer therapy was popularized by Linus Pauling. At high concentrations ascorbate is preferentially toxic to cancer cells. There is some evidence that large doses of vitamin C, either in multiple divided oral doses or intravenously, have beneficial effects in cancer therapy (Padayatty et al. 2004; Riordan et al. 2003). However, it was found that intravenous ascorbate may be a very beneficial adjuvant therapy for cancer with no negative side effects when administered properly.

Carotenoids

The carotenoids are a group of approximately 600 naturally-occurring pigments with diverse biological functions (Krinsky 1998). In plants and algae, carotenoids serve both photosynthetic and photoprotective role and in animals, carotenoids are effective chain-breaking antioxidants and singlet oxygen quenchers, and also serve as precursors for retinoids or vitamin A (Krinsky 1998). Carotenoids also have effects on cell communication and proliferation in animal (Wolf 1992). Since animals cannot synthesize carotenoids *de novo* and dietary sources are the only source for them to get carotenoids.

Even though, 40 or more naturally occurring carotenoids are found in the human diet, very few carotenoids are commonly found in human plasma and tissues, along with several of their isomers and various metabolites (Krinsky 1998). The most common of these dietary carotenoids are three hydrocarbon carotenoids (carotenes): α-carotene, β-carotene and lycopene, and three oxycarotenoids (xanthophylls): lutein, zeaxanthin and β-cryptoxanthin (Fig. 16.5) (Khachik et al. 1998). Intake of these compounds is principally through consumption of fruits and vegetables; the xanthophylls astaxanthin, on the other hand, is obtained principally from seafood such as salmon and shrimp. Astaxanthin occurs in these animals naturally, but it also occurs in farmed fish, shellfish and poultry as a result of its use as a feed additive (Lorenz and Cysewski 2000). Canthaxanthin, another potentially important xanthophyll, is also not generally considered a dietary carotenoid, but may be included in the human diet through its widespread use as a coloring agent in foods and animal feeds (Baker 2002). Nevertheless, all of these dietary carotenoids have demonstrated some anticarcinogenic activity in animal experiments (Nishino et al. 2002).

Tomatoes and tomato-based products are the major dietary sources for the red carotenoid lycopene and some fruits such as watermelon, grapefruit and guava also found to be a source of lycopene (Nguyen and Schwartz 1999). Lycopene is a very efficient biological singlet oxygen quencher and has exhibited tumor suppressive properties on animal and human cells in vitro and on mice *in vivo* (Gerster 1997). Lycopene is a natural pigment synthesized by plants and microorganisms and is a carotenoid, an acyclic isomer of ß-carotene. Lycopene is a highly unsaturated hydrocarbon containing 11 conjugated and 2 un-conjugated double bonds and the structure is given in Fig. 16.6. Lycopene is one of the most potent antioxidants with a singlet-oxygen-quenching ability twice as high as that of ß-carotene and ten times higher than that of –tocopherol (Di Mascio et al. 1989). It is the most predominant carotenoid in human plasma and its level is affected by several biological and lifestyle factors (Rao and Agarwal 1999). Two major hypotheses have been proposed to explain the anticarcinogenic and antiatherogenic activities of lycopene: nonoxidative and oxidative mechanisms. Based on nonoxidative mechanisms, the anticarcinogenic effects of lycopene have been suggested to be due to regulation of gap-junction communication in mouse embryo fibroblast cells (Zhang et al. 1991, 1992). Lycopene is hypothesized to suppress carcinogen-induced

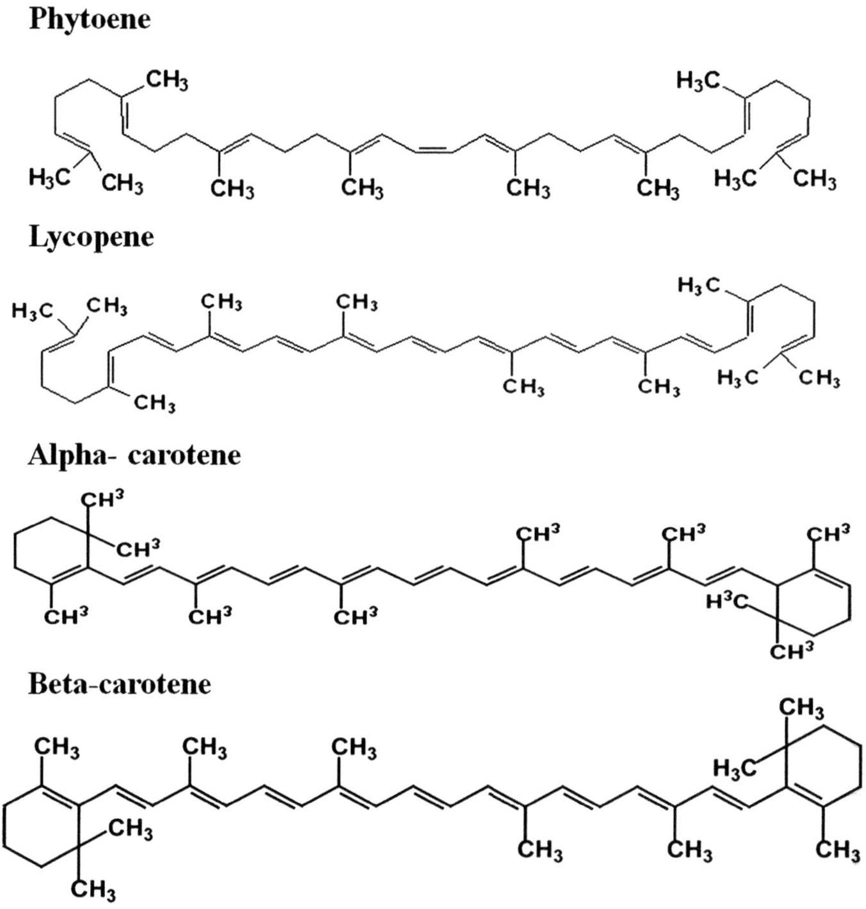

Phytoene

Lycopene

Alpha- carotene

Beta-carotene

Fig. 16.5 Structures of carotenoids

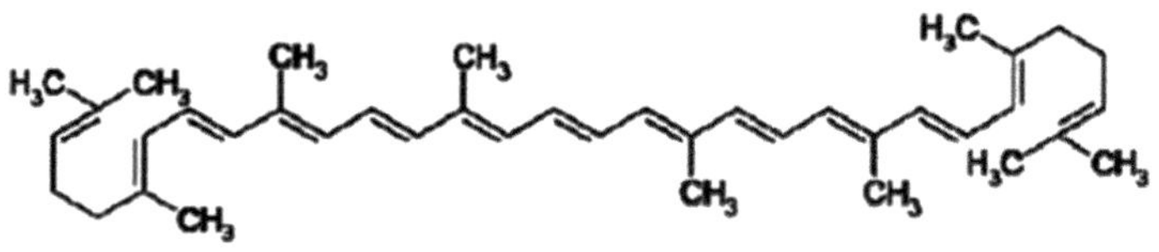

Fig. 16.6 Structures of lycopene

phosphorylation of regulatory proteins such as p53 and Rb antioncogenes and stop cell division at the G0-G1 cell cycle phase (Matsushima et al. 1995). Lycopene has been hypothesized to prevent carcinogenesis and atherogenesis by protecting critical cellular biomolecules, such as lipids, lipoproteins, proteins and DNA (Agarwal and Rao 1998).

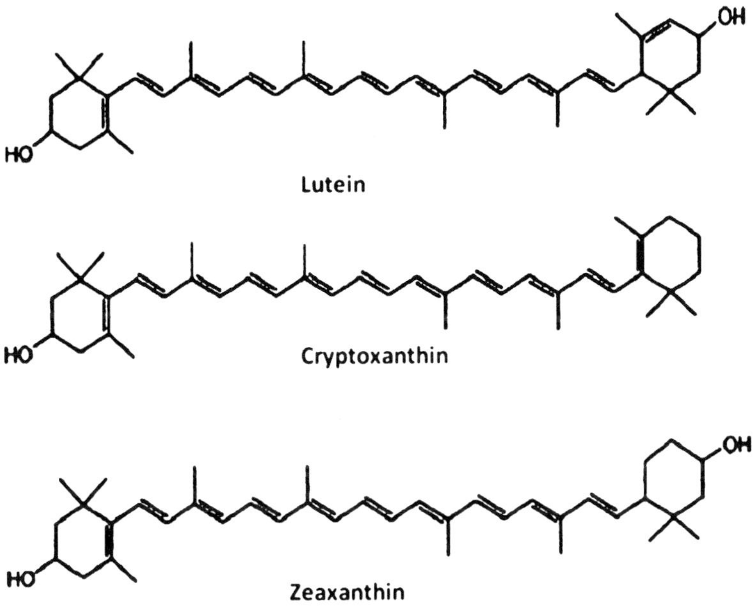

Lutein

Cryptoxanthin

Zeaxanthin

Fig. 16.7 Structures of xanthophylls

Lutein and zeaxanthin are yellow xanthophyll carotenoids commonly found in green and yellow vegetables and the structure are given in Fig. 16.7. Leafy green vegetables are main sources of lutein and orange peppers are rich in zeaxanthin (Landrum et al. 2002). A higher intake of lutein and zeaxanthin has been correlated with a lower incidence of lung cancer in humans (Voorrips et al. 2000). Lutein has also reported to inhibit carcinogenesis in rat colons and in the lungs of mice and inhibits mammary tumor growth in mice and in human cell cultures by regulating apoptosis. Similarly, zeaxanthin has been shown to reduce the formation of liver tumors in mice (Sumantran et al. 2000).

α-carotene and β-cryptoxanthin are major carotenoids present in human diet and have been inversely correlated with the incidence of human cervical cancer (Batieha et al. 1993). Dietary intake of β-cryptoxanthin is associated with reduced risk for lung cancer (Voorrips et al. 2000). Alpha-carotene has been demonstrated to have a potent preventive action against lung, skin and liver carcinogenesis (Murakoshi et al. 1992). β cryptoxanthin is found to be effective at inhibiting skin tumor formation in mice (Nishino et al. 2000). Canthaxanthin can suppress proliferation of human colon cancer cells and protect mouse embryo fibroblasts from transformation and protect mice from mammary and skin tumor development (Chew et al. 1999). Canthaxanthin has also proved effective at inhibiting both oral and colon carcinogenesis in rats. Although it is a potent antioxidant, the chemopreventive effects of canthaxanthin may also be related to its ability to up-regulate gene expression, resulting in enhanced gap junctional cell-cell communication (Hanusch et al. 1995). The chemopreventive effects of canthaxanthin may also be related to its ability to induce xenobiotic metabolizing enzymes (Jewell and O'Brien 1999). Several other naturally occurring carotenoids that are not considered significant in the human diet have shown potential as cancer chemopreventive agents. These include neoxanthin, fucoxanthin, phytofluene, ζ-carotene, phytoene, crocetin, capsanthin, peridinin and astaxanthin (Kotake-Nara et al. 2001).

The proposed mechanisms in the cancer chemopreventive actions of carotenoids can be grouped into three major categories: carotenoids can act as potent biological antioxidants, as enhancers of immune system function and as regulators of gene expression (Rousseau et al. 1992).

Dietary Fiber

Dietary fiber are generally defined as a group of endogenous compounds in plant foods that are resistant to human digestive enzymes, may play a beneficial, although still not fully defined, role in reducing cancer risk. Epidemiologic studies showed that cancer protective properties of dietary fiber and fiber-rich foods, and some indicate that fiber may modulate the risk-enhancing effects of dietary fat (Kritchevsky 1991). Dietary fiber is commonly defined as 'plant polysaccharides and lignin, which are resistant to hydrolysis by the digestive enzymes of man'. They are basically classified into two groups: soluble and insoluble dietary fibers. Soluble fibers are highly fermentable and are associated with carbohydrate and lipid metabolism, while insoluble fibers contribute to faecal bulk and reduce transit time. Pectin, cellulose and hemicellulose, with only trace amounts of lignin, are the predominant components of dietary fiber from most fruits and vegetables.

The mechanisms by which fiber can influence colon cancer include physical dilution of colon content, absorption of bile acids and carcinogens, decreased transit time, altered bile acid metabolism and the effects of fermentation, namely, the production of short-chain fatty acids, lowering of pH and stimulation of bacterial growth (Muir 1999). As with undigested carbohydrate and protein that reaches the colon undigested is metabolised by the colonic microflora to end products that include isoderivatives of SCFA (isobutyric and isovaleric), phenol, cresol, indoles, amines, ammonia and phenylated SCFA, many of which have adverse effect such as promotion of tumorigenesis by stimulating cell proliferation and favouring growth of malignant cells in preference to normal cells. Volatile phenols (p-cresol and phenol), produced from bacterial metabolism of the aromatic amino acids phenylalanine and tyrosine, are promoters of skin cancers and have been implicated in development of both bladder and bowel cancers (Muir 1999).

The risk of breast cancer, as well as other hormone-dependent cancers, may be influenced by dietary fiber through alteration of hormone production, metabolism, or actions at the cellular level (Rose 1993). Dietary fiber may influence estrogens primarily associated with breast cancer etiology through alteration of the microbial population and enzymes in the intestinal tract, reducing the deconjugation of estrogens and, thus, the amount available for reabsorption. Phytoestrogens, competes with estrogens for receptor-binding sites and thus potentially reducing breast cancer risk (Adlercreutz 1990).

Role of Diet as a Preventive Agent in Cancer

Epidemiologic data strongly recommend that higher intakes of vegetables, fruits, and whole grains are associated with reduced cancer risk. Based on many research studies, the relationship between high vegetable and fruit intake and reduced cancer risk appears to be strongest for cancers of the alimentary and respiratory tracts (cancers of the colon, lung, esophagus, and oral cavity) and weakest for hormone-related cancers (cancers of the breast, ovary, cervix, endometrium, and prostate) (Block et al. 1992). Many studies proved the protective role for vegetables and fruits indicate approximately twice the risk of cancer incidence for lowest vegetable and fruit intakes compared with highest intakes. The beneficial effect of vegetables, fruits, and whole grains may be due to either individual or combined effects of their constituents, including fiber, micronutrients, and phytochemicals. The additive and synergistic effects of phytochemicals in fruits and vegetables are responsible for these potent antioxidant and anticancer activities and that the benefit of a diet rich in fruits and vegetables is attributed to the complex mixture of phytochemicals present in whole foods.

Fruits and Cancer

During the 1990s, there was an increased enthusiasm for increasing consumption of fruits and vegetables with the expectation that this would substantially reduce the risk of many cancers. Potential reductions as large as 50% were suggested. This protection of cancer is mainly based on the bioactive compounds and antioxidants present in the fruits and vegetables.

Apples are a widely consumed, rich source of phytochemicals, and epidemiological studies have linked the consumption of apples with reduced risk of some cancers, cardiovascular disease, asthma, and diabetes. Apples have been found to have very strong antioxidant activity, inhibit cancer cell proliferation, decrease lipid oxidation, and lower cholesterol. Apples contain a variety of phytochemicals such as quercetin, catechin, phloridzin and chlorogenic acid, all of which are strong antioxidants. Several studies have specifically found the link between apple consumption with a reduced risk for cancer, especially lung cancer (Feskanich et al. 2000). Consumption of apples per day reduced the risk of lung cancer in women (Feskanich et al. 2000). Le Marchand et al. (2000) found an inverse association between lung cancer and quercetin intake although the trend was not statistically significant. When Caco-2 colon cancer cells were treated with apple extracts, cell proliferation was inhibited in a dose-dependent manner reaching a maximum inhibition of 43% at a dose of 50 mg/mL. The same trend was seen in Hep G2 liver cancer cells with maximal inhibition reaching 57% at a dose of 50 mg/mL (Le Marchand et al. 2000). Eberhardt et al. (2000) proposed that unique combinations of phytochemicals in the apples are responsible for inhibiting the growth of tumor cells. Apples had the third highest antiproliferative activity when compared to 11 other commonly consumed fruits (Sun et al. 2002). The antioxidant and antiproliferative activity of apple varied with its variety. At a dose of 50 mg/mL, Fuji apple extracts inhibited Hep G2 cell proliferation by 39% and Red Delicious extracts inhibited cell proliferation by 57%. Northern Spy apples had no effect on cell proliferation (Liu et al. 2001). Apples without peels were significantly less effective in inhibiting Hep G2 cell proliferation when compared to apples with the peel, suggesting that apple peels possess significant antiproliferative activity. Apples contain a large concentration of flavonoids, as well as a variety of other phytochemicals, and the concentration of these phytochemicals may depend on many factors, such as cultivar of the apple, harvest and storage of the apples, and processing of the apples. Apple peel contains more antioxidants compounds than apple flesh. The major antioxidants found in apples are quercetin-3-galactoside, quercetin-3-glucoside, quercetin-3-rhamnoside, catechin, epicatechin, procyanidin, cyanidin-3-galactoside, coumaric acid, chlorogenic acid, gallic acid, and phloridzin. The compounds most commonly found in apple peels are procyanidins, catechin, epicatechin, chlorogenic acid, phloridzin, and quercetin conjugates. Some of the antioxidants compounds found in the apple flesh are catechin, procyanidin, epicatechin, and phloridzin, but these compounds are found in much lower concentrations than in the peels. Quercetin conjugates are found exclusively in the peel of the apples. Chlorogenic acid tends to be higher in the flesh than in the peel (Escarpa and Gonzalez 1998). Apples with the peels were also better able to inhibit cancer cell proliferation when compared to apples without the peels (Eberhardt et al. 2000). It was reported that apple peels alone inhibited Hep G2 cell proliferation significantly more than whole apples (Wolfe et al. 2003).

Among small soft-fleshed colorful fruits, berries make up the largest proportion that is consumed in our diet. Berry fruits commonly consumed in North America include blackberries (*Rubus spp.*), black raspberries (*Rubus occidentalis*), blueberries (*Vaccinium corymbosum*), cranberries (*Vaccinium macrocarpon*), red raspberries (*Rubus idaeus*) and strawberries (*Fragaria* × *ananassa*). Other "niche-cultivated" berries and forest/wild berries such as bilberries, black currant, lingonberry, and cloudberry, are also popularly consumed in other regions of the world. There is also a growing trend in the consumption of exotic "berry-type" fruits and their products, including the pomegranate (*Punica granatum*), goji berries (*Lycium barbaru)* fruits of *Garcinia mangostana*, the Brazilian açaí berry (*Euterpe oleraceae*), and the Chilean maqui berry (*Aristotelia chilensis*). The major known bioactive compounds present in berries include vitamins A, C, and E and folic acid; calcium and selenium; β-carotene, R-carotene, and lutein; phytosterols such as β-sitosterol and stigmasterol; triterpene esters; and phenolic molecules such as anthocyanins, flavonols, flavanols, proanthocyanidins, ellagitannins, and phenolic acids like hydroxybenzoic and hydroxycinnamicacids (Seeram et al. 2006). Some recent studies have shown that berry extracts and their singly purified phenolic constituents inhibit cell proliferation, modulate cell cycle arrest, and induce apoptosis (programmed cell death) in cancer cells with little or no cytotoxic effects in normal cells (Seeram et al. 2006) Several berry extracts, including strawberry and raspberry, were recently evaluated for their effects on cell viability and expression of markers of cell proliferation and apoptosis in human HT29 colon cancer cells and it was hypothesized that the berry extracts inhibited cancer cell proliferation mainly via the p21WAF1 (a member of the cyclin kinase inhibitors) pathway (Wu et al. 2007). It was reported that freeze dried black raspberry ethanol extract suppressed cell proliferation without perturbing viability, inhibited translation of the complete angiogenic cytokine vascular endothelial growth factor, suppressed nitric oxide synthase activity, and induced both apoptosis and terminal differentiation (Rodrigo et al. 2006). Berry fruits also show potential in the inhibition of absorption of environmental carcinogens. The potential of red raspberry extracts to inhibit the absorption of environmental carcinogens such as polycyclic aromatic hydrocarbons (PAHs) using a Calu-3 cell monolayer model was studied (Mahadevan et al. 2005). It was reported that dietary black raspberry powder inhibited N-nitrosomethylbenzylamine (NMBA)-induced tumor development in the rat esophagus by inhibiting the formation of DNA adducts and reducing the proliferation rate of preneoplastic cells by the down-regulation of the expression of c-Jun, COX-2, and inducible nitric oxide synthase (Chen et al. 2006).

Cranberry fruit has a diverse phytochemical profile which contains three classes of flavonoids (flavonols, anthocyanins, and proanthocyanidins), catechins, hydroxycinnamic and other phenolic acids, and triterpenoids. This unique combination of phytochemicals found in cranberry fruit may produce synergistic health benefits. Possible chemopreventive mechanisms of action by cranberry phytochemicals include induction of apoptosis in tumor cells, reduced ornithine decarboxylase activity, decreased expression of matrix metalloproteinases associated with prostate tumor metastasis, and anti-inflammatory activities including inhibition of cyclooxygenases and these findings suggest a potential role for cranberry as a dietary chemopreventive dietary source (Neto 2007). Extracts of cranberry, bilberry, and other fruits were observed to inhibit ornithine decarboxylase (ODC) expression and induce the xenobiotic detoxification enzyme quinone reductase *in vitro* and extract of cranberry presscake inhibited proliferation of MCF-7 and MDA-MB-435 breast cancer cells (Ferguson et al. 2004). It was reported that water-soluble cranberry phenolic extracts prepared from commercial cranberry powder effectively inhibited proliferation of several human tumor cell lines (Sun and Liu 2006). Mixed anthocyanin rich extracts inhibited the induction of vascular endothelial growth factor by both hydrogen peroxide and tumor necrosis factor (TNF) and also resulted in decreased hemangioma formation and tumor growth. Proanthocyanidins and flavonoids from cranberry and other *Vaccinium* berries show some promise toward limiting processes involved in tumor invasion and metastasis by blocking the expression of MMPs involved in remodeling the extracellular matrix (Yu et al. 2009). Around 20 pure compounds from cranberries, including ursolic acid, quercetin, and

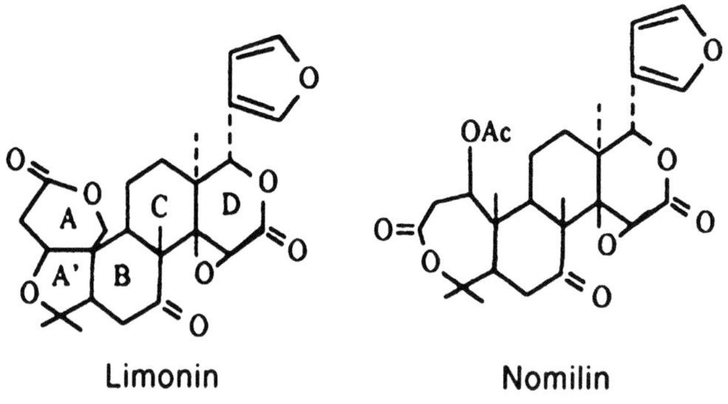

Fig. 16.8 Structures of limonin and nomilin

3,5,7,3′,4′-pentahydroxyflavonol-3-O-β-D-glucopyranoside identified and showed potent anti-proliferative activities against liver HepG2 and breast MCF7 cancer cell growth which was attributed to the ability of the extracts to initiate apoptosis and induce G1 phase arrest in the cell cycle (Yu et al. 2009).

Three major phenolics isolated from *Garcinia mangostana* fruit pericarp namely 1,3,6,7-tetrahydroxy-2,8-(3-methyl-2-butenyl) xanthone, 1,3,6-trihydroxy-7-methoxy-2,8-(3-methyl-2-butenyl) xanthone and epicatechin showed anticancer property against human breast cancer cells (MCF-7) and human colon cancer cells (LOVO) (Furusawa 2003). Antitumor potential of the noni fruit juice at animal level was studied and found that it could inhibit murine tumor growth with a definite curative potential (Baker 1994).

Citrus fruits, including oranges, lemons, limes and grapefruits, are a principal source of nutrients such as vitamin C, folate and dietary fibre, and other bioactive components, such as carotenoids and flavonoids, which are suggested to be responsible for the prevention of degenerative disease. Citrus fruits are particularly high in a class of phytochemicals known as the limonoids (Lam et al. 1994). The most prevalent limonoids are limonin and nomilin and the structures are shown in Fig. 16.8. It has been determined by *in vivo* studies that citrus limonoids and derivatives have certain biological activities that may be used as chemopreventive agents for cancer (Collins et al. 2003).

Studies on kiwifruit showed that it can provide a dual protection against oxidative DNA damage, enhancing antioxidant levels and stimulating DNA repair. It is probable that together these effects would decrease the risk of mutagenic changes leading to cancer (Wargovich 1997).

Vegetables and Cancer

Cruciferous vegetables such as cauliflower, broccoli, cabbage etc. are sources of isothiocyanates, chemicals that modulate the metabolism of a number of nitrosamine- carcinogens. Phytochemicals, such as organosulfur compounds from garlic and onion also known to modify the metabolic activation of procarcinogens (Morse et al. 1989). The isothiocyanates from crucifers modify the metabolism of an important carcinogenic class of carcinogens, the nitrosamines. Extensive structure-activity studies by these investigators have also shown that changing the carbon chain length of the isothiocyanate moiety correlates with tumor prevention theoretically by making the isothiocyanate more suitable insertion for into the cell due to increases in lipophilicity (Giovannucci et al. 2004). Lycopene-containing (Talalay and Fahey 2001), cruciferous (Milner 2001), and allium vegetables (FAO/WHO 2002) are inversely related to the risk of certain cancers. Potatoes and some fruit juices (often included with total vegetables and fruits) might actually increase the risk, as they have a high glycemic index and increase insulin secretion. Potato products contain high levels of acrylamide, formed during cooking at high temperatures, which has the ability to induce cancer and heritable mutations in animals (Block 1992).

In garlic and onion a cascade of organosulfur compounds are generated when precursor compounds are acted on by the enzyme allinase (Brady et al. 1991). The volatile sulfides and disulfides in onion and garlic have been extensively investigated for cancer preventive benefit. Diallyl sulfide (DAS) is one of the common volatiles in garlic and has been shown to be a potent inhibitor of cytochrome P450. It was found that diallys sulfide can compete as a substrate for cytochrome P450 oxidative reaction (Amagase et al. 2001). Isothiocyanatcs play dual role in the suppression of activation and in the detoxification of chemical carcinogens (Pinto and Rivlin 2001).

Garlic contains radioprotective antioxidants that are amplified in aged garlic extract (Kyolic), an odorless supplement made from organic garlic by a process of extraction and aging (Pinto and Rivlin 2001). The main antioxidant is the water-soluble S-allyl cysteine, which is highly effective in protecting cells from oxidant damage by radiation and anticancer drugs. The water-soluble organosulfur compound S-allyl mercaptocysteine, which is unique to aged garlic extract, induces apoptosis in human prostate, breast, and colon cancer cells as well as leukemia cells (Xiao et al. 2000). S-allyl mercaptocysteine activates caspase, inhibits antiapoptotic protein Bcl-2, and disrupts microtubules in the cancer cells, preventing further growth (Fowke et al. 2003).

Cruciferous vegetables (broccoli, cauliflower, cabbage, brussels sprouts) contain sulforophane, which has anti cancer properties. A case-control study in China found that intake of cruciferous vegetables, measured by urinary secretion of isothiocyanates, was inversely related to the risk of breast cancer, the quartile with the highest intake only had 50% of the risk of the lowest intake group (Zhang et al. 2000). It was reported that high intake of cruciferous vegetables (five or more servings/week Vs less than two servings/ week) was associated with a 33% lower risk of non- Hodgkin's lymphoma (Michaud et al. 1999). Another clinical study showed that high intake (five or more servings/week Vs 1 or less servings/wk) of cruciferous vegetables was associated with a statistically significant 51% decrease in bladder cancer (Cohen et al. 2000). Also, prostate cancer risk was found to be reduced statistically significant 41% by cruciferous vegetable consumption in a population-based case control study (London et al. 2000). It was found that men with detectable amounts of isothiocyanates in their urine (metabolic products that come from cruciferous vegetables) had a 35% decreased risk of lung cancer. Broccoli sprouts have a very high concentration of sulforophane since this compound originates in the seed and is not made in the plant as it grows (Fahey et al. 1997; Nadkarni and Nadkarni 1976).

Spices and Cancer

Spices are a group of esoteric food adjuncts, which have been in use for thousands of years. By virtue of their pleasing color, flavor or pungency, they transform food into attractive and appetizing meal. In addition to these organoleptic properties, few spices are also known to possess several medicinal properties (Joe and Lokesh 1994). Curcumin, one of the major spices used was found to inhibit the generation of ROS including superoxide dismutase and hydrogen peroxide in peritoneal macrophages (Deshpande and Maru 1995). Curcumin inhibited tumor initiation induced by benzo (a) pyrene and 7,12-dimethylbenz (a) anthracene and tumor promotion induced by phorbol esters (Naama et al. 2010). The ethanol extract of curcumin showed anticancer activity against the cell line of human hepato cellular liver carcinoma (Kaefer and Milner 2008). Spices have been known to be effective on cancers such as intestine cancer, liver cancer, colon cancer, stomach cancer, breast cancer, skin cancer, bladder cancer. Research work on the anticarcinogenic effect of spices such as turmeric, rosemary extract, sage extract, ginger, coriander seed, black pepper, cumin and garlic have been carried out by many research groups as shown in Table 16.3 (Zheng et al. 2004). The yellow pigment in turmeric, curcumin is a potent anti-inflammatory and cancer-preventive antioxidant in experimental systems, is widely used in Asian countries. Epidemiological studies have attributed the low rate of colon cancer in these countries to the high consumption of curcumin. Recent studies show that curcumin can induce apoptosis in colon cancer cells and multiple myeloma cells as well as ovarian cancer cells (Chauhan 2002). Curcumin has been found to suppress the activity of the antiapoptotic protein Bcl-2 in myeloma cells and in colon cancer cells (Zhou et al. 2003).

Phase I and Phase II enzymes have an important role in the cancer. Compounds in garlic, pepper, rosemary, turmeric, and cinnamon appear to influence phase I and phase II enzymes (Van Erk et al. 2004; Debersac et al. 2001). Multiple compounds in garlic, such as diallyl sulfide, diallyl sulfone, and diallyl sulfoxide may be involved in directly inhibiting CYP2E1 activity (Van Erk et al. 2004). Debersac et al. (2001) found that water-soluble rosemary extract and essential oil of rosemary, with a high content of 1,8-cineole (36.1%), induced CYP2B1 and multiple phase II enzymes, such as hepatic glutathione-S-transferases (GST), quinine reductase (QR), and UDP-glucuronosyl-transferase (UGT), especially UGT1A6, which are involved in critical detoxification pathways. The cause of the strong induction of phase II enzymes by spices may be due to the synergistic effects of a combination of

Table 16.3 Phytochemicals present in common spices and herbs

Spices and herbs	Phytochemicals
Turmeric	Curcumin, curcuminoids
Thyme	Thymol, carvacrol, cineole, α-pinene; apigenin, β-carotene, eugenol, limonene, ursolic acid, luteolin, gallic acid, caffeic acid, rosmarinic acid, carnosic acid
Saffron	Crocetin, crocin, β-carotene, safranal
Rosemary	Carnasol, carnosic acid, cineole, geraniol, α-pinene, β-carotene, apigenin, limonene, naringin, luteolin, caffeic acid, rosmarinic acid, rosmanol, vanillic acid
Basil	Eugenol, apigenin, limonene, ursolic acid, methyl cinnamate, 1,8-cineole, anthocyanins, carvacrol, cintronellol, farnesol, geraniol, kaempherol
Cardamom	Limonene, caffeic acid
Cinnamon	Cinnamic aldehyde, 2-hydroxycinnamaldehyde, eugenol
Cloves	Eugenol, isoeugenol, gallic acid
Coriander	Quercetin, caffeic acid, cineole, geraniol, borneol, 1,8-cineole, α-terpinene, β- carotene, βpinene,β-sitosterol, cinnamic acid, ferrulic acid, γ-terpinene, kaempferol, limonene, myrcene, p-coumaric acid, p-cymene, quercetin, rutin, vanillic acid
Mustard	Allyl isothiocyanate, β-carotene
Oregano	Apigenin, luteolin, myricetin, quercetin, caffeic acid
Parsley	Apigenin, luteolin, kaempferol, myricetin, quercetin, caffeic acid
Peppermint	Limonene, menthol, eriodictyol, hesperitin, apigenin, luteolin

phenolic compounds (Shen et al. 2006). Yellow pigments from turmeric, curcumin inhibited reactions catalyzed by CYP1A1, 1A2, and 2B1 in rat liver cells and induced phase II enzymes in the liver and kidney in rats, human melanoma cells, and GSTP1-1 in K562 and Jurkat leukemia cells. Shen et al. (Gangadeep et al. 2003) recently demonstrated *in vivo* that curcumin (1,000 mg/kg), along with transporter proteins and oxidative stress genes, could regulate phase I and II xenobiotic-metabolizing enzyme genes in mouse liver and small intestine through nuclear factor erythroid-2 (Nrf2) dependent pathways. *In vitro* studies indicate herbs, spices, and their bioactive components can inhibit, and sometimes induce, pathways that regulate cell division, cell proliferation, and detoxification, in addition to the inflammatory and immune response. It was found that low dose of cumin had 28.6% fewer forestomach tumors, and those consuming the higher dose of cumin had a 35.7% reduction in tumor incidence rate (Abdullaev 2002). Saffron and some of its bioactive components have also been shown to possess antitumor activity in different types of cultured malignant cells (Mukhtar and Ahmad 1999).

There are many factors which effects the complete studies on the role of spices and herb extracts such as lack of general terminology, lack of standardized spice and herb extracts and/or preparations, variability in the description of herbal and spice products used in studies, lack of proper information regarding the chemical profiles and active ingredients raise significant concerns about the studies in spices and herb extracts.

Tea and Cancer

Tea is the most popular beverage consumed by two-thirds of the world's population. Green tea, black tea, and Oolong tea are all derived from the leaves of *Camellia sinensis*. The chemical components of tea leave include polyphenols (catechins and flavonoides), alkaloids (caffeine, theobromine, theophylline, etc.), volatile oils, polysaccharides, amino acids, lipids, vitamins (e.g., vitamin C), inorganic elements (e.g., aluminium, fluorine and manganese), etc. However, the polyphenols are primarily responsible for the beneficial healthful properties of tea. Tea polyphenols, known as catechins, account for 30–42% of the dry weight of the solids in brewed green tea (Khan and Mukhtar 2007). The polyphenols content of green tea and black tea varies from 30% to 40% and 3% to 10%, respectively. Major catechins found in tea leaves are (-)-epigallocatechin-3-gallate (EGCG), (-)-epigallocatechin (EGC), (-)-epicatechin-3-gallate (ECG) and (-)-epicatechin (EC) and their structures are shown in Fig. 16.9. Catechin, gallocatechin, epigallocatechin digallates, epicatechin digallate, 3-O-methyl EC and EGC, catechin gallate, and gallocatechin gallate are present in smaller quantities. Flavonols, including quercetin, kaempferol, myricitin, and their glycosides are also present in tea. A typical tea beverage, with 1 g of leaf in 100 ml of water in three minute brew, usually comprised of 30–42% catechins and 3–6% caffeine (Kris-Etherton et al. 2002). The tea containing various antioxidants and phenolic compounds shown to have anti-cancer properties in laboratory conditions (Vasisht et al. 2003). Several population-based studies confirm about the cancer protective effects of tea (Ahmad et al. 1997). Various studies have demonstrated that green tea phenolics, especially EGCG can inhibit carcinogenesis and also the growth of established cancers at various organ sites (Kris-Etherton et al. 2002). EGCG induces apoptosis and cell cycle arrest in many cancer cells without affecting normal cells (Bettuzzi et al. 2006). Green tea catechins given in the form of capsules when given to men with high-grade prostate intraepithelial neoplasia (PIN) demonstrated cancer preventive activity by inhibiting the conversion of high grade PIN lesions to cancer (Beltz et al. 2006). Kumar et al. (2007) outlined the wide range of mechanisms by which epigallocatechin gallate (ECGC) and other green and black tea polyphenols inhibit cancer cell survival. Epidemiological studies have identified epigallocatechin gallate (EGCG) in green tea polyphenols (GTP), as the most potent chemopreventive agent that can induce apoptosis, suppress the formation and growth of human cancers including colorectal cancers (Katiyar et al. 1993). Green teas contain a number of polyphenolic catechins, polyphenolic agents. Green tea consumed by humans has been reported to inhibit a variety of chemically induced cancers. When green tea polyphenol fractions have been applied to mouse skin DMBA-initiated/TPA promoted skin tumorigenesis was suppressed (Yang and Wang 1993). Green tea polyphenols shown to suppress lung and forestomach tumors in A/J mice induced by benzo[a]pyrene and NNK induced lung cancer (Yang and Wang 1993). Epigallocatechin gallate (EGCG) was shown at low doses to inhibit NNK lung tumors in A/J mice. EGCG has been reported to be effective in inhibiting nitrosamine-induced liver cancer and has been shown to slow growth of skin papillomas in mice (Medić-Sarić et al. 2009).

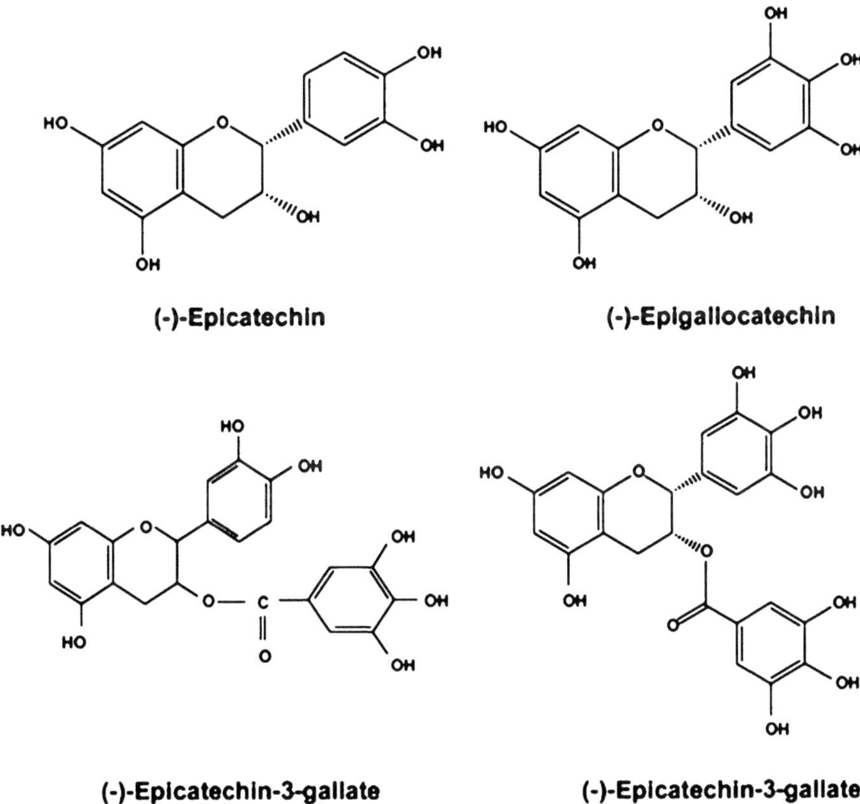

Fig. 16.9 Structures of major catechins found in tea

Wine and Cancer

Numerous studies indicate that moderate red wine consumption is associated with a protective effect against all-cause mortality. It is of interest to consider that red wine is one of the most abundant sources of polyphenols (Pandey and Rizvi 2009). Typically a glass of red wine contains about 100 mg polyphenols (Bruno and Sparapano 2007). Grape is a phenol-rich plant and these phenolics are mainly distributed in the skin, stem, leaf and seed of grape. The total phenolic content of grape skins varied with cultivar, soil composition, climate, geographic origin, and cultivation practices or exposure to diseases, such as fungal infections (Bell et al. 2000). In red wine, anthocyanins and flavonoids are the major two groups of phenolic compounds (Chacona et al. 2009). Phenolic compounds in grapes and wine are grouped within the following major classes: stilbenes, flavan-3-ols, flavonols, anthocyanins, hydroxybenzoic acids, procyanidins, hydroxycinnamic acids. Anthocyanins are the main polyphenolics in red grapes, while flavan-3-ols are more abundant in white varieties (Athar et al. 2009). Resveratrol is the most famous polyphenolic compound occurring in grapes and wine. Resveratrol has been shown to inhibit tumor initiation, promotion, and progression (Bhardwaj et al. 2007). Resveratrol acts at multiple levels, controlling the cell cycle progression, regulating the signs of apoptosis and survival pathways, inhibiting tumor growth and angiogenesis and modulating the activity of transcription factors related with the pathogenesis of cancer (Reagan-Shaw et al. 2008). Resveratrol also potentiates the apoptotic effects of cytokines, chemotherapeutic agents and gamma-radiation (Hudson et al. 2007). It has been reported that the grape skin extract induced prostate tumor cell lines apoptosis with high rates (Jung et al. 2006). Grape juice polyphenols also significantly inhibited carcinogen-induced DNA adducts formation in a rat model and inhibited DNA synthesis in breast cancer cells (Kim et al. 2006). Red wine polyphenols induced apoptosis–in dose dependent manner–in neoplastic cells of colon cancer *in vitro*, increasing caspase-3 activity and Bax expression (Lucas et al. 1957).

The beneficial health effects of wine polyphenols includes inhibiting some degenerative diseases, such as cardiovascular diseases, neurodegenerative disorders, diabetes, and certain types of cancers, reducing plasma oxidative stress and slowing ageing. Future large scale randomized clinical trials should be conducted to fully establish the role of individual wine polyphenol against human disease.

Other Dietary Sources

The use of medicinal mushrooms in the fight against cancer is known for a very long time in Korea, China, Japan etc. These mushrooms belonging to the family Polyporaceae have been effective against esophageal, stomach, prostate and lung cancers. Lucas et al. (1957) demonstrated the anti-tumor effect of higher basidiomyces (specifically extracts of fruiting bodies of *Boletus edulis*). An agent active against Ehrlich carcinoma of the mouse was isolated from *Lampteromyces japonicas* (Ikegawa et al. 1968). Daba and Ezeronye (2003) reported that an essence obtained from the fruit body of edible mushrooms exhibited remarkable host-mediatory anti-tumor activity against grafted cancer in animals. Kurashiga et al. (1997) reported that *Pleurotus ostreatus* mushrooms cultivated on date waste posses a potent antitumor activity against Ehrlich ascites carcinoma. Several studies have shown that B-D-glucan derived from *Grifola frondosa* (also known as Maitake) have strong antitumor activity in xenographs (Lin et al. 2002). Polysaccharide based carcinostatic (immunotherapy eutic) agents such Krestin, Lentinan and Sonifilan developed from mushroom are currently used in the treatment of cancer of the digestive organs, lung and breast, as well as cancer of the stomach and cervical cancer respectively (Kurashiga et al. 1997).

Flax seed and its lignan were found to reduce tumor growth (both in number and size of tumors), prevent metastasis, and even cause increased differentiation of mouse mammary tissue in suckling mice, making the offspring less susceptible to carcinogenesis even when not consuming any flax products. Diet supplemented with 5% flax inhibited the growth and development of prostate cancer in their experimental mouse model (Lin et al. 2002).

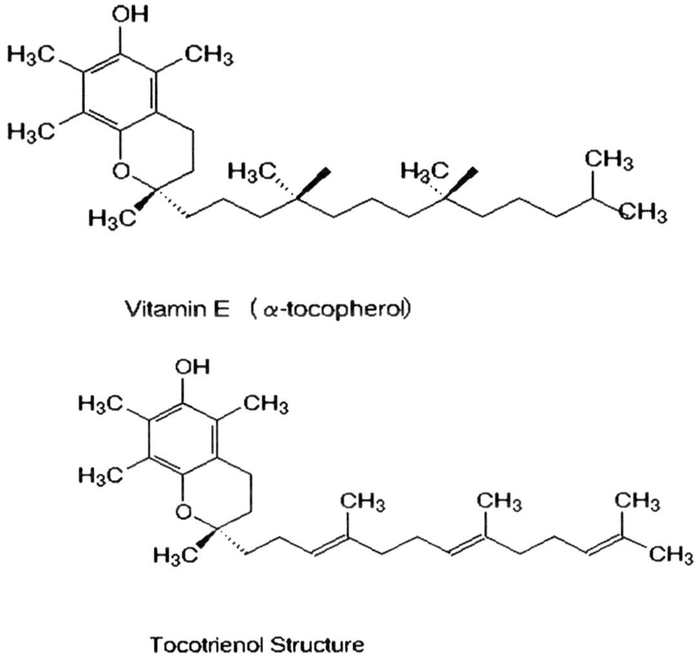

Vitamin E (α-tocopherol)

Tocotrienol Structure

Fig. 16.10 Structures of tocopherols and tocotrienols

Dietary fats and oils contain variable amounts of natural antioxidants that act to prevent spoilage, as well as maintain flavor and nutritional value and also shown to provide significant health benefits. Red palm oil is unique as compared to other dietary fats since palm oil contains the highest known concentrations of natural antioxidants, particularly provitamins A carotenes and vitamin E (Khor and Raajeswari 2001) and palm vitamin E is composed of 70–80% tocotrienols (McIntyre et al. 2000). Vitamin E represents a family of compounds that is further divided into two subclasses called tocopherols and tocotrienols. Tocopherols and tocotrienols have the same basic chemical structure characterized by a long phytyl tail attached to a chromane ring. Tocopherols have a saturated, whereas tocotrienols have an unsaturated phytyl tail, and individual isoforms of tocopherols and tocotrienols differ from each other based on the degree of methylation of the chromane ring (Fig. 16.10). Tocotrienols showed potent antiproliferative and apoptotic activity against breast cancer cells (McIntyre et al. 2000; Sylvester et al. 2001). The greater biopotency of tocotrienols versus tocopherols may be due to the reason that tocotrienols are more easily or preferentially taken up by neoplastic mammary epithelial cells (McIntyre et al. 2000). Neoplastic cells display greater sensitivity to the tocotrienol-induced apoptosis than normal mammary epithelial cells (McIntyre et al. 2000).

Olives contains many antioxidant compounds such as acteosides, hydroxytyrosol, tyrosol and phenyl propionic acids. Olive oil, especially extra virgin, contains smaller amounts of hydroxytyrosol and tyrosol, but also contains secoiridoids and lignans in abundance. Both olives and olive oil contain substantial amounts of other compounds deemed to be anticancer agents (e.g. squalene and terpenoids) as well as the peroxidation resistant lipid oleic acid (Sylvester et al. 2001). The consumption of live and olive oil in southern Europe represents an important contribution to the beneficial effects on health of the Mediterranean diet. Habitual high intakes of olives and extra virgin olive oil will provide a continuous supply of antioxidants, which may mediate their effects by reducing oxidative stress via inhibition of lipid peroxidation, thereby inhibiting formation of DNA adducts (Owen et al. 2004) factors that are currently linked to cancer.

Conclusion

Dietary modification by increasing the consumption of a variety of fruits, vegetables, and whole grains daily is a practical strategy for consumers to optimize their health and to reduce the risk of chronic diseases. Fruits and vegetables have strong antioxidant and anti-proliferative activities, and the major part of total antioxidant activity is from the combination of phytochemicals. The additive and synergistic effects of phytochemicals in fruits and vegetables are responsible for their potent antioxidant, anticancer activities and health benefits. The benefit of a diet rich in fruits, vegetables, and whole grains is attributed to the complex mixture of phytochemicals present in these and other whole foods. This explains why no single antioxidant can replace the combination of natural phytochemicals in fruits and vegetables and achieve their health benefits. Dietary improvement will be the most realistic to prevent cancer in the coming decades. A holistic approach integrating lifestyle and more specific improvements in the components and individuals of diet habits will provide a practical approach. Interdisciplinary research is highly recommended so that basic and preclinical studies can lead to translational research (from laboratory to patients). In conclusion, it is strongly recommended that this area of research which involves mainly the determination of its compositional analysis of phytochemicals present in the diet and its mechanism of action as chemopreventive agents of cancer and other degenerative disease continue to be explored, as this will lay the foundation for the development of diet-based strategies for the prevention and therapy of several types of human cancers.

Acknowledgements The authors are sincerely thankful to the Natural Sciences and Engineering Research Council of Canada (Discovery Grant 355254, Canada Research Chair), FQRNT (ENC 125216), MAPAQ (No. 809051) and Inde Initiative 2010 (Ministère de l'Éducation, du Loisir et du Sport) for financial support. The views or opinions expressed in this article are those of the authors.

References

Abdullaev FI (2002) Cancer preventive and tumoricidal properties of saffron (*Crocus sativus* L.). Exp Biol 227:20–25

Adlercreutz H (1990) Western diet and Western diseases: some hormonal and biochemical mechanisms and associations. Scand J Clin Lab Invest 50:3–23

Adom KK, Liu RH (2002) Antioxidant activity of grains. J Agric Food Chem 50:6182–6187

Agarwal S, Rao AV (1998) Tomato lycopene and low density lipoprotein oxidation: a human dietary intervention study. Lipids 33:981–984

Ahmad NDK, Feyes AL, Nieminen R, Agarwal H, Mukhtar H (1997) Green tea constituent epigallocatechin-3-gallate and induction of apoptosis and cell cycle arrest in human carcinoma cells. J Natl Cancer Inst 89:1881–1886

Ajila CM, Brar SK, Verma M, Tyagi RD, Valéro JR (2011) Solid-state fermentation of apple pomace using *Phanerocheate chrysosporium* – liberation and extraction of phenolic antioxidants. Food Chem 126(3):1071–1080

Amagase H, Petesch BL, Matsura H, Kasuga S, Itakura Y (2001) Intake of garlic and its bioactive compounds. J Nutr 131:955S–962S

Ames BN, Shigenaga MK, Gold LS (1993a) DNA lesions, inducible DNA repair, and cell division: the three key factors in mutagenesis and carcinogenesis. Environ Health Perspect 101:35–44

Ames BN, Shigenaga MK, Hagen TM (1993b) Oxidants, antioxidants, and the degenerative diseases of aging. Proc Natl Acad Sci U S A 90:7915

Athar M, Back JH, Kopelovich L, Bickers DR, Kim AL (2009) Multiple molecular targets of resveratrol: anti-carcinogenic mechanisms. Arch Biochem Biophys 486:95–102

Aylsworth CF, Cullum ME, Zile MH, Welsch CW (1986) Influence of dietary retinyl acetate on enhancement of DMBA-induced rat mammary carcinogenesis by high levels of dietary fat. J Natl Cancer Inst 76:339–345

Baker RA (1994) Potential dietary benefits of citrus pectin and fibre. Food Technol 11:133–139

Baker RTM (2002) Canthaxanthin in aquafeed applications: is there any risk? Trends Food Sci Technol 12:240

Batieha AM, Armenian HK, Norkus EP, Morris JS, Spate VE, Comstock GW (1993) Serum micronutrients and the subsequent risk of cervical cancer in a population-based nested case-control study. Biomark Prev 2:335–339

Bell JRC, Donovan JL, Wong R (2000) (+)-Catechin in human plasma after ingestion of a single serving of reconstituted red wine. Am J Clin Nutr 71:103–108

Beltz LA, Bayer DK, Moss AL, Simet IM (2006) Mechanisms of cancer prevention by green and black tea polyphenols. Anticancer Agents Med Chem 6(5):389–406

Bettuzzi S, Brausi M, Rizzi F, Castagnetti G, Peracchia G, Corti A (2006) Chemoprevention of human prostate cancer by oral administration of green tea catechins in volunteers with high-grade prostate intraepithelial neoplasia: a preliminary report from a one-year proof-of-principle study. Cancer Res 66:1234–1240

Bhardwaj A, Sethi G, Vadhan-Raj S, Bueso-Ramos C, Takada Y, Gaur U, Nair AS, Shishodia S, Aggarwal BB (2007) Resveratrol inhibits proliferation, induces apoptosis, and overcomes chemoresistance through down-regulation of STAT3 and nuclear factor-kappaB-regulated antiapoptotic and cell survival gene products in human multiple myeloma cells. Blood 109:2293–2302

Block E (1992) The organosulfur chemistry of the genus Allium: implications for the organic chemistry of sulfur. Angew Chem 31:1135–1178

Block G, Patterson B, Subar A (1992) Fruit, vegetables, and cancer prevention: a review of the epidemiological evidence. Nutr Cancer 18:1–29

Brady JF, Wang MH, Hong JY, Xiao F, Li Y, Yoo JS, Ning SM, Lee MJ, Fukuto JM, Gapac JM (1991) Modulation of rat hepatic microsomal monooxygenase enzymes and cytotoxicity by diallyl sulfide. Toxicol Appl Pharmacol 108:342–354

Bravo I (1998) Polyphenol chemistry, directory sources, metabolism and nutritional significance. Nutr Rev 56:317–325
Bruno G, Sparapano L (2007) Effects of three esca-associated fungi on *Vitis vinifera* L: changes in the chemical and biological profile of xylem sap from diseased cv. *Sangiovese* vines. Physiol Mol Plant Pathol 71:210–229
Chacona MR, Ceperuelo-Mallafrea V, Maymo-Masipa E, Mateo-Sanz JM, Arolac L, Guitiérrez C, Fernandez-Reald JM, Ardèvol A, Simón I, Vendrell J (2009) Grape-seed procyanidins modulate inflammation on human differentiated adipocytes *in vitro*. Cytokine 47:137–142
Chauhan DP (2002) Chemotherapeutic potential of curcumin for colorectal cancer. Curr Pharm Des 8:1695–1706
Chen T, Rose ME, Hwang H, Nines RG, Stoner GD (2006) Black raspberries inhibit N nitrosomethylbenzylamine (NMBA)- induced angiogenesis in rat esophagus parallel to the suppression of COX-2 and iNOS. Carcinogenesis 27:2301–2317
Chew BP, Park JS, Wong MW, Wong TS (1999) A comparison of the anticancer activities of dietary β-carotene, canthaxanthin and astaxanthin in mice *in vivo*. Anticancer Res 19:1849–1853
Chu YF, Sun J, Wu X, Liu RH (2002) Antioxidant and antiproliferative activities of vegetables. J Agric Food Chem 50:6910–6916
Cohen JH, Kristal AR, Stanford JL (2000) Fruit and vegetable intakes and prostate cancer risk. J Natl Cancer Inst 92:61–68
Collins AR, Harrington V, Drew J, Melvin R (2003) Molecular epidemiology and cancer prevention. Carcinogenesis 24(3):511–515
Daba AS, Ezeronye DO (2003) Anti-cancer effect of polysaccharides isolated from higher basidiomycetes mushrooms. Afr J Biotechnol 2(12):672–678
Davies KJA (1995) Oxidative stress: the paradox of aerobic life. Biochem Soc Symp 61:1–31
Debersac P, Heydel JM, Amiot MJ, Goudonnet H, Artur Y, Suschetet M, Siess MH (2001) Induction of cytochrome P450 and/or detoxication enzymes by various extracts of rosemary: description of specific patterns. Food Chem Toxicol 39(9):907–918
Del Rio D, Calani L, Scazzina F, Jechiu L, Cordero C, Brighenti F (2010) Bioavailability of catechins from ready-to-drink tea. Nutrition 26:528–533
Deshpande SS, Maru GB (1995) Effects of curcumin on the formation of benzo (a)pyrene derived DNA adducts in vitro. Cancer Lett 96:71–80
Dewanto V, Wu X, Liu RH (2002) Processed sweet corn has higher antioxidant activity. J Agric Food Chem 50:4959–4964
Di Mascio P, Kaiser S, Sies H (1989) Lycopene as the most effective biological carotenoid singlet oxygen quencher. Arch Biochem Biophys 274:532–538
Eberhardt M, Lee C, Liu RH (2000) Antioxidant activity of fresh apples. Nature 405:903–904
Eichholzer M, Luthy J, Moser U, Fowler B (2001) Folate and the risk of colorectal, breast and cervix cancer: the epidemiological evidence. Swiss Med Wkly 131:539–549
Escarpa A, Gonzalez M (1998) High-performance liquid chromatography with diode-array detection for the performance of phenolic compounds in peel and pulp from different apple varieties. J Chromat A 823:331–337
Fahey JW, Zhang Y, Talalay P (1997) Broccoli sprouts: an exceptionally rich source of inducers of enzymes that protect against chemical carcinogens. Proc Natl Acad Sci U S A 94:10367–10372
FAO/WHO (2002) Health implications of acrylamide in food. World Health Organization, Geneva
Ferguson P, Kurowska E, Freeman DJ, Chambers AF, Koropatnick DJ (2004) A flavonoid fraction from cranberry extract inhibits proliferation of human tumor cell lines. J Nutr 134:1529
Feskanich D, Ziegler R, Michaud D, Giovannucci E, Speizer F, Willett W, Colditz G (2000) Prospective study of fruit and vegetable consumption and risk of lung cancer among men and women. J Natl Cancer Inst 92:1812–1823
Fowke JH, Chung FL, Jin F, Qi D, Cai Q, Conaway C, Cheng JR, Shu XO, Gao YT, Zheng W (2003) Urinary isothiocyanate levels, brassica, and human breast cancer. Cancer Res 63: 3980–3986

Furusawa E (2003) Anti-cancer activity of noni fruit juice against tumors in mice. In: Nelson SC (ed) Proceedings of the 2002 Hawai'i noni conference, University of Hawaii at Manoa, College of Tropical Agriculture and Human Resources, Honolulu

Gangadeep DS, Mendiz E, Rao AR, Kale RK (2003) Chemopreventive effects of *Cuminum cyminum* in chemically induced forestomach and uterine cervix tumors in murine model systems. Nutr Cancer 47(2):171–180

Gerster H (1997) The potential role of lycopene for human health. J Am Coll Nutr 16:109–126

Giovannucci E (1999) Tomatoes, tomato-based products, lycopene, and cancer: review of the epidemiological literature. J Natl Cancer Inst 91:317–331

Giovannucci E (2002) Epidemiologic studies of folate and colorectal neoplasia: a review. J Nutr 132:2350S–2355S

Giovannucci E, Rimm EB, Liu Y, Willett WC (2004) Height, predictors of C-peptide and cancer risk in men. Int J Epidemiol 33:217–225

Halliwell B (1994) Free radicals, antioxidants, and human disease: curiosity, cause, or consequence? Lancet 344:721–724

Hanusch M, Stahl W, Schulz WA, Sies H (1995) Induction of gap junctional communication by 4-oxoretinoic acid generated from its precursor canthaxanthin. Arch Biochem Biophys 317: 423–428

Harborne JB, Baxter H, Moss GPA (1999) Handbook of bioactive compounds from plants. Taylor & Francis, London

Hollman PC, Arts ICW (2000) Flavonols, flavones and flavanols – nature, occurrence and dietary burden. J Sci Food Agric 80:1081–1093

Hollman PC, Katan MB (1999) Dietary flavonoids: intake, health effects and bioavailability. Food Chem Toxicol 37(9–10):937–942

Holt PR, Arber N, Halmos B, Forde K, Kissileff H, McGlynn KA, Moss SF, Fan K, Yang K, Lipkin M (2002) Colonic epithelial cell proliferation decreases with increasing levels of serum 25-hydroxy vitamin D. Cancer Epidemiol Biomarkers Prev 11:113–119

Huang MT, Ma W, Yen P, Xie JG, Han J, Frenkel K, Grunberger D, Conney AH (1996) Inhibitory effects of caffeic acid phenethyl ester (CAPE) on 12-O-tetradecanoylphorbol-13-acetate-induced tumor promotion in mouse skin and the synthesis of DNA, RNA and protein in HeLa cells. Carcinogenesis 17:761–765

Huang Z, Fasco MJ, Kaminsky LS (1997) Inhibition of estrone sulfatase in human liver microsomes by quercetin and other flavonoids. J Steroid Biochem Mol Biol 63:9–15

Hudson TS, Hartle DK, Hursting SD, Nunez NP, Wang TTY, Young HA, Arany P, Green JE (2007) Inhibition of prostate cancer growth by muscadine grape skin extract and resveratrol through distinct mechanisms. Cancer Res 67:8396–8405

Ikegawa T, Nakanishi M, Uehara N, Chihara G, Fukuoka F (1968) Antitumor action of some basidiomycetes, especially *Phellinus lintens*. Gann 59:155–157

Ip C (1982) Dietary vitamin E intake and mammary carcinogenesis in rats. Carcinogenesis 3: 1453–1456

Jacobs EJ, Connell CJ, Patel AV, Chao A, Rodriguez C, Seymour J, McCullough M, Calle EE, Thun MJ (2001) Vitamin C and vitamin E supplement use and colorectal cancer mortality in a large American Cancer Society cohort. Cancer Causes Control 12:927–934

Jewell C, O'Brien NM (1999) Effect of dietary supplementation with carotenoids on xenobiotic metabolizing enzymes in the liver, lung, kidney and small intestine of the rat. Br J Nutr 81: 235–242

Joe B, Lokesh BR (1994) Role of capsaicin, curcumin and dietary n-fatty acids in lowering the generation of reactive oxygen species in rat peritoneal macrophages. Biochem Biophys Acta 1224:255–263

John EM, Schwartz GG, Dreon DM, Koo J (1999) Vitamin D and breast cancer risk: the NHANES I epidemiologic follow-up study, 1971–1975 to 1992. National Health and Nutrition Examination Survey. Cancer Epidemiol Biomarkers Prev 8:399–406

Jung K, Wallig M, Singletary K (2006) Purple grape juice inhibits 7, 12-dimethylbenz- [a] anthracene (DMBA)-induced rat mammary tumorigenesis and *in vivo* DMBADNA adduct formation. Cancer Lett 233:279–288

Kaefer CM, Milner JA (2008) The role of herbs and spices in cancer prevention. J Nutr Biochem 19:347–361

Katiyar SK, Agarwal R, Zaim MT, Mukhtar H (1993) Protection against N-nitrosodiethylamine and benzo[a]pyrene-induced forestomach and lung tumorigenesis in A/J mice by green tea. Carcinogenesis 145:849–855

Keijer J, Bekkenkamp-Grovenstein M, Venema D, Dommels YEM (2011) Bioactive food components, cancer cell growth limitation and reversal of glycolytic metabolism. Biochim Biophys Acta 1807:697–706

Khachik F, Askin FB, Lai K (1998) Distribution, bioavailability, and metabolism of carotenoids in humans. In: Bidlack WR et al (eds) Phytochemicals: a new paradigm. Technomic Publishing Company, Lancaster

Khan N, Mukhtar H (2007) Tea polyphenols for health promotion. Life Sci 81:519–533

Khor HT, Raajeswari R (2001) Red palm oil, vitamin A, and the antioxidant enzymes. In: Nesaretnam K, Packer L (eds) Micronutrients and health: molecular biological mechanisms. AOCS Press, Champaign

Kim MJ, Kim YJ, Park HJ, Chung JH, Leem KH, Kim HK (2006) Apoptotic effect of red wine polyphenols on human colon cancer SNU-C4 cells. Food Chem Toxicol 44:898–902

Kimmick GG, Bell RA, Bostick CM (1997) Vitamin E and breast cancer. Nutr Cancer 27:109–117

King P, Ma G, Miao W, Jia Q, McDougall B, Reinecke ME, Cornell C, Kuan J, Kim T, Robinson W (1999) Structure-activity relationships: analogues of the dicaffeoylquinic and dicaffeoyltartaric acids as potent inhibitors of human immunodeficiency virus type 1 integrase and replication. J Med Chem 42:497–509

Koshihara Y, Neichi T, Murota S, Laob A, Fujimoto S, Tatsuno T (1984) Caffeic acid is a selective inhibitor for leukotriene biosynthesis. Biochem Biophys Acta 792:92–97

Kotake-Nara E, Kushiro M, Zhang H, Sugawara T, Miyashita K, Nagao A (2001) Carotenoids affect proliferation of human prostate cancer cells. J Nutr 131:3303–3306

Krinsky NI (1998) The antioxidant and biological properties of the carotenoids. Ann NY Acad Sci 854:443–447

Krinsky NI, Johnson EJ (2005) Carotenoid actions and their relation to health and disease. Mol Aspects Med 26:459–516

Kris-Etherton PM, Hecker KD, Bonanome A, Coval SM, Binkoski AE, Hilpert KF, Griel AE, Etherton TD (2002) Bioactive compounds in foods: their role in the prevention of cardiovascular disease and cancer. Am J Med 113(9B):71S–88S

Kritchevsky D (1991) Evaluation of publicly available scientific evidence regarding certain nutrient disease relationships: dietary fiber and cancer (prepared for food safety and applied nutrition, FDA, DHHS). Life Sciences Research Office, FASEB, Washington, DC

Kumar N, Shibata D, Helm J, Coppola D, Malafa M (2007) Green tea polyphenols in the prevention of colon cancer. Front Biosci 12:2309–2315

Kurashiga S, Akuzawa Y, Eudo F (1997) Effect of *Lentinus edodes*, *Grifola Frondosa* and *Pleurotus ostreatus* administration on cancer outbreak and activities of macrophages and lymphocytes in mice treated with a carcinogen. Immunopharmacol Immunotoxicol 19: 175–185

Lam LKT, Zang J, Hasegawa S (1994) Citrus limonoid reduction of chemically induced tumorigenesis. Food Technol 48:104–108

Lamson D, Brignall M (2000) Antioxidants and cancer III: quercetin. Altern Med Rev 5:196–209

Landrum JT, Bone RA, Herrero C (2002) Astaxanthin, β-cryptoxanthin, lutein, and zeaxanthin, in phytochemicals. In: Meskin MS et al (eds) Nutrition and health. CRC Press, Boca Raton

Le Marchand L, Murphy S, Hankin J, Wilkens L, Kolonel L (2000) Intake of flavonoids and lung cancer. J Natl Cancer Inst 92:154–160

Lin X, Gingrich JR, Bao W, Li J, Haroon ZA, Demark-Wahnefried W (2002) Effect of flaxseed supplementation on prostatic carcinoma in transgenic mice. Urology 60:919–924

Lipkin M, Newmark HL (1999) Vitamin D, calcium and prevention of breast cancer: a review. J Am Coll Nutr 18:392S–397S

Liu RH, Eberhardt M, Lee C (2001) Antioxidant and antiproliferative activities of selected New York apple cultivars. NY Fruit Q 9:15–17

London SJ, Yuan JM, Chung FL, Gao YT, Coetzee GA, Ross RK, Yu MC (2000) Isothiocyanates, glutathione S-transferase M1 and T1 polymorphisms, and lung-cancer risk: a prospective study of men in Shanghai, China. Lancet 356:724–729

Lorenz RT, Cysewski GR (2000) Commercial potential for *Haematococcus* microalgae as a natural source of astaxanthin. Trends Biotechnol 18:160–167

Lucas EH, Montesano R, Pepper MS, Hafner M, Sablon E (1957) Tumor inhibitors in *Boletus edulis* and other holobasidiomycetes. Antibiot Chemother 7:1–4

Mahadevan B, Mata JE, Albershardt DJ, Stevens JF, Pereira CB, Rodriguez-Proteau R, Baird WM (2005) The effects of red raspberry extract on PAH transport across Calu-3 cell monolayer, an *in vitro* cell model. Int J Cancer Prev 2:129–141

Matsushima NR, Shidoji Y, Nishiwaki S, Yamada T, Moriwaki H, Muto Y (1995) Suppression by carotenoids of microcystin-induced morphological changes in mouse hepatocytes. Lipids 30:1029–1034

McIntyre BS, Briski KP, Tirmenstein MA, Fariss MW, Gapor A, Sylvester PW (2000) Antiproliferative and apoptotic effects of tocopherols and tocotrienols on normal mouse mammary epithelial cells. Lipids 35:171–180

Medić-Sarić M, Rastija V, Bojić M, Males Z (2009) From functional food to medicinal product: systematic approach in analysis of polyphenolics from propolis and wine. Nutr J 8:33

Mertens-Talcott S, Talcott S, Percival S (2003) Low concentration of quercetin and ellagic acid synergistically influence proliferation, cytotoxicity and apoptosis in MOLT-4 human leukemia cells. J Nutr 133:2669–2674

Michaud DS, Spiegelman D, Clinton SK, Rimm EB, Willett WC, Giovannucci EL (1999) Fruit and vegetable intake and incidence of bladder cancer in a male prospective cohort. J Natl Cancer Inst 91:605–613

Milner JA (2001) A historical perspective on garlic and cancer. J Nutr 131:1027S–11031S

Molina M, Sanchez-Reus I, Iglesias I, Benedi J (2003) Quercetin, a flavonoid antioxidant, prevents and protects against ethanol induced oxidative stress in mouse liver. Biol Pharm Bull 26: 1398–1402

Moon RC (1994) Vitamin A, retinoids and breast cancer. Adv Exp Med Biol 364:101–107

Morse MA, Elkind KI, Amin SG, Hecht SS, Chung FL (1989) Effects of alkyl chain length on the inhibition of NNK-induced lung neoplasia in A/J mice by arylalkyl isothiocyanates. Carcinogenesis 10:1757–1759

Mudnic I, Modun D, Rastija V, Vukovic J, Brizic I, Katalinic V, Kozina B, Medic-Saric M, Boban M (2010) Antioxidative and vasodilatory effects of phenolic acids in wine. Food Chem 119:1205–1210

Muir JG (1999) Location of colonic fermentation events: importance of combining resistant starch with dietary fibre. Asia Pac J Clin Nutr 8:S14–S21

Mukhtar H, Ahmad N (1999) Cancer chemoprevention: future holds in multiple agents. Toxicol Appl Pharmacol 158:207–210

Murakoshi M, Nishino H, Satomi Y, Takayasu J, Hasegawa T, Tokuda H, Iwashima A, Okuzumi J, Okabe H, Kitano H et al (1992) Potent preventive action of α-carotene against carcinogenesis: spontaneous liver carcinogenesis and promoting stage of lung and skin carcinogenesis in mice are suppressed more effectively by α-carotene than by β-carotene. Cancer Res 52:6583–6587

Naama JH, Al-Temimi AA, Hussain Al-Amiery AAH (2010) Study the anticancer activities of ethanolic curcumin extract. Afr J Pure Appl Chem 4(5):68–73

Nadkarni KM, Nadkarni AK (1976) Indian Materia Medica, 3rd edn. Popular Prakashan Ltd, Bombay

Neto CC (2007) Cranberry and its phytochemicals: a review of *in vitro* anticancer studies. J Nutr 137:186S–193S

Nguyen ML, Schwartz SJ (1999) Lycopene: chemical and biological properties. Food Technol 53:38–45

Nishino H, Murakosh M, Ii T, Takemura M, Kuchide M, Kanazawa M, Mou XY, Wada S, Masuda M, Ohsaka Y, Yogosawa S, Satomi Y, Jinno K (2000) Cancer prevention by carotenoids and curcumins. In: Bidlack WR et al (eds) Phytochemicals as bioactive agents. Technomic Publishing Company, Lancaster

Nishino H, Murakosh M, Ii T, Takemura M, Kuchide M, Kanazawa M, Mou XY, Wada S, Masuda M, Ohsaka Y, Yogosawa S, Satomi Y, Jinno K (2002) Carotenoids in cancer chemoprevention. Cancer Metastasis Rev 21:257–264

Owen RW, Haubner R, Wurtele G, Hull WE, Spiegelhalder B, Bartsch H (2004) Olives and olive oil in cancer prevention. Eur J Cancer Prev 13:319–326

Padayatty SJ, Sun H, Wang Y, Riordan HD, Hewitt SM, Katz A, Wesley RA, Levine M (2004) Vitamin C pharmacokinetics: implications for oral and intravenous use. Ann Intern Med 140:533–537

Pandey KB, Rizvi SI (2009) Protective effect of resveratrol on formation of membrane protein carbonyls and lipid peroxidation in erythrocytes subjected to oxidative stress. Appl Physiol Nutr Metab 34:1093–1097

Papas AM (1998) Diet and antioxidant status. In: Papas AM (ed) Antioxidant status, diet, nutrition and health. CRC Press, Boca Raton

Peng I, Kuo S (2003) Flavonoid structure affects inhibition of lipid peroxidation in caco-2 intestinal cells at physiological conditions. J Nutr 133:2184–2187

Percival M (1998) Antioxidants. Clin Nutr Insight 31:1–4

Peters U, McGlynn KA, Chatterjee N, Gunter E, Garcia-Closas M, Rothman N, Sinha R (2001) Vitamin D, calcium and vitamin D receptor polymorphism in colorectal adenomas. Cancer Epidemiol Biomarkers Prev 10:1267–1274

Pietta PG (2000) Flavonoids as antioxidants. J Nat Prod 63:1035–1042

Pinto JT, Rivlin RS (2001) Antiproliferative effects of allium derivatives from garlic. J Nutr 131:1058S–1060S

Rao AV, Agarwal S (1999) Role of lycopene as antioxidant carotenoid in the prevention of chronic diseases: a review. Nutr Res 19:305–323

Reagan-Shaw S, Mukhtar H, Ahmad N (2008) Resveratrol imparts photoprotection of normal cells and enhances the efficacy of radiation therapy in cancer cells. Photochem Photobiol 84: 415–421

Riordan HD, Hunninghake RB, Riordan NH, Jackson JJ, Meng X, Taylor P, Casciari JJ, Gonzalez MJ, Miranda-Massari JR, Mora EM, Rosario N, Rivera A (2003) Intravenous ascorbic acid: protocol for its application and use. P R Health Sci J 2:287–290

Rodrigo KA, Rawal Y, Renner RJ, Schwartz SJ, Tian Q, Larsen PE, Mallery SR (2006) Suppression of the tumorigenic phenotype in human oral squamous cell carcinoma cells by an ethanol extract derived from freeze-dried black raspberries. Nutr Cancer 54:58–68

Rose DP (1993) Diet, hormones, and cancer. Annu Rev Public Health 14:1–17

Rousseau EJ, Davison AJ, Dunn B (1992) Protection by β-carotene and related compounds against oxygen-mediated cytotoxicity and genotoxicity: implications for carcinogenesis and anticarcinogenesis. Free Radic Biol Med 13:407–433

Ryan D, Robar Ds K, Enzier P, Antolovich M (1999) Applications of mass spectrometry to plant phenols. Trends Anal Chem 18:362–372

Salah N, Miller NJ, Paganga G, Tijburg L, Bolwell GP, Rice-Evans C (1995) Polyphenolic flavanols as scavengers of aqueous phase radicals and as chain-breaking antioxidants. Arch Biochem Biophys 322:339–346

Seeram NP, Adams LS, Zhang Y, Sand D, Heber D (2006) Blackberry, black raspberry, blueberry, cranberry, red raspberry and strawberry extracts inhibit growth and stimulate apoptosis of human cancer cells *in vitro*. J Agric Food Chem 54:9329–9339

Shahidi F, Naczk M (1995) Food phenolics: sources, chemistry, effects, and applications. Technomic Publishing Co, Lancaster

Shen G, Xu C, Hu R, Jain MR, Gopalkrishnan A, Nair S, Huang MT, Chan JY, Kong AN (2006) Modulation of nuclear factor E2-related factor 2-mediated gene expression in mice liver and small intestine by cancer chemopreventive agent curcumin. Mol Cancer Ther 5(1):39–51

Singh R, Akhtar N, Haqqi TM (2010) Green tea polyphenol epigallocatechi3-gallate: inflammation and arthritis. Life Sci 86:907–918

Sumantran VN, Zhang R, Lee DS, Wicha MS (2000) Differential regulation of apoptosis in normal versus transformed mammary epithelium by lutein and retinoic acid. Cancer Epidemiol Biomarkers Prev 9:257–263

Sun J, Liu RH (2006) Cranberry phytochemical extracts induce cell cycle arrest and apoptosis in human MCF-7 breast cancer cells. Cancer Lett 241:124–134

Sun J, Chu Y, Wu X, Liu RH (2002) Antioxidant and antiproliferative activities of common fruits. J Agric Food Chem 50:7449–7454

Sylvester PW, McIntyre BS, Gapor A, Briski KP (2001) Vitamin E inhibition of normal mammary epithelial cell growth is associated with a reduction in protein kinase Ca activation. Cell Prolif 34:347–357

Tagliazucchi D, Verzelloni E, Conte A (2010) Contribution of melanoidins to the antioxidant activity of traditional balsamic vinegar during aging. J Food Biochem 34(5):1061–1078

Talalay P, Fahey JW (2001) Phytochemicals from cruciferous plants protect against cancer by modulating carcinogen metabolism. J Nutr 131:3027S–3033S

Tangrea J, Helzlsouer K, Pietinen P, Taylor P, Hollis B, Virtamo J, Albanes D (1997) Serum levels of vitamin D metabolites and the subsequent risk of colon and rectal cancer in Finnish men. Cancer Causes Control 8:615–625

Terao J (2008) Highlight on polyphenols and health. Arch Biochem Biophys 476:101

Trueba GP, Sánchez GM, Giuliani A (2004) Oxygen free radical and antioxidant defense mechanism in cancer. Front Biosci 9:2029–2244

Van Erk MJ, Teuling E, Staal YC, Huybers S, Van Bladeren PJ, Aarts JM, Van Ommen B (2004) Time- and dose-dependent effects of curcumin on gene expression in human colon cancer cells. J Carcinog 3(1):8

Vasisht K, Sharma PD, Karan M, Rakesh D, Vyas S, Sethi S, Manktala R (2003) In study to promote the industrial exploitation of green tea polyphenols in India. ICS-UNIDO, Trieste

Voorrips LE, Voorrips LE, Goldbohm A, Brants HAM, Poppel GAFC, Sturmans F, Hermus RJJ, Brandt PAV et al (2000) A prospective cohort study on antioxidant and folate intake and male lung cancer risk. Cancer Epidemiol Biomarkers Prev 9:357–365

Waladkhani AR, Clemens MR (1998) Effect of dietary phytochemicals on cancer development. Int J Mol Med 1:747–753

Wargovich MJ (1997) Experimental evidence for cancer preventive elements in foods. Cancer Lett 114:11–17

Welsch CW (1987) Enhancement of mammary tumorigenesis by dietary fat; review of potential mechanisms. Am J Clin Nutr 45:192–202

Wolf G (1992) Retinoid and carotenoids as inhibitors of carcinogenesis and inducers of cell-cell communication. Nutr Rev 50:270–274

Wolfe K, Wu X, Liu RH (2003) Antioxidant activity of apple peels. J Agric Food Chem 51: 609–614

Wong RWK, Hägg U, Samaranayake L, Yuen MKC, Seneviratne CJ, Kao R (2010) Antimicrobial activity of Chinese medicine herbs against common bacteria in oral biofilm – a pilot study. Int J Oral Maxillofac Surg 39:599–605

World Cancer Research Fund/American Institute for Cancer Research (2007) Food, nutrition, physical activity and the prevention of cancer: a global perspective. American Institute of Cancer Research, Washington, DC

World Health Organization (2003) News release. http://www.who.int/mediacentre/news/releases/2003/pr27/en. Cited 3 Apr 2003

Woude H, Gliszczynska-Swiglo A, Struijs K, Smeets A, Alink GM, Rietjens IMCM (2003) Biphasic modulation of cell proliferation by quercetin at concentrations physiologically relevant in humans. Cancer Lett 200:41–47

Wu QK, Koponen JM, Mykkänen HM, Törrönen AR (2007) Berry phenolic extracts modulate the expression of p21(WAF1) and Bax but not Bcl-2 in HT-29 colon cancer cells. J Agric Food Chem 55:1156–1163

Xiao D, Pinto JT, Soh J, Deguchi A, Gundersen GG, Palazzo AF, Yoon J, Shirin H, Weinstein IB (2000) Induction of apoptosis by the garlic derived compound S-allylmercaptocysteine (SAMC) is associated with microtubule depolymerization and c-Jun NH2-terminal kinase 1 activation. Cancer Res 63:6825–6837

Yang CS, Wang ZY (1993) Tea and cancer. J Natl Cancer Inst 85:1038–1049

Yu L, Zhao M, Yang B (2009) Weidong Bai a immunomodulatory and anticancer activities of phenolics from *Garcinia mangostana* fruit pericarp. Food Chem 116:969–973

Zhang LX, Cooney RV, Bertram JS (1991) Carotenoids enhance gap junctional communication and inhibit lipid peroxidation in C3H/10T1/2 cells: relationship to their cancer chemopreventive action. Carcinogenesis 12:2109–2114

Zhang LX, Cooney RV, Bertram JS (1992) Carotenoids up-regulate connexin43 gene expression independent of their provitamin A or antioxidant properties. Cancer Res 52:5707–5712

Zhang SM, Hunter DJ, Rosner BA, Giovannucci EL, Colditz GA, Speizer FE, Willett WC (2000) Intakes of fruits, vegetables, and related nutrients and the risk of non-Hodgkin's lymphoma among women. Cancer Epidemiol Biomarkers Prev 9:477–485

Zheng L, Tong Q, Wu C (2004) Growth inhibitory effects of curcumin on ovary cells and its mechanism. J Huazhong Univ Sci Technolog Med Sci 24:55–58

Zhou S, Gao Y, Jiang W, Huang M, Xu A, Paxton JW (2003) Interactions of herbs with cytochrome P450. Drug Metab Rev 35(1):35–98

Chapter 17
Curcumin: Structure, Biology and Clinical Applications

Sharmila Shankar and Rakesh K. Srivastava

Contents

S. Shankar (✉)
Department of Pathology and Laboratory Medicine, The University of Kansas Cancer Center, The University of Kansas Medical Center, 3901 Rainbow Boulevard, Kansas City, KS 66160, USA
e-mail: sshankar@kumc.edu

R.K. Srivastava
Department of Pharmacology, Toxicology and Therapeutics, and Medicine, The University of Kansas Cancer Center, The University of Kansas Medical Center, 3901 Rainbow Boulevard, Kansas City, KS 66160, USA
e-mail: rsrivastava@kumc.edu

S. Shankar and R.K. Srivastava (eds.), *Nutrition, Diet and Cancer*,
DOI 10.1007/978-94-007-2923-0_17,

Abstract Curcumin, the principal polyphenolic curcuminoid derived from the rhizome *Curcuma longa*, is present in an Indian spice, turmeric. Curcumin possesses antitumor, antioxidant, and anti-inflammatory properties, and has been studied as a cancer chemopreventive agent. Curcumin is extensively studied, evaluated and accepted for its wide range of medicinal properties. The therapeutic activities of curcumin for a wide variety of diseases such as diabetes, allergies, arthritis and other chronic and inflammatory diseases have been known for a long time. The mechanisms of therapeutic action of curcumin include inhibition of several cell signaling pathways at multiple levels, immune-modulation, effects on cellular enzymes such as cyclooxygenase and glutathione S-transferases and effects on angiogenesis and metastasis. It has ability to affect gene transcription and induce cell cycle arrest and apoptosis. Although curcumin is a highly pleiotropic molecule with an excellent safety profile targeting multiple diseases, it could not achieve its optimum therapeutic outcome in clinical trials, largely due to its low solubility and poor bioavailability. Based on the results of the clinical trials, curcumin can be developed as a therapeutic drug through improvement in formulations or delivery systems, enabling its enhanced absorption and cellular uptake. In this review article, we provide a comprehensive outlook for the therapeutic potential of curcumin, and discuss future strategies and potential challenges involved in the use of curcumin.

Introduction

Epidemiological data support the concept that naturally occurring compounds in the human diet are devoid of toxicity and have numerous long lasting beneficial effects on human health. Curcumin [1,7-bis(4-hydroxy-3-methoxyphenyl)-1,6-hepatadiene-3,5-dione; diferulolylmethane], a major constituent of turmeric derived from the rhizomes of *Curcuma spp*., has been reported to have several pharmacological effects including antitumor, anti-inflammatory and antioxidant properties (Piper et al. 1998; Plummer et al. 2001; Susan and Rao 1992). It increases the level of glutathione-S-transferase and, thus, upregulates the synthesis of glutathione (Piper et al. 1998; Sharma et al. 2001). Recent studies have also suggested that it can inhibit tumor metastasis, invasion and angiogenesis (Aggarwal et al. 2006c; Bae et al. 2006; Lin et al. 2007; Singh and Khar 2006; Yoysungnoen et al. 2006). Other beneficial effects of curcumin include wound-healing, antiviral, anti-infectious, and antiamyloidogenic properties. It is used as a flavoring and coloring agent, as a food preservative, and also has been used in Ayurvedic medicine for over 6,000 years. Crude curcumin has a natural yellow hue and its components include curcumin, demethoxycurcumin, and bisdemethoxycurcumin. Oral administration of curcumin has been shown to inhibit leukemia and solid tumors including breast, prostate, skin, colon, stomach, duodenum, head and neck, and soft palate, through induction of apoptosis (Dikshit et al. 2006; Khor et al. 2006; Okunieff et al. 2006; Parodi et al. 2006; Sharma et al. 2006; Valentine et al. 2006; Yoysungnoen et al. 2006). However, the molecular mechanisms by which it inhibits growth and induces apoptosis in cancer cells are not well understood.

Curcumin induces apoptosis in cancer cells by inhibiting Akt activity, and inducing Bax and Bak genes upstream of mitochondria (Shankar and Srivastava 2007a, b). Furthermore, curcumin inhibits NFκB activity in cancer cells (Divya and Pillai 2006; Singh and Khar 2006) and sensitizes cancer cells to chemotherapy and radiotherapy (Aggarwal et al. 2006a; Chirnomas et al. 2006; Du et al. 2006; HemaIswarya and Doble 2006; Kamat et al. 2007; Kunnumakkara et al. 2007; Wahl et al. 2007).

The process of malignant transformation involves the sequential acquisition of a number of genetic and epigenetic alterations as a result of increasing genomic instability caused by defects in checkpoint controls (Hahn and Weinberg 2002; Nowak et al. 2002). These alterations allow cancer cells to acquire the capabilities to become self-sufficient in mitogenic signals, deregulate the control of cell cycle, escape from apoptosis, and obtain unlimited replication potential via the reactivation of telomerase (Artandi and DePinho 2000; Blasco 2002; Hanahan and Weinberg 2000). Within a growing tumor mass, the genetic changes during tumor progression also enable cancer cells to gain the ability to induce angiogenesis, invade neighboring tissues, and metastasize to distinct organs (Folkman 2003). The new chemopreventive agents or therapeutic strategies that inhibit angiogenesis, metastasis and invasion can be considered for future clinical development.

Derivatives and Analogues

In recent years, several analogs of curcumin have been prepared. However, some of them are more potent and exhibit better pharmacokinetic and pharmacodynamic properties than others. There are three main analogs of curcumin: (I) Diferuloylmethane/Curcumin (II) Demethoxycurcumin and (III) Bisdemethoxycurcumin (Fig. 17.1). New analogs appear to be better than curcumin in terms of solubility, stability, half-life and bioavailability. Furthermore, curcumin and its analogs are being conjugated with nanoparticles to improve their delivery and bioavailability.

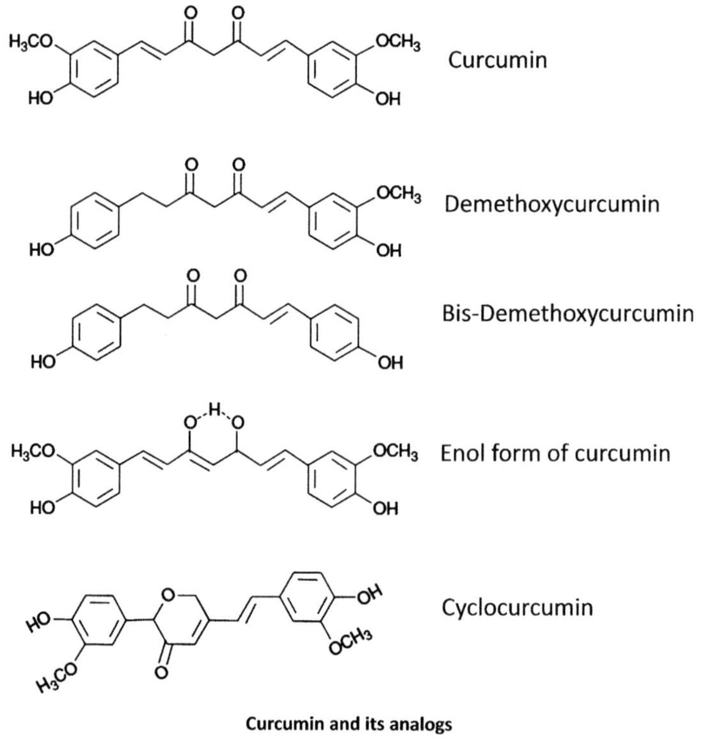

Curcumin

Demethoxycurcumin

Bis-Demethoxycurcumin

Enol form of curcumin

Cyclocurcumin

Curcumin and its analogs

Fig. 17.1 Structures of curcumin and its analogs. Curcumin, demethoxycurcumin, bis-demethoxycurcumin, enol form of curcumin, and cyclocurcumin

Mechanism of Action

Bcl-2 Family Members

The Bcl-2 family of proteins plays a key role in regulating apoptosis at the level of mitochondrial cytochrome c release (Srivastava et al. 1999a, b). Once released from mitochondria, cytochrome c interacts with Apaf-1, leading to caspase-9 activation and subsequent cleavage and activation of caspase-3, spurring the demise of the cell. Antiapoptotic Bcl-2 proteins, such as Bcl-2 and Bcl-X_L, function to prevent cytochrome c release by counteracting the effects of proapoptotic members, which are divided into two subgroups based on the presence of Bcl-2 homology (BH) domains: the BH3-only family (e.g. Bid and Bim) and the BH123 multidomain proteins (e.g. Bax and Bak). The BH3-only family activates the multidomain proteins, mainly Bax and Bak, either directly or indirectly by engaging the antiapoptotic proteins (Kandasamy et al. 2003; Kuwana and Newmeyer 2003; Willis et al. 2003). The exact mechanism of direct activation remains unclear, but it appears that Bax and Bak interact with certain BH3-only molecules, such as Bid, inducing them to undergo conformational changes, oligomerize, and permeabilize membranes which causes release of apoptogenic molecules from mitochondria to cytosol (Kuwana and Newmeyer 2003; Wei et al. 2000). Previous studies including those from our laboratories, indicated that curcumin-induced apoptosis in different cellular systems was associated with induction of Bax and Bak protein expression. Alternatively, the indirect mechanism involves BH3-only-family members binding to and occupying the antiapoptotic proteins, thereby derepressing Bax and Bak (Kuwana and Newmeyer 2003; Willis et al. 2003). Neutralization or removal of antiapoptotic proteins may be necessary to initiate proapoptotic signals and, ultimately, Bax or Bak activation. However, release from antiapoptotic molecules may not be sufficient to activate Bax or Bak without an additional activation step. These findings lead to an emerging model, where not only do apoptotic signals often converge on the multidomain proteins, but the activation of these proteins is regulated on multiple levels to determine precisely when to engage an apoptotic program and commit a cell to die.

Defect in apoptosis may contribute to tumor progression and treatment resistance. Apoptosis signaling may be disrupted by deregulated expression and/or function of antiapoptotic or proapoptotic molecules. Bcl-2 family members are important regulators of apoptosis that include antiapoptotic (Bcl-2, Bcl-X_L and Mcl-1), proapoptotic (Bax and Bak) and the BH-3-domain-only (Bim, Bid, and Bik) proteins. Bax and Bak are multidomain proteins that function as an obligate gateway for the activation of apoptosis via the mitochondrial and endoplasmic reticulum pathway (Kandasamy et al. 2003; Oakes et al. 2005; Wei et al. 2001). In contrast to the BH-3-only proteins, which function as transducers of the apoptotic signals upstream of mitochondria, Bax and Bak also contain BH-1 and BH-2 domains and function at the mitochondrial outer membrane to release holocytochrome c in response to diverse stimuli (Scorrano and Korsmeyer 2003). Consequently, we and others have shown that mouse embryonic fibroblasts (MEFs) lacking both Bax and Bak exhibited marked resistance to diverse pro-apoptotic insults, and loss of either Bax and Bak alone exerts no measurable protective effects (Kandasamy et al. 2003; Wei et al. 2001). Furthermore, mice deleted for either bax or bak alone are viable, showing either defects in only a few discrete lineage (in the case of Bax) or no defects (in the case of Bak) (Lindsten et al. 2000). In contrast, mice lacking both Bax and Bak die in early embryogenesis due to failure of apoptosis in multiple developing tissues (Lindsten et al. 2000). Overall, these findings suggest that Bax and Bak are critical for apoptosis induction.

We have recently demonstrated that curcumin downregulated the expression of Bcl-2, and Bcl-X_L and upregulated the expression of p53, Bax, Bak, PUMA, Noxa, and Bim at mRNA and protein levels in prostate cancer cells (Shankar and Srivastava 2007b). Curcumin upregulated the expression, phosphorylation, and acetylation of p53 in androgen-dependent LNCaP cells (Shankar and Srivastava 2007b). The ability of curcumin to regulate gene transcription was also evident as it caused acetylation of histone H3 and H4 in LNCaP cells (Shankar and Srivastava 2007b). Furthermore, treatment of LNCaP cells with curcumin resulted in translocation of Bax and p53 to mitochondria, production of reactive oxygen species, drop in mitochondrial membrane potential, release of mitochondrial proteins (cytochrome c, Smac/DIABLO and Omi/HtrA2), and activation of caspase-3 leading to apoptosis (Shankar and Srivastava 2007b). In another study, we have demonstrated that deletion of Bax and Bak genes completely inhibited curcumin-induced cytochrome c and Smac/DIABLO release in mouse embryonic fibroblasts (Shankar and Srivastava 2007a). Tumor tissues derived from curcumin treated mice showed that curcumin inhibited the expression of Bcl-2 and Bcl-X_L, and induced the expression of Bax and Bak. The combination of curcumin and TRAIL was more effective in regulating Bcl-2 family members than single agent alone. These studies suggest that curcumin can engage cell-intrinsic pathway of apoptosis by regulating the expression of Bcl-2 family of proteins.

Matrix Metalloproteinases

Matrix metalloproteinases (MMPs) are a family of neutral endopeptidases that require Zn + 2 or Ca + 2 for their degradation of most or all of the constituent macromolecules of the extracellular matrix. The MMPs gene family consists of 20 structurally related members. MMPs are divided into subgroups including gelatinases, collagenases, stromelysins, membrane type MMPs and others (Decock et al. 2011; Deryugina and Quigley 2010; Hua et al. 2011; Raffo et al. 2011). MMPs are known to be involved in both physiological and pathological processes such as differentiation, inflammation, wound healing, rheumatoid arthritis, tumor invasion and other fibrotic manifestations. MMP9 (gelatinase B) has been implicated in both angiogenesis and potentiation of the invasive character of the producer cells (Raffo et al. 2011). Analysis of the 5'-flanking sequence of its encoding gene revealed the binding sites for transcription factors including AP-1 and NF-kB. Curcumin has been demonstrated to inhibit angiogenesis as well as tumor invasion through inhibition of MMPs in various cancers (Swarnakar et al. 2005). FGF-2, as an angiogenic factor, can induce MMP9 expression that is dependent on AP-1, but not NF-kB activation. In the presence of curcumin, the FGF-2 induced limbal vessel dilatation and corneal anginogenesis was not observed in corneal micropocket assay. These studies suggest that curcumin can inhibit tumor growth by inhibiting angiogenesis and metastasis.

MAP Kinases

MAPK pathway has received increasing attention as a target molecule for cancer therapy. The MAPK cascades include extracellular signal-regulated protein kinases (ERKs), c-Jun N-terminal kinases/stress-activated protein kinases (JNKs/ SAPKs), and p38 kinases. ERKs are believed to play a critical role in transmitting signals initiated by growth-inducing tumor promoters, including 12- O-tetradecanoylphorbol-13-acetate (TPA), epidermal growth factor (EGF), and platelet-derived growth factor (PDGF) (Huang et al. 2010; Katz et al. 2007; Min et al. 2011). On the other hand, stress-related tumor promoters, such as ultraviolet (UV) irradiation and arsenic, potently activate JNKs/SAPKs and p38 kinases. The MAPK pathway consists of a cascade in which a MAP3K activates a MAP2K that activates a MAPK (ERK, JNK, and p38), resulting in the activation of NF-kB, cell growth, and cell survival (Keshet and Seger 2010). The curcumin have been shown to modulate the MAP kinases. The ability of curcumin to modulate the MAPK signaling pathway might contribute to the inhibition of inflammation by curcumin. Curcumin is reported to attenuate experimental colitis through a reduction in the activity of p38 MAPK (Salh et al. 2003). It is also found that curcumin inhibits JNK activation induced by various agonists including PMA plus ionomycin, anisomycin, UV-C, gamma radiation, TNFα, and sodium orthovanadate (Chen and Tan 1998).

PI3 Kinase/Akt

Phosphatidylinositol-3 kinase (PI3K) is a heterodimeric enzyme composed of one 110-kDa catalytic subunit and another 85-kDa regulatory subunit and serves as a major signaling component downstream of growth factor receptor tyrosine kinases (Cantley 2002; Luo et al. 2003). PI3K catalyzes the production of the lipid secondary messenger phosphatidylinositol-3,4,5-triphosphate, which in turn activates a wide range of downstream targets, including the serine/threonine kinase AKT (Luo et al. 2003). Full activation of AKT/PKB is PI3K dependent and requires both recruitment to the plasma membrane and phosphorylation on two key residues, Thr^{308} and Ser^{473} (Cantley 2002; Lawlor and Alessi 2001). The PI3K/AKT pathway regulates multiple cellular processes, including cell proliferation, differentiation, survival, growth, motility and angiogenesis. We and others have shown that the activated PI3K/AKT pathway provides major survival signals to prostate and many other cancer cells (Chen et al. 2001; Datta et al. 1999; Downward 2004; Kandasamy and Srivastava 2002). Constitutive activation of AKT is frequently described in many types of human cancers (Khwaja 1999). Furthermore, the ectopic expression of AKT induces cell survival and malignant transformation, whereas the inhibition of AKT activity stimulates apoptosis in a range of mammalian cells (Beresford et al. 2001, Chen et al. 2001, Kandasamy and Srivastava 2002; Lei et al. 2005; Michl and Downward 2005; Yuan and Whang 2002). Recent studies have identified the substrates of AKT that are involved in the pro-cell survival effects, which thus far include glycogen synthase kinase-3, mTOR, FKHR, MDM2, p21, HIF-1, IKK, Bad, and caspase-9 (Datta et al. 1997; Khwaja 1999; Lentzsch et al. 2004; Schmidt et al. 2002). Phosphatase and tensin homologue deleted on chromosome 10 (PTEN) is a phospholipid phosphatase that dephosphorylates phosphatidylinositol 3,4,5-triphosphate (Maehama and Dixon 1999; Myers et al. 1998) and inhibits PI3K-dependent activation of AKT. The mutation or loss of PTEN leads to constitutively activated AKT. Overexpression of PTEN into PTEN-deficient breast, prostate, lung and glial cancer cells resulted in a decrease in activated AKT (Davies et al. 1998; Li et al. 1997; Wu et al. 1998). These observations establish AKT as an attractive target for cancer therapy, both alone and in conjunction with standard cancer chemotherapies, as a means of reducing the apoptotic threshold and preferentially killing cancer cells.

Although AKT has been shown to affect nuclear p53 function, the current study provides strong evidence that AKT may serve a more antiapoptotic role by interfering with the mitochondrial accumulation of p53. We have shown that AKT activation by constitutively active AKT inhibits mitochondrial p53 accumulation whereas inhibition of AKT function by PTEN, dominant negative AKT or inhibitors of PI3K (LY294002 and Wortmannin) and AKT promotes curcumin-induced mitochondrial import of p53. This suggests that AKT may regulate Smac release and apoptosis by attenuating the mitochondrial actions of p53. Because mitochondrial p53 accumulation is correlated with p53-induced apoptosis and not cell cycle arrest (Mihara et al. 2003), this strongly suggests that prevention of mitochondrial accumulation of p53 by AKT may be a critical intermediary step in the process of curcumin-induced apoptosis.

Wnt/β-Catenin

Wnt/β-catenin pathway modulates cell proliferation, differentiation, migration, apoptosis and stem cell self-renewal (Barker and Clevers 2000; Clevers 2004; Dodge and Lum 2011; Polakis 2000; Smalley and Dale 1999; Wend et al. 2010). Wnt ligands are lipid-modified secreted glycoproteins that regulate embryonic development, cell fate specification, and the homeostasis of self-renewing adult tissues. Wnt/β-catenin signaling is also implicated in the maintenance of cancer stem cells (CSCs) of leukemia, breast, colon, melanoma, lung and liver cancers. Overexpression of β-catenin in stem cell survival pathway mediates the resistance of mouse mammary stem/progenitor cells to radiation (Woodward et al. 2007). Wnt/β-catenin signaling promoted expansion of the hepatic progenitor cell population when it is overexpressed in transplanted rat oval cells and when it is transiently expressed in adult mice (Yang et al. 2008). Elimination of β-catenin abrogated the chemoresistant cell population endowed with progenitor-like features (Yang et al. 2008). β-Catenin, the essential mediator of canonical Wnt signaling, participates in two distinct functions in the cell, depending on its cellular localization. Membrane-localized β-catenin is sequestered by the epithelial cell–cell adhesion protein E-cadherin to maintain cell–cell adhesion (Nelson and Nusse 2004). On the other hand, cytoplasmic accumulation of β-catenin and its subsequent nuclear translocation, followed by cooperation with the transcription factors T cell factor/lymphoid enhancer factor (TCF/LEF) as a transcription activator, eventually leads to activation of Wnt target genes such as c-Jun, c-Myc, fibronectin and cyclin D1 (Clevers 2006; He et al. 1998; Lin et al. 2000; Liu et al. 2005; Mann et al. 1999; Tetsu and McCormick 1999). Binding of Wnt proteins, a family of secreted proteins, to Frizzled receptors results in the cytoplasmic accumulation of β-catenin (Schweizer and Varmus 2003). In the absence of Wnt signaling, β-catenin forms a multiprotein complex with glycogen synthase kinase 3β (GSK3β), adenomatous polyposis coli, casein kinase1α and axin (Takahashi-Yanaga and Sasaguri 2008). When β-catenin is phosphorylated at Ser33/Ser37/ Thr41 by GSK3β, it is immediately subject to ubiquitin-proteasome degradation (Liu et al. 2002; Takahashi-Yanaga and Sasaguri 2008). The link between PI3K/Akt and Wnt/β-catenin pathway has been well established. Activated Akt (i.e., phospho-Akt Ser473) phosphorylates Ser9 on GSK3β, which may decrease the activity of GSK3β, thereby stabilizing β-catenin (Cohen 2003; Cohen and Frame 2001; Pap and Cooper 1998). Furthermore, PI3K/Akt pathway is important in regulating the mammary stem/progenitor cells by promoting β-catenin downstream events through phosphorylation of GSK3β (Korkaya et al. 2009).

Curcumin induced caspase-3-mediated cleavage of β-catenin, leading to inactivation of Wnt/β-catenin signaling in HCT116 intestinal cancer cells (Jaiswal et al. 2002). Curcumin decreased β-catenin/TCF transcription activity in all tested cancer cell lines, including gastric, colon and intestinal cancer cells, which was attributed to the reduced amount of nuclear β-catenin and TCF-4 proteins (Park et al. 2005). In a recent study, the expression of Wnt receptor Frizzled-1 was potently suppressed by curcumin (Yan et al. 2005). Curcumin attenuated response of β-catenin to Wnt-3a in colon cancer cells through down-regulation of p300, a positive regulator of Wnt/β-catenin signaling (Ryu et al. 2008).

Hedgehog

The Hedgehog (Hh) pathway is a conserved signalling system essential for embryonic development and for the maintenance of self-renewal pathways in stem cells and progenitor cells (Cerdan and Bhatia 2010; Katoh and Katoh 2009; Kelleher 2011; Merchant and Matsui 2010; Pece et al. 2011; Takebe et al. 2011). The hedgehog pathway plays a crucial role in regulating self-renewal of normal and malignant human mammary, pancreatic and prostate stem cells (Hsieh et al. 2011; Kelleher 2011; Klarmann et al. 2009; Liu et al. 2006; Sarkar et al. 2010; Thayer et al. 2003; Ulasov et al. 2011). Another recent study revealed the essential role of hedgehog-Gli signaling in controlling the self-renewal behavior of human glioma CSCs and tumorigenicity (Katoh and Katoh 2009; Natsume et al. 2011; Zbinden et al. 2010). In the absence of hedgehog ligands (Sonic Hedgehog, Desert Hedgehog and Indian Hedgehog), their transmembrane receptor Patched (Ptch) associates with Smoothened (Smo) and blocks Smo function (Traiffort et al. 2010). When secreted hedgehog ligands bind to Ptch, Smo is released, triggering dissociation of transcription factors, Gli1, Gli2 and Gli3 from Fused (Fu) and suppressor of Fused (SuFu), leading to transcription of an array of genes, such as cyclin D, cyclin E, Myc and elements of EGF pathway (Cohen 2003; Pasca di Magliano and

Hebrok 2003). Sonic hedgehog pathway is also linked to transcription factor NF-κB signaling. It was suggested that overexpression of sonic hedgehog is activated by NF-κB in pancreatic cancer and pancreatic cancer cell proliferation is accelerated by NF-κB in part through sonic hedgehog overexpression (Nakashima et al. 2006). Sonic hedgehog was characterized as a novel NF-κB target gene by mapping the minimal NF-κB consensus site to position +139 of sonic hedgehog promoter (Kasperczyk et al. 2009). Canonical Hh signaling promotes the expression of target genes through the oncogene GLI transcription factors. There is now increasing evidence suggesting that 'non-canonical' Hh signalling mechanisms, some of which are independent of GLI-mediated transcription, may be important in cancer and development.

Curcumin has been shown to inhibit the Shh-Gli1 signaling pathway by down-regulating the Shh protein and its downstream targets GLI1 and PTCH1 in various cancers (Elamin et al. 2010; Mimeault and Batra 2011). Furthermore, curcumin reduced the levels of beta-catenin, the activate/phosphorylated form of Akt and NF-kappaB, which led to downregulating the three common key effectors, namely C-myc, N-myc, and Cyclin D1. Consequently, apoptosis was triggered by curcumin through the mitochondrial pathway via downregulation of Bcl-2, a downstream anti-apoptotic effector of the Shh signaling. Importantly, the resistant cells that exhibited no decrease in the levels of Shh and Bcl-2, were sensitized to curcumin by the addition of the Shh antagonist, cyclopamine. Furthermore, curcumin enhances the killing efficiency of nontoxic doses of cisplatin and gamma-rays. In addition, piperine, an enhancer of curcumin bioavailability in humans, potentiates the apoptotic effect of curcumin against several cancer cells (Garg et al. 2005; Li et al. 2011; Manoharan et al. 2009; Shaikh et al. 2009). This effect was mediated through strong downregulation of Bcl-2. Therefore, it can be suggested that curcumin represents great promise as Shh-targeted therapy for cancers.

Notch

Notch receptor or ligand overexpression is associated with Drosophila eye tumors that exhibit hallmarks of mammalian cancers such as uncontrolled overgrowth, invasion, and metastasis (Ferres-Marco et al. 2006; Martinez and Cavalli 2010; Martinez et al. 2009; Palomero et al. 2007), providing a powerful model for the genetic dissection of the regulatory circuits controlling tissue homeostasis, growth and cancer by Notch signalling pathway. The activation of the Notch pathway is an ancient mechanism to control the growth of numerous tissues and organs (Artavanis-Tsakonas et al. 1995; Artavanis-Tsakonas and Muskavitch 2010), and recent evidence indicates this pathway is often recruited to stimulate growth of many solid tumors and leukemic stem cells and to orchestrate angiogenesis and/or the reprogramming of cancer cells via epithelial–mesenchymal transition (EMT) (Bailey et al. 2007; Miele 2006; Miele et al. 2006).

In Drosophila, there is a single Notch receptor and two genes that encode the ligands Delta and Serrate (Ser) (Martinez and Cavalli 2010). Four different Notch receptors (NOTCH1–4) and five canonical ligands of the Delta (DLL1, 2, and 4) and Ser (JAGGED/JAG1, 2) families have been characterized in humans. In all phyla, Notch binding of its ligand triggers receptor activation through a round of two consecutive cleavages, one extracellular and the other intracellular. The latter requires the activity of the ADAM protease family and γ-secretase. Subsequently the intracellular domain of Notch is released, which then translocates to the nucleus to form a transcriptional activator in complex with the DNA binding protein, CSL (CBF1/RBP-J in mammals, Suppressor of Hairless in Drosophila, and LAG-1 in Caenorhabditis elegans), and with the co-activator Mastermind-like proteins (Artavanis-Tsakonas et al. 1995). Timely ligand-receptor activation and signal strength requires not only spatiotemporal regulation of ligand genes but also post-transcriptional regulation of ligand levels via ligand endocytosis, ubiquitination, and endosome sorting (Bray 2006; Kopan and Ilagan 2009). The importance of ligand regulation is highlighted in humans in which the loss of one gene copy or gain of Notch ligand are directly linked to developmental syndromes and age-related diseases including cancer (Kopan and Ilagan 2009). Significantly, high JAG1 protein correlates with the metastasis, shorter survival time, and recurrence in human carcinomas, including prostate (Santagata et al. 2004). High JAG1 has been shown to induce invasion and migration through EMT in breast and prostate cancer cell lines (Chen et al. 2010; Ferrari-Toninelli et al. 2010; Kettunen et al. 2001; Lindner et al. 2001; Noseda et al. 2004; Pang et al. 2010; Santagata et al. 2004; Six et al. 2004; Vallejo et al. 2011; Weller et al. 2006; Yang and Proweller 2011; Yeh et al. 2009; Zhang et al. 2010). However, how the tightly regulated NOTCH pathway activation is subverted in carcinogenesis remains poorly understood, particularly since activating mutations of NOTCH pathway components are rarely detected in solid tumors.

Recent studies have demonstrated that Notch-activated genes and pathways can drive tumor growth through the expansion of CSCs (Bigas et al. 2010; D'Souza et al. 2008; Dikic and Schmidt 2010; Guo et al. 2011; Radtke et al. 2010; Stockhausen et al. 2010). Notch pathway is believed to be dysregulated in CSCs, ultimately leading to uncontrolled CSC self-renewal. For example, Notch pathway was shown to play an important role in the self-renewal function of malignant breast cancer CSCs (Farnie and Clarke 2007; Guo et al. 2011; Harrison et al. 2010; Kakarala and Wicha 2008; Li et al. 2011). NOTCH pathway activates downstream target genes such as c-Myc, cyclin D1, p21, NF-κB (Brennan et al. 2009; Cohen et al. 2010; D'Altri et al. 2011; Das et al. 2010; Ling et al. 2010; Mazumdar et al. 2009; Okuhashi et al. 2010; Ronchini and Capobianco 2001; Sharma et al. 2007; Stahl et al. 2006; Tanaka et al. 2009; Wei et al. 2010). NOTCH1 has been reported to cross-talk with NF-κB pathway in diverse cellular situations (Chen et al. 2007; Jang et al. 2004; Nickoloff et al. 2002; Oswald et al. 1998; Shin et al. 2006; Wang et al. 2001, 2006b). It has also been demonstrated that NOTCH-1 is necessary for expression of several NF-κB subunits (Cheng et al. 2001; Jang et al. 2004) and stimulates NF-κB promoter activity (Jang et al. 2004). These studies directly link NOTCH pathway with NF-κB to regulate various physiological functions.

Antiproliferative effects of curcumin has been associated with down-regulation of NOTCH-1 and NF-κB in various cancers (Chen et al. 2007; Howells et al. 2010; Li et al. 2011; Sarkar et al. 2009; Wang et al. 2006a, 2008). Curcumin-induced inactivation of NF-κB DNA-binding activity was potentially mediated by Notch-1 signaling pathway (Wang et al. 2006a). Taken together, these studies suggest that the down-regulation of NOTCH-1 and/or NF-κB by curcumin could be an effective approach for inhibiting tumorigenesis.

Cyclooxygenases

Cyclooxygenases are prostaglandin H synthase, which convert arachidonic acid released by membrane phospholipids into prostaglandins (Aggarwal et al. 2006b; Subbaramaiah and Dannenberg 2003). Two isoforms of prostaglandin H synthase, COX-1 and COX-2 are identified. COX-1 is constitutively expressed in many tissues, but the expression of COX-2 is regulated by mitogens, tumor promoters, cytokines, and growth factors. COX-2 is overexpressed in practically all premalignant and malignant condition involving the liver, colon, pancreas, lung, breast, bladder, skin, stomach, head and neck, and esophagus (Subbaramaiah and Dannenberg 2003). Many transcription factors have been shown to stimulate COX-2 transcription. Curcumin was one of the first chemopreventive phytochemicals shown to possess significant COX-2 inhibiting activity through the suppression of NF-kB. COX-2 inhibitors will be particularly useful in the treatment of breast cancers through inhibition of HER-2/neu activity and aromatase activity (Subbaramaiah and Dannenberg 2003). Preclinical studies have shown that curcumin suppresses COX-2 activity through the suppression of NF-kB-inducing kinase (NIK) and IkBa kinase (IKK) enzymes (Plummer et al. 1999).

Recently, it has been observed that difluorinated-curcumin (CDF) together with 5-fluorouracil and oxaliplatin (5-FU + Ox) were more potent than curcumin in reducing CD44 and CD166 in chemo-resistant colon cancer cells, accompanied by inhibition of growth, induction of apoptosis and disintegration of colonospheres (Kanwar et al. 2011). These changes were associated with down-regulation of the membrane transporter ABCG2 and attenuation of EGFR, IGF-1R, and NFκB signaling consistent with inactivation of β-catenin, COX-2, c-Myc and Bcl-X_L and activation of the pro-apoptotic Bax. This study suggests that CDF together with the conventional chemotherapeutics could be an effective treatment strategy for preventing the emergence of chemo-resistant colon cancer cells by eliminating cancer stem cells.

Epidermal Growth Factor Receptors

The epidermal growth factor receptor (EGFR) is a 170 kDa receptor tyrosine kinase. Upon EGF stimulation, EGFR dimerizes and becomes enzymatically active, and these results in a cascade of cellular events, including phosphorylation and activation of its substrates (Dasari and Messersmith 2010; Lo 2010). This enzymatic activation of EGFR is essential to propagate the EGF-induced signaling that culminates in DNA synthesis and cell division. The inhibitory effect of curcumin on the ligand-induced activation of EGFR was observed and this might explain the antiproliferative effect of curcumin on EGF stimulated cells (Korutla et al. 1995; Korutla and Kumar 1994). Furthermore, curcumin inhibited EGFR expression in pancreatic, lung, colon and prostate cancers (Chen et al. 2006; Dorai et al. 2000; Kim et al. 2006; Lee et al. 2011; Lev-Ari et al. 2006). Curcumin potentiates antitumor activity of gefitinib in cell lines and xenograft mice model of NSCLC through inhibition of proliferation, EGFR phosphorylation, and induction EGFR ubiquitination and apoptosis (Lee et al. 2011). In addition, curcumin attenuates gefitinib-induced gastrointestinal adverse effects via altering p38 activation. These findings provide a novel treatment strategy that curcumin as an adjuvant to increase the spectrum of the usage of gefitinib and overcome the gefitinib inefficiency in NSCLC patients.

Transcription Factors

NFκB

The NFκB family of transcription factors has been shown to be constitutively activated in various human malignancies, including a number of solid tumors and leukemias, lymphomas (Karin 2006b). NFκB is shown to contribute to development and/or progression of malignancy by regulating the expression of genes involved in cell growth and proliferation, anti-apoptosis, angiogenesis, and metastasis (Karin 2006b). Prostate cancer cells have been reported to have constitutive NFκB activity due to increased activity of the IκB kinase complex (Aggarwal et al. 2006c). Furthermore, an inverse correlation between androgen receptor (AR) status and NFκB activity was observed in prostate cancer cell lines (Peant et al. 2007). In prostate cancer cells, NFκB may promote cell growth and proliferation by regulating expression of genes such as c-myc, cyclin D1, and IL-6 (Karin 2006a, b), and inhibit apoptosis through activation of expression of anti-apoptotic genes, such as Bcl-2. NFκB-mediated expression of genes involved in angiogenesis (IL-8, VEGF), and invasion and metastasis (MMP9, uPA, uPA receptor) may further contribute to the progression of prostate cancer. Constitutive NFκB activity has also been demonstrated in primary prostate cancer tissue samples and suggested to have prognostic importance for a subset of primary tumors. We have shown that curcumin inhibits the activation of NFκB and its gene products (e.g. VEGF, Bcl-2,

Bcl-X_L, uPA, cyclin D1, MMP-2, MMP-9, COX-2 and IL-8) in xenografted tumors, which play significant roles in invasion, metastasis and angiogenesis (Shankar et al. 2007a, b). All these events will significantly contribute to the anti-proliferative and antitumor activities of curcumin. The inhibitory effect of curcumin on NF-κB signal transduction pathway may be mediated via the various components of the HDACs and p300/Notch 1 signal molecules, and may represent a novel therapeutic option for cancer. These findings suggest that NFκB may play a role in human cancer development and/or progression, and curcumin can inhibit these processes through regulation of NFκB-dependent gene products.

STAT

STAT proteins are signaling molecules with dual functions that were discovered during studies on interferon (IFN) gamma-dependent gene expression (Darnell et al. 1994). Of the seven STAT proteins identified so far, constitutively activated STAT3 and STAT5 have been implicated in multiple myeloma, lymphomas, and several solid tumors, making these proteins logical targets for cancer therapy. These STAT proteins contribute to cell survival and growth by preventing apoptosis through increased expression of antiapoptotic proteins, such as bcl-2 and bcl-X_L. STAT3 was shown to be a direct activator of the *VEGF* gene, which is responsible for increased angiogenesis. Elevated STAT3 activity has been detected in head and neck squamous cell carcinoma, leukemias, lymphomas, multiple myeloma, and pancreatic, prostate and breast cancers (Arthan et al. 2010; Hazan-Halevy et al. 2010; Li et al. 2010; Lin et al. 2010a; Liu et al. 2010; Madoux et al. 2010; Pandey et al. 2010; Ramakrishnan et al. 2010; Sandur et al. 2010; Scuto et al. 2011; Yang et al. 2010).

Curcumin has been shown to inhibit interleukin (IL) 6-induced STAT3 phosphorylation and consequent STAT3 nuclear translocation. It was even more efficient than JAK2 inhibitor AG490. Overall, curcumin is a potent inhibitor of STAT3 phosphorylation and therefore, it suppresses proliferation of cancer cells (Aggarwal et al. 2006a; Glienke et al. 2010; Goel and Aggarwal 2010; Lin et al. 2010a, b; Rezende et al. 2009; Seo et al. 2010; Weissenberger et al. 2010). Curcumin has been shown to inhibit cellular proliferation and the expression of STAT5 mRNA, and to downregulate the activation of STAT5 in chronic myelogenous leukemia cells and solid tumors (Bhattacharyya et al. 2007; Bill et al. 2009; Blasius et al. 2006; Lin et al. 2004; Rajasingh et al. 2006). These studies suggest curcumin exerts its antitumor activity through inhibition of JAK/STAT pathway.

AP-1

AP-1 is associated with activation of NF-κB and has been closely linked with proliferation and transformation of tumor cells (Karin 2006b). Curcumin suppresses the JNK activation hence suppresses the phosphorylation of c-jun and ultimately suppresses the activation of AP-1 (Huang et al. 1991). It also interacts with the

AP-1-DNA binding motif, thereby inhibiting activation of AP-1 (Haase et al. 2008). It suppresses AP-1-DNA binding and transcriptional activity in an HTLV-1-infected T-cell line. It inhibited the growth of these cells by inducing cell cycle arrest followed by apoptosis. Curcumin has been inhibited hydrogen peroxide induced heparin affin regulatory peptide *(HARP)* and LNCaP cell proliferation and migration (Polytarchou et al. 2005). It is also reported to downregulate AP-1 binding activity in cancer cells (Balasubramanian and Eckert 2007; Balogun et al. 2003b; Cai et al. 2011; Sharma et al. 2010).

Nrf2

Transcription factor NrF-2 normally exists in an inactive state as a result of binding to a cytoskeleton-associated protein, Keap1. It can be activated by redox-dependent stimuli. Nrf-2 translocates to the nucleus, bind to the antioxidant-responsive element (ARE), and initiate the transcription of genes coding for detoxifying enzymes and cytoprotective proteins. Nrf-2-ARE signaling pathway plays a key role in activating cellular antioxidant. The same response is also triggered by curcumin. It stimulated concentration and time dependently expression of Nrf-2. This effect is associated with increased Ho-1 protein expression and hemoxygenase activity. The *ho-1* gene expression is stimulated by curcumin through inactivating Nrf-2-Keap1 complex, leading to increased Nrf-2 binding to resident *ho-1* ARE (Balogun et al. 2003a, b). It has been known that curcumin activates ARE-mediated gene expression in human monocytes through PKC delta (Rushworth et al. 2006). It has been also found to exert anti-inflammatory and anticarcinogenic effects by up-regulating the selenoprotein gastrointestinal glutathione peroxidase by activating the Nrf-2/Keap1syatem (Banning et al. 2005).

Apoptosis

Anticancer drugs or irradiation induce the release of mitochondrial proteins such as cytochrome c, second mitochondria-derived activator of caspases (Smac)/ direct inhibitor of apoptosis protein (IAP) binding protein with low isoelectric point (DIABLO), apoptosis inducing factor (AIF) and endonucleases G. Cytochrome c together with apoptosis protease activating factor (Apaf-1) and procaspase-9 forms the apoptosome complex (Liu et al. 1996). Caspase-9 subsequently activates caspase-3 that can cleave several caspase substrates leading to apoptosis (Zou et al. 1997). Smac/DIABLO contains an NH_2-terminal 55-amino-acid mitochondrial import sequence (Du et al. 2000; Verhagen et al. 2001). Once released into the cytosol, Smac docks to IAPs within the baculovirus IAP repeat domains via an NH_2-terminal motif, thereby eliminating the inhibitory effects of IAPs on caspase-3, caspase-7, and caspase-9 (Verhagen and Vaux 2002). In addition, the interaction of Smac with IAPs results in a rapid ubiquitination and subsequent degradation of released Smac, which is mediated by the ubiquitin-protein ligase (E3) function of some IAPs (Du et al. 2000; MacFarlane et al. 2002). Recent studies have shown that mitochondrial Smac release is suppressed by Akt, Bcl-2, and Bcl-X_L, but promoted by Bax, Bad, and Bid (Du et al. 2000; Kandasamy et al. 2003; Verhagen et al. 2000).

Binding of TRAIL to its receptors TRAIL-R1/DR4 and TRAIL-R2/DR5, both of which contain a cytoplasmic region of 80 amino acids designated as the "death domain", activated the extrinsic apoptosis pathway. Death receptors DR4 and DR5 can recruit the initiator caspases, caspase-8 and caspase-10, by a homotypic interaction between the death effector domains of the adapter molecule Fas-associated death domain (FADD) protein and the prodomain of the initiator caspase, thereby forming the death-inducing signaling complex (DISC). The formation of active DISC is essential for TRAIL to transmit apoptotic signals. We and others have shown that tumor-selective targeting molecules such as tumor necrosis factor (TNF)-related apoptosis-inducing ligand (TRAIL) induces apoptosis in prostate cancer cells, both *in vitro* and *in vivo* (Shankar et al. 2004, 2005; Shankar and Srivastava 2004; Srivastava 2001). Data on experimental animals and primates led us to believe that TRAIL has great promise as a selective anticancer agent (Ashkenazi et al. 1999; Shankar et al. 2004, 2005). We have recently demonstrated that TRAIL induces apoptosis in several prostate cancer cells lines, but it was ineffective in inducing apoptosis in LNCaP cells (Chen et al. 2001; Shankar et al. 2004, 2005). Chemopreventive agent curcumin has been shown to sensitize TRAIL-resistant prostate cancer cells *in vitro* (Deeb et al. 2003, 2005; Jung et al. 2006). However, the ability of curcumin to sensitize TRAIL-resistant cells *in vivo* has not yet been demonstrated.

Cell Cycle

Inappropriate and/or accelerated rates of cell proliferation are hallmark of cancer. The molecular regulatory network of the cell cycle and apoptosis are tightly intertwined (Hahn and Weinberg 2002; Nowak et al. 2002) The known molecular regulatory networks of the cell cycle and apoptosis are quite complex and can overlap. During malignant transformation, a number of genetic and epigenetic alterations occurs as a result of increasing genomic instability caused by defects in checkpoint controls (Hahn and Weinberg 2002; Nowak et al. 2002) These alterations allow cancer cells to acquire the capabilities to become self-sufficient in mitogenic signals, deregulate the control of cell cycle, escape from apoptosis, and obtain unlimited replication potential.

The transition from one cell cycle phase to another occurs in an orderly fashion and is regulated by different cellular proteins. Key regulatory proteins are the cyclin-dependent kinases (CDK), a family of serine/threonine protein kinases that are activated at specific points of the cell cycle. Until now, nine CDK have been identified and, of these, five are active during the cell cycle, i.e. during G1 (CDK4, CDK6 and CDK2), S (CDK2), G2 and M (CDK1). When activated, CDK induce downstream processes by phosphorylating selected proteins (Morgan 1995; Pines 1995) CDK protein levels remain stable during the cell cycle, in contrast to their activating proteins, the cyclins. Cyclin protein levels rise and fall during the cell cycle and in this way they periodically activate CDK (Evans et al. 1983). Different cyclins are required at different phases of the cell cycle. The three D type cyclins (cyclin D1, cyclin D2, cyclin D3) bind to CDK4 and CDK6, and CDK-cyclin D complexes are essential for entry in G1 (Sherr 1994) Unlike the other cyclins, cyclin D is not expressed periodically, but is synthesized as long as growth factor stimulation persists (Assoian 1997). Another G1 cyclin is cyclin E which associates with CDK2 to regulate progression from G1 into S phase (Ohtsubo et al. 1995). Cyclin A binds with CDK2 and this complex is required during S phase (Girard et al. 1991; Walker and Maller 1991). In late G2 and early M, cyclin A complexes with CDK1 to promote entry into M phase. Mitosis is further regulated by cyclin B in complex with CDK1 (Arellano and Moreno 1997; Azuine and Bhide 1994). Cyclins A and B contain a destruction box and cyclins D and E contain a PEST sequence [segment rich in proline (P), glutamic acid (E), serine (S) and threonine (T) residues]; these are protein sequences required for efficient ubiquitin-mediated cyclin proteolysis at the end of a cell cycle phase (Glotzer et al. 1991).

In addition to cyclin binding, CDK activity is also regulated by phosphorylation on conserved threonine and tyrosine residues. Full activation of CDK1 requires phosphorylation of threonine 161 (threonine 172 in CDK4 and threonine 160 in CDK2), brought about by the CDK7-cyclin H complex, also called CAK. These phosphorylations induce conformational changes and enhance the binding of cyclins (Jeffrey et al. 1995; Paulovich and Hartwell 1995). The Wee1 and Myt1 kinases phosphorylate CDK1 at tyrosine-15 and/or threonine-14, thereby inactivating the kinase. Dephosphorylation at these sites by the enzyme Cdc25 is necessary for activation of CDK1 and further progression through the cell cycle (Lew and Kornbluth 1996). Alterations of CDK molecules in cancer have been reported, although with low frequency. CDK4 overexpression, that occurs as a result of amplification, has been identified in cell lines, melanoma, sarcoma and glioma (Wolfel et al. 1995). CDK1 and CDK2 have been reported to be overexpressed in a subset of colon adenomas, a greater overexpression was seen in focal carcinomas in adenomatous tissue (Kim et al. 1999; Yamamoto et al. 1998).

CDK activity can be counteracted by cell cycle inhibitory proteins, called CDK inhibitors (CKI) which bind to CDK alone or to the CDK-cyclin complex and regulate CDK activity. Two distinct families of CDK inhibitors have been discovered, the INK4 family and CIP/KIP family (Sherr and Roberts 1995) The INK4 family includes p15 (INK4b), p16 (INK4a), p18 (INK4c), p19 (INK4d), which specifically inactivate G1 CDK (CDK4 and CDK6). These CKI form stable complexes with the CDK enzyme before cyclin binding, preventing association with cyclin D (Carnero and Hannon 1998). The second family of inhibitors, the CIP/KIP family, includes p21 (WAF1/CIP1), p27 (KIP1), p57 (KIP2). These inhibitors inactivate CDK-cyclin complexes (Harper et al. 1995; Koff 2006). They inhibit the G1 CDK-cyclin complexes, and to a lesser extent, CDK1-cyclin B complexes (Hengst and Reed 1998). CKI are regulated both by internal and external signals:

the expression of p21/WAF1/CIP1 is under transcriptional control of the *p53* tumour suppressor gene.(el-Deiry et al. 1993). p27/KIP1 binds to CDK2 and cyclin E complexes to prevent cell cycle progression from G1 to S phase (Harper et al. 1995; Koff 2006; Lees 1995). Cell cycle deregulation associated with cancer occurs through mutation of proteins important at different levels of the cell cycle. In cancer, mutations have been observed in genes encoding CDK, cyclins, CDK-activating enzymes, CKI, CDK substrates, and checkpoint proteins (McDonald and El-Deiry 2000; Sherr 1996). Mutations in *CDK4* and *CDK6* genes resulting in loss of CKI binding have also been identified (Easton et al. 1998).

The retinoblastoma tumor suppressor protein (pRB) is a negative regulator of cell proliferation (Classon and Harlow 2002). The antiproliferative activity of pRB is mediated by its ability to inhibit the transcription of genes that are required for cell cycle progression. This transcriptional regulatory function of pRB is achieved through several distinct mechanisms, which are best illustrated by its interaction with the E2F family and the inhibition of E2F-regulated gene expression. The binding of E2F to pRB requires the large pocket of pRB (amino acids 379–870). The ability of pRB to inhibit cellular proliferation is counterbalanced by the action of CDKs (Sherr and Roberts 1999; Taya 1997). pRB is phosphorylated in a cell cycle-dependent manner by CDKs. In quiescent and early G1 cells, pRB exists in a predominantly unphosphorylated state. As cells progress toward S phase, pRB becomes phosphorylated. The initial phosphorylation of pRB is most likely catalyzed by CDK4-cyclin D or CDK6-cyclin D complexes. Subsequently, CDK2-cyclin E and CDK2-cyclin A phosphorylate pRB (Ortega et al. 2002; Sherr 2002). pRB is rapidly dephosphorylated during mitosis (Ludlow et al. 1993). Inactivation of pRB by phosphorylation leads to the dissociation and activation of E2F, allowing the expression of many genes required for cell cycle progression and S phase entry. It has been shown that CDK4-cyclin D1, but not CDK2-cyclin E, specifically phosphorylated Ser780 in pRB, which cannot bind to E2F-1 (Kitagawa et al. 1996).

Proliferation arrest is the main effect of curcumin on cancer cells from different origins. Using different prostate cancer cell lines, it has been suggested that curcumin induces disruption of the G1/S transition of the cell cycle (Aggarwal et al. 2007a; Shenouda et al. 2004). We have recently shown that curcumin caused a growth arrest at G1/S stage in both androgen-sensitive LNCaP and androgen-insensitive PC-3 cells (Srivastava et al. 2007). The G1/S phase arrest by curcumin was associated with the induction of p21/WAF1, p27/KIP1, and p16, and inhibition of cyclin D1, cyclin E, Cdk4 and cdk 6 (Srivastava et al. 2007). The ability of curcumin to induce cdk inhibitors p21 and p27 and inhibit cyclin D1 expression was also confirmed in our xenograft experiment. In support of our data, it has been demonstrated that curcumin induces the degradation of cyclin E expression through ubiquitin-dependent pathway and up-regulates p21 and p27 in several cancer cell lines (Aggarwal et al. 2007a). Moreover, deregulated expression of cyclin E was found to be correlated with chromosome instability (Spruck et al. 1999), malignant transformation (Haas et al. 1997), tumor progression (Rosen et al. 2006), and patient survival (Keyomarsi et al. 2002). Overall, these data suggest that curcumin induces growth arrest at G1/S stage of cell cycle.

Curcumin inhibited hyper-phosphorylation of pRB and enhanced hypo-phosphorylation of pRb in both PC-3 and LNCaP cell lines. Similarly, curcumin induced the expression of p16/INK4a, p21/WAF1/CIP1 and p27/KIP1, and inhibited the expression of cyclin D1 in LNCaP xenografts implanted in nude mice (Shankar et al. 2007). Curcumin also inhibited LNCaP tumor growth, metastasis and angiogenesis *in vivo* (Srivastava et al. 2007), suggesting its clinical utility for anticancer therapy and/or prevention. The G1/S phase arrest by curcumin was associated with the induction of CDK inhibitors p16/INK4a, p21/WAF1/CIP1, and p27/KIP1, and inhibition of hyper-phosphorylated state of pRb protein *in vitro*. The ability of curcumin to induce CDK inhibitors p21/WAF1/CIP1 and p27/KIP1 was also confirmed in our xenograft experiment (Shankar et al. 2007). Most importantly, we have demonstrated a link between cell cycle and apoptosis as CDK inhibitor p21/WAF1/CIP1 blocked curcumin-induced apoptosis.

The p27/KIP1 binds to CDK2 and cyclin E complexes to prevent cell cycle progression from G1 to S phase. p27/KIP1 also acts as a tumor suppressor and its expression is often disrupted in human cancers. Studies in mice have shown that loss of p27/KIP1 increases tumor incidence and tumor growth rate in either specific genetic backgrounds, or when mice are challenged with carcinogens (Fero et al. 1998; Ophascharoensuk et al. 1998). Decreased p27/KIP1 levels have been correlated with tumor aggressiveness and poor patient survival (Loda et al. 1997; Lu et al. 1999; Migita et al. 2002; Mineta et al. 1999; Ponce-Castaneda et al. 1995; Porter et al. 1997). Although p27/KIP1 is characterized as a tumor suppressor, inactivating point mutations with loss of heterozygosity are rarely observed in human cancer. The abundance of p27/KIP1 protein is largely controlled through a variety of post-transcriptional regulatory mechanisms (Alessandrini et al. 1997; Chu et al. 2007; Grimmler et al. 2007; Kardinal et al. 2006), among which are sequestration by cyclin D/CDK4 complexes, accelerated protein destruction and cytoplasmic retention. In certain types of cancers, such as colorectal cancer, high expression levels of Skp2 and Cks1, specific p27/KIP1 ubiquitin ligase subunits, were strongly associated with low p27/KIP1 expression and aggressive tumor behavior (Hershko and Shapira 2006). p27/KIP1 protein level changes during cell cycle progression, accumulating when cells progress through G1 and sharply decreasing just before cells enter S phase (Kaldis 2007). Additionally, p27/KIP1 protein levels rise when cells exit cell cycle to G0, and decreases when cells enter the cell cycle again (Kaldis 2007). These alterations in p27/KIP1 levels are mainly caused by regulation at the protein degradation level (Alessandrini et al. 1997; Chu et al. 2007; Grimmler et al. 2007; Kardinal et al. 2006). However, several studies have indicated that p27/KIP1 can also be regulated at the level of translation (Chiarle et al. 2000; Chilosi et al. 2000; Hengst and Reed 1996; Millard et al. 1997). Similarly, induction of p19(INK4d) expression contributed to cell cycle arrest by vitamin D(3) and retinoids (Tavera-Mendoza et al. 2006).

Cyclins are tightly regulated in different stages of cell cycle. In support of our data, it has been demonstrated that curcumin induces the degradation of cyclin E expression through ubiquitin-dependent pathway (Aggarwal et al. 2007a). Moreover, deregulated expression of cyclin E was found to be correlated with chromosome instability (Spruck et al. 1999), malignant transformation (Haas et al. 1997), tumor progression (Rosen et al. 2006), and patient survival (Keyomarsi et al. 2002). Cyclin E expression increases with increasing stage and grade of the cancers including breast, head and neck, prostate, colon, and lung cancer, and acute lymphoblastic and acute myeloid leukemias (Gong et al. 1994; Iida et al. 1997; Keyomarsi et al. 2002; Kitahara et al. 1995; Muller-Tidow et al. 2001; Rosen et al. 2006; Scuderi et al. 1996), suggesting its potential use as a prognostic marker. The down-regulation of cyclin E by curcumin correlates with the decrease in the proliferation of human prostate cancer cells. The suppression of cyclin E expression was not cell type dependent as down-regulation occurred in androgen-sensitive LNCaP and -insensitive PC-3 prostate cancer cells. Curcumin-induced down-regulation of cyclin E was reversed by proteasome inhibitor lactacystin, an inhibitor of 26S proteasome, suggesting the role of ubiquitin-dependent proteasomal pathway.

Cyclin D acts as a growth sensor and provides a link between mitogenic stimuli and the cell cycle. Cyclin D1 binds to CDK4 and CDK6 in early G1. Aberrant cyclin D1 expression has been reported in many human cancers. Cyclin *D1* gene amplification occurs in breast, esophageal, bladder, lung and squamous cell carcinomas (Hall and Peters 1996), and parathyroid adenomas (Motokura et al. 1991). Cyclin D2 and cyclin D3 have also been reported to be overexpressed in some tumours (Hunter and Pines 1994; Keyomarsi et al. 1995; Leach et al. 1993). The suppression of cyclin D1 by curcumin led to inhibition of CDK4-mediated phosphorylation of Rb protein. The present study has demonstrated that curcumin-induced down-regulation of cyclin D1 was inhibited by lactacystin, suggesting that curcumin represses cyclin D1 expression by promoting proteolysis. Similarly, recent studies have demonstrated that curcumin can regulate cyclin D1 expression through transcriptional and posttranslational modifications (Aggarwal and Shishodia 2006; Aggarwal et al. 2007b), and this may contribute to the antiproliferative effects of curcumin against various cell types. Overall, these data suggest that downregulation of cyclins may be useful for cancer therapy and prevention.

The transition of the G1 to the S phase of the cell cycle marks an irreversible commitment to DNA synthesis and proliferation and is strictly regulated by positive and negative growth-regulatory signals. The G1-S transition is controlled by the Rb-E2F pathway, which links growth-regulatory pathways to a transcription program required for DNA synthesis, cell cycle progression and cell division (Brugarolas et al. 1999; Dyson 1998; Weinberg 1995). This transcription program is activated by the E2F transcription factors and repressed by E2F-Rb complexes (Nevins et al. 1997). E2F overexpression or Rb inactivation is sufficient to induce S phase entry, whereas Rb overexpression can arrest cycling cells in G1, suggesting that the Rb-E2F pathway is central to the control of the G1-S transition (Dyson 1998; Weinberg 1995). Mitogenic signal causes sequential activation of the CDK-cyclin complexes CDK4/6-cyclin D and CDK2-cyclin E, which hyper-phosphorylate pRb and thereby cause the release of active E2F (Dyson 1998; Weinberg 1995). pRB-deficient cells are hypersensitive to DNA damage-induced apoptosis.(Almasan et al. 1995; Knudsen et al. 2000). On the other hand, E2F-1 has a role distinct from other

E2Fs in the regulation of apoptosis (DeGregori et al. 1997). Loss of E2F-1 reduces tumorigenesis and extends the lifespan of Rb1(+/−) mice (Yamasaki et al. 1998). E2F-1 has been found to induce the expression of many apoptotic genes(Attwooll et al. 2004) and thus mediate the response of chemopreventive agents.

Overall, these studies provide the molecular mechanisms through which curcumin contributes to the antiproliferative and antitumor activities. The down-regulation of cyclin E, cyclin D1, and hyper-phosphorylation of pRb, and up-regulation of CDK inhibitors $p16^{/INK4a}$, $p21^{/WAF1/CIP1}$ and $p27^{/KIP1}$ may contribute to the antiproliferative effects of curcumin against various cancer. These events may be responsible for growth arrest followed by apoptosis in cancer cells. Curcumin chemosensitizes and radiosensitizes the effects by down-regulating the MDM2 oncogene through the PI3K/mTOR/ETS2 pathway (Li et al. 2007). Thus, targeting of cyclins and/or CDKs by curcumin may be considered beneficial for cancer therapy or prevention.

Metastasis and Angiogenesis

Entry of malignant cells into the vasculature (i.e. intravasation) requires proteolytic remodeling of the extracellular matrix so that tumor cells may pass through the local stroma and penetrate the vessel wall. The circulatory system then provides a means of transporting tumor cells to distant sites where they extravasate and establish metastatic lesions. Matrix metalloproteinase (MMP) is up-regulated in many tumor types and has been implicated in tumor progression and metastasis (Bailey et al. 2007; Dreesen and Brivanlou 2007; Lopez-Otin and Matrisian 2007; Lynch 2011). MMP is critical for pericellular degradation of the extracellular matrix, thereby promoting tumor cell invasion and dissemination. To grow efficiently *in vivo*, tumor cells induce angiogenesis in both primary solid tumors and metastatic foci. Curcumin significantly inhibited the growth of TRAIL-resistant LNCaP xenografts and sensitized these xenografts to undergo apoptosis by TRAIL (Shankar et al. 2007b, 2008). Tumor tissues derived from curcumin treated mice showed that curcumin inhibited proliferation (PCNA and Ki67 staining), induced apoptosis (TUNEL staining), metastasis (uPA, MMP-2 and MMP-9 staining), and angiogenesis (CD31 and VEGF staining). Curcumin also inhibited VEGFR2-positive circulating endothelial cells. Treatment of LNCaP xenografted mice with TRAIL alone had no effect on tumor growth, apoptosis, metastasis and angiogenesis. *In vitro* studies demonstrated the role of ERK MAP kinase on the inhibitory effects of curcumin in capillary tube formation and endothelial cell migration. These data suggest that curcumin can inhibit tumor growth by inhibiting apoptosis, metastasis and angiogenesis.

Activation of death receptor pathway by TRAIL play a major role in apoptosis. The upregulation of death receptors by chemotherapeutic and chemopreventive drugs, irradiation and chemopreventive agents have been shown to enhance or sensitize cancer cells to TRAIL treatment (Srivastava 2001). TRAIL-resistant

LNCaP cells can be sensitized by chemotherapeutic and chemopreventive drugs, and irradiation *in vitro* and *in vivo* through upregulation of death receptors DR4 and/or DR5 (Shankar et al. 2004, 2005). These finding suggest that upregulation of death receptors DR4 and DR5 by curcumin may be one of the mechanisms by which curcumin enhances the therapeutic potential of TRAIL.

Clinical Significance of Curcumin

Curcumin is known to possess antioxidant, anti-inflammatory, antiviral, antibacterial, antifungal, anticancer and antidiabetic activities and is also beneficial in allergies, arthritis, and alzheimer's disease. Here, we present a brief update on the mechanisms of curcumin action in various diseases.

Antioxidant Activity of Curcumin

Oxidative stress plays a major role in the pathogenesis of various diseases including cancer, diabetes, cardiovascular diseases, neuronal cell injury and hypoxia. Curcumin exhibits strong antioxidant activity that is comparable to ascorbic acid and vitamin E. Curcumin is a potent scavenger of a variety of reactive oxygen species including superoxide anion radicals, hydroxyl radicals (Reddy and Lokesh 1994) and nitrogen dioxide radicals (Sreejayan and Rao 1997; Unnikrishnan and Rao 1995a; Unnikrishnan and Rao 1995b). It was also shown to inhibit lipid peroxidation *in vivo* (Reddy and Lokesh 1992; Sreejayan and Rao 1994). It has protected oxidative cell injury of kidney cells (LLC-PK1) by inhibiting lipid degradation, lipid peroxidation and cytolysis (Cohly et al. 1998; Dikshit et al. 1995). Curcumin treatment showed beneficial effects on renal injury by its ability to inhibit the expression of the apoptosis-related genes Fas and Fas-L (Jones et al. 2000; Jones and Shoskes 2000). In short, curcumin appears to have a significant potential in the treatment of multiple diseases that are a result of oxidative stress. These protective effects of curcumin are attributed mainly to its antioxidant properties and should be further exploited to develop novel drugs.

Neuroprotective Activity of Curcumin

Several reports suggest that curcumin has potential against Alzheimer's disease, a disease characterized by the amyloid-induced inflammation in the brain. It is suggested that dietary supplementation with curcumin may be beneficial in neurodegenerative diseases including Alzheimer's disease (Giri et al. 2004; Lim et al. 2001; Yang et al. 2005). The effect of curcumin in Alzheimer's disease is mediated through the downmodulation of cytokine (i.e., TNF-α and IL-1β) and chemokine (i.e., MIP-1b, MCP- 1, and IL-8) activity in peripheral blood monocytes and reduces amyloid-β plaque formation.

Anti-inflammatory Activity of Curcumin

Curcumin has been known to possess anti-inflammatory activity since thousands of years. It suppresses the activation of NF-kB that regulates pro-inflammatory genes. It down-regulates the expression of COX-2 enzyme and inhibits the expression of pro-inflammatory enzyme 5-LOX. The curcumin induces down-regulation of various inflammatory cytokines viz., TNF, IL-1, IL-6, IL-8 and chemokines (Surh 2002).

Curcumin in Cardiovascular Disorders

With several recent studies focusing on the beneficial effects of polyphenol-based dietary components such as red wine on vascular health, curcumin has been shown to improve several aspects of cardiovascular health. The key findings are: (I) Curcumin has potent cholesterol lowering ability mediated through increased expression of LDL receptors. The increased LDL receptors will result into increased uptake of LDL-cholesterol from plasma and (II) It also reduces triglycerides and inhibits platelet aggregation. Curcumin treatment resulted in a significant decrease in early atherosclerotic lesions (fatty streaks) in rabbits fed high fat and cholesterol diets. Curcumin has established antioxidant and anti-inflammatory activities that offer promise in the treatment of cardiovascular diseases. For example, it can inhibit lipid peroxidation; reduce creatinine kinase and lactate dehydrogenase levels; and restore reduced glutathione, glutathione peroxidase, and superoxide dismutase to normal levels. Curcumin can also downregulate the expression of myocardial TNF-α and MMP-2 and upregulate the expression of eNOS mRNA (Cheng et al. 2005; Dikshit et al. 1995; Nirmala and Puvanakrishnan 1996a; b; Yao et al. 2004).

Curcumin in Cancer Therapy

Anti-cancerous property of curcumin is the also one of the most significant medicinal property of curcumin. The extensive research has been done on these areas and several research papers have been published. The extensive reviews of curcumin and cancer can be found elsewhere (Aggarwal et al. 2006a; Bemis et al. 2006; Bengmark 2006; Bengmark et al. 2009; Kunnumakkara et al. 2008; Shanmugam et al. 2011; Thomasset et al. 2007). Curcumin has been found to inhibit growth of oral and hepatic cancers. It inhibited polyp formation in rodents and cell death in colon cancers. It has also inhibited the growth of head and neck tumor cells *in vitro*, as well increased cell death. It has been shown to increased sensitivity to a specific chemotherapy (IFN-γ) in non-small cell lung cancer that without curcumin was relatively insensitive. Curcumin was able to target breast stem/progenitor cells, as evidenced by suppressed mammosphere formation along serial passage and by a decrease in the percent of ALDH-positive cells (Kakarala et al. 2010). By comparison, curcumin had little impact on differentiated cells (Kakarala et al. 2010). By utilizing a TCF-LEF reporter assay system in MCF7 cells, it was confirmed that the effect of curcumin on breast cancer stem/progenitor cells was mediated through its potent inhibitory effect on Wnt/β-catenin signaling pathway.

Wound Healing Property of Curcumin

Tissue repair and wound healing are complex processes that involve inflammation, granulation and tissue remodeling. Injury initiates a complex series of events that involves interactions of multiple cell types, various cytokines, growth factors, their mediators and the extra-cellular matrix proteins (ECM). Many studies have evaluated the effect of curcumin on enhancement of wound healing (Maheshwari et al. 2006). Curcumin treated wound biopsies showed a large number of infiltrating cells such as macrophage, neutrophils and fibroblasts as compared to untreated wound. The presence of myofibroblast in curcumin treated wound demonstrated faster wound contraction (Sidhu et al. 1998). Migration of various cells represents potential sources of growth factors required for the regulation of biological processes during wound healing. Curcumin treatment resulted in enhanced fibronectin (FN) and collagen expression (Sidhu et al. 1998). Furthermore, the treatment led to an increased formation of granulation tissue including greater cellular content, neo-vascularization and a faster re-epithelialization of wound in both diabetic as well as hydrocortisone impaired wounds (Sidhu et al. 1999) by regulating the expression of TGF-β1, its receptors and nitric oxide synthase during wound healing (Mani et al. 2002). Systemic administration of curcumin has shown its beneficial effects by the enhancement of muscle regeneration after trauma in vivo by modulating NF-κB activity (Thaloor et al. 1999). Curcumin incorporated collagen matrix treatment showed increased wound reduction, enhanced cell proliferation and efficient free radical scavenging as compared with control and collagen treated rats (Gopinath et al. 2004). It has also been studied for antiulcer activity in acute ulcer model in rat by preventing glutathione depletion, lipid peroxidation and protein oxidation. Both oral and intraperitoneal administration of curcumin blocked gastric ulceration in a dose dependent manner. It accelerated the healing process and protected gastric ulcer through attenuation of MMP-9 activity and amelioration of MMP-2 activity (Swarnakar et al. 2005). Thus it is well established that curcumin treatment results in faster closure of wounds, better regulation of granulation tissue formation and induction of growth factors.

Neuroprotective Property of Curcumin

Inflammation in Alzheimer's disease (AD) patients is characterized by increased cytokines and activated microglia. Several studies suggest reduced AD risk associates with long-term use of nonsteroidal anti-inflammatory drugs (NSAIDs). Beta-amyloid-induced oxidative toxicity on neuronal cells is a principal route in AD, and its toxicity occurs after fibril formation. Epidemiological studies have raised the possibility that curcumin used by Asian Indian population is involved for the significantly lower prevalence of AD in India compared to United States. 500 ppm dose of curcumin placed in rat diets for 2 months could prevent deficits in memory, as tested with the Morris Water Maze analysis after an intracerebroventricular infusion of the amyloid β peptide. Moreover, the amyloid β peptide deposits in 9 month old female rat were also attenuated (Frautschy and Cole 2010). Curcumin can exist in an equilibrium between keto and enol tautomers, binds to beta-amyloid fibrils/aggregates. The keto-enol tautomerism of curcumin derivatives may be a novel target for the design of amyloid-binding agents that can be used both for therapy and for amyloid detection in Alzheimer's disease. These observations suggest that curcumin has potential to inhibit the amyloid β fibril formation (Kim et al. 2005).

Role of Curcumin in Diabetes

Curcumin has been reported to suppress blood glucose levels, increase the antioxidant status of pancreatic β- cells, and enhance the activation of PPAR-γ in diabetes (Arun and Nalini 2002; Srinivasan 1972). Curcumin has been observed to lower blood sugar levels in diabetic patients (Lin and Chen 2011). Curcumin administration also reduced the serum levels of cholesterol and lipid peroxides in ten healthy human volunteers receiving 500 mg of curcumin daily for 7 days. A significant decrease in the level of serum lipid peroxides (33%), an increase in high-density lipoproteins (HDL) cholesterol (29%), and a decrease in total serum cholesterol (12%) were noted. Daily administration of 10 mg of curcumin for 30 days to eight human subjects increased HDL cholesterol and decreased LDL cholesterol (Ramirez Bosca et al. 2000). The same research group also investigated the effect of curcumin in human subjects with atherosclerosis, in which 10 mg curcumin was administered twice a day for 15 days to 16 men and 14 women. Curcumin significantly lowered the levels of plasma fibrinogen in both men and women. A recent study conducted an interventional, randomized, double-blind, controlled trial to investigate the effects of curcumin administration at escalating doses (low dose three times 15 mg/day, moderate dose three times 30 mg/ day, and high dose three times 60 mg/day) on total cholesterol level, LDL cholesterol level, HDL cholesterol level, and triglyceride level in 75 acute coronary syndrome (ACS) patients (Alwi et al. 2008). Based on 63 patient's results, it is concluded that the administration of low-dose curcumin showed a trend of reduction in total cholesterol level and LDL cholesterol level in ACS patients (Alwi et al. 2008). Moreover, curcumin in physiological concentration was reported to induce the expression of ABCG1 in the human hepatoma cell line HepG2, thus increasing HDL-dependent lipid efflux and plasma HDL cholesterol levels.

Hyperglycemia leads to increased oxidative stress resulting in endothelial dysfunction. A randomized, parallel-group, placebo-controlled, 8-week study was performed to evaluate the effects of NCB-02 (a standardized preparation of curcuminoids), atorvastatin, and placebo on endothelial function and its biomarkers in patients with type 2 diabetes mellitus. In this study, 72 patients with type 2 diabetes were randomized to receive NCB-02 (two capsules containing curcumin 150 mg twice daily), atorvastatin 10 mg once daily, or placebo for 8 weeks. NCB-02 had a favorable effect, comparable with that of atorvastatin, on endothelial dysfunction in association with reductions in inflammatory cytokines and markers of oxidative stress. Patients receiving NCB-02 showed significant reductions in the levels of malondialdehyde, endothelin-1 (ET-1), IL-6, and TNFα. Recently, the effect of curcumin has been investigated in the activities of drug-metabolizing enzymes such as CYP1A2, CYP2A6, N-acetyltransferase (NAT2), and xanthine oxidase (XO) in 16 healthy male Chinese volunteers, using caffeine as a probe drug. After 14 days, in the curcumin-treated (1,000 mg/day) group, CYP1A2 activity was decreased by 28.6%, while CYP2A6 activity was increased by 48.9%. Curcumin–phosphatidylcholine complex (Meriva / Norflo) was evaluated in 50 patients with osteoarthritis at dosages corresponding to 200 mg of curcumin per diem. After 3 months of treatment, C-reactive protein (CRP) levels significantly decreased in the subpopulation with high CRP, while control group experienced only a modest improvement in these parameters in the CRP plasma concentration. It has been suggested that Meriva is clinically effective in the treatment of osteoarthritis and could be taken into consideration for clinical use. In addition, the same curcumin–phosphatidylcholine complex has been investigated among inflammatory conditions such as chronic anterior uveitis relapses in a 12-month follow-up clinical trial.

Curcumin's ability to lower blood glucose and cholesterol and its antioxidant nature make it a potential therapeutic for the treatment of obesity-related diseases. Recent evidence has shown that curcumin plays a key role in the protection against various obesity-related cancers including pancreatic cancer. Curcumin (8,000 mg/day) in concomitant administration with gemcitibine intravenously (1,000 mg/m/week) was observed in 17 patients of advanced pancreatic cancer for 4 weeks. According to a join report of the Food and Agriculture Organization and the World Health Organization on food additives, the recommended maximum daily intake of curcumin is 0–1 mg/kg body weight, but several clinical studies dealing with its efficacy suggested that it is safe and well tolerated even when intake is as high as 12 g/day. However, high doses of curcumin caused side effects such as gastrointestinal upset, chest tightness, inflamed skin, and skin rashes. The chronic use of curcumin can cause liver toxicity, and individuals with hepatic disease, persons misusing alcohol, and those who take prescription medications that are metabolized by liver should probably avoid curcumin. Curcumin is not recommended for persons with biliary tract obstruction, because it stimulates bile secretion. Nevertheless, the multifaceted pharmacological nature of curcumin and its pharmacokinetics in obesity remains unknown and additional research is needed to understand it's therapeutic benefits.

Future Prospects

In recent decades, a rapid increase in the costs of health care has increased the importance of naturally occurring phytochemicals in plants for the prevention and treatment of human diseases, including obesity. The modulation of several cellular transduction pathways by curcumin has recently been extended to elucidate the molecular basis for obesity and obesity-related metabolic diseases. Current knowledge suggests that the potential complementary effect of curcumin may occur through several mechanisms including suppression of inflammatory proteins, uptake of glucose, stimulation of catabolic pathways in adipose tissues, liver, and other tissues, inhibition of angiogenesis in adipose tissues, inhibition of differentiation of adipocytes, stimulation of apoptosis of mature adipocytes, and reduction in chronic inflammation associated with adiposity. Numerous studies confirm its potential role *in vitro* and in animals, yet further human studies, in particular clinical trials, are required to confirm the therapeutic nature of curcumin in obesity and insulin resistance. Expanded use of molecular technologies such as DNA microarrays and proteomics will help to identify newly molecular targets of curcumin and individuals at high risk of obesity-related metabolic diseases. Recent studies have successfully demonstrated the enhanced *in vitro* and *in vivo* anticancer activity of encapsulated curcumin with several types of nanoparticles such as poly(lactic-co-glycolide) (PLGA), β-cyclodextrin, ploy(β-cyclodextrin), cellulose, fibrinogen and hydrogel. Encapsulating hydrophobic drugs on polymer is a promising method for sustained and controlled drug delivery with improved bioavailability of curcumin. Future trials should also include suitably planned pharmacodynamic studies, because the effective dose required for modulating these metabolic responses is unclear at the present. It is important to note that high doses of curcumin in supplement form may have adverse effects. At present, there is not sufficient data to support recommending long-term, safe usage for the prevention and treatment of obesity. Future translational and clinical research overlapping metabolism with the aim to unravel the role of curcumin in obesity-related comorbidities is highly warranted. On behalf of such studies, one might be able to gain insights into curcumin mechanisms at a clinical level and assess, within a short period, the potential success or failure of long-term interventions.

Acknowledgements This work was supported by the grants from the National Institutes of Health, Kansas Bioscience Authority, and the Department of Defense, US Army. We thank all the lab members for critically reading the manuscript.

References

Aggarwal BB, Shishodia S (2006) Molecular targets of dietary agents for prevention and therapy of cancer. Biochem Pharmacol 71:1397–1421

Aggarwal BB, Sethi G, Ahn KS, Sandur SK, Pandey MK, Kunnumakkara AB, Sung B, Ichikawa H (2006a) Targeting signal-transducer-and-activator-of-transcription-3 for prevention and therapy of cancer: modern target but ancient solution. Ann N Y Acad Sci 1091:151–169

Aggarwal BB, Shishodia S, Sandur SK, Pandey MK, Sethi G (2006b) Inflammation and cancer: how hot is the link? Biochem Pharmacol 72:1605–1621

Aggarwal S, Ichikawa H, Takada Y, Sandur SK, Shishodia S, Aggarwal BB (2006c) Curcumin (diferuloylmethane) down-regulates expression of cell proliferation and antiapoptotic and metastatic gene products through suppression of IkappaBalpha kinase and Akt activation. Mol Pharmacol 69:195–206

Aggarwal BB, Banerjee S, Bharadwaj U, Sung B, Shishodia S, Sethi G (2007a) Curcumin induces the degradation of cyclin E expression through ubiquitin-dependent pathway and up-regulates cyclin-dependent kinase inhibitors p21 and p27 in multiple human tumor cell lines. Biochem Pharmacol 73:1024–1032

Aggarwal BB, Sundaram C, Malani N, Ichikawa H (2007b) Curcumin: the Indian solid gold. Adv Exp Med Biol 595:1–75

Alessandrini A, Chiaur DS, Pagano M (1997) Regulation of the cyclin-dependent kinase inhibitor p27 by degradation and phosphorylation. Leukemia 11:342–345

Almasan A, Yin Y, Kelly RE, Lee EY, Bradley A, Li W, Bertino JR, Wahl GM (1995) Deficiency of retinoblastoma protein leads to inappropriate S-phase entry, activation of E2F-responsive genes, and apoptosis. Proc Natl Acad Sci U S A 92:5436–5440

Alwi I, Santoso T, Suyono S, Sutrisna B, Suyatna FD, Kresno SB, Ernie S (2008) The effect of curcumin on lipid level in patients with acute coronary syndrome. Acta Med Indones 40: 201–210

Arellano M, Moreno S (1997) Regulation of CDK/cyclin complexes during the cell cycle. Int J Biochem Cell Biol 29:559–573

Artandi SE, DePinho RA (2000) Mice without telomerase: what can they teach us about human cancer? Nat Med 6:852–855

Artavanis-Tsakonas S, Muskavitch MA (2010) Notch: the past, the present, and the future. Curr Top Dev Biol 92:1–29

Artavanis-Tsakonas S, Matsuno K, Fortini ME (1995) Notch signaling. Science 268:225–232

Arthan D, Hong SK, Park JI (2010) Leukemia inhibitory factor can mediate Ras/Raf/MEK/ERK-induced growth inhibitory signaling in medullary thyroid cancer cells. Cancer Lett 297:31–41

Arun N, Nalini N (2002) Efficacy of turmeric on blood sugar and polyol pathway in diabetic albino rats. Plant Foods Hum Nutr 57:41–52

Ashkenazi A, Pai RC, Fong S, Leung S, Lawrence DA, Marsters SA, Blackie C, Chang L, McMurtrey AE, Hebert A, DeForge L, Koumenis IL, Lewis D, Harris L, Bussiere J, Koeppen H, Shahrokh Z, Schwall RH (1999) Safety and antitumor activity of recombinant soluble Apo2 ligand. J Clin Invest 104:155–162

Assoian RK (1997) Control of the G1 phase cyclin-dependent kinases by mitogenic growth factors and the extracellular matrix. Cytokine Growth Factor Rev 8:165–170

Attwooll C, Lazzerini Denchi E, Helin K (2004) The E2F family: specific functions and overlapping interests. EMBO J 23:4709–4716

Azuine MA, Bhide SV (1994) Adjuvant chemoprevention of experimental cancer: catechin and dietary turmeric in forestomach and oral cancer models. J Ethnopharmacol 44:211–217

Bae MK, Kim SH, Jeong JW, Lee YM, Kim HS, Kim SR, Yun I, Bae SK, Kim KW (2006) Curcumin inhibits hypoxia-induced angiogenesis via down-regulation of HIF-1. Oncol Rep 15:1557–1562

Bailey JM, Singh PK, Hollingsworth MA (2007) Cancer metastasis facilitated by developmental pathways: Sonic hedgehog, Notch, and bone morphogenic proteins. J Cell Biochem 102: 829–839

Balasubramanian S, Eckert RL (2007) Curcumin suppresses AP1 transcription factor-dependent differentiation and activates apoptosis in human epidermal keratinocytes. J Biol Chem 282:6707–6715

Balogun E, Foresti R, Green CJ, Motterlini R (2003a) Changes in temperature modulate heme oxygenase-1 induction by curcumin in renal epithelial cells. Biochem Biophys Res Commun 308:950–955

Balogun E, Hoque M, Gong P, Killeen E, Green CJ, Foresti R, Alam J, Motterlini R (2003b) Curcumin activates the haem oxygenase-1 gene via regulation of Nrf2 and the antioxidant-responsive element. Biochem J 371:887–895

Banning A, Deubel S, Kluth D, Zhou Z, Brigelius-Flohe R (2005) The GI-GPx gene is a target for Nrf2. Mol Cell Biol 25:4914–4923

Barker N, Clevers H (2000) Catenins, Wnt signaling and cancer. Bioessays 22:961–965

Bemis DL, Katz AE, Buttyan R (2006) Clinical trials of natural products as chemopreventive agents for prostate cancer. Expert Opin Investig Drugs 15:1191–1200

Bengmark S (2006) Curcumin, an atoxic antioxidant and natural NFkappaB, cyclooxygenase-2, lipooxygenase, and inducible nitric oxide synthase inhibitor: a shield against acute and chronic diseases. JPEN J Parenter Enteral Nutr 30:45–51

Bengmark S, Mesa MD, Gil A (2009) Plant-derived health: the effects of turmeric and curcuminoids. Nutr Hosp 24:273–281

Beresford SA, Davies MA, Gallick GE, Donato NJ (2001) Differential effects of phosphatidylinositol-3/Akt-kinase inhibition on apoptotic sensitization to cytokines in LNCaP and PCc-3 prostate cancer cells. J Interferon Cytokine Res 21:313–322

Bhattacharyya S, Mandal D, Saha B, Sen GS, Das T, Sa G (2007) Curcumin prevents tumor-induced T cell apoptosis through Stat-5a-mediated Bcl-2 induction. J Biol Chem 282: 15954–15964

Bigas A, Robert-Moreno A, Espinosa L (2010) The Notch pathway in the developing hematopoietic system. Int J Dev Biol 54:1175–1188

Bill MA, Bakan C, Benson DM Jr, Fuchs J, Young G, Lesinski GB (2009) Curcumin induces proapoptotic effects against human melanoma cells and modulates the cellular response to immunotherapeutic cytokines. Mol Cancer Ther 8:2726–2735

Blasco MA (2002) Telomerase beyond telomeres. Nat Rev Cancer 2:627–633

Blasius R, Reuter S, Henry E, Dicato M, Diederich M (2006) Curcumin regulates signal transducer and activator of transcription (STAT) expression in K562 cells. Biochem Pharmacol 72: 1547–1554

Bray SJ (2006) Notch signalling: a simple pathway becomes complex. Nat Rev Mol Cell Biol 7:678–689

Brennan C, Momota H, Hambardzumyan D, Ozawa T, Tandon A, Pedraza A, Holland E (2009) Glioblastoma subclasses can be defined by activity among signal transduction pathways and associated genomic alterations. PLoS One 4:e7752

Brugarolas J, Moberg K, Boyd SD, Taya Y, Jacks T, Lees JA (1999) Inhibition of cyclin-dependent kinase 2 by p21 is necessary for retinoblastoma protein mediated G1 arrest after gamma-irradiation. Proc Natl Acad Sci U S A 96:1002–1007

Cai K, Qi D, Hou X, Wang O, Chen J, Deng B, Qian L, Liu X, Le Y (2011) MCP-1 upregulates amylin expression in murine pancreatic beta cells through ERK/JNK-AP1 and NF-kappaB related signaling pathways independent of CCR2. PLoS One 6:e19559

Cantley LC (2002) The phosphoinositide 3-kinase pathway. Science 296:1655–1657

Carnero A, Hannon GJ (1998) The INK4 family of CDK inhibitors. Curr Top Microbiol Immunol 227:43–55

Cerdan C, Bhatia M (2010) Novel roles for Notch, Wnt and Hedgehog in hematopoesis derived from human pluripotent stem cells. Int J Dev Biol 54:955–963

Chen YR, Tan TH (1998) Inhibition of the c-Jun N-terminal kinase (JNK) signaling pathway by curcumin. Oncogene 17:173–178

Chen X, Thakkar H, Tyan F, Gim S, Robinson H, Lee C, Pandey SK, Nwokorie C, Onwudiwe N, Srivastava RK (2001) Constitutively active Akt is an important regulator of TRAIL sensitivity in prostate cancer. Oncogene 20:6073–6083

Chen A, Xu J, Johnson AC (2006) Curcumin inhibits human colon cancer cell growth by suppressing gene expression of epidermal growth factor receptor through reducing the activity of the transcription factor Egr-1. Oncogene 25:278–287

Chen Y, Shu W, Chen W, Wu Q, Liu H, Cui G (2007) Curcumin, both histone deacetylase and p300/CBP-specific inhibitor, represses the activity of nuclear factor kappa B and Notch 1 in Raji cells. Basic Clin Pharmacol Toxicol 101:427–433

Chen J, Imanaka N, Griffin JD (2010) Hypoxia potentiates Notch signaling in breast cancer leading to decreased E-cadherin expression and increased cell migration and invasion. Br J Cancer 102:351–360

Cheng P, Zlobin A, Volgina V, Gottipati S, Osborne B, Simel EJ, Miele L, Gabrilovich DI (2001) Notch-1 regulates NF-kappaB activity in hemopoietic progenitor cells. J Immunol 167: 4458–4467

Cheng H, Liu W, Ai X (2005) Protective effect of curcumin on myocardial ischemia reperfusion injury in rats. Zhong Yao Cai 28:920–922

Chiarle R, Budel LM, Skolnik J, Frizzera G, Chilosi M, Corato A, Pizzolo G, Magidson J, Montagnoli A, Pagano M, Maes B, De Wolf-Peeters C, Inghirami G (2000) Increased proteasome degradation of cyclin-dependent kinase inhibitor p27 is associated with a decreased overall survival in mantle cell lymphoma. Blood 95:619–626

Chilosi M, Chiarle R, Lestani M, Menestrina F, Montagna L, Ambrosetti A, Prolla G, Pizzolo G, Doglioni C, Piva R, Pagano M, Inghirami G (2000) Low expression of p27 and low proliferation index do not correlate in hairy cell leukaemia. Br J Haematol 111:263–271

Chirnomas D, Taniguchi T, de la Vega M, Vaidya AP, Vasserman M, Hartman AR, Kennedy R, Foster R, Mahoney J, Seiden MV, D'Andrea AD (2006) Chemosensitization to cisplatin by inhibitors of the Fanconi anemia/BRCA pathway. Mol Cancer Ther 5:952–961

Chu I, Sun J, Arnaout A, Kahn H, Hanna W, Narod S, Sun P, Tan CK, Hengst L, Slingerland J (2007) p27 phosphorylation by Src regulates inhibition of cyclin E-Cdk2. Cell 128:281–294

Classon M, Harlow E (2002) The retinoblastoma tumour suppressor in development and cancer. Nat Rev Cancer 2:910–917

Clevers H (2004) Wnt breakers in colon cancer. Cancer Cell 5:5–6

Clevers H (2006) Wnt/beta-catenin signaling in development and disease. Cell 127:469–480

Cohen MM Jr (2003) The hedgehog signaling network. Am J Med Genet A 123A:5–28

Cohen P, Frame S (2001) The renaissance of GSK3. Nat Rev Mol Cell Biol 2:769–776

Cohen B, Shimizu M, Izrailit J, Ng NF, Buchman Y, Pan JG, Dering J, Reedijk M (2010) Cyclin D1 is a direct target of JAG1-mediated Notch signaling in breast cancer. Breast Cancer Res Treat 123:113–124

Cohly HH, Taylor A, Angel MF, Salahudeen AK (1998) Effect of turmeric, turmerin and curcumin on H2O2-induced renal epithelial (LLC-PK1) cell injury. Free Radic Biol Med 24:49–54

D'Altri T, Gonzalez J, Aifantis I, Espinosa L, Bigas A (2011) Hes1 expression and CYLD repression are essential events downstream of Notch1 in T-cell leukemia. Cell Cycle 10: 1031–1036

Darnell JE Jr, Kerr IM, Stark GR (1994) Jak-STAT pathways and transcriptional activation in response to IFNs and other extracellular signaling proteins. Science 264:1415–1421

Das D, Lanner F, Main H, Andersson ER, Bergmann O, Sahlgren C, Heldring N, Hermanson O, Hansson EM, Lendahl U (2010) Notch induces cyclin-D1-dependent proliferation during a specific temporal window of neural differentiation in ES cells. Dev Biol 348:153–166

Dasari A, Messersmith WA (2010) New strategies in colorectal cancer: biomarkers of response to epidermal growth factor receptor monoclonal antibodies and potential therapeutic targets in phosphoinositide 3-kinase and mitogen-activated protein kinase pathways. Clin Cancer Res 16:3811–3818

Datta SR, Dudek H, Tao X, Masters S, Fu H, Gotoh Y, Greenberg ME (1997) Akt phosphorylation of BAD couples survival signals to the cell-intrinsic death machinery. Cell 91:231–241
Datta SR, Brunet A, Greenberg ME (1999) Cellular survival: a play in three Akts. Genes Dev 13:2905–2927
Davies MA, Lu Y, Sano T, Fang X, Tang P, LaPushin R, Koul D, Bookstein R, Stokoe D, Yung WK, Mills GB, Steck PA (1998) Adenoviral transgene expression of MMAC/PTEN in human glioma cells inhibits Akt activation and induces anoikis. Cancer Res 58:5285–5290
Decock J, Thirkettle S, Wagstaff L, Edwards DR (2011) Matrix metalloproteinases: protective roles in cancer. J Cell Mol Med 15:1254–1265
Deeb D, Xu YX, Jiang H, Gao X, Janakiraman N, Chapman RA, Gautam SC (2003) Curcumin (diferuloyl-methane) enhances tumor necrosis factor-related apoptosis-inducing ligand-induced apoptosis in LNCaP prostate cancer cells. Mol Cancer Ther 2:95–103
Deeb DD, Jiang H, Gao X, Divine G, Dulchavsky SA, Gautam SC (2005) Chemosensitization of hormone-refractory prostate cancer cells by curcumin to TRAIL-induced apoptosis. J Exp Ther Oncol 5:81–91
DeGregori J, Leone G, Miron A, Jakoi L, Nevins JR (1997) Distinct roles for E2F proteins in cell growth control and apoptosis. Proc Natl Acad Sci U S A 94:7245–7250
Deryugina EI, Quigley JP (2010) Pleiotropic roles of matrix metalloproteinases in tumor angiogenesis: contrasting, overlapping and compensatory functions. Biochim Biophys Acta 1803:103–120
Dikic I, Schmidt MH (2010) Notch: implications of endogenous inhibitors for therapy. Bioessays 32:481–487
Dikshit M, Rastogi L, Shukla R, Srimal RC (1995) Prevention of ischaemia-induced biochemical changes by curcumin & quinidine in the cat heart. Indian J Med Res 101:31–35
Dikshit P, Goswami A, Mishra A, Chatterjee M, Jana NR (2006) Curcumin induces stress response, neurite outgrowth and prevent NF-kappaB activation by inhibiting the proteasome function. Neurotox Res 9:29–37
Divya CS, Pillai MR (2006) Antitumor action of curcumin in human papillomavirus associated cells involves downregulation of viral oncogenes, prevention of NFkB and AP-1 translocation, and modulation of apoptosis. Mol Carcinog 45:320–332
Dodge ME, Lum L (2011) Drugging the cancer stem cell compartment: lessons learned from the hedgehog and Wnt signal transduction pathways. Annu Rev Pharmacol Toxicol 51:289–310
Dorai T, Gehani N, Katz A (2000) Therapeutic potential of curcumin in human prostate cancer. II. Curcumin inhibits tyrosine kinase activity of epidermal growth factor receptor and depletes the protein. Mol Urol 4:1–6
Downward J (2004) PI 3-kinase, Akt and cell survival. Semin Cell Dev Biol 15:177–182
Dreesen O, Brivanlou AH (2007) Signaling pathways in cancer and embryonic stem cells. Stem Cell Rev 3:7–17
D'Souza B, Miyamoto A, Weinmaster G (2008) The many facets of Notch ligands. Oncogene 27:5148–5167
Du C, Fang M, Li Y, Li L, Wang X (2000) Smac, a mitochondrial protein that promotes cytochrome c-dependent caspase activation by eliminating IAP inhibition. Cell 102:33–42
Du B, Jiang L, Xia Q, Zhong L (2006) Synergistic inhibitory effects of curcumin and 5-fluorouracil on the growth of the human colon cancer cell line HT 29. Chemotherapy 52:23 28
Dyson N (1998) The regulation of E2F by pRB-family proteins. Genes Dev 12:2245–2262
Easton J, Wei T, Lahti JM, Kidd VJ (1998) Disruption of the cyclin D/cyclin-dependent kinase/INK4/retinoblastoma protein regulatory pathway in human neuroblastoma. Cancer Res 58:2624–2632
Elamin MH, Shinwari Z, Hendrayani SF, Al-Hindi H, Al-Shail E, Khafaga Y, Al-Kofide A, Aboussekhra A (2010) Curcumin inhibits the Sonic Hedgehog signaling pathway and triggers apoptosis in medulloblastoma cells. Mol Carcinog 49:302–314
el-Deiry WS, Tokino T, Velculescu VE, Levy DB, Parsons R, Trent JM, Lin D, Mercer WE, Kinzler KW, Vogelstein B (1993) WAF1, a potential mediator of p53 tumor suppression. Cell 75: 817–825

Evans T, Rosenthal ET, Youngblom J, Distel D, Hunt T (1983) Cyclin: a protein specified by maternal mRNA in sea urchin eggs that is destroyed at each cleavage division. Cell 33: 389–396
Farnie G, Clarke RB (2007) Mammary stem cells and breast cancer–role of Notch signalling. Stem Cell Rev 3:169–175
Fero ML, Randel E, Gurley KE, Roberts JM, Kemp CJ (1998) The murine gene p27Kip1 is haplo-insufficient for tumour suppression. Nature 396:177–180
Ferrari-Toninelli G, Bonini SA, Uberti D, Buizza L, Bettinsoli P, Poliani PL, Facchetti F, Memo M (2010) Targeting Notch pathway induces growth inhibition and differentiation of neuroblastoma cells. Neuro Oncol 12:1231–1243
Ferres-Marco D, Gutierrez-Garcia I, Vallejo DM, Bolivar J, Gutierrez-Avino FJ, Dominguez M (2006) Epigenetic silencers and Notch collaborate to promote malignant tumours by Rb silencing. Nature 439:430–436
Folkman J (2003) Fundamental concepts of the angiogenic process. Curr Mol Med 3:643–651
Frautschy SA, Cole GM (2010) Why pleiotropic interventions are needed for Alzheimer's disease. Mol Neurobiol 41:392–409
Garg AK, Buchholz TA, Aggarwal BB (2005) Chemosensitization and radiosensitization of tumors by plant polyphenols. Antioxid Redox Signal 7:1630–1647
Girard F, Strausfeld U, Fernandez A, Lamb NJ (1991) Cyclin A is required for the onset of DNA replication in mammalian fibroblasts. Cell 67:1169–1179
Giri RK, Rajagopal V, Kalra VK (2004) Curcumin, the active constituent of turmeric, inhibits amyloid peptide-induced cytochemokine gene expression and CCR5-mediated chemotaxis of THP-1 monocytes by modulating early growth response-1 transcription factor. J Neurochem 91:1199–1210
Glienke W, Maute L, Wicht J, Bergmann L (2010) Curcumin inhibits constitutive STAT3 phosphorylation in human pancreatic cancer cell lines and downregulation of survivin/BIRC5 gene expression. Cancer Invest 28:166–171
Glotzer M, Murray AW, Kirschner MW (1991) Cyclin is degraded by the ubiquitin pathway. Nature 349:132–138
Goel A, Aggarwal BB (2010) Curcumin, the golden spice from Indian saffron, is a chemosensitizer and radiosensitizer for tumors and chemoprotector and radioprotector for normal organs. Nutr Cancer 62:919–930
Gong J, Ardelt B, Traganos F, Darzynkiewicz Z (1994) Unscheduled expression of cyclin B1 and cyclin E in several leukemic and solid tumor cell lines. Cancer Res 54:4285–4288
Gopinath D, Ahmed MR, Gomathi K, Chitra K, Sehgal PK, Jayakumar R (2004) Dermal wound healing processes with curcumin incorporated collagen films. Biomaterials 25:1911–1917
Grimmler M, Wang Y, Mund T, Cilensek Z, Keidel EM, Waddell MB, Jakel H, Kullmann M, Kriwacki RW, Hengst L (2007) Cdk-inhibitory activity and stability of p27Kip1 are directly regulated by oncogenic tyrosine kinases. Cell 128:269–280
Guo S, Liu M, Gonzalez-Perez RR (2011) Role of Notch and its oncogenic signaling crosstalk in breast cancer. Biochim Biophys Acta 1815:197–213
Haas K, Johannes C, Geisen C, Schmidt T, Karsunky H, Blass-Kampmann S, Obe G, Moroy T (1997) Malignant transformation by cyclin E and Ha-Ras correlates with lower sensitivity towards induction of cell death but requires functional Myc and CDK4. Oncogene 15: 2615–2623
Haase MG, Klawitter A, Bierhaus A, Yokoyama KK, Kasper M, Geyer P, Baumann M, Baretton GB (2008) Inactivation of AP1 proteins by a nuclear serine protease precedes the onset of radiation-induced fibrosing alveolitis. Radiat Res 169:531–542
Hahn WC, Weinberg RA (2002) Modelling the molecular circuitry of cancer. Nat Rev Cancer 2:331–341
Hall M, Peters G (1996) Genetic alterations of cyclins, cyclin-dependent kinases, and Cdk inhibitors in human cancer. Adv Cancer Res 68:67–108
Hanahan D, Weinberg RA (2000) The hallmarks of cancer. Cell 100:57–70

Harper JW, Elledge SJ, Keyomarsi K, Dynlacht B, Tsai LH, Zhang P, Dobrowolski S, Bai C, Connell-Crowley L, Swindell E et al (1995) Inhibition of cyclin-dependent kinases by p21. Mol Biol Cell 6:387–400

Harrison H, Farnie G, Brennan KR, Clarke RB (2010) Breast cancer stem cells: something out of notching? Cancer Res 70:8973–8976

Hazan-Halevy I, Harris D, Liu Z, Liu J, Li P, Chen X, Shanker S, Ferrajoli A, Keating MJ, Estrov Z (2010) STAT3 is constitutively phosphorylated on serine 727 residues, binds DNA, and activates transcription in CLL cells. Blood 115:2852–2863

He TC, Sparks AB, Rago C, Hermeking H, Zawel L, da Costa LT, Morin PJ, Vogelstein B, Kinzler KW (1998) Identification of c-MYC as a target of the APC pathway. Science 281:1509–1512

HemaIswarya S, Doble M (2006) Potential synergism of natural products in the treatment of cancer. Phytother Res 20:239–249

Hengst L, Reed SI (1996) Translational control of p27Kip1 accumulation during the cell cycle. Science 271:1861–1864

Hengst L, Reed SI (1998) Inhibitors of the Cip/Kip family. Curr Top Microbiol Immunol 227: 25–41

Hershko DD, Shapira M (2006) Prognostic role of p27Kip1 deregulation in colorectal cancer. Cancer 107:668–675

Howells LM, Sale S, Sriramareddy SN, Irving GR, Jones DJ, Ottley CJ, Pearson DG, Mann CD, Manson MM, Berry DP, Gescher A, Steward WP, Brown K (2010) Curcumin ameliorates oxaliplatin-induced chemoresistance in HCT116 colorectal cancer cells in vitro and in vivo. Int J Cancer 129(2):476–486

Hsieh A, Ellsworth R, Hsieh D (2011) Hedgehog/GLI1 regulates IGF dependent malignant behaviors in glioma stem cells. J Cell Physiol 226:1118–1127

Hua H, Li M, Luo T, Yin Y, Jiang Y (2011) Matrix metalloproteinases in tumorigenesis: an evolving paradigm. Cell Mol Life Sci 68(23):3853–3868

Huang TS, Lee SC, Lin JK (1991) Suppression of c-Jun/AP-1 activation by an inhibitor of tumor promotion in mouse fibroblast cells. Proc Natl Acad Sci U S A 88:5292–5296

Huang P, Han J, Hui L (2010) MAPK signaling in inflammation-associated cancer development. Protein Cell 1:218–226

Hunter T, Pines J (1994) Cyclins and cancer. II: cyclin D and CDK inhibitors come of age. Cell 79:573–582

Iida H, Towatari M, Tanimoto M, Morishita Y, Kodera Y, Saito H (1997) Overexpression of cyclin E in acute myelogenous leukemia. Blood 90:3707–3713

Jaiswal AS, Marlow BP, Gupta N, Narayan S (2002) Beta-catenin-mediated transactivation and cell-cell adhesion pathways are important in curcumin (diferuylmethane)-induced growth arrest and apoptosis in colon cancer cells. Oncogene 21:8414–8427

Jang MS, Miao H, Carlesso N, Shelly L, Zlobin A, Darack N, Qin JZ, Nickoloff BJ, Miele L (2004) Notch-1 regulates cell death independently of differentiation in murine erythroleukemia cells through multiple apoptosis and cell cycle pathways. J Cell Physiol 199:418–433

Jeffrey PD, Russo AA, Polyak K, Gibbs E, Hurwitz J, Massague J, Pavletich NP (1995) Mechanism of CDK activation revealed by the structure of a cyclinA-CDK2 complex. Nature 376:313–320

Jones EA, Shoskes DA (2000) The effect of mycophenolate mofetil and polyphenolic bioflavonoids on renal ischemia reperfusion injury and repair. J Urol 163:999–1004

Jones EA, Shahed A, Shoskes DA (2000) Modulation of apoptotic and inflammatory genes by bioflavonoids and angiotensin II inhibition in ureteral obstruction. Urology 56:346–351

Jung EM, Park JW, Choi KS, Park JW, Lee HI, Lee KS, Kwon TK (2006) Curcumin sensitizes tumor necrosis factor-related apoptosis-inducing ligand (TRAIL)-mediated apoptosis through CHOP-independent DR5 upregulation. Carcinogenesis 27(10):2008–2017

Kakarala M, Wicha MS (2008) Implications of the cancer stem-cell hypothesis for breast cancer prevention and therapy. J Clin Oncol 26:2813–2820

Kakarala M, Brenner DE, Korkaya H, Cheng C, Tazi K, Ginestier C, Liu S, Dontu G, Wicha MS (2010) Targeting breast stem cells with the cancer preventive compounds curcumin and piperine. Breast Cancer Res Treat 122:777–785

Kaldis P (2007) Another piece of the p27Kip1 puzzle. Cell 128:241–244

Kamat AM, Sethi G, Aggarwal BB (2007) Curcumin potentiates the apoptotic effects of chemotherapeutic agents and cytokines through down-regulation of nuclear factor-kappaB and nuclear factor-kappaB-regulated gene products in IFN-alpha-sensitive and IFN-alpha-resistant human bladder cancer cells. Mol Cancer Ther 6:1022–1030

Kandasamy K, Srivastava RK (2002) Role of the phosphatidylinositol 3′-kinase/PTEN/Akt kinase pathway in tumor necrosis factor-related apoptosis-inducing ligand-induced apoptosis in non-small cell lung cancer cells. Cancer Res 62:4929–4937

Kandasamy K, Srinivasula SM, Alnemri ES, Thompson CB, Korsmeyer SJ, Bryant JL, Srivastava RK (2003) Involvement of proapoptotic molecules Bax and Bak in tumor necrosis factor-related apoptosis-inducing ligand (TRAIL)-induced mitochondrial disruption and apoptosis: differential regulation of cytochrome c and Smac/DIABLO release. Cancer Res 63:1712–1721

Kanwar SS, Yu Y, Nautiyal J, Patel BB, Padhye S, Sarkar FH, Majumdar AP (2011) Difluorinated-curcumin (CDF): a novel curcumin analog is a potent inhibitor of colon cancer stem-like cells. Pharm Res 28:827–838

Kardinal C, Dangers M, Kardinal A, Koch A, Brandt DT, Tamura T, Welte K (2006) Tyrosine phosphorylation modulates binding preference to cyclin-dependent kinases and subcellular localization of p27Kip1 in the acute promyelocytic leukemia cell line NB4. Blood 107: 1133–1140

Karin M (2006a) NF-kappaB and cancer: mechanisms and targets. Mol Carcinog 45:355–361

Karin M (2006b) Nuclear factor-kappaB in cancer development and progression. Nature 441: 431–436

Kasperczyk H, Baumann B, Debatin KM, Fulda S (2009) Characterization of sonic hedgehog as a novel NF-kappaB target gene that promotes NF-kappaB-mediated apoptosis resistance and tumor growth in vivo. FASEB J 23:21–33

Katoh Y, Katoh M (2009) Hedgehog target genes: mechanisms of carcinogenesis induced by aberrant hedgehog signaling activation. Curr Mol Med 9:873–886

Katz M, Amit I, Yarden Y (2007) Regulation of MAPKs by growth factors and receptor tyrosine kinases. Biochim Biophys Acta 1773:1161–1176

Kelleher FC (2011) Hedgehog signaling and therapeutics in pancreatic cancer. Carcinogenesis 32:445–451

Keshet Y, Seger R (2010) The MAP kinase signaling cascades: a system of hundreds of components regulates a diverse array of physiological functions. Methods Mol Biol 661:3–38

Kettunen E, Nissen AM, Ollikainen T, Taavitsainen M, Tapper J, Mattson K, Linnainmaa K, Knuutila S, El-Rifai W (2001) Gene expression profiling of malignant mesothelioma cell lines: cDNA array study. Int J Cancer 91:492–496

Keyomarsi K, Conte D Jr, Toyofuku W, Fox MP (1995) Deregulation of cyclin E in breast cancer. Oncogene 11:941–950

Keyomarsi K, Tucker SL, Buchholz TA, Callister M, Ding Y, Hortobagyi GN, Bedrosian I, Knickerbocker C, Toyofuku W, Lowe M, Herliczek TW, Bacus SS (2002) Cyclin E and survival in patients with breast cancer. N Engl J Med 347:1566–1575

Khor TO, Keum YS, Lin W, Kim JH, Hu R, Shen G, Xu C, Gopalakrishnan A, Reddy B, Zheng X, Conney AH, Kong AN (2006) Combined inhibitory effects of curcumin and phenethyl isothiocyanate on the growth of human PC-3 prostate xenografts in immunodeficient mice. Cancer Res 66:613–621

Khwaja A (1999) Akt is more than just a Bad kinase. Nature 401:33–34

Kim JH, Kang MJ, Park CU, Kwak HJ, Hwang Y, Koh GY (1999) Amplified CDK2 and cdc2 activities in primary colorectal carcinoma. Cancer 85:546–553

Kim H, Park BS, Lee KG, Choi CY, Jang SS, Kim YH, Lee SE (2005) Effects of naturally occurring compounds on fibril formation and oxidative stress of beta-amyloid. J Agric Food Chem 53:8537–8541

Kim JH, Xu C, Keum YS, Reddy B, Conney A, Kong AN (2006) Inhibition of EGFR signaling in human prostate cancer PC-3 cells by combination treatment with beta-phenylethyl isothiocyanate and curcumin. Carcinogenesis 27:475–482

Kitagawa M, Higashi H, Jung HK, Suzuki-Takahashi I, Ikeda M, Tamai K, Kato J, Segawa K, Yoshida E, Nishimura S, Taya Y (1996) The consensus motif for phosphorylation by cyclin D1-Cdk4 is different from that for phosphorylation by cyclin A/E-Cdk2. EMBO J 15: 7060–7069

Kitahara K, Yasui W, Kuniyasu H, Yokozaki H, Akama Y, Yunotani S, Hisatsugu T, Tahara E (1995) Concurrent amplification of cyclin E and CDK2 genes in colorectal carcinomas. Int J Cancer 62:25–28

Klarmann GJ, Hurt EM, Mathews LA, Zhang X, Duhagon MA, Mistree T, Thomas SB, Farrar WL (2009) Invasive prostate cancer cells are tumor initiating cells that have a stem cell-like genomic signature. Clin Exp Metastasis 26:433–446

Knudsen KE, Booth D, Naderi S, Sever-Chroneos Z, Fribourg AF, Hunton IC, Feramisco JR, Wang JY, Knudsen ES (2000) RB-dependent S-phase response to DNA damage. Mol Cell Biol 20:7751–7763

Koff A (2006) How to decrease p27Kip1 levels during tumor development. Cancer Cell 9:75–76

Kopan R, Ilagan MX (2009) The canonical Notch signaling pathway: unfolding the activation mechanism. Cell 137:216–233

Korkaya H, Paulson A, Charafe-Jauffret E, Ginestier C, Brown M, Dutcher J, Clouthier SG, Wicha MS (2009) Regulation of mammary stem/progenitor cells by PTEN/Akt/beta-catenin signaling. PLoS Biol 7:e1000121

Korutla L, Kumar R (1994) Inhibitory effect of curcumin on epidermal growth factor receptor kinase activity in A431 cells. Biochim Biophys Acta 1224:597–600

Korutla L, Cheung JY, Mendelsohn J, Kumar R (1995) Inhibition of ligand-induced activation of epidermal growth factor receptor tyrosine phosphorylation by curcumin. Carcinogenesis 16:1741–1745

Kunnumakkara AB, Guha S, Krishnan S, Diagaradjane P, Gelovani J, Aggarwal BB (2007) Curcumin potentiates antitumor activity of gemcitabine in an orthotopic model of pancreatic cancer through suppression of proliferation, angiogenesis, and inhibition of nuclear factor-kappaB-regulated gene products. Cancer Res 67:3853–3861

Kunnumakkara AB, Anand P, Aggarwal BB (2008) Curcumin inhibits proliferation, invasion, angiogenesis and metastasis of different cancers through interaction with multiple cell signaling proteins. Cancer Lett 269:199–225

Kuwana T, Newmeyer DD (2003) Bcl-2-family proteins and the role of mitochondria in apoptosis. Curr Opin Cell Biol 15:691–699

Lawlor MA, Alessi DR (2001) PKB/Akt: a key mediator of cell proliferation, survival and insulin responses? J Cell Sci 114:2903–2910

Leach FS, Elledge SJ, Sherr CJ, Willson JK, Markowitz S, Kinzler KW, Vogelstein B (1993) Amplification of cyclin genes in colorectal carcinomas. Cancer Res 53:1986–1989

Lee JY, Lee YM, Chang GC, Yu SL, Hsieh WY, Chen JJ, Chen HW, Yang PC (2011) Curcumin induces EGFR degradation in lung adenocarcinoma and modulates p38 activation in intestine: the versatile adjuvant for gefitinib therapy. PLoS One 6:e23756

Lees E (1995) Cyclin dependent kinase regulation. Curr Opin Cell Biol 7:773–780

Lei H, Furlong PJ, Ra JH, Mullins D, Cantor R, Fraker DL, Spitz FR (2005) AKT activation and response to interferon-beta in human cancer cells. Cancer Biol Ther 4:709–715

Lentzsch S, Chatterjee M, Gries M, Bommert K, Gollasch H, Dorken B, Bargou RC (2004) PI3-K/AKT/FKHR and MAPK signaling cascades are redundantly stimulated by a variety of cytokines and contribute independently to proliferation and survival of multiple myeloma cells. Leukemia 18:1883–1890

Lev-Ari S, Starr A, Vexler A, Karaush V, Loew V, Greif J, Fenig E, Aderka D, Ben-Yosef R (2006) Inhibition of pancreatic and lung adenocarcinoma cell survival by curcumin is associated with increased apoptosis, down-regulation of COX-2 and EGFR and inhibition of Erk1/2 activity. Anticancer Res 26:4423–4430

Lew DJ, Kornbluth S (1996) Regulatory roles of cyclin dependent kinase phosphorylation in cell cycle control. Curr Opin Cell Biol 8:795–804

Li J, Yen C, Liaw D, Podsypanina K, Bose S, Wang SI, Puc J, Miliaresis C, Rodgers L, McCombie R, Bigner SH, Giovanella BC, Ittmann M, Tycko B, Hibshoosh H, Wigler MH, Parsons R (1997) PTEN, a putative protein tyrosine phosphatase gene mutated in human brain, breast, and prostate cancer. Science 275:1943–1947

Li M, Zhang Z, Hill DL, Wang H, Zhang R (2007) Curcumin, a dietary component, has anticancer, chemosensitization, and radiosensitization effects by down-regulating the MDM2 oncogene through the PI3K/mTOR/ETS2 pathway. Cancer Res 67:1988–1996

Li T, Wang W, Chen H, Ye L (2010) Evaluation of anti-leukemia effect of resveratrol by modulating STAT3 signaling. Int Immunopharmacol 10:18–25

Li Y, Wicha MS, Schwartz SJ, Sun D (2011) Implications of cancer stem cell theory for cancer chemoprevention by natural dietary compounds. J Nutr Biochem 22(9):799–806

Lim GP, Chu T, Yang F, Beech W, Frautschy SA, Cole GM (2001) The curry spice curcumin reduces oxidative damage and amyloid pathology in an Alzheimer transgenic mouse. J Neurosci 21:8370–8377

Lin J, Chen A (2011) Curcumin diminishes the impacts of hyperglycemia on the activation of hepatic stellate cells by suppressing membrane translocation and gene expression of glucose transporter-2. Mol Cell Endocrinol 333:160–171

Lin SY, Xia W, Wang JC, Kwong KY, Spohn B, Wen Y, Pestell RG, Hung MC (2000) Beta-catenin, a novel prognostic marker for breast cancer: its roles in cyclin D1 expression and cancer progression. Proc Natl Acad Sci U S A 97:4262–4266

Lin SK, Kok SH, Yeh FT, Kuo MY, Lin CC, Wang CC, Goldring SR, Hong CY (2004) MEK/ERK and signal transducer and activator of transcription signaling pathways modulate oncostatin M-stimulated CCL2 expression in human osteoblasts through a common transcription factor. Arthritis Rheum 50:785–793

Lin YG, Kunnumakkara AB, Nair A, Merritt WM, Han LY, Armaiz-Pena GN, Kamat AA, Spannuth WA, Gershenson DM, Lutgendorf SK, Aggarwal BB, Sood AK (2007) Curcumin inhibits tumor growth and angiogenesis in ovarian carcinoma by targeting the nuclear factor-kappaB pathway. Clin Cancer Res 13:3423–3430

Lin L, Deangelis S, Foust E, Fuchs J, Li C, Li PK, Schwartz EB, Lesinski GB, Benson D, Lu J, Hoyt D, Lin J (2010a) A novel small molecule inhibits STAT3 phosphorylation and DNA binding activity and exhibits potent growth suppressive activity in human cancer cells. Mol Cancer 9:217

Lin L, Hutzen B, Zuo M, Ball S, Deangelis S, Foust E, Pandit B, Ihnat MA, Shenoy SS, Kulp S, Li PK, Li C, Fuchs J, Lin J (2010b) Novel STAT3 phosphorylation inhibitors exhibit potent growth-suppressive activity in pancreatic and breast cancer cells. Cancer Res 70:2445–2454

Lindner V, Booth C, Prudovsky I, Small D, Maciag T, Liaw L (2001) Members of the Jagged/Notch gene families are expressed in injured arteries and regulate cell phenotype via alterations in cell matrix and cell-cell interaction. Am J Pathol 159:875–883

Lindsten T, Ross AJ, King A, Zong WX, Rathmell JC, Shiels HA, Ulrich E, Waymire KG, Mahar P, Frauwirth K, Chen Y, Wei M, Eng VM, Adelman DM, Simon MC, Ma A, Golden JA, Evan G, Korsmeyer SJ, MacGregor GR, Thompson CB (2000) The combined functions of proapoptotic Bcl-2 family members Bak and Bax are essential for normal development of multiple tissues. Mol Cell 6:1389–1399

Ling H, Sylvestre JR, Jolicoeur P (2010) Notch1-induced mammary tumor development is cyclin D1-dependent and correlates with expansion of pre-malignant multipotent duct-limited progenitors. Oncogene 29:4543–4554

Liu ZG, Hsu H, Goeddel DV, Karin M (1996) Dissection of TNF receptor 1 effector functions: JNK activation is not linked to apoptosis while NF-kappaB activation prevents cell death. Cell 87:565–576

Liu C, Li Y, Semenov M, Han C, Baeg GH, Tan Y, Zhang Z, Lin X, He X (2002) Control of beta-catenin phosphorylation/degradation by a dual-kinase mechanism. Cell 108:837–847

Liu S, Dontu G, Wicha MS (2005) Mammary stem cells, self-renewal pathways, and carcinogenesis. Breast Cancer Res 7:86–95

Liu S, Dontu G, Mantle ID, Patel S, Ahn NS, Jackson KW, Suri P, Wicha MS (2006) Hedgehog signaling and Bmi-1 regulate self-renewal of normal and malignant human mammary stem cells. Cancer Res 66:6063–6071

Liu S, Ma Z, Cai H, Li Q, Rong W, Kawano M (2010) Inhibitory effect of baicalein on IL-6-mediated signaling cascades in human myeloma cells. Eur J Haematol 84:137–144

Lo HW (2010) EGFR-targeted therapy in malignant glioma: novel aspects and mechanisms of drug resistance. Curr Mol Pharmacol 3:37–52

Loda M, Cukor B, Tam SW, Lavin P, Fiorentino M, Draetta GF, Jessup JM, Pagano M (1997) Increased proteasome-dependent degradation of the cyclin-dependent kinase inhibitor p27 in aggressive colorectal carcinomas. Nat Med 3:231–234

Lopez-Otin C, Matrisian LM (2007) Emerging roles of proteases in tumour suppression. Nat Rev Cancer 7:800–808

Lu CD, Morita S, Ishibashi T, Hara H, Isozaki H, Tanigawa N (1999) Loss of p27Kip1 expression independently predicts poor prognosis for patients with resectable pancreatic adenocarcinoma. Cancer 85:1250–1260

Ludlow JW, Glendening CL, Livingston DM, DeCarprio JA (1993) Specific enzymatic dephosphorylation of the retinoblastoma protein. Mol Cell Biol 13:367–372

Luo J, Manning BD, Cantley LC (2003) Targeting the PI3K-Akt pathway in human cancer: rationale and promise. Cancer Cell 4:257–262

Lynch CC (2011) Matrix metalloproteinases as master regulators of the vicious cycle of bone metastasis. Bone 48:44–53

MacFarlane M, Merrison W, Bratton SB, Cohen GM (2002) Proteasome-mediated degradation of Smac during apoptosis: XIAP promotes Smac ubiquitination in vitro. J Biol Chem 277: 36611–36616

Madoux F, Koenig M, Sessions H, Nelson E, Mercer BA, Cameron M, Roush W, Frank D, Hodder P (2010) Modulators of STAT transcription factors for the targeted therapy of cancer (STAT3 inhibitors). Probe Reports from the NIH Molecular Libraries Program [Internet]. Bethesda (MD): National Center for Biotechnology Information (US)

Maehama T, Dixon JE (1999) PTEN: a tumour suppressor that functions as a phospholipid phosphatase. Trends Cell Biol 9:125–128

Maheshwari RK, Singh AK, Gaddipati J, Srimal RC (2006) Multiple biological activities of curcumin: a short review. Life Sci 78:2081–2087

Mani H, Sidhu GS, Kumari R, Gaddipati JP, Seth P, Maheshwari RK (2002) Curcumin differentially regulates TGF-beta1, its receptors and nitric oxide synthase during impaired wound healing. Biofactors 16:29–43

Mann B, Gelos M, Siedow A, Hanski ML, Gratchev A, Ilyas M, Bodmer WF, Moyer MP, Riecken EO, Buhr HJ, Hanski C (1999) Target genes of beta-catenin-T cell-factor/lymphoid-enhancer-factor signaling in human colorectal carcinomas. Proc Natl Acad Sci U S A 96:1603–1608

Manoharan S, Balakrishnan S, Menon VP, Alias LM, Reena AR (2009) Chemopreventive efficacy of curcumin and piperine during 7,12-dimethylbenz[a]anthracene-induced hamster buccal pouch carcinogenesis. Singapore Med J 50:139–146

Martinez AM, Cavalli G (2010) Uncovering a tumor-suppressor function for Drosophila polycomb group genes. Cell Cycle 9:215–216

Martinez AM, Schuettengruber B, Sakr S, Janic A, Gonzalez C, Cavalli G (2009) Polyhomeotic has a tumor suppressor activity mediated by repression of Notch signaling. Nat Genet 41: 1076–1082

Mazumdar J, Dondeti V, Simon MC (2009) Hypoxia-inducible factors in stem cells and cancer. J Cell Mol Med 13:4319–4328

McDonald ER 3rd, El-Deiry WS (2000) Cell cycle control as a basis for cancer drug development (review). Int J Oncol 16:871–886

Merchant AA, Matsui W (2010) Targeting Hedgehog–a cancer stem cell pathway. Clin Cancer Res 16:3130–3140

Michl P, Downward J (2005) Mechanisms of disease: PI3K/AKT signaling in gastrointestinal cancers. Z Gastroenterol 43:1133–1139

Miele L (2006) Notch signaling. Clin Cancer Res 12:1074–1079

Miele L, Golde T, Osborne B (2006) Notch signaling in cancer. Curr Mol Med 6:905–918

Migita T, Oda Y, Naito S, Tsuneyoshi M (2002) Low expression of p27(Kip1) is associated with tumor size and poor prognosis in patients with renal cell carcinoma. Cancer 94:973–979

Mihara M, Erster S, Zaika A, Petrenko O, Chittenden T, Pancoska P, Moll UM (2003) p53 has a direct apoptogenic role at the mitochondria. Mol Cell 11:577–590

Millard SS, Yan JS, Nguyen H, Pagano M, Kiyokawa H, Koff A (1997) Enhanced ribosomal association of p27(Kip1) mRNA is a mechanism contributing to accumulation during growth arrest. J Biol Chem 272:7093–7098

Mimeault M, Batra SK (2011) Potential applications of curcumin and its novel synthetic analogs and nanotechnology-based formulations in cancer prevention and therapy. Chin Med 6:31

Min L, He B, Hui L (2011) Mitogen-activated protein kinases in hepatocellular carcinoma development. Semin Cancer Biol 21:10–20

Mineta H, Miura K, Suzuki I, Takebayashi S, Misawa K, Ueda Y, Ichimura K (1999) p27 expression correlates with prognosis in patients with hypopharyngeal cancer. Anticancer Res 19:4407–4412

Morgan DO (1995) Principles of CDK regulation. Nature 374:131–134

Motokura T, Bloom T, Kim HG, Juppner H, Ruderman JV, Kronenberg HM, Arnold A (1991) A novel cyclin encoded by a bcl1-linked candidate oncogene. Nature 350:512–515

Muller-Tidow C, Metzger R, Kugler K, Diederichs S, Idos G, Thomas M, Dockhorn-Dworniczak B, Schneider PM, Koeffler HP, Berdel WE, Serve H (2001) Cyclin E is the only cyclin-dependent kinase 2-associated cyclin that predicts metastasis and survival in early stage non-small cell lung cancer. Cancer Res 61:647–653

Myers MP, Pass I, Batty IH, Van der Kaay J, Stolarov JP, Hemmings BA, Wigler MH, Downes CP, Tonks NK (1998) The lipid phosphatase activity of PTEN is critical for its tumor suppressor function. Proc Natl Acad Sci U S A 95:13513–13518

Nakashima H, Nakamura M, Yamaguchi H, Yamanaka N, Akiyoshi T, Koga K, Yamaguchi K, Tsuneyoshi M, Tanaka M, Katano M (2006) Nuclear factor-kappaB contributes to Hedgehog signaling pathway activation through sonic hedgehog induction in pancreatic cancer. Cancer Res 66:7041–7049

Natsume A, Kinjo S, Yuki K, Kato T, Ohno M, Motomura K, Iwami K, Wakabayashi T (2011) Glioma-initiating cells and molecular pathology: implications for therapy. Brain Tumor Pathol 28:1–12

Nelson WJ, Nusse R (2004) Convergence of Wnt, beta-catenin, and cadherin pathways. Science 303:1483–1487

Nevins JR, Leone G, DeGregori J, Jakoi L (1997) Role of the Rb/E2F pathway in cell growth control. J Cell Physiol 173:233–236

Nickoloff BJ, Qin JZ, Chaturvedi V, Denning MF, Bonish B, Miele L (2002) Jagged-1 mediated activation of notch signaling induces complete maturation of human keratinocytes through NF-kappaB and PPARgamma. Cell Death Differ 9:842–855

Nirmala C, Puvanakrishnan R (1996a) Effect of curcumin on certain lysosomal hydrolases in isoproterenol-induced myocardial infarction in rats. Biochem Pharmacol 51:47–51

Nirmala C, Puvanakrishnan R (1996b) Protective role of curcumin against isoproterenol induced myocardial infarction in rats. Mol Cell Biochem 159:85–93

Noseda M, McLean G, Niessen K, Chang L, Pollet I, Montpetit R, Shahidi R, Dorovini-Zis K, Li L, Beckstead B, Durand RE, Hoodless PA, Karsan A (2004) Notch activation results in phenotypic and functional changes consistent with endothelial-to-mesenchymal transformation. Circ Res 94:910–917

Nowak MA, Komarova NL, Sengupta A, Jallepalli PV, Shih Ie M, Vogelstein B, Lengauer C (2002) The role of chromosomal instability in tumor initiation. Proc Natl Acad Sci U S A 99: 16226–16231

Oakes SA, Scorrano L, Opferman JT, Bassik MC, Nishino M, Pozzan T, Korsmeyer SJ (2005) Proapoptotic BAX and BAK regulate the type 1 inositol trisphosphate receptor and calcium leak from the endoplasmic reticulum. Proc Natl Acad Sci U S A 102:105–110

Ohtsubo M, Theodoras AM, Schumacher J, Roberts JM, Pagano M (1995) Human cyclin E, a nuclear protein essential for the G1-to-S phase transition. Mol Cell Biol 15:2612–2624

Okuhashi Y, Nara N, Tohda S (2010) Effects of gamma-secretase inhibitors on the growth of leukemia cells. Anticancer Res 30:495–498

Okunieff P, Xu J, Hu D, Liu W, Zhang L, Morrow G, Pentland A, Ryan JL, Ding I (2006) Curcumin protects against radiation-induced acute and chronic cutaneous toxicity in mice and decreases mRNA expression of inflammatory and fibrogenic cytokines. Int J Radiat Oncol Biol Phys 65:890–898

Ophascharoensuk V, Fero ML, Hughes J, Roberts JM, Shankland SJ (1998) The cyclin-dependent kinase inhibitor p27Kip1 safeguards against inflammatory injury. Nat Med 4:575–580

Ortega S, Malumbres M, Barbacid M (2002) Cyclin D-dependent kinases, INK4 inhibitors and cancer. Biochim Biophys Acta 1602:73–87

Oswald F, Liptay S, Adler G, Schmid RM (1998) NF-kappaB2 is a putative target gene of activated Notch-1 via RBP-Jkappa. Mol Cell Biol 18:2077–2088

Palomero T, Sulis ML, Cortina M, Real PJ, Barnes K, Ciofani M, Caparros E, Buteau J, Brown K, Perkins SL, Bhagat G, Agarwal AM, Basso G, Castillo M, Nagase S, Cordon-Cardo C, Parsons R, Zuniga-Pflucker JC, Dominguez M, Ferrando AA (2007) Mutational loss of PTEN induces resistance to NOTCH1 inhibition in T-cell leukemia. Nat Med 13:1203–1210

Pandey MK, Sung B, Aggarwal BB (2010) Betulinic acid suppresses STAT3 activation pathway through induction of protein tyrosine phosphatase SHP-1 in human multiple myeloma cells. Int J Cancer 127:282–292

Pang RT, Leung CO, Ye TM, Liu W, Chiu PC, Lam KK, Lee KF, Yeung WS (2010) MicroRNA-34a suppresses invasion through downregulation of Notch1 and Jagged1 in cervical carcinoma and choriocarcinoma cells. Carcinogenesis 31:1037–1044

Pap M, Cooper GM (1998) Role of glycogen synthase kinase-3 in the phosphatidylinositol 3-Kinase/Akt cell survival pathway. J Biol Chem 273:19929–19932

Park CH, Hahm ER, Park S, Kim HK, Yang CH (2005) The inhibitory mechanism of curcumin and its derivative against beta-catenin/Tcf signaling. FEBS Lett 579:2965–2971

Parodi FE, Mao D, Ennis TL, Pagano MB, Thompson RW (2006) Oral administration of diferuloyl-methane (curcumin) suppresses proinflammatory cytokines and destructive connective tissue remodeling in experimental abdominal aortic aneurysms. Ann Vasc Surg 20:360–368

Pasca di Magliano M, Hebrok M (2003) Hedgehog signalling in cancer formation and maintenance. Nat Rev Cancer 3:903–911

Paulovich AG, Hartwell LH (1995) A checkpoint regulates the rate of progression through S phase in S. cerevisiae in response to DNA damage. Cell 82:841–847

Peant B, Diallo JS, Lessard L, Delvoye N, Le Page C, Saad F, Mes-Masson AM (2007) Regulation of IkappaB kinase epsilon expression by the androgen receptor and the nuclear factor-kappaB transcription factor in prostate cancer. Mol Cancer Res 5:87–94

Pece S, Confalonieri S, Romano PR, Di Fiore PP (2011) NUMB-ing down cancer by more than just a NOTCH. Biochim Biophys Acta 1815:26–43

Pines J (1995) Cyclins, CDKs and cancer. Semin Cancer Biol 6:63–72

Piper JT, Singhal SS, Salameh MS, Torman RT, Awasthi YC, Awasthi S (1998) Mechanisms of anticarcinogenic properties of curcumin: the effect of curcumin on glutathione linked detoxification enzymes in rat liver. Int J Biochem Cell Biol 30:445–456

Plummer SM, Holloway KA, Manson MM, Munks RJ, Kaptein A, Farrow S, Howells L (1999) Inhibition of cyclo-oxygenase 2 expression in colon cells by the chemopreventive agent curcumin involves inhibition of NF-kappaB activation via the NIK/IKK signalling complex. Oncogene 18:6013–6020

Plummer SM, Hill KA, Festing MF, Steward WP, Gescher AJ, Sharma RA (2001) Clinical development of leukocyte cyclooxygenase 2 activity as a systemic biomarker for cancer chemopreventive agents. Cancer Epidemiol Biomarkers Prev 10:1295–1299

Polakis P (2000) Wnt signaling and cancer. Genes Dev 14:1837–1851

Polytarchou C, Hatziapostolou M, Papadimitriou E (2005) Hydrogen peroxide stimulates proliferation and migration of human prostate cancer cells through activation of activator protein-1 and up-regulation of the heparin affin regulatory peptide gene. J Biol Chem 280:40428–40435

Ponce-Castaneda MV, Lee MH, Latres E, Polyak K, Lacombe L, Montgomery K, Mathew S, Krauter K, Sheinfeld J, Massague J et al (1995) p27Kip1: chromosomal mapping to 12p12-12p13.1 and absence of mutations in human tumors. Cancer Res 55:1211–1214

Porter PL, Malone KE, Heagerty PJ, Alexander GM, Gatti LA, Firpo EJ, Daling JR, Roberts JM (1997) Expression of cell-cycle regulators p27Kip1 and cyclin E, alone and in combination, correlate with survival in young breast cancer patients. Nat Med 3:222–225

Radtke F, Fasnacht N, Macdonald HR (2010) Notch signaling in the immune system. Immunity 32:14–27

Raffo D, Pontiggia O, Simian M (2011) Role of MMPs in metastatic dissemination: implications for therapeutic advances. Curr Pharm Biotechnol 1; 12(11):1937–1947

Rajasingh J, Raikwar HP, Muthian G, Johnson C, Bright JJ (2006) Curcumin induces growth-arrest and apoptosis in association with the inhibition of constitutively active JAK-STAT pathway in T cell leukemia. Biochem Biophys Res Commun 340:359–368

Ramakrishnan V, Kimlinger T, Haug J, Timm M, Wellik L, Halling T, Pardanani A, Tefferi A, Rajkumar SV, Kumar S (2010) TG101209, a novel JAK2 inhibitor, has significant in vitro activity in multiple myeloma and displays preferential cytotoxicity for CD45+ myeloma cells. Am J Hematol 85:675–686

Ramirez Bosca A, Soler A, Carrion-Gutierrez MA, Pamies Mira D, Pardo Zapata J, Diaz-Alperi J, Bernd A, Quintanilla Almagro E, Miquel J (2000) An hydroalcoholic extract of Curcuma longa lowers the abnormally high values of human-plasma fibrinogen. Mech Ageing Dev 114: 207–210

Reddy AC, Lokesh BR (1992) Studies on spice principles as antioxidants in the inhibition of lipid peroxidation of rat liver microsomes. Mol Cell Biochem 111:117–124

Reddy AC, Lokesh BR (1994) Effect of dietary turmeric (Curcuma longa) on iron-induced lipid peroxidation in the rat liver. Food Chem Toxicol 32:279–283

Rezende LF, Vieira AS, Negro A, Langone F, Boschero AC (2009) Ciliary neurotrophic factor (CNTF) signals through STAT3-SOCS3 pathway and protects rat pancreatic islets from cytokine-induced apoptosis. Cytokine 46:65–71

Ronchini C, Capobianco AJ (2001) Induction of cyclin D1 transcription and CDK2 activity by Notch(ic): implication for cell cycle disruption in transformation by Notch(ic). Mol Cell Biol 21:5925–5934

Rosen DG, Yang G, Deavers MT, Malpica A, Kavanagh JJ, Mills GB, Liu J (2006) Cyclin E expression is correlated with tumor progression and predicts a poor prognosis in patients with ovarian carcinoma. Cancer 106:1925–1932

Rushworth SA, Ogborne RM, Charalambos CA, O'Connell MA (2006) Role of protein kinase C delta in curcumin-induced antioxidant response element-mediated gene expression in human monocytes. Biochem Biophys Res Commun 341:1007–1016

Ryu MJ, Cho M, Song JY, Yun YS, Choi IW, Kim DE, Park BS, Oh S (2008) Natural derivatives of curcumin attenuate the Wnt/beta-catenin pathway through down-regulation of the transcriptional coactivator p300. Biochem Biophys Res Commun 377:1304–1308

Salh B, Assi K, Templeman V, Parhar K, Owen D, Gomez-Munoz A, Jacobson K (2003) Curcumin attenuates DNB-induced murine colitis. Am J Physiol Gastrointest Liver Physiol 285: G235–G243

Sandur SK, Pandey MK, Sung B, Aggarwal BB (2010) 5-hydroxy-2-methyl-1,4-naphthoquinone, a vitamin K3 analogue, suppresses STAT3 activation pathway through induction of protein tyrosine phosphatase, SHP-1: potential role in chemosensitization. Mol Cancer Res 8:107–118

Santagata S, Demichelis F, Riva A, Varambally S, Hofer MD, Kutok JL, Kim R, Tang J, Montie JE, Chinnaiyan AM, Rubin MA, Aster JC (2004) JAGGED1 expression is associated with prostate cancer metastasis and recurrence. Cancer Res 64:6854–6857

Sarkar FH, Li Y, Wang Z, Kong D (2009) Cellular signaling perturbation by natural products. Cell Signal 21:1541–1547

Sarkar FH, Li Y, Wang Z, Kong D (2010) Novel targets for prostate cancer chemoprevention. Endocr Relat Cancer 17:R195–R212

Schmidt M, Fernandez de Mattos S, van der Horst A, Klompmaker R, Kops GJ, Lam EW, Burgering BM, Medema RH (2002) Cell cycle inhibition by FoxO forkhead transcription factors involves downregulation of cyclin D. Mol Cell Biol 22:7842–7852

Schweizer L, Varmus H (2003) Wnt/Wingless signaling through beta-catenin requires the function of both LRP/Arrow and frizzled classes of receptors. BMC Cell Biol 4:4

Scorrano L, Korsmeyer SJ (2003) Mechanisms of cytochrome c release by proapoptotic BCL-2 family members. Biochem Biophys Res Commun 304:437–444

Scuderi R, Palucka KA, Pokrovskaja K, Bjorkholm M, Wiman KG, Pisa P (1996) Cyclin E overexpression in relapsed adult acute lymphoblastic leukemias of B-cell lineage. Blood 87:3360–3367

Scuto A, Krejci P, Popplewell L, Wu J, Wang Y, Kujawski M, Kowolik C, Xin H, Chen L, Kretzner L, Yu H, Wilcox WR, Yen Y, Forman S, Jove R (2011) The novel JAK inhibitor AZD1480 blocks STAT3 and FGFR3 signaling, resulting in suppression of human myeloma cell growth and survival. Leukemia 25:538–550

Seo JH, Jeong KJ, Oh WJ, Sul HJ, Sohn JS, Kim YK, Cho do Y, Kang JK, Park CG, Lee HY (2010) Lysophosphatidic acid induces STAT3 phosphorylation and ovarian cancer cell motility: their inhibition by curcumin. Cancer Lett 288:50–56

Shaikh J, Ankola DD, Beniwal V, Singh D, Kumar MN (2009) Nanoparticle encapsulation improves oral bioavailability of curcumin by at least 9-fold when compared to curcumin administered with piperine as absorption enhancer. Eur J Pharm Sci 37:223–230

Shankar S, Srivastava RK (2004) Enhancement of therapeutic potential of TRAIL by cancer chemotherapy and irradiation: mechanisms and clinical implications. Drug Resist Updat 7: 139–156

Shankar S, Srivastava RK (2007a) Bax and Bak genes are essential for maximum apoptotic response by curcumin, a polyphenolic compound and cancer chemopreventive agent derived from turmeric, Curcuma longa. Carcinogenesis 28:1277–1286

Shankar S, Srivastava RK (2007b) Involvement of Bcl-2 family members, phosphatidylinositol 3′-kinase/AKT and mitochondrial p53 in curcumin (diferulolylmethane)-induced apoptosis in prostate cancer. Int J Oncol 30:905–918

Shankar S, Singh TR, Srivastava RK (2004) Ionizing radiation enhances the therapeutic potential of TRAIL in prostate cancer in vitro and in vivo: intracellular mechanisms. Prostate 61:35–49

Shankar S, Chen X, Srivastava RK (2005) Effects of sequential treatments with chemotherapeutic drugs followed by TRAIL on prostate cancer in vitro and in vivo. Prostate 62:165–186

Shankar S, Chen Q, Sarva K, Siddiqui I, Srivastava RK (2007a) Curcumin enhances the apoptosis-inducing potential of TRAIL in prostate cancer cells: molecular mechanisms of apoptosis, migration and angiogenesis. J Mol Signal 2:10

Shankar S, Chen Q, Siddiqui I, Sarva K, Srivastava RK (2007b) Sensitization of TRAIL-resistant LNCaP cells by resveratrol (3, 4′, 5 tri-hydroxystilbene): molecular mechanisms and therapeutic potential. J Mol Signal 2:7

Shankar S, Ganapathy S, Chen Q, Srivastava RK (2008) Curcumin sensitizes TRAIL-resistant xenografts: molecular mechanisms of apoptosis, metastasis and angiogenesis. Mol Cancer 7:16

Shanmugam MK, Kannaiyan R, Sethi G (2011) Targeting cell signaling and apoptotic pathways by dietary agents: role in the prevention and treatment of cancer. Nutr Cancer 63:161–173

Sharma RA, Ireson CR, Verschoyle RD, Hill KA, Williams ML, Leuratti C, Manson MM, Marnett LJ, Steward WP, Gescher A (2001) Effects of dietary curcumin on glutathione S-transferase and malondialdehyde-DNA adducts in rat liver and colon mucosa: relationship with drug levels. Clin Cancer Res 7:1452–1458

Sharma S, Kulkarni SK, Agrewala JN, Chopra K (2006) Curcumin attenuates thermal hyperalgesia in a diabetic mouse model of neuropathic pain. Eur J Pharmacol 536:256–261

Sharma VM, Draheim KM, Kelliher MA (2007) The Notch1/c-Myc pathway in T cell leukemia. Cell Cycle 6:927–930

Sharma M, Manoharlal R, Puri N, Prasad R (2010) Antifungal curcumin induces reactive oxygen species and triggers an early apoptosis but prevents hyphae development by targeting the global repressor TUP1 in Candida albicans. Biosci Rep 30:391–404

Shenouda NS, Zhou C, Browning JD, Ansell PJ, Sakla MS, Lubahn DB, Macdonald RS (2004) Phytoestrogens in common herbs regulate prostate cancer cell growth in vitro. Nutr Cancer 49:200–208

Sherr CJ (1994) G1 phase progression: cycling on cue. Cell 79:551–555

Sherr CJ (1996) Cancer cell cycles. Science 274:1672–1677

Sherr CJ (2002) D1 in G2. Cell Cycle 1:36–38

Sherr CJ, Roberts JM (1995) Inhibitors of mammalian G1 cyclin-dependent kinases. Genes Dev 9:1149–1163

Sherr CJ, Roberts JM (1999) CDK inhibitors: positive and negative regulators of G1-phase progression. Genes Dev 13:1501–1512

Shin HM, Minter LM, Cho OH, Gottipati S, Fauq AH, Golde TE, Sonenshein GE, Osborne BA (2006) Notch1 augments NF-kappaB activity by facilitating its nuclear retention. EMBO J 25:129–138

Sidhu GS, Singh AK, Thaloor D, Banaudha KK, Patnaik GK, Srimal RC, Maheshwari RK (1998) Enhancement of wound healing by curcumin in animals. Wound Repair Regen 6:167–177

Sidhu GS, Mani H, Gaddipati JP, Singh AK, Seth P, Banaudha KK, Patnaik GK, Maheshwari RK (1999) Curcumin enhances wound healing in streptozotocin induced diabetic rats and genetically diabetic mice. Wound Repair Regen 7:362–374

Singh S, Khar A (2006) Biological effects of curcumin and its role in cancer chemoprevention and therapy. Anticancer Agents Med Chem 6:259–270

Six EM, Ndiaye D, Sauer G, Laabi Y, Athman R, Cumano A, Brou C, Israel A, Logeat F (2004) The notch ligand Delta1 recruits Dlg1 at cell-cell contacts and regulates cell migration. J Biol Chem 279:55818–55826

Smalley MJ, Dale TC (1999) Wnt signalling in mammalian development and cancer. Cancer Metastasis Rev 18:215–230

Spruck CH, Won KA, Reed SI (1999) Deregulated cyclin E induces chromosome instability. Nature 401:297–300

Sreejayan N, Rao MN (1994) Curcuminoids as potent inhibitors of lipid peroxidation. J Pharm Pharmacol 46:1013–1016

Sreejayan N, Rao MN (1997) Nitric oxide scavenging by curcuminoids. J Pharm Pharmacol 49:105–107

Srinivasan M (1972) Effect of curcumin on blood sugar as seen in a diabetic subject. Indian J Med Sci 26:269–270

Srivastava RK (2001) TRAIL/Apo-2 L: mechanisms and clinical applications in cancer. Neoplasia 3:535–546

Srivastava RK, Sasaki CY, Hardwick JM, Longo DL (1999a) Bcl-2-mediated drug resistance: inhibition of apoptosis by blocking nuclear factor of activated T lymphocytes (NFAT)-induced Fas ligand transcription. J Exp Med 190:253–265

Srivastava RK, Sollott SJ, Khan L, Hansford R, Lakatta EG, Longo DL (1999b) Bcl-2 and Bcl-X(L) block thapsigargin-induced nitric oxide generation, c-Jun NH(2)-terminal kinase activity, and apoptosis. Mol Cell Biol 19:5659–5674

Srivastava RK, Chen Q, Siddiqui I, Sarva K, Shankar S (2007) Linkage of curcumin-induced cell cycle arrest and apoptosis by cyclin-dependent kinase inhibitor p21(/WAF1/CIP1). Cell Cycle 6(23):2953–2961

Stahl M, Ge C, Shi S, Pestell RG, Stanley P (2006) Notch1-induced transformation of RKE-1 cells requires up-regulation of cyclin D1. Cancer Res 66:7562–7570

Stockhausen MT, Kristoffersen K, Poulsen HS (2010) The functional role of Notch signaling in human gliomas. Neuro Oncol 12:199–211

Subbaramaiah K, Dannenberg AJ (2003) Cyclooxygenase 2: a molecular target for cancer prevention and treatment. Trends Pharmacol Sci 24:96–102

Surh YJ (2002) Anti-tumor promoting potential of selected spice ingredients with antioxidative and anti-inflammatory activities: a short review. Food Chem Toxicol 40:1091–1097

Susan M, Rao MN (1992) Induction of glutathione S-transferase activity by curcumin in mice. Arzneimittelforschung 42:962–964

Swarnakar S, Ganguly K, Kundu P, Banerjee A, Maity P, Sharma AV (2005) Curcumin regulates expression and activity of matrix metalloproteinases 9 and 2 during prevention and healing of indomethacin-induced gastric ulcer. J Biol Chem 280:9409–9415

Takahashi-Yanaga F, Sasaguri T (2008) GSK-3beta regulates cyclin D1 expression: a new target for chemotherapy. Cell Signal 20:581–589

Takebe N, Harris PJ, Warren RQ, Ivy SP (2011) Targeting cancer stem cells by inhibiting Wnt, Notch, and Hedgehog pathways. Nat Rev Clin Oncol 8:97–106

Tanaka M, Setoguchi T, Hirotsu M, Gao H, Sasaki H, Matsunoshita Y, Komiya S (2009) Inhibition of Notch pathway prevents osteosarcoma growth by cell cycle regulation. Br J Cancer 100:1957–1965

Tavera-Mendoza LE, Wang TT, White JH (2006) p19INK4D and cell death. Cell Cycle 5:596–598

Taya Y (1997) RB kinases and RB-binding proteins: new points of view. Trends Biochem Sci 22:14–17

Tetsu O, McCormick F (1999) Beta-catenin regulates expression of cyclin D1 in colon carcinoma cells. Nature 398:422–426

Thaloor D, Miller KJ, Gephart J, Mitchell PO, Pavlath GK (1999) Systemic administration of the NF-kappaB inhibitor curcumin stimulates muscle regeneration after traumatic injury. Am J Physiol 277:C320–C329

Thayer SP, di Magliano MP, Heiser PW, Nielsen CM, Roberts DJ, Lauwers GY, Qi YP, Gysin S, Fernandez-del Castillo C, Yajnik V, Antoniu B, McMahon M, Warshaw AL, Hebrok M (2003) Hedgehog is an early and late mediator of pancreatic cancer tumorigenesis. Nature 425: 851–856

Thomasset SC, Berry DP, Garcea G, Marczylo T, Steward WP, Gescher AJ (2007) Dietary polyphenolic phytochemicals–promising cancer chemopreventive agents in humans? A review of their clinical properties. Int J Cancer 120:451–458

Traiffort E, Angot E, Ruat M (2010) Sonic Hedgehog signaling in the mammalian brain. J Neurochem 113:576–590

Ulasov IV, Nandi S, Dey M, Sonabend AM, Lesniak MS (2011) Inhibition of Sonic hedgehog and Notch pathways enhances sensitivity of CD133(+) glioma stem cells to temozolomide therapy. Mol Med 17:103–112

Unnikrishnan MK, Rao MN (1995a) Curcumin inhibits nitrogen dioxide induced oxidation of hemoglobin. Mol Cell Biochem 146:35–37

Unnikrishnan MK, Rao MN (1995b) Inhibition of nitrite induced oxidation of hemoglobin by curcuminoids. Pharmazie 50:490–492

Valentine SP, Le Nedelec MJ, Menzies AR, Scandlyn MJ, Goodin MG, Rosengren RJ (2006) Curcumin modulates drug metabolizing enzymes in the female Swiss Webster mouse. Life Sci 78:2391–2398

Vallejo DM, Caparros E, Dominguez M (2011) Targeting Notch signalling by the conserved miR-8/200 microRNA family in development and cancer cells. EMBO J 30:756–769

Verhagen AM, Vaux DL (2002) Cell death regulation by the mammalian IAP antagonist Diablo/Smac. Apoptosis 7:163–166

Verhagen AM, Ekert PG, Pakusch M, Silke J, Connolly LM, Reid GE, Moritz RL, Simpson RJ, Vaux DL (2000) Identification of DIABLO, a mammalian protein that promotes apoptosis by binding to and antagonizing IAP proteins. Cell 102:43–53

Verhagen AM, Coulson EJ, Vaux DL (2001) Inhibitor of apoptosis proteins and their relatives: IAPs and other BIRPs. Genome Biol 2: REVIEWS3009

Wahl H, Tan L, Griffith K, Choi M, Liu JR (2007) Curcumin enhances Apo2L/TRAIL-induced apoptosis in chemoresistant ovarian cancer cells. Gynecol Oncol 105:104–112

Walker DH, Maller JL (1991) Role for cyclin A in the dependence of mitosis on completion of DNA replication. Nature 354:314–317

Wang J, Shelly L, Miele L, Boykins R, Norcross MA, Guan E (2001) Human Notch-1 inhibits NF-kappa B activity in the nucleus through a direct interaction involving a novel domain. J Immunol 167:289–295

Wang Z, Zhang Y, Banerjee S, Li Y, Sarkar FH (2006a) Notch-1 down-regulation by curcumin is associated with the inhibition of cell growth and the induction of apoptosis in pancreatic cancer cells. Cancer 106:2503–2513

Wang Z, Zhang Y, Li Y, Banerjee S, Liao J, Sarkar FH (2006b) Down-regulation of Notch-1 contributes to cell growth inhibition and apoptosis in pancreatic cancer cells. Mol Cancer Ther 5:483–493

Wang Z, Desmoulin S, Banerjee S, Kong D, Li Y, Deraniyagala RL, Abbruzzese J, Sarkar FH (2008) Synergistic effects of multiple natural products in pancreatic cancer cells. Life Sci 83:293–300

Wei MC, Lindsten T, Mootha VK, Weiler S, Gross A, Ashiya M, Thompson CB, Korsmeyer SJ (2000) tBID, a membrane-targeted death ligand, oligomerizes BAK to release cytochrome c. Genes Dev 14:2060–2071

Wei MC, Zong WX, Cheng EH, Lindsten T, Panoutsakopoulou V, Ross AJ, Roth KA, MacGregor GR, Thompson CB, Korsmeyer SJ (2001) Proapoptotic BAX and BAK: a requisite gateway to mitochondrial dysfunction and death. Science 292:727–730

Wei P, Walls M, Qiu M, Ding R, Denlinger RH, Wong A, Tsaparikos K, Jani JP, Hosea N, Sands M, Randolph S, Smeal T (2010) Evaluation of selective gamma-secretase inhibitor PF-03084014 for its antitumor efficacy and gastrointestinal safety to guide optimal clinical trial design. Mol Cancer Ther 9:1618–1628

Weinberg RA (1995) The retinoblastoma protein and cell cycle control. Cell 81:323–330

Weissenberger J, Priester M, Bernreuther C, Rakel S, Glatzel M, Seifert V, Kogel D (2010) Dietary curcumin attenuates glioma growth in a syngeneic mouse model by inhibition of the JAK1,2/STAT3 signaling pathway. Clin Cancer Res 16:5781–5795

Weller M, Krautler N, Mantei N, Suter U, Taylor V (2006) Jagged1 ablation results in cerebellar granule cell migration defects and depletion of Bergmann glia. Dev Neurosci 28:70–80

Wend P, Holland JD, Ziebold U, Birchmeier W (2010) Wnt signaling in stem and cancer stem cells. Semin Cell Dev Biol 21:855–863

Willis S, Day CL, Hinds MG, Huang DC (2003) The Bcl-2-regulated apoptotic pathway. J Cell Sci 116:4053–4056

Wolfel T, Hauer M, Schneider J, Serrano M, Wolfel C, Klehmann-Hieb E, De Plaen E, Hankeln T, Meyer zum Buschenfelde KH, Beach D (1995) A p16INK4a-insensitive CDK4 mutant targeted by cytolytic T lymphocytes in a human melanoma. Science 269:1281–1284

Woodward WA, Chen MS, Behbod F, Alfaro MP, Buchholz TA, Rosen JM (2007) WNT/beta-catenin mediates radiation resistance of mouse mammary progenitor cells. Proc Natl Acad Sci U S A 104:618–623

Wu X, Senechal K, Neshat MS, Whang YE, Sawyers CL (1998) The PTEN/MMAC1 tumor suppressor phosphatase functions as a negative regulator of the phosphoinositide 3-kinase/Akt pathway. Proc Natl Acad Sci U S A 95:15587–15591

Yamamoto H, Monden T, Miyoshi H, Izawa H, Ikeda K, Tsujie M, Ohnishi T, Sekimoto M, Tomita N, Monden M (1998) Cdk2/cdc2 expression in colon carcinogenesis and effects of cdk2/cdc2 inhibitor in colon cancer cells. Int J Oncol 13:233–239

Yamasaki L, Bronson R, Williams BO, Dyson NJ, Harlow E, Jacks T (1998) Loss of E2F-1 reduces tumorigenesis and extends the lifespan of Rb1(+/-)mice. Nat Genet 18:360–364

Yan C, Jamaluddin MS, Aggarwal B, Myers J, Boyd DD (2005) Gene expression profiling identifies activating transcription factor 3 as a novel contributor to the proapoptotic effect of curcumin. Mol Cancer Ther 4:233–241

Yang K, Proweller A (2011) Vascular smooth muscle Notch signals regulate endothelial cell sensitivity to angiogenic stimulation. J Biol Chem 286:13741–13753

Yang Y, Hou H, Haller EM, Nicosia SV, Bai W (2005) Suppression of FOXO1 activity by FHL2 through SIRT1-mediated deacetylation. EMBO J 24:1021–1032

Yang W, Yan HX, Chen L, Liu Q, He YQ, Yu LX, Zhang SH, Huang DD, Tang L, Kong XN, Chen C, Liu SQ, Wu MC, Wang HY (2008) Wnt/beta-catenin signaling contributes to activation of normal and tumorigenic liver progenitor cells. Cancer Res 68:4287–4295

Yang J, Ikezoe T, Nishioka C, Furihata M, Yokoyama A (2010) AZ960, a novel Jak2 inhibitor, induces growth arrest and apoptosis in adult T-cell leukemia cells. Mol Cancer Ther 9: 3386–3395

Yao QH, Wang DQ, Cui CC, Yuan ZY, Chen SB, Yao XW, Wang JK, Lian JF (2004) Curcumin ameliorates left ventricular function in rabbits with pressure overload: inhibition of the remodeling of the left ventricular collagen network associated with suppression of myocardial tumor necrosis factor-alpha and matrix metalloproteinase-2 expression. Biol Pharm Bull 27:198–202

Yeh TS, Wu CW, Hsu KW, Liao WJ, Yang MC, Li AF, Wang AM, Kuo ML, Chi CW (2009) The activated Notch1 signal pathway is associated with gastric cancer progression through cyclooxygenase-2. Cancer Res 69:5039–5048

Yoysungnoen P, Wirachwong P, Bhattarakosol P, Niimi H, Patumraj S (2006) Effects of curcumin on tumor angiogenesis and biomarkers, COX-2 and VEGF, in hepatocellular carcinoma cell-implanted nude mice. Clin Hemorheol Microcirc 34:109–115

Yuan XJ, Whang YE (2002) PTEN sensitizes prostate cancer cells to death receptor-mediated and drug-induced apoptosis through a FADD-dependent pathway. Oncogene 21:319–327

Zbinden M, Duquet A, Lorente-Trigos A, Ngwabyt SN, Borges I, Ruiz i Altaba A (2010) NANOG regulates glioma stem cells and is essential in vivo acting in a cross-functional network with GLI1 and p53. EMBO J 29:2659–2674

Zhang Z, Wang H, Ikeda S, Fahey F, Bielenberg D, Smits P, Hauschka PV (2010) Notch3 in human breast cancer cell lines regulates osteoblast-cancer cell interactions and osteolytic bone metastasis. Am J Pathol 177:1459–1469

Zou H, Henzel WJ, Liu X, Lutschg A, Wang X (1997) Apaf-1, a human protein homologous to C. elegans CED-4, participates in cytochrome c-dependent activation of caspase-3. Cell 90: 405–413

Chapter 18
Obesity, Cancer and Psychopathology: Can Vegetarian Diet Be of Help?

Vikas Kumar, Ajit Kumar Thakur, and Shyam Sunder Chatterjee

Contents

Abstract High body mass index, low fruit and vegetable intake, physical inactivity, tobacco use, alcohol use and unsafe sex are six behaviorally modifiable risk factors potentially involved in increased cancer rates observed during recent years. Numerous epidemiological and experimental data are now beginning to point out

---

V. Kumar (✉) • A.K. Thakur
Neuropharmacology Research Laboratory, Department of Pharmaceutics, Institute of Technology, Banaras Hindu University, Varanasi 221 005, Uttar Pradesh, India
e-mail: vikas.phe@itbhu.ac.in; ajit.thakur.phe09@itbhu.ac.in

S.S. Chatterjee
Retired Head of Pharmacology Research Laboratories, Dr. Willmar Schwabe GmbH & Co. KG., Stettiner Str. 1, D-76138 Karlsruhe, Germany
e-mail: shyam.chatterjee@web.de

S. Shankar and R.K. Srivastava (eds.), *Nutrition, Diet and Cancer*,
DOI 10.1007/978-94-007-2923-0_18,

that the functions of the central nervous system may also be detrimentally effected by these risk factors, and that complex psychobiological processes are involved in obesity associated comorbidities. Several phytochemicals commonly consumed with fruits and vegetables are known since long to possess chemopreventive as well as beneficial effects on cognitive functions. However, as yet little concentrated efforts have been made to properly understand the health benefits of diverse combinations of phytochemicals commonly consumed with every day meals. Available information on health benefits of some vegetables in obesity associated carcinogenesis are summarized and discussed in short in this chapter. It is concluded that at old fashioned holistic pharmacological approaches could be helpful for identifying effective safe and affordable nutraceuticals and drug leads urgently needed for combating oncological problems associated with obesity.

Introduction

The epidemic of obesity has become pandemic, defined as an epidemic occurring over a wide geographic area and affecting an exceptionally high proportion of the population. The rise in obesity rates was first noted in the US, but has spread to other industrialized nations and it is now being documented even in developing countries. Obesity is characterized by excessive generalized deposition of fat in the body. Since fat cannot be determined directly (except in research centers), indirect measures like body-mass-index, waist circumference, waist/hip ratio, skin fold thickness, and bioimpedance etc. are commonly used to define obesity. The most widely used index for such purposes is the body mass index (BMI, also called Quetelet's index) calculated by dividing the body weight in kilograms by the square of the person's height in meters (kg/m^2). BMI also provides one way to estimate diverse health risks commonly associated with obesity. According to the World Health Organization (Table 18.1) a BMI of 18.5–24.9 is considered normal weight, 25–29.9 overweight and $\geq$30 is obese (WHO 2000). It is well known that obesity increases the risks of almost all non communicable diseases, and that dietary measures together with appropriate physical activity is a feasible means for preventing obesity-associated medical conditions. Adverse metabolic effects of excess body fat are known to accelerate atherogenesis and increase the risk of coronary heart disease, stroke, and early death. Obesity has long been recognized to be an important cause of type 2 diabetes mellitus, hypertension,

Table 18.1 Body mass index and popular description in WHO classification

BMI (kg/m^2)	WHO classification	Popular description
$<$18.5	Underweight	Thin
18.5–24.9	Normal range	'Healthy' or 'Normal'
25.0–29.9	Grade 1 overweight	Overweight
30.0–39.9	Grade 2 overweight	Obesity
$\geq$40.0	Grade 3 overweight	Morbid obesity

and dyslipidemia (NIH 1998; NTFPTO 2000). Evidence accumulating during more recent decades suggests also that increased adiposity may increase incidence and/or death rates from a wide variety of human cancers, including colon and rectum, esophagus, kidney, pancreas, gallbladder, ovary, cervix, liver, prostate, and certain hematopoietic cancers (WHO 2000). Obesity is often considered to be a problem of the belly rather than of the brain. It is now becoming increasingly apparent though, that complex psychobiological processes involving gut microbiota, gut-brain axis and mental functions play important roles in its etiology and progression (McAllister et al. 2009; Bruce-Keller et al. 2009).

Obesity is a risk factor for numerous psychopathological conditions including dementia, intracranial hypertension, stroke, and sleep disorders (Knecht et al. 2008; Bellanger and Bray 2005). One especially costly and debilitating deficit of aging is the loss of cognitive function and the onset of dementia. All cognitive disorders, including dementia, become more common with age. Despite its strong association with age, dementia has been proposed as a mainly preventable condition with a large number of modifiable risk factors, including obesity, metabolic syndrome, and cardiovascular disease (Haan and Wallace 2004). In terms of brain function, obesity may disrupt cognition. Several studies have reported deficits in learning, memory, and executive functioning in obese when compared to non-obese patients (Elias et al. 2003, 2005; Waldstein and Katzel 2006). Other studies of young and middle-aged healthy adults have confirmed the association of obesity with behavioral declines in executive function (Gunstad et al. 2007). Overall, current evidence suggests that obesity and the consequences of obesity, including midlife hypertension, diabetes, and cerebrovascular disease, contribute significantly to cognitive decline and accelerate the development of dementia (Qiu et al. 2007). Although the physiologic mechanisms whereby obesity adversely affects the brain are not understood, both experimental and human studies have shown that obesity is associated with increased oxidative stress, which has been implicated in cognitive declines seen in neurodegenerative diseases (Ames et al. 1993; Liu et al. 2002), which can indeed be regulated by dietary constituents (Mattson et al. 2003).

Psychiatric problems are often encountered in cancer patients as well. The most common mental health problems of such patients are anxiety, depression and adjustment problems related to cancer diagnosis, treatment modalities, and terminal phase of the lethal condition (Greer 1983; Lovestone and Fahy 1991). In general, these problems are considered to be of major importance in palliative care, health benefits of which are known since long. It is now becoming exceedingly apparent though, that considerable cancer survival benefits can be achieved by such interventions also (Temel et al. 2010; Spiegel 2011). These findings are in agreement with more recent observations made in experimental animals, demonstrating cancer survival benefits of environmental enrichment (Pang and Hannan 2010). Diet is one of the major environmental factors implicated in the genesis and progression of both obesity and cancer, and beneficial effects of diverse environmental factors on mental health is now well recognized (Gomez-Pinilla 2008; Diener and Chan 2011).

Although to date little concentrated efforts have been made to identify specific dietary measures for combating mental health problems of diagnosed cancer patients, there is now considerable epidemiological evidences pointing out protective associations between vegetables and/or fruits and several cancers. Vegetarian diets may play a beneficial role in promoting health and preventing obesity (Fraser 1999; Rosell et al. 2006; Phillips et al. 2004). Ecologic, observational and laboratory studies generally agree that eating a diet high in vegetable and other plant-based food; low in animal fats and low in salt content, along with maintaining a healthy weight and being physically active can reduce the risk of cancer and other chronic diseases (WCRF/AICR 2007; Schaefer 2002). However, dietary customs and habit in different parts of the globe vary considerably according to their cultural background, religious belief, and diverse other socio-economic reasons. India is one of the few countries where there is a tradition to link vegetarianism with medicine. Ayurveda, i.e. one of the oldest known holistic health care systems currently widely practiced in India and other countries, provides dietary guidance and prescriptions that have been developed over millennia to prevent and treat multiple ailments, including cancer and diabetes (Sinha et al. 2003). For the past 70 years, the Indian Council of Medical Research (ICMR) has produced information on nutrition requirements specific to the population of India. Approximately every 10 years, the ICMR updates nutrition recommendations based on evolving information from surveys conducted by the National Institute of Nutrition (NIN), Hyderabad, India (Vijayaraghavan and Rao 1998).

The NIN has also conducted studies on several aspects of diet-cancer interrelationships. These include studies on metabolic susceptibility, case-control approach to determine the risk factors and intervention studies to determine the role of nutrients and non-nutrient components on preneoplastic events. Extensive work demonstrating antimutagenic/anticarcinogenic potential of some commonly consumed spices and vegetables, such as turmeric, mustard, green leafy and allium species of vegetables, have been carried out during more recent decades. These studies strongly suggest that besides avoiding risk factors such as smoking and alcoholism and exposure to genotoxicants, dietary intervention for cancer prevention is also needed to control further spread of the disease. Public education and awareness about the beneficial effects of consuming a healthy diet including plenty of fresh vegetables and fruits with spices such as turmeric in adequate amounts to prevent cancer are required (Krishnaswamy and Polasa 1995). Analogous, but not identical, recommendations are also valid for other countries (Scarborough et al. 2010; Kushi et al. 2006) and suggestions that dietary advice on prescription in clinical setting could be an useful means for preventing cancer and other lethal diseases are also well known (Johansson 2011). Current state of knowledge on possibilities offered by food, nutrition, physical activity for cancer prevention in global perspective has recently been reviewed by 'World Cancer Research Fund' and 'American Institute of Cancer Research' (WCRF/AICR 2007).

Obesity and Cancer

Epidemiology of Obesity and Cancer Risk

The relationships between excess body weight and mortality from all causes and from cardiovascular disease have since long been known and well-established by epidemiologic studies (Manson et al. 1995; Willett et al. 1995; Lindsted and Singh 1998; Stevens et al. 1998; Calle et al. 1999). Excess weight is also known to be associated with an increased risk of morbidity, including cardiovascular diseases, type 2 diabetes mellitus, hypertension, dyslipidemia, glucose intolerance, and osteoarthritis (NIH 1998; NTFPTO 2000). The association of overweight and obesity with most of these non-cancerous outcomes is generally stronger than the association with cancer. In populations experiencing temporal increases in the prevalence of obesity, increases in hypertension, hyperlipidemia and diabetes emerge earlier than increases in cancer outcomes. As the incidence and mortality of specific types of cancer are less common than noncancerous outcomes, the relationship between obesity and carcinogenicity in a particular body site has been more difficult to study. Moreover, a biologic mechanism that clearly links obesity to forms of cancer without an endocrine component could not yet be established (Renehan 2010). The International Agency for Research on Cancer (IARC) Working Group (Vainio and Bianchini 2002) on the Evaluation of Cancer-Preventive Strategies recently published a comprehensive evaluation of the available literature on weight and cancer that considered epidemiological, clinical and experimental data. Their report concluded that avoidance of weight gain reduces the risk of developing cancers of the colon, breast (in postmenopausal women), endometrium, kidney (renal cell) and oesophagus (adenocarcinoma). These conclusions are based on epidemiological studies of overweight and/or obese individuals compared with leaner individuals, and not on studies of individuals who have lost weight. Unfortunately, few individuals manage to maintain a significant weight loss after intentional weight reduction, making it extremely difficult to examine cancer outcomes in populations of weight losers. Consequently, the IARC report and, more recently, the World Cancer Research Fund (WCRF) have concluded that, among the different cancer sites, this association is positive for esophageal adenocarcinoma, pancreas, colorectal, post-menopausal breast, endometrial, kidney cancer, and probably the risk of gallbladder cancer as well (WCRF/AICR 2007). These reports concluded that there is inadequate evidence that weight loss reduces the risk of cancer. However, there have been many studies that have added evidence for the association between adiposity and cancer risk. Attributable fractions of cancer were estimated for overweight ($25 \leq$ BMI <30 kg/m^2, BMI $=27$) and obese (BMI ≥ 30 kg/m^2 BMI $=32$) persons compared to those of normal weight (BMI 20–25 kg/m^2 BMI $=22$) according to the WHO guidelines for a healthy physical status (WHO 2000). The relative risk of developing certain cancer types in European Union with relation to BMI is shown in Table 18.2 (Bergström et al. 2001). A landmark study on the relationship between cancer and obesity was conducted by the American

Table 18.2 Proportion of cancer cases attributable to overweight and obesity in the European Union, by cancer sites

	Men		Women	
Type of Cancer	Overweight ($25 \leq BMI < 30$)	Obese ($BMI \geq 30$)	Overweight ($25 \leq BMI < 30$)	Obese ($BMI \geq 30$)
Breast	–	–	4.1	4.5
Colon	6.9	4.2	5.0	5.7
Endometrium	–	–	17.2	22.0
Prostate	2.9	1.6	–	–
Kidney	15.2	10.3	11.1	13.4
Gallbladder	14.7	10.1	10.7	13.0
All cancer sites	2.1	1.3	2.9	3.5

Cancer Society over a 13-year period from 1959 to 1972. After adjusting for the effects of age and cigarette smoking, people whose body weight was 40% higher than average had an overall increased risk of cancer death (33% increase in men and a 55% increase in women). Overweight males experienced significantly higher rates of colorectal and prostate cancer; whereas, overweight women experienced higher rates of gallbladder, breast, cervical, endometrial, uterine and ovarian cancers (Lew and Garfinkel 1979). The relationship between obesity and the risks for various forms of cancer in a population-based cohort of 28,129 hospital patients (8,165 men, 19,964 women) in Sweden from 1965 to 1993 have also been evaluated. Cancer risk was estimated using the standardized incidence ratio (with 95% confidence interval), which is the ratio of the observed number of cancers to that expected. Overall, a 33% excess incidence of cancer was seen in obese persons, 25% in men and 37% in women (Wolk et al. 2001). Numerous reviews consistently pointing out strong association between obesity and cancer have appeared during more recent years (Hemminki et al. 2011; Renehan et al. 2010) and it is now well recognized that more precise understanding of the biological processes linking obesity and cancer is necessary for obtaining more sustainable progress towards prevention and cure of cancer (Renehan et al. 2008; Renehan 2011).

Biological Relationship Between Obesity and Cancer

Although importance of central nervous system, and specially the hypothalamus, in regulating bodily energy balance has been known since long, it was only during 1970s that the role of adipose tissue in central obesity associated co-morbidities started becoming more evident. Extensive efforts made during the past two decades have clearly pointed out the crucial role of adipose tissue in regulating numerous functions of diverse bodily organs including those of the brain. Despite extensive efforts and considerable progress though, our current understanding of the biological processes involved in etiology, pathogenesis, and progression of obesity associated cancers and other comorbidities still remain to be far from being definitive. It is now apparent though, that adipose tissue constitutes an active endocrine and metabolic organ that can have far-reaching effects on the functions of other tissues, and that neuronal signals are also involved in the its proper functioning (Rajala and Scherer 2003). In response to endocrine and metabolic signals from other organs, adipose tissue responds by either increasing or decreasing the release of free fatty acids an energy-providing fuel for skeletal muscle and other tissues. Adipose tissue is also important in the regulation of energy balance and lipid metabolism through the release of peptide hormones such as leptin, adiponectin, resistin and tumour necrosis factor-α (TNF-α). Increased release of free fatty acids, resistin and TNFα by adipose tissue and reduced release of adiponectin give rise to insulin resistance, a metabolic state characterized by reduced metabolic response of tissues (muscle, liver, adipose) to insulin, and to compensatory hyperinsulinaemia (Reaven 1988). Taken together, these findings have led to the suggestion that adipose tissue could be considered as a "third brain" (Chaldakov et al. 2009) which can regulate diverse biological processes associated with paracrine and endocrine functions of the adipose tissue (Chaldakov et al. 2010).

Some Proposed Mechanisms

It is now evident that inflammatory responses play decisive roles at different stages of tumor development, including initiation, promotion, malignant conversion, invasion and metastasis, and that inflammation also affects immune surveillance and response to available therapies (Grivennikov et al. 2010). Although involvements of diverse biological mechanisms in such processes have been identified or proposed (Calle and Kaaks 2004; Roberts et al. 2010), successful translation of such knowledge in terms prevention and therapy have not yet been possible. Some biological mediators and processes that could potentially be involved in reported pharmacological activity profiles of phytochemicals consumed with food will be discussed in short in the following.

Hormones and Growth Factors

Energy expenditure, appetite regulation, metabolism and thermo genesis, are all under hormonal control. Recent evidence, particularly from several mutant mouse models in which specific hormonal factors have been altered, have provided evidence that insulin, insulin-like growth factor-1 (IGF-1), glucocorticoids and several adipose-derived factors (such as leptin and adiponectin) associated with inflammation and energy metabolism which is potential mechanism in cancer and tumorigenesis (Hursting et al. 2007, 2010).

Insulin

Insulin, particularly under conditions of chronic hyperinsulinemia and insulin resistance, increases risk for cancer at several sites (Calle et al. 2003; Belfiore and Roberta 2011). As yet it is unclear though, whether the tumor-enhancing effects of insulin are due to direct effects involving the insulin receptor on pre-neoplastic cells, or alternatively due to indirect effects on IGF-1, estrogens and/or other hormones. Certainly, high circulating levels of insulin promote the hepatic synthesis of IGF-1 and decrease the production of IGF binding protein-1, thus increasing the biologic activity of IGF-1 (Calle and Kaaks 2004). Furthermore, both insulin and IGF-1 act in vitro as growth factors to promote cancer cell proliferation and decrease apoptosis (Yakar et al. 2005). Insulin resistance, a state of reduced responsiveness of tissues to the physiological actions of insulin, results in a compensatory rise in plasma insulin levels and is affected by both adiposity and physical activity. Intra-abdominal obesity is associated with insulin resistance (Abate 1996), whereas physical activity improves insulin sensitivity (Grimm 1999). A growing body of epidemiologic evidence suggests that type-2 diabetes, usually characterized by hyperinsulinemia and insulin resistance for long periods, is associated with increased risks of endometrial, colon, pancreas, kidney and postmenopausal breast cancers (Calle and Kaaks 2004).

IGF-1

IGF-1 is a mitogen so named because of its sequence homology to pro-insulin. IGF-1 plays a central role in regulating cell cycle progression from G1 to S phase by activating the phosphatidylinositol 3-kinase (PI3K)/Akt signal transduction pathway and modulating cyclin- dependent kinases (Sara and Hall 1990; Baserga 1994; Bellanger and Bray 2005). IGF-1 can also significantly suppress apoptosis in a variety of cell types, and cells overexpressing IGF-1 receptor show decreased apoptosis (Dunn et al. 1998; Resnicoff et al. 1995). IGF-1 is thus a major endocrine and paracrine regulator of tissue growth and metabolism. IGF-1's involvement in cancer was first suspected when in vitro studies consistently showed that supplementation of culture media with IGF-1 enhances the growth of a variety of cancer cell lines (Macaulay 1992; LeRoith et al. 1995; Singh et al. 1996; Fenton et al. 2005). There is also abundant epidemiologic evidence supporting the hypothesis that IGF-1 is involved in several types of human cancers (Hankinson et al. 1998; Chan et al. 1998; Wolk et al. 2001; Yu et al. 1999; Ma et al. 1999; Giovannucci et al. 2000; Petridou et al. 1999). IGF-1 may be acting either directly on cell via its receptor, IGF-1 receptor, or indirectly through interaction with other cancer-related molecules such as the tumor suppressor p53 (Buckbinder et al. 1995; Takahashi and Suzuki 1993). Levels of circulating IGF-1 are determined primarily by growth hormone-regulated hepatic synthesis, which is influenced by dietary intake of energy and protein

(Hursting et al. 1993). To a lesser extent, IGF-1 synthesis can also occur in extra hepatic tissues, but this involves a complex integration of signals involving growth hormone, other hormones and growth factors and IGF binding proteins, which determine the local availability of IGF-1 and systemic half-life (LeRoith et al. 1995).

Downstream targets of the IGF-1 receptor and insulin receptor comprise a signaling network that regulates cellular growth and metabolism predominately through induction of the PI3K/Akt pathway (Pollak et al. 2004). The importance of this signaling cascade in human cancers has recently been highlighted by the observation that it is one of the most commonly altered pathways in human epithelial tumors. Engagement of the PI3K/Akt pathway allows both intracellular and environmental cues, such as energy availability and growth factor supply, to affect cell growth, proliferation, survival and metabolism. Activation of receptor tyrosine kinases and/or the Ras proto-oncogene stimulates PI3K to produce the lipid second messenger, phosphatidyl-inositol-3,4,5-*tris*phosphate. Phosphatidyl-inositol-3,4,5-*tris*phosphate recruits and anchors Akt to the cell membrane where it can be further phosphorylated and activated (Pollak et al. 2004; Yuan and Cantley 2008; Engelman 2009; Franke 2008). Akt is a cyclic adenosine 3',5'-monophosphate-dependent, cyclic guanosine-monophosphate dependent protein kinase C that when constitutively active is sufficient for cellular transformation by stimulating cell cycle progression and cell survival as well as inhibiting apoptosis (Brazil et al. 2004; Guertin and Sabatini 2005). Ultimately, activation of mTOR results in cell growth, cell proliferation and resistance to apoptosis (Hursting et al. 2007; Lin et al. 2010). An important convergent point for these signaling cascades is the tumor suppressor, tuberous sclerosis complex (TSC) (Astrinidis and Henske 2005; Inoki et al. 2005; Tee and Blenis 2005). Briefly, the TSC binds to and sequesters Rheb, a G-protein required for mTOR activation, thus inhibiting mTOR and downstream targets. However, phosphorylation of the TSC elicits inactivation and Rheb is released, allowing for direct interaction with adenosine triphosphate (ATP) and subsequent activation of mTOR (Fig. 18.1). Alternatively, when the TSC is inhibited, Rheb is able to phosphorylate and activate mTOR (Woods et al. 1998).

Leptin

Leptin, originally identified in 1994 as the 16 kDa product of the *ob* gene (Zhang et al. 1994) may also be important in central nervous system (CNS) responses to obesity. Leptin is a peptide hormone secreted from adipocytes that is involved with appetite control and energy metabolism through its effects on the hypothalamus. Leptin is best known for its action as an afferent adiposity signal to the brain that suppresses appetite and increases energy expenditure (Friedman and Halaas 1998). Leptin enters the brain via a saturable transport mechanism (Banks et al. 1996) and it is known that leptin acts on hypothalamic centers to regulate feeding behavior. Leptin receptors are widely expressed in numerous extra-hypothalamic regions of the brain, including the hippocampus, cerebellum, amygdale, and brain

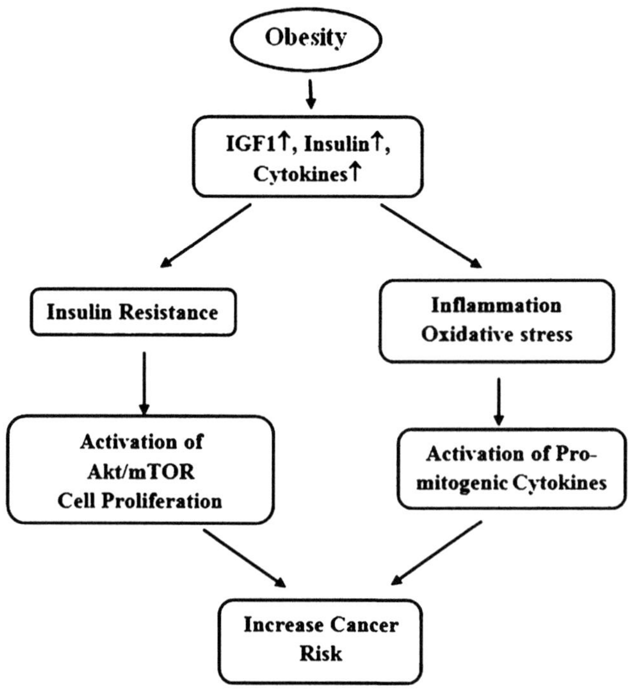

Fig. 18.1 Insulin, insulin-like growth factor-1 (IGF-1), glucocorticoids and several adipose-derived factors (such as leptin and adiponectin) associated with inflammation and cell proliferation

stem (Elmquist et al. 1998; Tartaglia et al. 1995; Fei et al. 1997). While the full extant of leptin's actions on the brain have not been characterized, the past decade of research has not only revealed that leptin receptors are widely expressed in the CNS, but has also identified numerous additional functions for this hormone in the brain (Harvey 2007).

In the non-obese state, rising leptin levels result in decreased appetite through a series of neuroendocrine changes. The obese state is associated with high circulating levels of leptin (Woods et al. 1998; Zhang and Leibel 1998; Lonnqvist et al. 1997; Montague et al. 1997) suggesting that the obese may develop leptin resistance. This resistance appears to explain much of the inability of exogenous leptin administration to prevent weight gain and may result in a higher 'set point' for body weight (Brennan and Mantzoros 2006). The limited number of studies to date is suggestive of an association between circulating leptin levels and cancer risk, with the most consistent findings thus far for colon (Stattin et al. 2004) and prostate cancer (Chang et al. 2001; Saglam et al. 2003). In vitro, leptin stimulates proliferation of multiple types of preneoplastic and neoplastic cells (but not 'normal') cells (Fenton et al. 2005) and in animal models it appears to promote angiogenesis and tumor invasion (Bouloumie et al. 1998). The primary physiologic role of leptin may be the regulation of energy homeostasis by providing a signal to the central nervous system regarding the size of fat stores, as circulating leptin levels correlate strongly with adipose tissue levels in animals and humans (Ostlund et al. 1996). The canonical pathway that transduces leptin's signal from its receptor is the Janus kinase 2/signal transducer and activator of transcription three pathway (Villanueva and Myers 2008). Leptin may also exerts its metabolic effects, at least in part, by activating AMPK in muscle and liver, thus decreasing several anabolic pathways (including glucose-regulated transcription and fatty acid and triglyceride synthesis) and increasing several ATP producing catabolic pathways. Furthermore, leptin plays a role in regulating the hypothalamus/pituitary/adrenal axis and thus influences IGF-1 synthesis (Rajala and Scherer 2003). In addition, there is emerging evidence of cross talk between the Janus kinase/signal transducer and activator of transcription family of transcription factors, the insulin/ IGF-1/Akt pathway and AMPK (Gonzalez et al. 2006). Finally, leptin functions as an inflammatory cytokine and appears to influence immune function, possibly by triggering release of interleukin-6 (IL-6) and other obesity-related cytokines (Fenton et al. 2005; Loffreda et al. 1998). Thus, although not well-studied to date, leptin can certainly be positioned as a central player in the energy balance and cancer association.

Adiponectin

Adiponectin is a 28 kDa peptide hormone produced by adipocytes and intimately involved in the regulation of insulin sensitivity and carbohydrate and lipid metabolism. The link between adiponectin and cancer risk is not well-characterized, although there is a report that adiponectin infusion inhibits endothelial proliferation and inhibits transplanted fibrosarcoma growth (Bråkenhielm et al. 2004). Plasma levels of adiponectin, in contrast with other adipokines, are decreased in response to several metabolic impairments, including type 2 diabetes, dyslipidemia and extreme obesity. Recent findings suggest leptin and adiponectin interact antagonistically to influence carcinogenesis (Grossmann et al. 2008; Ray et al. 2007).

Steroid Hormones

Steroid hormones including estrogens, androgens, progesterone and adrenal steroids, reportedly play a role in the relationship between energy balance and certain types of cancer (Fig. 18.2). Adipose tissue is the main site of estrogen synthesis in men and postmenopausal (or otherwise ovarian hormone deficient) women, through the ability of aromatase (a P450 enzyme present in adipose tissue) to convert androgenic precursors produced in the adrenals and gonads to estrogens. Moreover, adipose tissue is the second major source of circulating IGF-1, after liver. The increased insulin and bioactive IGF-1 levels that typically accompany increased adiposity can feedback to reduce levels of sex hormone-binding globulin,

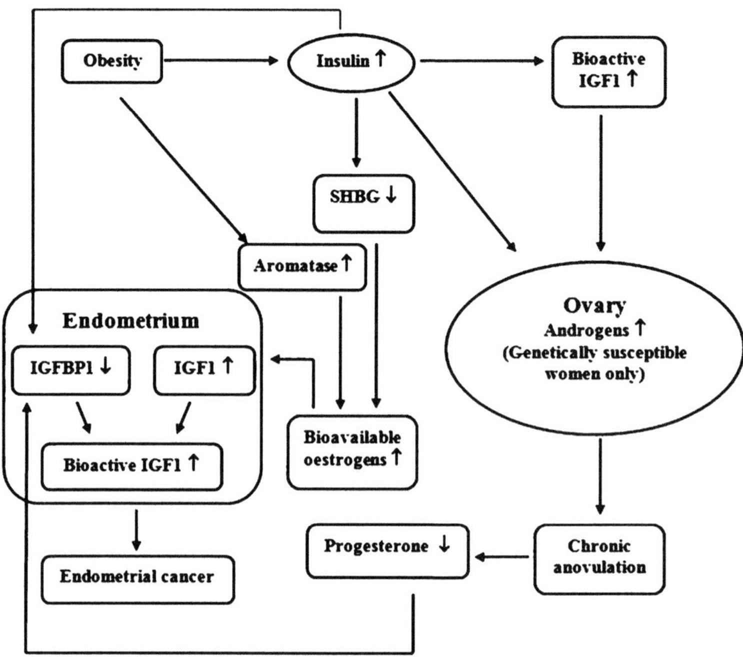

Fig. 18.2 Effect of obesity on hormones and endometrial cancer. Obesity can increase risk of endometrial cancer through several parallel endocrine pathways

resulting in an increased fraction of bio-available estradiol in both men and women (Calle et al. 2003). The epidemiologic literature clearly suggests that the increased bioavailability of sex steroids that accompanies increased adiposity is strongly associated with risk of endometrial and postmenopausal breast cancers (Kaaks et al. 2002) and may impact colon and other cancers as well. Overweight women are known to have increased risk of endometrial cancer and breast cancer after menopause due to increased levels of circulating estrogen. Glucocorticoid hormones have long been known to inhibit tumor promotion (Boutwell 1964). Obesity is associated with increased insulin levels, which lead to increases in insulin-like growth factor-1 (IGF-1) activity and, in some individuals, an increased androgen production by the ovaries. An excessive increase in ovarian androgen production inhibits ovulation (chronic anovulation), which leads to progesterone deficiency. Increased adiposity also increases aromatase activity, leading to increased levels of bioavailable oestrogen levels in postmenopausal women. Oestrogens increase endometrial cell proliferation and inhibit apoptosis, partially by stimulating the local synthesis of IGF-1 in endometrial tissue. Progesterone normally counteracts these effects through various mechanisms, in part by promoting synthesis of IGF-binding protein-1 (IGFBP-1) the most abundant IGFBP in endometrial tissue.

Among premenopausal women, the lack of progesterone, because of ovarian androgen production and continuous anovulation, leads to reduced production of

IGFBP-1 by the endometrium. Loss of progesterone production therefore seems to be the most important physiological risk factor for cancer in premenopausal women. After menopause (and in the absence of exogenous oestrogen production), when ovarian progesterone synthesis has ceased altogether, the more central risk factor seems to be obesity-related increases in bioavailable oestrogen levels. In addition to oestrogens and progesterone, insulin itself could also promote endometrial cancer development by reducing concentrations of sex-hormone-binding globulin (SHBG) in the blood, which would increase the levels of bio-available oestrogens that can diffuse into endometrial tissue (Calle and Kaaks 2004).

Inflammation

The association between chronic inflammation and cancer is well established (Coussens and Werb 2002) as is the link between obesity and inflammation (Hursting et al. 2003). In obesity, increased release from adipose tissue of free fatty acids (FFA), tumour-necrosis factor (TNF-α) and resistin, and reduced release of adiponectin lead to the development of insulin resistance and compensatory, chronic hyperinsulinaemia. Increased insulin levels, in turn, lead to reduced liver synthesis and blood levels of insulin-like growth factor binding protein-1 (IGFBP-1), and probably also reduce IGFBP-1 synthesis locally in other tissues (Fig. 18.3). Increased fasting levels of insulin in the plasma are generally also associated with reduced levels of IGFBP-2 in the blood. This results in increased levels of bio-available IGF-1. Insulin and IGF-1 signal through the insulin receptors (IRs) and IGF-1 receptor (IGF-1R), respectively, to promote cellular proliferation and inhibit apoptosis in many tissue types (Calle and Kaaks 2004). In general, acute inflammation is a process that is beneficial to the host by providing protection from invading pathogens and initiating wound healing. In the acute phase response, the pro-inflammatory cytokines tumor necrosis factor-alpha (TNF-α) and IL-1β are produced locally at the site of infection by macrophages. These cytokines stimulate the release of IL-6, which has been shown to have both pro- and anti-inflammatory effects (Tilg et al. 1997) and the secretion of C-reactive protein by the liver into the blood and increased release from adipose tissue of free fatty acids and resistin (Ceciliani et al. 2002; Mittendorfer et al. 2009; Park et al. 2005). Following clearance of the infection, the production of IL-1β and TNF-α is dampened by the production and release of IL-1 receptor antagonist and soluble TNF-α receptors, respectively, thus altering signal transduction via these receptors (Dinarello 2000). Additionally, IL-10, an anti-inflammatory cytokine produced by T-lymphocytes, works by inhibiting the production of IL-6 and by deactivating pro-inflammatory macrophages (Moore et al. 1993; Pretolani 1999). In contrast to the acute inflammatory response, chronic (low grade) systemic inflammation, which typically accompanies obesity, has been described as a perpetual inflammatory

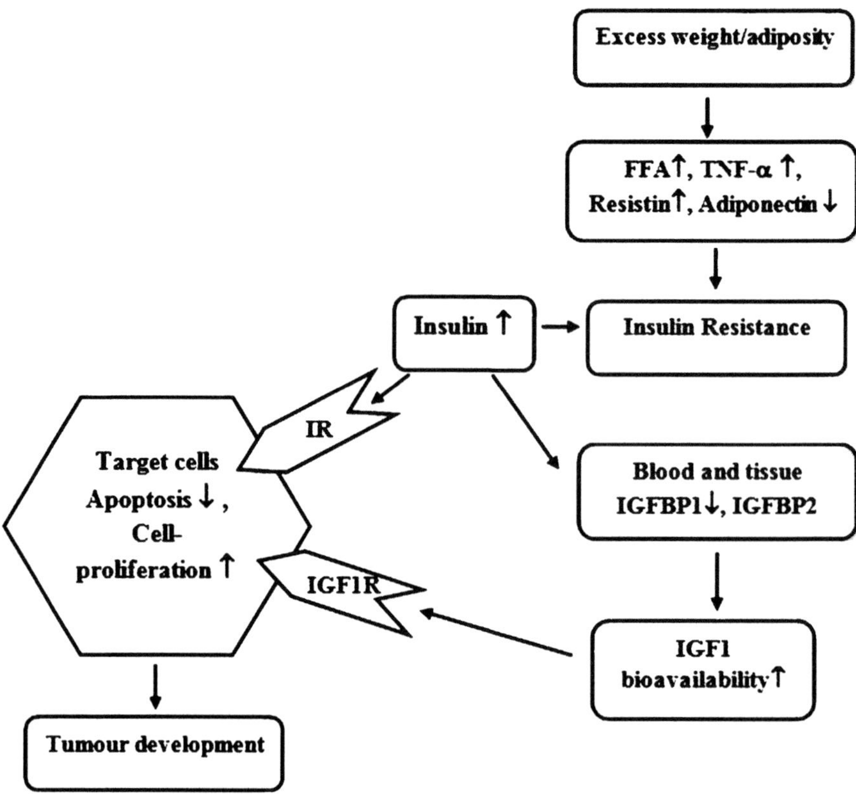

Fig. 18.3 Effects of obesity and chronic inflammation. In obesity, increased release from adipose tissue of free fatty acids (*FFA*), tumour-necrosis factor (*TNF-α*) and resistin, and reduced release of adiponectin lead to the development of insulin resistance and compensatory, chronic hyperinsulinaemia and promote cellular proliferation and tumour development

process in which there is a two to three fold increase in the circulating levels of TNF-α IL-1β, IL-6, IL-1 receptor antagonist, soluble TNF-α receptors and C-reactive protein. Unlike acute inflammation, the origin of the cytokine cascade that accompanies obesity is not believed to be due to the presence of a foreign pathogen.

The cause of elevated cytokines with chronic systemic inflammation is not well understood, although adipocytes as well as immune cells (such as macrophages) within adipose tissue of obese subjects are known sources of pro-inflammatory mediators such as IL-6, IL-1β and TNF-α. In addition, the type of macrophage present in the adipose tissue may also affect the extent and degree of the inflammatory response. Adipose tissue macrophages are recruited in response to the adipocyte enlargement that occurs due to excessive nutrient intake (Lumeng et al. 2007).

Obesity and Psychopathology

Obesity is the most common chronic physical illness in modern society, and depression is the most prevalent psycho-pathological condition. Despite the high prevalence of these conditions, exploration of any association between them has been limited. A number of mechanisms exist through which depression and obesity may be linked. Symptoms of depression correlate significantly with reported body image dissatisfaction (Friedman et al. 2002; Sarwer et al. 1998; Smith et al. 1999). Severely obese person may understandably experience many of the symptoms of depression. The stigmatization and discrimination experienced by obese subjects cause major psychosocial distress (Kaminsky and Gadaleta 2002; Rand and Macgregor 1990) and major psychosocial disturbance (Stunkard and Wadden 1992) which may cause or aggravate a depressive illness. In addition, repeated failed attempts to lose weight are the norm, and this failure may be accompanied by thoughts of guilt, hopelessness, and poor self-esteem (Wooley and Garner 1991). Obesity is associated with a high prevalence of binge eating disorder, which is frequently accompanied by depression and seen more commonly in those attempting to lose weight (de Zwaan 2001; Smith et al. 1998). Serious health consequences and physical disability often accompany severe obesity, and these in turn may aggravate depression. Research relating obesity to psychological disorders and emotional distress is based on clinical studies and community studies of patients seeking treatment. Overweight people seeking weight loss treatment may, in clinic settings, show emotional disturbances (Stunkard and Rush 1974; Prather and Williamson 1988; Fitzgibbon et al. 1993). In a review of dieting and depression, there was a high incidence of emotional illness symptoms in outpatients treated for obesity (Stunkard and Rush 1974). People's negative attitudes toward the obese often translate into discrimination in employment opportunities (Larkin and Pines 1979; Pingitore et al. 1994; Roe and Eickwort 1976), college acceptance, less financial aid from their parents in paying for college (Crandall and Biernat 1990; Crandall 1991), job earnings (Sargent and Blanchflower 1994) and opportunities for marriage (Gortmaker et al. 1993). While the consequences of obesity on metabolic and cardiovascular physiology are well established, epidemiological and experimental data are beginning to establish that the central nervous system may also be detrimentally affected by obesity and obesity-induced metabolic dysfunction. In particular, available data show that obesity in human populations is associated with cognitive decline and enhanced vulnerability to brain injury, while experimental studies in animal models confirm a profile of heightened vulnerability and decreased cognitive function.

Obesity is an increasingly prevalent public health problem, with approximately half the current US population overweight or obese. Although many studies have shown that obesity is associated with numerous medical complications and increased all-cause mortality (Allison and Pi-Sunyer 1995) much less is known about its association with clinical depression and suicidal tendencies. Clinical

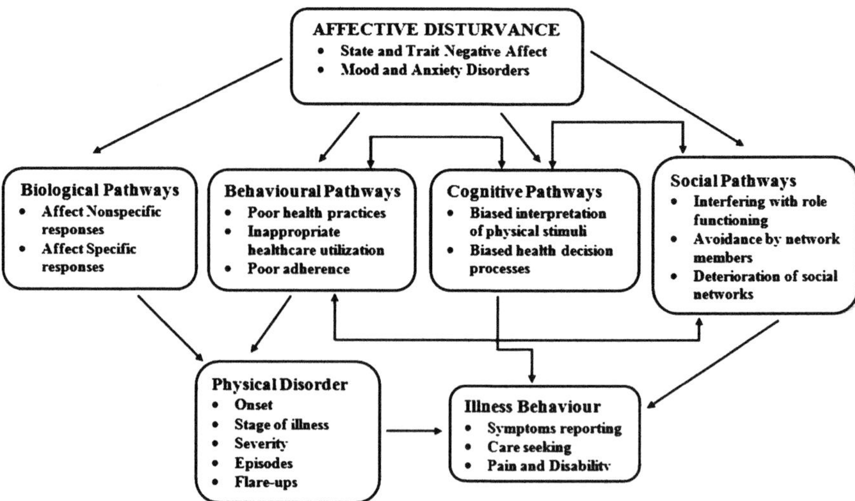

Fig. 18.4 Pathways linking affective disturbances to physical disorders

observations since the turn of the century have postulated a possible association between obesity and depression (Faith et al. 1997). These observations have received some support from epidemiologic studies suggesting a relationship between being overweight and having increased psychiatric symptoms (Moore et al. 1962; Istvan et al. 1992). Obesity is a risk factor for stroke, dementia, intracranial hypertension, and sleep disorders (Bellanger and Bray 2005) and mild to moderately symptoms of depression are often encountered in obese patients, or in patients with eating disorders (Musante et al. 1998; Porzelius et al. 1995; Tanco et al. 1998; Telch and Agras 1994; Troisi et al. 2001). A recent systematic review and meta-analysis on the longitudinal relationship between depression and obesity (Luppino et al. 2010) confirms reciprocal link between the two disorders. Thus, obesity seems to increase the risk of depression, and depression could be predictive of obesity as well. This inference is in agreement with those made in a prospective cohort study with four measures of common mental disorders (Kivimäki et al. 2009).

Taken together, these and numerous other preclinical and clinical observations clearly point out that proper management of mental health problems is necessary not only for palliative care but also for prevention of obesity and associated medical conditions. A conceptual framework proposed during mid 1990s (Cohen and Rodriguez 1995) and summarized in the Fig. 18.4, could be an useful starting point not only for gaining more precise information on biological pathways potentially involved in co-morbidity of physical and psychological health problems, but also for discovering preventive and curative measures against diverse spectrums of co-morbidities.

Dietary Prevention and Therapy

The World Cancer Report predicts that worldwide new cases of cancer will increase by 50% by 2020 and will present a huge challenge for health and cancer support services. It is estimated that eating healthily, staying physically active and maintaining a healthy body weight could reduce cancer risk (Wolin et al. 2010). It is now well established that a plant-based diet including fiber rich foods and a wide range of vitamins and minerals may offer cancer protection, while obesity and low levels of physical activity may increase cancer risk. In the past, chemoprotective ability of nutrients has been widely debated, but there is now consistent and clearer experimental evidences suggesting such potentials of vegetables and fruits. Fruit and vegetables are high in fiber, vitamins and minerals and phytochemicals (plant compounds that are biologically active in humans). There is now considerable evidence that combinations of these constituents of vegetables and fruits work together to protect against cancer genesis, and can also afford protection against diverse pathologies associated with obesity and cancer. It has been estimated that diets containing substantial and varied amounts of fruit and vegetables will prevent 20% or more of all cases of cancer (WCRF/AICR 2007). An important mechanism underpinning the association relates to oxidative stress, a process which can damage DNA. Inability to repair such oxidative damages ultimately leads to cancer, and it is now well established that diverse types of naturally occurring and other antioxidants can afford protection against cellular oxidative damages. Some well known dietary antioxidants with demonstrated chemopreventive potentials are:

- Carotenoids – a group of over 600 yellow-orange pigments that give color to a variety of fruit and vegetables such as carrots, apricots and pink grapefruit. Examples include b-carotene, a precursor of vitamin A, and lycopene which is found in tomatoes.
- Vitamins, particularly C and E – vitamin C is found in many fruits and vegetables such as citrus fruits, spinach and tomatoes. Vitamin E is mainly found in vegetable oils, nuts and seeds.
- Flavonoids and polyphenolics – a group of more than 2,000 compounds that are found in fruit and vegetables, as well as in coffee, tea, beer and wine. Flavonoids like Quercetin, catechins and other flavonoids have been linked to anti-cancer activity. Quercetin is found in berries, apples and broccoli. Catechins are present in green and black tea.
- Selenium – a trace element important for the body's antioxidant defenses. It is found mainly in nuts, particularly Brazil nuts, but it is also in cereal grains and fish.

Plants have since long been used in the treatment of cancer (Hartwell 1982) and the US National Cancer Institute collected about 35,000 plant samples from 20 countries and has screened around 114,000 extracts for anticancer activity (Shoeb 2006). Current interest of modern therapeutic researchers in edible plants was triggered only by epidemiological observations made during mid 1970s (Armstrong

Table 18.3 Protective effects of some phytochemicals consumed with food against cancer growth (DeWeerdt 2011)

Phytochemical	Food material	Cancer type	Studied in
Anthocyanins (A class of Flavonoid)	Cranberry and other berries	Various	In vitro; human cell lines (Ferguson et al. 2004)
Isothiocyanates	Brocccoli	Breast	Human female (Ambrosone et al. 2004)
Resveratrol	Red wine	Glioma (brain)	Rats with gliomas (Tseng et al. 2004)
Lycopene	Tomato	Prostrate	Human male (Etminan et al. 2004)
Curcumin	Turmeric; curry	Pancreas	Mice; human (Perkins et al. 2002; Cruz-Correa et al. 2006)

and Doll 1975) suggesting that eating more fruits and vegetables could reduce risk of several cancers. Extensive efforts made since then have identified several phytochemicals commonly consumed with food as potential chemopreventive agents. A few experimentally better studied food items together with their major identified bioactive constituents are summarized in Table 18.3. However, many questions concerning more realistic use of this knowledge for preventive or therapeutic purposes still remain unanswered (DeWeerdt 2011). Concentrated efforts are now being made in several laboratories to more rationally evaluate and clinically verify their therapeutic potentials. Till now these efforts have not only revealed the complexities of the issues involved in evaluating therapeutic potentials of edible plants and food, but also have pointed out novel possibilities for discovering hits and leads potentially useful for combating obesity associated cancer and other comorbidities.

Presently, dietary therapies consist of high potassium, low sodium diet, with no fats or oils, and minimal animal proteins. Juices of raw fruits and vegetables and of raw liver are often used to facilitate rehabilitation of the liver. For diverse reasons iodine and niacin supplementation are also often recommended. Caffeine enemas cause dilation of bile ducts, which facilitates excretion of toxic cancer breakdown products by the liver and dialysis of toxic products from blood across the colonic wall. The therapy must be used as an integrated whole (Gerson 1978). The incidence and mortality of hormone-related cancers such as breast, endometrial, and prostate cancer vary around the world, being higher in the Western world than in Asian countries (Parkin et al. 2005). Phytoestrogens are natural estrogen-like substances in plant foods and their two major classes are isoflavones and lignans. The two most important isoflavones are genistein and daidzein and their richest dietary source is soybeans. Animal and in vitro studies have provided evidence that phytoestrogens may play a significant inhibitory role during the initiation and promotion of breast and prostate cancer (Magee and Rowland 2004). The epidemiologic evidence for a protective role of phytoestrogens on breast and prostate cancer has been reviewed (Peeters et al. 2003; Boccardo et al. 2006; McCann et al. 2005).

The IARC concluded that in experimental animals, there is limited but sufficient evidence for a cancer-preventive effect of avoidance of weight gain by calorie restriction, based on studies of spontaneous and chemically induced cancers of the mammary gland, liver, pituitary gland (adenoma), and pancreas, for chemically induced cancers of the colon, skin (nonmelanoma), and prostate, and for spontaneous and genetically induced lymphoma. An association between overweight and obesity and cancer at many sites is consistent with animal studies showing that caloric restriction dramatically decreases spontaneous and carcinogen-induced tumor incidence, multiplicity, and size (Dunn et al. 1998; Hursting et al. 1997). Possible mechanisms involved in these observations include altered carcinogen metabolism, decreased oxidative DNA damage, greater DNA repair capacity (IARC, 2002) and a reduction of IGF-1 levels in calorie-restricted animals (Dunn et al. 1997). Wide spread uses of diverse dietary practices in palliative care and as adjuvant therapies are now quite well accepted and recommended by most modern oncological practitioners around the globe.

Carcinogenesis is a multistage process; cells susceptible to genetic changes (initiation) and epigenetic changes (promotions) may gain a growth advantage and undergo clonal expansion. Genetic changes are considered to result from interactions between DNA and a carcinogen/mutagen, which can be metabolised into an electrophilic intermediate and bind to DNA. If repair of the damage does not occur, replication of DNA can lead to permanent DNA lesion and in presence of a tumor promotor to preneoplastic cells, neoplastic cells and finally metastases (Harris 1991). At each stage of the carcinogenic process a possibility of intervention exists. One possible anticarcinogenic intervention is via modulation of metabolism of carcinogenic/mutagenic compounds, thereby preventing the formation of electrophilic intermediates. This modulation of metabolism comprises inhibition of activation of promutagens/procarcinogens, induction of detoxifying mechanisms, and stimulation of activation coordinated with detoxification and blocking of reactive metabolites (De Flora et al. 1993). Involved in this modulation are phase 1 and phase 2 biotransformation enzymes (Jakoby 1980). Phase 1 involves oxidation, reduction and hydrolysis reactions, thereby making xenobiotics more hydrophilic (which can result in inhibition of activation but also inactivation of the compound) as well as susceptible to detoxification. The most important phase 1 enzymes are the cytochrome P450 enzymes. Phase 2 metabolisms, a detoxifying mechanism, comprises conjugation reactions making phase 1 metabolites, more polar and readily excretable. Examples of phase 2 enzymes are glutathione S-transferases and UDP-glucuronyl transferases. Alteration of biotransformation enzyme activities is supposed to be involved, at least partly, in the alteration of the toxicity, mutagenicity and tumorigenicity of specific chemicals (NCM 1994).

Isothiocyanates and indoles, both glucosinolate hydrolysis products, are considered to be able to modulate biotransformation enzyme activities (McDanell et al. 1988; NCM 1994; Boone et al. 1990; Zhang and Talalay 1994). Plant of Brassicaseae family contains glucosinolates, glycosides, flavonoids, phenolic compounds, sterols and triterpene alcohols and other phytoconstituents (Sang et al. 1984; Hill et al. 1987; Kim et al. 2002; Yokozawa et al. 2002; Yoon et al. 2007).

Many studies showed an inverse association between the consumption of various Brassica vegetables and cancer risk. The results of the epidemiological studies agree with results of experimental studies in which Brassica vegetables reduced mammary tumor incidence, hepatic tumor size, number of tumors per liver, tumor frequency and the number of pulmonary metastases when given to rodents before or after a carcinogen insult (Wattenberg 1983; Wattenberg et al. 1989; Stoewsand et al. 1978, 1988; Bresnick et al. 1990; Boyd et al. 1982; Scholar et al. 1989; Srisangam et al. 1980). The relatively high glucosinolate content of Brassica has been suggested to partly cause the anticarcinogenic effects, because certain hydrolysis products of glucosinolates, namely indoles and isothiocyanates, have shown anticarcinogenic properties. The possible anticarcinogenic activity of isothiocyanates and indoles appears to stem mainly from their ability to influence phase 1 and 2 biotransformation enzyme activities (Zhang and Talalay 1994; Boone et al. 1990; McDanell et al. 1988). Phase 1 and 2 biotransformation enzymes are involved in the modulation of metabolism of carcinogenic/mutagenic compounds, thereby preventing the formation of electrophilic intermediates (Jakoby 1980). Electrophilic intermediates can bind to DNA. If repair of the damage does not occur, replication of DNA can lead to permanent DNA lesion and in presence of a tumor promotor, to preneoplastic cells, neoplastic cells, and finally metastases (Harris 1991). Phase 1 involves oxidation, reduction, and hydrolysis reactions, thereby making xenobiotics more hydrophilic (which can result in inhibition of activation but also in activation of the compound) as well as susceptible to detoxification. Phase 2 metabolisms, a detoxifying mechanism, comprises conjugation reactions making phase 1 metabolites more polar and readily excretable (Jakoby 1980). Indoles thereby also affect estradiol metabolism, which is P450 dependent, and may reduce the risk of estrogen-dependent diseases such as mammary cancer (Davis et al. 1993). Besides modulators of biotransformation enzymes isothiocyanates are seen as suppressing agents (Wattenberg 1992). Suppressing agents act during the promotion phase of the neoplastic process via prevention of the evolution of the neoplastic process in cells.

Glucosinolates and some of their metabolites have also been shown to be mutagenic and weakly genotoxic effects (Conaway et al. 2002; Mawson et al. 1994a, b; Mithen et al. 2000; Burel et al. 2001). A recent preclinical study in our laboratories demonstrated beneficial effect of *Brassica juncea leaf* extract in co-morbid anxiety and depression associated with diabesity, i.e. a metabolic disorder commonly encountered in obese individuals (Thakur and Kumar 2010a, b). This extract also demonstrated significant nootropic and anti-oxidant activity in diabetic and non-diabetic rats (unpublished data). Crude juice extracts of a number of Brassica vegetables all caused genotoxic effects in the absence of metabolic activation measured as point mutations in Salmonella strains, repairable DNA damage in *E. coli* K-12 cells, and clastogenic effects in cultured mammalian cells. In mammalian cells, chromosomal aberrations and sister chromatid exchanges were also described (Kassie et al. 1999). A high oral dose of Allyl isothiocyanate (AITC) in corn oil given five times/ week by gavage for 103 weeks in F344 rats resulted in increased incidences of epithelial hyperplasia and transitional-cell papillomas of the urinary bladder in males, whereas in females subcutaneous fibrosarcomas were observed at the same dose. The reviewers concluded that under the conditions of this bioassay, AITC was carcinogenic for male F344/N rats, causing transitional-cell papillomas in the urinary bladder. Evidence for associating allyl isothiocyanate with subcutaneous fibrosarcomas in female F344/N rats was vague (NTP 1982). In contrast, phenylethyl isothiocyanate was shown to be an inhibitor of tumor formation at several sites in rats and in lungs of A/J mice in various assays (Chung et al. 1996; Stoner et al. 2002; Adam-Rodwell et al. 1993; Rao et al. 1995). However, investigations with indole-3-carbinol present in cruciferous vegetables gave conflicting results: when administered before or at the same time as a chemical carcinogen, it was found to inhibit the developments of cancers of the breast, stomach, colon, lung and liver (Guo et al. 1995). In contrast, in other studies in which indole-3-carbinol was administered after the carcinogen (post initiation) an enhancement of cancer of the liver, thyroid, colon and uterus was observed in rats (Stoner et al. 2002; Kim et al. 1994; Yoshida et al. 2004). The exact mechanisms underlying these controversial results are not entirely elucidated and the therapeutic use of these compounds has been questioned. This is in contrast to the increasing epidemiological evidences that higher intake of cruciferous vegetables is associated with a decreased cancer risk in humans (Higdon et al. 2007).

Since Brassica vegetables are one of the very first and better clinically studies food material as cancer preventing possibility, it has been discussed here in some details. Analogous contradictory, or not easily interpretable, information on numerous other edible phytochemicals and other food components are littered throughout the literature of modern nutritional medicine and food sciences. In view of the situation the findings summarized in a recent systematic review and meta-analysis of available information on epidemiological studies on fruits and vegetables are not surprising (Key 2011). Although this study does not completely negate preventive potentials of fruits and vegetables, it revealed only their marginal, and questionable, benefits in reducing cancer incidents in general. Critical analysis of the situation have clearly pointed out that the questions concerning how much and how often of which fruits and vegetables will be necessary for cancer prevention has to be solved first before their beneficial effects can be properly evaluated (Moiseeva and Manson 2009). Unfortunately, till now little concentrated efforts have been made to more rationally answer such and diverse other related questions. Close collaborative efforts between nutritional scientists trained in diverse sub-disciplines of modern medicine and diverse types of food industries will be necessary for better clarification of the situation.

Future Perspective

A vast majority of numerous putative etiological factors involved in obesity associated medical conditions identified to date (McAllister et al. 2009) can be effectively controlled or modulated by human behavior. Many of them concerning dietary, physical and sexual activities, and tobacco and alcohol abuses related risk factors are more efficiently modifiable only by each individual person only. Available therapeutic, nutritional, and behavioral preventive recommendations are either ineffective, or not safe enough, or are not assessable and affordable to a vast majority of world population (Holman and White 2011). Despite such knowledge though, as yet little systematic concentrated efforts have been made to identify therapeutic leads and pharmacological targets potentially useful for modifying behaviors involved in choices of appropriate food and physical activities. It is now well established though, that structurally diverse secondary plant metabolites commonly consumed with food have modulating effects on brain functions and behavior as well (Morris et al. 2006; Macready et al. 2009) and that food synergy plays important roles in their modes of actions (Jacobs et al. 2009). Proper uses of such knowledge for evaluating therapeutic potentials of fruits and vegetables according to current concepts of evidence based medicine will be possible only when well known facts on food and psychobiological processes are kept in mind. Some such facts are:

- All edibles are not equal in their chemical composition, and it their combination of different doses and consumption modalities that dictate the ultimate biological effects of food.
- Contents of bio-active constituents, their bioavailability, and metabolism of a given vegetable or fruit is dependant only on growing and harvesting conditions used but also on the cooking and other processing methods used.
- Some phyto-nutrients are difficult to access or are costly. Some are found in small quantities in bulky foodstuffs, whereas some others commonly consumed in larger quantities could have inhibitory effects on beneficial effects of others.
- Human microbiome spectrum varies considerably amongst diverse populations, and a vast majority of known edible phytochemicals are metabolized by gut micro-biota. Analogous is also the case for human genomes which also dictate bioavailability and metabolic spectrum of almost all chemicals consumed.
- In epidemiological studies it is difficult, if not impossible, to give due attention to the fact that diet as a whole, ant not specific phytochemicals consumed with it, dictates the efficacy of the phytochemicals studied. This is mainly because only a few of the innumerable possible bioactive food components and body metabolites can yet be reasonably quantified.

Although detailed discussions on these and many other analogous facts are beyond the scope of this chapter, it must be mentioned that reductionist logic commonly used by modern researchers have to wait long before problems arising from such facts can be more reasonably solved or tackled. Consequently, more holistic and approximating strategies for combating the situation seem to be an urgent therapeutic necessity. During more recent years a few such strategies based on post modern concepts of system biology and network biology have been proposed. Most of them necessitate extensive uses of complex and expensive technologies not commonly available, or affordable, in many laboratories interested in evaluating therapeutic potentials of fruits and vegetables. For avoiding problems arising from these, and many other facts, widespread uses of the old fashioned, and more holistic, pharmacological screen procedures using laboratory animals could be a more rational and feasible approach not only for identifying more healthy vegetables and fruits but also for identifying more economically affordable and culturally better acceptable therapies against obesity and cancer. Hereupon due attention has to be paid to the psychobiological processes associated with, or caused by, these conditions, and attempts should be made to more properly clarify numerous questions very recently pointed out in a review on existing preclinical research problems hampering more appropriate therapeutic uses of plant derived edibles (Martin et al. 2011).

Concluding Remarks

It is common knowledge that food and eating habits have crucial effects on human health and Ayurveda and all other traditionally known or modern integrative health care systems consistently recommend their proper uses and control for maintaining healthy life. Till recently, most such recommendations were based on diverse random observations made during thousands of years of history of human civilization. During more recent years, diverse types of preclinical information on potential health benefits of food have accumulated, and it is now apparent also that food can also be useful for modulating personal food choices, eating habits, and sedentary behavior necessary for combating obesity, cancer and numerous other comorbidities associated with these conditions. Efforts to more reasonably understand health benefits of fruits and vegetables will certainly necessitate closer cooperation and understanding between medical scientists and researchers with the food industry. Better definition and more critical fundamental analysis of the role of food industries in obesity associated and other health problems is just the first essential step for combating the spreading epidemics of the twenty-first century.

References

Abate N (1996) Insulin resistance and obesity. The role of fat distribution pattern. Diabetes Care 19(3):292–294

Adam-Rodwell G, Morse MA, Stoner GD (1993) The effects of phenethyl isothiocyanate on benzo[a]pyrene-induced tumors and DNA adducts in A/J mouse lung. Cancer Lett 71(1–3): 35–42

Allison DB, Pi-Sunyer FX (1995) Obesity treatment: examining the premises. Endocr Pract 1(5):353–364

Ambrosone CB, McCann SE, Freudenheim JL, Marshall JR, Zhang Y, Shields PG (2004) Breast cancer risk in premenopausal women is inversely associated with consumption of broccoli, a source of isothiocyanates, but is not modified by GST genotype. J Nutr 134(5):1134–1138

Ames BN, Shigenaga MK, Hagen TM (1993) Oxidants, antioxidants, and the degenerative diseases of aging. Proc Natl Acad Sci U S A 90(17):7915–7922

Armstrong B, Doll R (1975) Environmental factors and cancer incidence and mortality in different countries, with special reference to dietary practices. Int J Cancer 15(4):617–631
Astrinidis A, Henske EP (2005) Tuberous sclerosis complex: linking growth and energy signaling pathways with human disease. Oncogene 24(50):7475–7481
Banks WA, Kastin AJ, Huang W, Jaspan JB, Maness LM (1996) Leptin enters the brain by a saturable system independent of insulin. Peptides 17(2):305–311
Baserga R (1994) Oncogenes and the strategy of growth factors. Cell 79(6):927–930
Belfiore A, Roberta M (2011) The insulin receptor and cancer. Endocr Relat Cancer 18(4): R125–R147
Bellanger TM, Bray GA (2005) Obesity related morbidity and mortality. J La State Med Soc 157(1):S42–S49
Bergström A, Pisani P, Tenet V, Wolk A, Adami HO (2001) Overweight as an avoidable cause of cancer in Europe. Int J Cancer 91(3):421–430
Boccardo F, Puntoni M, Guglielmini P, Rubagotti A (2006) Enterolactone as a risk factor for breast cancer: a review of the published evidence. Clin Chim Acta 365(1–2):58–67
Boone CW, Kelloff GJ, Malone WE (1990) Identification of candidate cancer chemopreventive agents and their evaluation in animal models and human clinical trials: a review. Cancer Res 50(1):2–9
Bouloumie A, Drexler HC, Lafontan M, Busse R (1998) Leptin, the product of Ob gene, promotes angiogenesis. Circ Res 83(10):1059–1066
Boutwell RK (1964) Some biological aspects of skin carcinogenisis. Prog Exp Tumor Res 4: 207–250
Boyd JN, Babish JG, Stoewsand GS (1982) Modification of beet and cabbage diets of aflatoxin B1-induced rat plasma alpha-foetoprotein elevation, hepatic tumorigenesis, and mutagenicity of urine. Food Chem Toxicol 20(1):47–52
Bråkenhielm E, Veitonmäki N, Cao R, Kihara S, Matsuzawa Y, Zhivotovsky B, Funahashi T, Cao Y (2004) Adiponectin-induced antiangiogenesis and antitumor activity involve caspase-mediated endothelial cell apoptosis. Proc Natl Acad Sci U S A 101(8):2476–2481
Brazil DP, Yang ZZ, Hemmings BA (2004) Advances in protein kinase B signalling: AKTion on multiple fronts. Trends Biochem Sci 29(5):233–242
Brennan AM, Mantzoros CS (2006) Drug insight: the role of leptin in human physiology and pathophysiology – emerging clinical applications. Nat Clin Pract Endocrinol Metab 2(6): 318–327
Bresnick E, Birt DF, Wolterman K, Wheeler M, Markin RS (1990) Reduction in mammary tumorigenesis in the rat by cabbage and cabbage residue. Carcinogenesis 11(7):1159–1163
Bruce-Keller AJ, Keller JN, Morrison CD (2009) Obesity and vulnerability of the CNS. Biochim Biophys Acta 1792(5):395–400
Buckbinder L, Talbott R, Velasco-Miguel S, Takenaka I, Faha B, Seizinger BR, Kley N (1995) Induction of the growth inhibitor IGF-binding protein 3 by p53. Nature 377(6550):646–649
Burel C, Boujard T, Kaushik SJ, Boeuf G, Mol KA, Van der Geyten S, Darras VM, Kühn ER, Pradet-Balade B, Quérat B, Quinsac A, Krouti M, Ribaillier D (2001) Effects of rapeseed mealglucosinolates on thyroid metabolism and feed utilization in rainbow trout. Gen Comp Endocrinol 124(3):343–358
Calle EE, Kaaks R (2004) Overweight, obesity and cancer: epidemiological evidence and proposed mechanisms. Nat Rev Cancer 4(8):579–591
Calle EE, Thun MJ, Petrelli JM, Rodriguez C, Heath CW Jr (1999) Body-mass index and mortality in a prospective cohort of U.S. adults. N Engl J Med 341:1097–1105
Calle EE, Rodriguez C, Walker-Thurmond K, Thun MJ (2003) Overweight, obesity, and mortality from cancer in a prospectively studied cohort of U.S. adults. N Engl J Med 348(17):1625–1638
Ceciliani F, Giordano A, Spagnolo V (2002) The systemic reaction during inflammation: the acute-phase proteins. Protein Pept Lett 9(3):211–223
Chaldakov GN, Tonchev AB, Manni L, Hristova MG, Nikolova V, Fiore M, Vyagova D, Peneva VN, Aloe L (2009) The adipose tissue as a third brain. Obes Metab 5:94–96

Chaldakov GN, Fiore M, Tonchev AB, Aloe L (2010) Neuroadipology: a novel component of neuroendocrinology. Cell Biol Int 34:1051–1053

Chan JM, Stampfer MJ, Giovannucci E, Gann PH, Ma J, Wilkinson P, Hennekens CH, Pollak M (1998) Plasma insulin-like growth factor-I and prostate cancer risk: a prospective study. Science 279(5350):563–566

Chang S, Hursting SD, Contois JH, Strom SS, Yamamura Y, Babaian RJ, Troncoso P, Scardino PS, Wheeler TM, Amos CI, Spitz MR (2001) Leptin and prostate cancer. Prostate 46(1):62–67

Chung FL, Kelloff G, Steele V, Pittman B, Zang E, Jiao D, Rigotty J, Choi CI, Rivenson A (1996) Chemopreventive efficacy of arylalkyl isothiocyanates and Nacetylcysteine for lung tumorigenesis in Fischer rats. Cancer Res 56:772–778

Cohen S, Rodriguez MS (1995) Pathways linking affective disturbances and physical disorders. Health Psychol 14(5):374–380

Conaway CC, Yang YM, Chung FL (2002) Isothiocyanates as cancer chemopreventive agents: their biological activities and metabolism in rodents and humans. Curr Drug Metab 3(3):233–255

Coussens LM, Werb Z (2002) Inflammation and cancer. Nature 420(6917):860–867

Crandall CS (1991) Do heavy-weight students have more difficulty paying for college? Pers Soc Psychol Bull 17:606–611

Crandall CS, Biernat M (1990) The ideology of anti-fat attitudes. J Appl Soc Psychol 20:227–243

Cruz-Correa M, Shoskes DA, Sanchez P, Zhao R, Hylind LM, Wexner SD, Giardiello FM (2006) Combination treatment with curcumin and quercetin of adenomas in familial adenomatous polyposis. Clin Gastroenterol Hepatol 4(8):1035–1038

Davis DL, Bradlow HL, Wolff M, Woodruff T, Hoel DG, Anton-Culver H (1993) Anton-Culver, medical hypothesis: xeno-estrogens as preventable causes of breast cancer. Environ Health Perspect 101(5):372–377

De Flora S, Izzotti A, Bennicelli C (1993) Mechanisms of antimutagenesis and anticarcinogenesis: role in primary prevention. Basic Life Sci 61:1–16

de Zwaan M (2001) Binge eating disorder and obesity. Int J Obes Relat Metab Disord 25(suppl 1): S51–S55

DeWeerdt S (2011) Food: the omnivore's labyrinth. Nature 471(7339):S22–S24

Diener E, Chan MY (2011) Happy people live longer: subjective well-being contributes to health and longevity. Appl Psychol Health Well-Being Int Assoc Appl Psychol. Blackwell Publishing Ltd., UK 3(1):1–43

Dinarello CA (2000) The role of the interleukin-1-receptor antagonist in blocking inflammation mediated by interleukin-1. N Engl J Med 343(10):732–734

Dunn SE, Kari FW, French J, Leininger JR, Travlos G, Wilson R, Barrett JC (1997) Dietary restriction reduces insulin-like growth factor I levels, which modulates apoptosis, cell proliferation, and tumor progression in p53-deficient mice. Cancer Res 57(21):4667–4672

Dunn SE, Ehrlich M, Sharp NJ, Reiss K, Solomon G, Hawkins R, Baserga R, Barrett JC (1998) A dominant negative mutant of the insulin-like growth factor-I receptor inhibits the adhesion, invasion, and metastasis of breast cancer. Cancer Res 58:3353–3361

Elias MF, Elias PK, Sullivan LM, Wolf PA, D'Agostino RB (2003) Lower cognitive function in the presence of obesity and hypertension: the Framingham Heart Study. Int J Obes Relat Metab Disord 27:260–268

Elias MF, Elias PK, Sullivan LM, Wolf PA, D'Agostino RB (2005) Obesity, diabetes and cognitive deficit: the Framingham Heart Study. Neurobiol Aging 26(suppl 1):11–16

Elmquist JK, Bjørbaek C, Ahima RS, Flier JS, Saper CB (1998) Distributions of leptin receptor mRNA isoforms in the rat brain. J Comp Neurol 395(4):535–547

Engelman JA (2009) Targeting PI3K signalling in cancer: opportunities, challenges and limitations. Nat Rev Cancer 9(8):550–562

Etminan M, Takkouche B, Caamano-Isorna F (2004) The role of tomato products and lycopene in the prevention of prostate cancer: a meta-analysis of observational studies. Cancer Epidemiol Biomarkers Prev 13(3):340–345

Faith MS, Allison DB, Geliebter A (1997) Emotional eating and obesity: theoretical considerations and practical recommendations. In: Dalton S (ed) Overweight and weight management: the health professional's guide to understanding and practice. Aspen, Gaithersburg, pp 439–465. ISBN 9780834206366

Fei H, Okano HJ, Li C, Lee GH, Zhao C, Darnell R, Friedman JM (1997) Anatomic localization of alternatively spliced leptin receptors (Ob-R) in mouse brain and other tissues. Proc Natl Acad Sci U S A 94:7001–7005

Fenton JI, Hord NG, Lavigne JA, Perkins SN, Hursting SD (2005) Leptin, insulin-like growth factor-1, and insulin-like growth factor-2 are mitogens in ApcMin/+ but not Apc+/+ colonic epithelial cell lines. Cancer Epidemiol Biomarkers Prev 14(7):1646–1652

Ferguson PJ, Kurowska E, Freeman DJ, Chambers AF, Koropatnick DJ (2004) A flavonoid fraction from cranberry extract inhibits proliferation of human tumor cell lines. J Nutr 134(6): 1529–1535

Fitzgibbon ML, Stolley MR, Kirschenbaum DS (1993) Obese people who seek treatment have different characteristics than those who do not seek treatment. Health Psychol 12(5):342–345

Franke TF (2008) PI3K/Akt: getting it right matters. Oncogene 27(50):6473–6488

Fraser GE (1999) Associations between diet and cancer, ischemic heart disease, and allcause mortality in non-Hispanic white California Seventh-day Adventists. Am J Clin Nutr 20(suppl 3): 532s–538s

Friedman JM, Halaas JL (1998) Leptin and the regulation of body weight in mammals. Nature 395(6704):763–770

Friedman KE, Reichmann SK, Costanzo PR, Musante GJ (2002) Body image partially mediates the relationship between obesity and psychological distress. Obes Res 10(1):33–41

Gerson M (1978) The cure of advanced cancer by diet therapy: a summary of 30 years of clinical experimentation. Physiol Chem Phys 10(5):449–464

Giovannucci E, Pollak MN, Platz EA, Willett WC, Stampfer MJ, Majeed N, Colditz GA, Speizer FE, Hankinson SE (2000) A prospective study of plasma insulin-like growth factor-1 and binding protein-3 and risk of colorectal neoplasia in women. Cancer Epidemiol Biomarkers Prev 9(4):345–349

Gomez-Pinilla F (2008) The influences of diet and exercise on mental health through hormesis. Ageing Res Rev 7(1):49–62

Gonzalez RR, Cherfils S, Escobar M, Yoo JH, Carino C, Styer AK, Sullivan BT, Sakamoto H, Olawaiye A, Serikawa T, Lynch MP, Rueda BR (2006) Leptin signaling promotes the growth of mammary tumors and increases the expression of vascular endothelial growth factor (VEGF) and its receptor type two (VEGF-R2). J Biol Chem 281(36):26320–26328

Gortmaker SL, Must A, Perrin JM, Sobol AM, Dietz WH (1993) Social and economic consequences of overweight in adolescence and young adulthood. N Engl J Med 329:1008–1012

Greer S (1983) Cancer and the mind. Maudsley Bequest Lecture delivered before the Royal College of Psychiatrists, February 1983. Br J Psychiatry 143:535–543

Grimm JJ (1999) Interaction of physical activity and diet: implications for insulin-glucose dynamics. Public Health Nutr 2(3A):363–368

Grivennikov SI, Greten FR, Karin M (2010) Immunity, inflammation, and cancer. Cell 140(6): 883–899

Grossmann ME, Nkhata KJ, Mizuno NK, Ray A, Cleary MP (2008) Effects of adiponectin on breast cancer cell growth and signaling. Br J Cancer 98(2):370–379

Guertin DA, Sabatini DM (2005) An expanding role for mTOR in cancer. Trends Mol Med 11(8):353–361

Gunstad J, Paul RH, Cohen RA, Tate DF, Spitznagel MB, Gordon E (2007) Elevated body mass index is associated with executive dysfunction in otherwise healthy adults. Compr Psychiatry 48(1):57–61

Guo D, Schut HA, Davis CD, Snyderwine EG, Bailey GS, Dashwood RH (1995) Protection by chlorophyllin and indole-3-carbinol against 2-amino-1-methyl-6-phenylimidazo[4,5-b]pyridine (PhIP)-induced DNA adducts and colonic aberrant crypts in the F344 rat. Carcinognesis 16(12):2931–2937

Haan MN, Wallace R (2004) Can dementia be prevented? Brain aging in a population-based context. Annu Rev Public Health 25:1–24

Hankinson SE, Willett WC, Colditz GA, Hunter DJ, Michaud DS, Deroo B, Rosner B, Speizer FE, Pollak M (1998) Circulating concentrations of insulin-like growth factor-I and risk of breast cancer. Lancet 351(9113):1393–1396

Harris CC (1991) Chemical and physical carcinogenesis: advances and perspectives for the 1990s. Cancer Res 51(suppl 18):5023s–5044s

Hartwell JL (1982) Plants used against cancer: a survey. Quarterman Publications, Lawrence, pp 438–439. ISBN 0880001305

Harvey J (2007) Leptin regulation of neuronal excitability and cognitive function. Curr Opin Pharmacol 7(6):643–647

Hemminki K, Sundquist J, Sundquist K (2011) Obesity and familial obesity and risk of cancer. Eur J Cancer Prev 20(5):438–443

Higdon JV, Delage B, Williams DE, Dashwood RH (2007) Cruciferous vegetables and human cancer risk: epidemiologic evidence and mechanistic basis. Pharmacol Res 55(3):224–236

Hill CB, Williams PH, Carlson DG, Tookey HL (1987) Variation in glucosinolates in oriental brassica vegetables. J Am Soc Hortic Sci 112(2):309–313

Holman DW, White MC (2011) Dietary behaviors related to cancer prevention among pre-adolescents and adolescents: the gap between recommendations and reality. Nutr J 10:60

Hursting SD, Switzer BR, French JE, Kari FW (1993) The growth hormone: insulin-like growth factor 1 axis is a mediator of diet restriction-induced inhibition of mononuclear cell leukemia in Fischer rats. Cancer Res 53(12):2750–2757

Hursting SD, Perkins SN, Brown CC, Haines DC, Phang JM (1997) Calorie restriction induces a p53-independent delay of spontaneous carcinogenesis in p53-deficient and wild-type mice. Cancer Res 57(14):2843–2846

Hursting SD, Lavigne JA, Berrigan D, Perkins SN, Barrett JC (2003) Calorie restriction, aging, and cancer prevention: mechanisms of action and applicability to humans. Annu Rev Med 54: 131–152

Hursting SD, Nunez NP, Varticovski L, Vinson C (2007) The obesity-cancer link: lessons learned from a fatless mouse. Cancer Res 67(6):2391–2393

Hursting SD, Smith SM, Lashinger LM, Harvey AE, Perkins SN (2010) Calories and carcinogenesis: lessons learned from 30 years of calorie restriction research. Carcinogenesis 31(1):83–89

Inoki K, Corradetti MN, Guan KL (2005) Dysregulation of the TSC-mTOR pathway in human disease. Nat Genet 37(1):19–24

Istvan J, Zavela K, Weidner G (1992) Body weight and psychological distress in the NHANES I. Int J Obes Relat Metab Disord 16(12):999–1003

Jacobs DR, Gross MD, Tapsell LC (2009) Food synergy: an operational concept for understanding nutrition. Am J Clin Nutr 89(5):1543S–1548S

Jakoby WB (1980) Enzymatic basis of detoxification, vol I and II. Academic, New York (Vol I-0123800013), (Vol II-0123800021)

Johansson G (2011) Dietary advice on prescription: a novel approach to dietary counseling. Int J Qual Stud Health Well-being 6(2). doi:10.3402/qhw.v6i2.7136

Kaaks R, Lukanova A, Kurzer MS (2002) Obesity, endogenous hormones, and endometrial cancer risk: a synthetic review. Cancer Epidemiol Biomarkers Prev 11(12):1531–1543

Kaminsky J, Gadaleta D (2002) A study of discrimination within the medical community as viewed by obese patients. Obes Surg 12(1):14–18

Kassie F, Pool-Zobel B, Parzefall W, Knasmuller S (1999) Genotoxic effects of benzyl isothiocyanate, a natural chemopreventive agent. Mutagenesis 14(6):595–604

Key TJ (2011) Fruits and vegetables and cancer risk. Br J Cancer 104(1):6–11

Kim DJ, Lee KK, Han BS, Ahn B, Bae JH, Jang JJ (1994) Biphasic modifying effect of indole-3-carbinol on diethylnitrosamine- induced preneoplastic glutathione S-transferase placenta form-positive liver cell foci in Sprague Dawley rat. Jpn J Cancer Res 85(6):578–583

Kim JE, Jung MJ, Jung HA, Woo JJ, Cheigh HS, Chung HY, Choi JS (2002) A new kaempferol 7-O-triglucoside from the leaves of Brassica juncea L. Arch Pharm Res 25(5):621–624

Kivimäki M, Lawlor DA, Singh-Manoux A, Batty GD, Ferrie JE, Shipley MJ, Nabi H, Sabia S, Marmot MG, Jokela M (2009) Common mental disorder and obesity: insight from four repeat measures over 19 years: prospective Whitehall II cohort study. BMJ 339:b3765. doi:10.1136/bmj.b3765

Knecht S, Ellger T, Levine JA (2008) Obesity in neurobiology. Prog Neurobiol 84:85–103

Krishnaswamy K, Polasa K (1995) Diet, nutrition & cancer–the Indian scenario. Indian J Med Res 102:200–209

Kushi LH, Byers T, Doyle C, Bandera EV, McCullough M, McTiernan A, Gansler T, Andrews KS, Thun MJ, American Cancer Society, Nutrition and Physical Activity Guidelines Advisory Committee (2006) American cancer society guidelines on nutrition and physical activity for cancer prevention: reducing the risk of cancer with healthy food choices and physical activity. CA Cancer J Clin 56(5):254–281

Larkin JC, Pines HA (1979) No fat persons need apply: experimental studies of the overweight stereotype and hiring preference. Work Occup 6(3):312–327

LeRoith D, Baserga R, Helman L, Roberts CT (1995) Insulin-like growth factors and cancer. Ann Intern Med 122(1):54–59

Lew EA, Garfinkel L (1979) Variations in mortality by weight among 750,000 men and women. J Chron Dis 32(8):563–576

Lin J, Wang J, Greisinger AJ, Grossman HB, Forman MR, Dinney CP, Hawk ET, Wu X (2010) Energy balance, the PI3K-AKT-mTOR pathway genes, and the risk of bladder cancer. Cancer Prev Res (Phila) 3(4):505–517

Lindsted KD, Singh PN (1998) Body mass and 26 y risk of mortality among men who never smoked: a re-analysis among men from the Adventist Mortality Study. Int J Obes Relat Metab Disord 22(6):544–548

Liu J, Head E, Gharib AM, Yuan W, Ingersoll RT, Hagen TM, Cotman CW, Ames BN (2002) Memory loss in old rats is associated with brain mitochondrial decay and RNA/DNA oxidation: partial reversal by feeding acetyl-L-carnitine and/or R-alpha-lipoic acid. Proc Natl Acad Sci U S A 99(4):2356–2361

Loffreda S, Yang SQ, Lin HZ, Karp CL, Brengman ML, Wang DJ, Klein AS, Bulkley GB, Bao C, Noble PW, Lane MD, Diehl AM (1998) Leptin regulates proinflammatory immune responses. FASEB J 12(1):57–65

Lonnqvist F, Wennlund A, Arner P (1997) Relationship between circulating leptin and peripheral fat distribution in obese subjects. Int J Obes Relat Metab Disord 21(4):255–260

Lovestone S, Fahy T (1991) Psychological factors in breast cancer. BMJ 302(6787):1219–1220

Lumeng CN, Deyoung SM, Bodzin JL, Saltiel AR (2007) Increased inflammatory properties of adipose tissue macrophages recruited during diet-induced obesity. Diabetes 56(1):16–23

Luppino FS, de Witt LM, Stijnen T, Cuijpers P, Penninx BW, Zitman FG (2010) Overweight, obesity, and depression: a systematic review and meta-analysis of longitudinal studies. Arch Gen Psychiatry 67(3):220–229

Ma J, Pollak MN, Giovannucci E, Chan JM, Tao Y, Hennekens CH, Stampfer MJ (1999) Prospective study of colorectal cancer risk in men and plasma levels of insulin-like growth factor (IGF)-I and IGF-binding protein-3. J Natl Cancer Inst 91(7):620–625

Macaulay VM (1992) Insulin-like growth factors and cancer. Br J Cancer 65(3):311–320

Macready AL, Kennedy OB, Ellis JA, Williams CM et al (2009) Flavonoids and cognitive function: a review of human randomized control trial studies and recommendations for future studies. Gene Nutr 4(4):227–242

Magee PJ, Rowland IR (2004) Phyto-oestrogens, their mechanism of action: current evidence for a role in breast and prostate cancer. Br J Nutr 91(4):513–531

Manson JE, Willett WC, Stampfer MJ, Colditz GA, Hunter DJ, Hankinson SE, Hennekens CH, Speizer FE (1995) Body weight and mortality among women. N Engl J Med 333(11):677–685

Martin C, Butelli E, Petroni K, Tonelli C (2011) How can research on plants contribute to promoting human health? Plant Cell 23(5):1685–1699

Mattson MP, Duan W, Guo Z (2003) Meal size and frequency affect neuronal plasticity and vulnerability to disease: cellular and molecular mechanisms. J Neurochem 84(3):417–431

Mawson R, Heaney RK, Zdunczyk Z, Kozłowska H (1994a) Rapeseed meal glucosinolates and their antinutritional effects. Part 3. Animal growth and performance. Nahrung 38(2):167–177

Mawson R, Heaney RK, Zdunczyk Z, Kozłowska H (1994b) Rapeseed meal glucosinolates and their antinutritional effects. Part 4. Goitrogenicity and internal organs abnormalities in animals. Nahrung 38(2):178–191

McAllister EJ, Dhurandhar NV, Keith SW, Aronne LJ, Barger J, Baskin M, Benca RM, Biggio J, Boggiano MM, Eisenmann JC, Elobeid M, Fontaine KR, Gluckman P, Hanlon EC, Katzmarzyk P, Pietrobelli A, Redden DT, Ruden DM, Wang C, Waterland RA, Wright SM, Allison DB (2009) Ten putative contributors to the obesity epidemic. Crit Rev Food Sci Nutr 49(10): 868–913

McCann MJ, Gill CI, McGlynn H, Rowland IR (2005) Role of mammalian lignans in the prevention and treatment of prostate cancer. Nutr Cancer 52(1):1–14

McDanell R, McLean AE, Hanley AB, Heaney RK, Fenwick GR (1988) Chemical and biological properties of indole glucosinolates (glucobrassicins): a review. Food Chem Toxicol 26(1): 59–70

Mithen RF, Dekker M, Verkerk R, Rabot S, Johnson IT (2000) The nutritional significance, biosynthesis and bioavailability of glucosinolates in human food. J Sci Food Agric 80(7): 967–984

Mittendorfer B, Magkos F, Fabbrini E, Mohammed BS, Klein S (2009) Relationship between body fat mass and free fatty acid kinetics in men and women. Obesity (Silver Spring) 17(10): 1872–1877

Moiseeva EP, Manson MM (2009) Dietary chemopreventive phytochemicals: too little or too much? Cancer Prev Res (Phila) 2:611–616

Montague CT, Prins JB, Sanders L, Digby JE, O'Rahilly S (1997) Depot- and sex-specific differences in human leptin mRNA expression: implications for the control of regional fat distribution. Diabetes 46(3):342–347

Moore ME, Stunkard A, Srole L (1962) Obesity, social class, and mental illness. JAMA 181: 962–966

Moore KW, O'Garra A, de Waal MR, Vieira P, Mosmann TR (1993) Interleukin-10. Annu Rev Immunol 11:165–190

Morris MC, Evans DA, Tangney CC, Bienias JL, Wilson RS (2006) Association of vegetables and fruit consumption with age related cognitive functions. Neurology 67(8):1370–1376

Musante GJ, Costanzo PR, Friedman KE (1998) The comorbidity of depression and eating dysregulation processes in a diet-seeking obese population: a matter of gender specificity. Int J Eat Disord 23(1):65–75

National Institutes of Health (NIH) (1998) Clinical guidelines on the identification, evaluation, and treatment of overweight and obesity in adults. The evidence report. Obes Res 6(suppl 2): 51S–209S

National Task Force on the Prevention and Treatment of Obesity (NTFPTO) (2000) Overweight, obesity, and health risk. Arch Intern Med 160(7):898–904

National Toxicology Program (NTP) (1982) Carcinogenesis bioassay of allyl isothiocyanate (CAS No. 57-06-7) in F344N rats and B6C3F1 mice (gavage study). Technical report series no. 234. NIH publication no. 83–1790

Nordic Council of Ministers (NCM) (1994) Naturally occurring antitumourigens, vol 2, Organic isothiocyanates. TemaNord, Copenhagen. ISBN 9291204560

Ostlund RE, Yang JW, Klein S, Gingerich R (1996) Relation between plasma leptin concentration and body fat, gender, diet, age, and metabolic covariates. J Clin Endocrinol Metab 81(11): 3909–3913

Pang TY, Hannan AJ (2010) Environmental enrichment: a cure for cancer? It's all in mind. J Mol Cell Biol 2:302–304

Park J, Rho HK, Kim KH, Choe SS, Lee YS, Kim JB (2005) Overexpression of glucose-6-phosphate dehydrogenase is associated with lipid dysregulation and insulin resistance in obesity. Mol Cell Biol 25(12):5146–5157

Parkin DM, Bray F, Ferlay J, Pisani P (2005) Global cancer statistics, 2002. CA Cancer J Clin 55(2):74–108

Peeters PH, Keinan-Boker L, van der Schouw YT, Grobbee DE (2003) Phytoestrogens and breast cancer risk. Review of the epidemiological evidence. Breast Cancer Res Treat 77(2):171–183

Perkins S, Verschoyle RD, Hill K, Parveen I, Threadgill MD, Sharma RA, Williams ML, Steward WP, Gescher AJ (2002) Chemopreventive efficacy and pharmacokinetics of curcumin in the min/+ mouse, a model of familial adenomatous polyposis. Cancer Epidemiol Biomarkers Prev 11(6):535–540

Petridou E, Dessypris N, Spanos E, Mantzoros C, Skalkidou A, Kalmanti M, Koliouskas D, Kosmidis H, Panagiotou JP, Piperopoulou F, Tzortzatou F, Trichopoulos D (1999) Insulin-like growth factor-I and binding protein-3 in relation to childhood leukaemia. Int J Cancer 80(4):494–496

Phillips F, Hackett AF, Stratton G, Billington D (2004) Effects of changing from a mixed to self-selected vegetarian diet on anthropometric measurements in UK adults. J Hum Nutr Diet 17(3):249–255

Pingitore R, Dugoni BL, Tindale RS, Spring B (1994) Bias against overweight job applicants in a simulated employment interview. J Appl Psychol 79(6):909–917

Pollak MN, Schernhammer ES, Hankinson SE (2004) Insulin-like growth factors and neoplasia. Nat Rev Cancer 4(7):505–518

Porzelius LK, Houston C, Smith M, Arfken C, Fisher E (1995) Comparison of a standard behavioral weight loss treatment and a binge eating weight loss treatment. Behav Ther 26(1):119–134

Prather RC, Williamson DA (1988) Psychopathology associated with bulimia, binge eating, and obesity. Int J Eat Disord 7:177–184

Pretolani M (1999) Interleukin-10: an anti-inflammatory cytokine with therapeutic potential. Clin Exp Allergy 29(9):1164–1171

Qiu C, De Ronchi D, Fratiglioni L (2007) The epidemiology of the dementias: an update. Curr Opin Psychiatry 20(4):380–385

Rajala MW, Scherer PE (2003) Minireview: the adipocyte at the crossroads of energy homeostasis, inflammation, and atherosclerosis. Endocrinology 144(9):3765–3773

Rand CS, Macgregor AM (1990) Morbidly obese patients' perceptions of social discrimination before and after surgery for obesity. South Med J 83(12):1390–1395

Rao CV, Rivenson A, Simi B, Zang E, Hamid R, Kelloff GJ, Steele V, Reddy BS (1995) Enhancement of experimental colon carcinogenesis by dietary 6-phenylhexyl isothiocyanates. Cancer Res 55(19):4311–4318

Ray A, Nkhata KJ, Cleary MP (2007) Effects of leptin on human breast cancer cell lines in relationship to estrogen receptor and HER2 status. Int J Oncol 30(6):1499–1509

Reaven GM (1988) Banting lecture (1988). Role of insulin resistance in human disease. Diabetes 37(12):1595–1607

Renehan AG (2010) Obesity and cancer. In: Leff T, Granneman JG (eds) Adipose tissue in health and disease. Wiley-VCH Verlag GmbH & Co. KGaA, Weinheim. ISBN 9783527629527

Renehan AG (2011) The epidemiology of overweight/obesity and cancer. In: McTiernan A (ed) Physical activity, dietary calories restriction, and cancer, vol 3, Energy balance and cancer. Springer, New York, pp 5–23

Renehan AG, Roberts DL, Dive C (2008) Obesity and cancer: pathophysiological and biological mechanisms. Arch Physiol Biochem 114(1):71–83

Renehan AG, Soerjomataram I, Leitzmann MF (2010) Interpreting the epidemiological evidence linking obesity and cancer: a framework for population-attributable risk estimations in Europe. Eur J Cancer 46(14):2581–2592

Resnicoff M, Abraham D, Yutanawiboonchai W, Rotman HL, Kajstura J, Rubin R, Zoltick P, Baserga R (1995) The insulin-like growth factor I receptor protects tumor cells from apoptosis in vivo. Cancer Res 55(11):2463–2469

Roberts DL, Dive C, Renehan AG (2010) Biological mechanisms linking obesity and cancer risk: new perspectives. Annu Rev Med 61:301–316

Roe DA, Eickwort KR (1976) Relationships between obesity and associated health factors with unemployment among low income women. J Am Med Womens Assoc 31(5):193–194
Rosell M, Appleby P, Spencer E, Key T (2006) Weight gain over 5 years in 21,966 meat-eating, fish-eating, vegetarian, and vegan men and women in EPIC-Oxford. Int J Obes (Lond) 30(9):1389–1396
Saglam K, Aydur E, Yilmaz M, Goktaş S (2003) Leptin influences cellular differentiation and progression in prostate cancer. J Urol 169(4):1308–1311
Sang JP, Minchinton IR, Johnstone PK, Truscott RJ (1984) Glucosinolates profiles in the seed, root and leaf tissue of cabbage, mustard, rapeseed, radish and swede. Can J Plant Sci 64:77–93
Sara VR, Hall K (1990) Insulin-like growth factors and their binding proteins. Physiol Rev 70(3):591–614
Sargent JD, Blanchflower DG (1994) Obesity and stature in adolescence and earnings in young adulthood. Analysis of a British birth cohort. Arch Pediatr Adolesc Med 148(7):681–687
Sarwer DB, Wadden TA, Foster GD (1998) Assessment of body image dissatisfaction in obese women: specificity, severity, and clinical significance. J Consult Clin Psychol 66(4):651–654
Scarborough P, Nnoaham KE, Clarke D, Capewell S, Rayner M (2010) Modelling the impact of a healthy diet on cardiovascular disease and cancer mortality. J Epidemiol Community Health. doi:10.1136/jech.2010.114520
Schaefer EJ (2002) Lipoproteins, nutrition and heart disease. Am J Clin Nutr 75(2):191–212
Scholar EM, Wolterman K, Birt DF, Bresnick E (1989) The effect of diets enriched in cabbage and collards on mtLrine pulmonary metastasis. Nutr Cancer 12(2):121–126
Shoeb M (2006) Anticancer agents from medicinal plants. Bangladesh J Pharmacol 1:35–41
Singh P, Dai B, Yallampalli U, Lu X, Schroy PC (1996) Proliferation and differentiation of a human colon cancer cell line (CaCo2) is associated with significant changes in the expression and secretion of insulin-like growth factor (IGF) IGF-II and IGF binding protein-4: role of IGF-II. Endocrinology 137(5):1764–1774
Sinha R, Anderson DE, McDonald SS, Greenwald P (2003) Cancer risk and diet in India. J Postgrad Med 49(3):222–228
Smith DE, Marcus MD, Lewis CE, Fitzgibbon M, Schreiner P (1998) Prevalence of binge eating disorder, obesity, and depression in a biracial cohort of young adults. Ann Behav Med 20(3):227–232
Smith DE, Thompson JK, Raczynski JM, Hilner JE (1999) Body image among men and women in a biracial cohort: the CARDIA study. Int J Eat Disord 25(1):71–82
Spiegel D (2011) Mind matters in cancer survival. JAMA 305(5):502–503
Srisangam C, Hendricks DG, Sharma RP, Salunkhe DK, Mahoney AW (1980) Effects of dietary cabbage on the tumorigenicity of 1,2-dimethylhydrazine in mice. J Food Saf 2(4):235–245
Stattin P, Lukanova A, Biessy C, Söderberg S, Palmqvist R, Kaaks R, Olsson T, Jellum E (2004) Obesity and colon cancer: does leptin provide a link? Int J Cancer 109(1):149–152
Stevens J, Plankey MW, Williamson DF, Thun MJ, Rust PF, Palesch Y, O'Neil PM (1998) The body mass index-mortality relationship in white and African American women. Obesity 6(4): 268–277
Stoewsand GS, Babish JB, Wimberly HC (1978) Inhibition of hepatic toxicities from polybrominated biphenyls and aflatoxin B1 in rats fed cauliflower. J Environ Pathol Toxicol 2(2):399–406
Stoewsand GS, Anderson JL, Munson L (1988) Protective effect of dietary Brussels sprouts against mammary carcinogenesis in Sprague-Dawley rats. Cancer Lett 39(2):199–207
Stoner G, Casto B, Ralston S, Roebuck B, Pereira C, Bailey G (2002) Development of a multi-organ rat model for evaluating chemopreventive agents: efficacy of indole-3-carbinol. Carcinogenesis 23(2):265–272
Stunkard AJ, Rush J (1974) Dieting and depression reexamined: a critical review of reports of untoward responses during weight reduction for obesity. Ann Int Med 81(4):526–533
Stunkard AJ, Wadden TA (1992) Psychological aspects of severe obesity. Am J Clin Nutr 55(suppl 2):524s–532s

Takahashi K, Suzuki K (1993) Association of insulin-like growth-factor-I-induced DNA synthesis with phosphorylation and nuclear exclusion of p53 in human breast cancer MCF-7 cells. Int J Cancer 55(3):453–458

Tanco S, Linden W, Earle T (1998) Well-being and morbid obesity in women: a controlled therapy evaluation. Int J Eat Disord 23(3):325–339

Tartaglia LA, Dembski M, Weng X, Deng N, Culpepper J, Devos R, Richards GJ, Campfield LA, Clark FT, Deeds J, Muir C, Sanker S, Moriarty A, Moore KJ, Smutko JS, Mays GG, Wool EA, Monroe CA, Tepper RI (1995) Identification and expression cloning of a leptin receptor, OB-R. Cell 83(7):1263–1271

Tee AR, Blenis J (2005) mTOR, translational control and human disease. Semin Cell Dev Biol 16(1):29–37

Telch CF, Agras WS (1994) Obesity, binge eating and psychopathology: are they related? Int J Eat Disord 15(1):53–61

Temel JS, Greer JA, Muzikansky A, Gallagher ER, Admane S, Jackson VA, Dahlin CM, Blinderman CD, Jacobsen J, Pirl WF, Billings JA, Lynch TJ (2010) Early palliative care for patients with metastatic non-small-cell lung cancer. N Engl J Med 363(8):733–742

Thakur AK, Kumar V (2010a) Beneficial effect of Brassica juncea in co-morbid anxiety associated with alloxan induced diabetes in rats. Indian J Pharmacol 42(suppl 2):S223

Thakur AK, Kumar V (2010b) Beneficial effect of Brassica juncea in co-morbid depression associated with alloxan induced diabetes in rodents. Poster presented during international conference on recent advances in pharmaceutical sciences, 22–23 Dec 2010. Organized by the Department of Pharmaceutics, Institute of Technology, Banaras Hindu University, Varanasi

Tilg H, Dinarello CA, Mier JW (1997) IL-6 and APPs: anti-inflammatory and immunosuppressive mediators. Immunol Today 18(9):428–432

Troisi A, Scucchi S, San Martino L, Montera P, d'Amore A, Moles A (2001) Age specificity of the relationship between serum cholesterol and mood in obese women. Physiol Behav 72(3): 409–413

Tseng SH, Lin SM, Chen JC, Su YH, Huang HY, Chen CK, Lin PY, Chen Y (2004) Resveratrol suppresses the angiogenesis and tumor growth of gliomas in rats. Clin Cancer Res 10(6): 2190–2202

Vainio H, Bianchini F (eds) (2002) IARC handbook of cancer prevention, vol 6, Weight control and physical activity. IARC Press, Lyon. ISBN 9789283230069

Vijayaraghavan K, Rao DH (1998) Diet & nutrition situation in rural India. Indian J Med Res 108:243–253

Villanueva EC, Myers MG (2008) Leptin receptor signaling and the regulation of mammalian physiology. Int J Obes (Lond) 32(Suppl 7):S8–S12

Waldstein SR, Katzel LI (2006) Interactive relations of central versus total obesity and blood pressure to cognitive function. Int J Obes (Lond) 30(1):201–207

Wattenberg LW (1983) Inhibition of neoplasia by minor dietary constituents. Cancer Res 43(suppl 5):2448s–2453s

Wattenberg LW (1992) Inhibition of carcinogenesis by minor dietary constituents. Cancer Res 52(suppl 7):2085s–2091s

Wattenberg LW, Sachafer HW, Water L, Davis DW (1989) Inhibition of mammary tumor formation by broccoli and cabbage. Proc Am Assoc Cancer Res 30:181–188

Willett WC, Manson JE, Stampfer MJ, Colditz GA, Rosner B, Speizer FE, Hennekens CH (1995) Weight, weight change, and coronary heart disease in women. Risk within the 'normal' weight range. JAMA 273(6):461–465

Wolin KY, Carson K, Colditz GA (2010) Obesity and cancer. Oncologist 15(6):556–565

Wolk A, Gridley G, Svensson M, Nyrén O, McLaughlin JK, Fraumeni JF, Adam HO (2001) A prospective study of obesity and cancer risk (Sweden). Cancer Causes Control 12(1):13–21

Woods SC, Seeley RJ, Porte D, Schwartz MW (1998) Signals that regulate food intake and energy homeostasis. Science 280(5368):1378–1383

Wooley SC, Garner DM (1991) Obesity treatment: the high cost of false hope. J Am Diet Assoc 91(10):1248–1251

World Cancer Research Fund / American Institute for Cancer Research (WCRF/AICR) (2007) Food, nutrition, physical activity, and the prevention of cancer: a global perspective. AICR, Washington, DC. ISBN 9780972252225

World Health Organization (WHO) (2000) Obesity: preventing and managing the global epidemic. World Health Organization technical reprints series no. 894, i–xii, pp 1–253. ISBN: 9789241208949

Yakar S, Leroith D, Brodt P (2005) The role of the growth hormone/insulin-like growth factor axis in tumor growth and progression: lessons from animal models. Cytokine Growth Factor Rev 16(4–5):407–420

Yokozawa T, Kim HY, Cho EJ, Choi JS, Chung HY (2002) Antioxidant effects of isorhamnetin 3,7-di-O-beta-D-glucopyranoside isolated from mustard leaf (Brassica juncea) in rats with streptozotocin-induced diabetes. J Agric Food Chem 50(19):5490–5495

Yoon BH, Jung JW, Lee JJ, Cho YW, Jang CG, Jin C, Oh TH, Ryu JH (2007) Anxiolytic-like effects of sinapic acid in mice. Life Sci 81(3):234–240

Yoshida M, Katashima S, Ando J, Tanaka T, Uematsu F, Nakae D, Maekawa A (2004) Dietary indole-3-carbinol promotes endometrial adenocarcinoma development in rats initiated with Nethyl- N′-nitro-N-nitrosoguanidine, with induction of cytochrome P450s in the liver and consequent modulation of estrogen metabolism. Carcinogenesis 25(11):2257–2264

Yu H, Spitz MR, Mistry J, Gu J, Hong WK, Wu X (1999) Plasma levels of insulin-like growth factor-I and lung cancer risk: a case-control analysis. J Natl Cancer Inst 91(2):151–156

Yuan TL, Cantley LC (2008) PI3K pathway alterations in cancer: variations on a theme. Oncogene 27(41):5497–5510

Zhang Y, Leibel R (1998) Molecular physiology of leptin and its receptor. Growth Genet Horm 14:17–35

Zhang Y, Talalay P (1994) Anticarcinogenic activities of organic isothiocyanates: chemistry and mechanisms. Cancer Res 5(suppl 7):1976s–1981s

Zhang Y, Proenca R, Maffei M, Barone M, Leopold L, Friedman JM (1994) Positional cloning of the mouse obese gene and its human homologue. Nat Neurosci 372(6505):425–432

Chapter 19
Dietary Phytochemicals as Epigenetic Modulators in Cancer

Vijay S. Thakur Ph.D. and Sanjay Gupta Ph.D.

Contents

V.S. Thakur Ph.D. • S. Gupta Ph.D. (✉)
Department of Urology & Nutrition, Case Western Reserve University,
10900 Euclid Avenue, Cleveland, OH 44106, USA

University Hospitals Case Medical Center, 11100 Euclid Avenue, Cleveland, OH, USA
e-mail: vst2@case.edu; sanjay.gupta@case.edu

S. Gupta Ph.D.
Case Comprehensive Cancer Center, Cleveland, OH 44106, USA
e-mail: sanjay.gupta@case.edu

S. Shankar and R.K. Srivastava (eds.), *Nutrition, Diet and Cancer*,
DOI 10.1007/978-94-007-2923-0_19,

Abstract Epigenetics refers to heritable changes in gene expression that are not attributable to changes in DNA sequence, but rather depend on alterations in DNA methylation, chromatin structure or microRNA profiles. Although epigenetic changes are heritable in somatic cells, these modifications are potentially reversible and make them attractive and promising targets in the prevention and therapy of cancer. Dietary phytochemicals, especially present in fruits, vegetables and beverages have recently shown considerable promise in affecting gene expression via reversible epigenetic mechanisms. These agents include tea polyphenols, genistein, curcumin, sulforaphane, isothiocynates, lycopene, resveratrol, quercetin, indol-3-carbinol, ellagitannin and organosulfur compounds. This chapter discusses the impact of environment, lifestyle and dietary factors on epigenetic alterations and presents considerable evidence that modulation of epigenetic targets by dietary phytochemicals is associated with the prevention and therapy of cancer. This chapter also emphasizes that an increased understanding of the anticancer effects of dietary phytochemicals offer new epigenetic targets and promising agents with more opportunities for prevention, and perhaps therapy of cancer.

Abbreviations

Akt	v-akt murine thymoma viral oncogene homolog 1
AM	allyl mercaptan
AP-1	Activator Protein-1
AR	androgen receptor
Bax	BCL2-associated X protein
Bcl2	B-cell CLL/lymphoma 2
Bcl-xL	B-cell lymphoma-extra large
Bmi-1	B-cell-specific Moloney murine leukemia virus integration site 1
BRCA1	breast cancer 1 early onset
CBP	CREB-binding protein
CCND2	cyclin D2
Cdc25A	cell division cycle 25 homolog A
Cdk	cyclin-dependent kinase
CDX-2	caudal-related homeodomain protein 2
c-Kit	v-kit Hardy-Zuckerman 4 feline sarcoma viral oncogene homolog
COMT	catechol-O-methyltransferase
COX-2	cyclooxygenase-2
CYLD	cylindromatosis (turban tumor syndrome)
DADS	diallyl disulfide
DAS	diallyl sulfide
DATS	diallyl trisulfide
DHFR	dihydrofolate reductase

DMBA	7,12-dimethylbenz(a)anthracene
DNMT	DNA methyltransferase
DNMT-3 L	DNA (cytosine-5)-methyltransferase 3-like
E2F	E2F transcription factor
EC	[−]-epicatechin
ECG	[−]-epicatechin-3-gallate
EGC	[−]-epigallocatechin
EGCG	[−]-epigallocatechin-3-gallate
EGFR	epidermal growth factor receptor
ER	estrogen receptor
ERβ	estrogen receptor beta
ERBB2	human epidermal growth factor receptor 2
ERα	estrogen receptor alpha
EZH-2	enhancer of zeste homolog 2
FOXO3a	forkhead box protein O3
GCN5	SAGA complex histone acetyltransferase catalytic subunit Gcn5
GSTP1	glutathione-S-transferase pi 1
HATs	histone acetyl transferases
HDACs	histone deacetylase
HER-2	human epidermal growth factor receptor 2
HIF-1 α	hypoxia inducible factor 1 alpha subunit
HKMTs	histone lysine methyltransferases
hMLH1	human mutL homolog 1
HOX family proteins	homeobox family proteins
HSP90	heat shock protein 90
hTERT	human telomerase reverse transcriptase
IP-10	TNF-induced interferon-gamma-inducible protein 10
K	Lysine
LEF	lymphoid enhancer factor
LOI	loss of imprinting
MBD	methylated DNA binding domain proteins
MCL1	induced myeloid leukemia cell differentiation protein Mcl-1
MCM-2	minichromosome maintenance gene
MGMT-O(6)	methylguanine-DNA methyltransferase
MIP-2	macrophage inflammatory protein 2
miRNA	microRNA
MMP	matrix metalloproteinase
MTA-2	metastasis associated 1 family member 2
NF-κB	nuclear factor kappa-light-chain-enhancer of activated B cells
Notch1	notch homolog 1 translocation-associated (Drosophila)
NuRD	nucleosome remodeling complex
OSCs	organosulfur compounds
p16INK4a	cyclin-dependent kinase 4 inhibitor A

p21WAF1/CIP1	cyclin-dependent kinase inhibitor 1A
p53	tumor protein 53
PARP	Poly ADP-ribose polymerase
PCAF	K(lysine) acetyltransferase 2B
PcG	polycomb group proteins
PDCD4	programmed cell death 4
PEITC	phenethyl isothiocyanate
PRMTs	arginine methyltransferases
PRPS1	phosphoribosyl pyrophosphate synthetase 1
PTEN	phosphatase and tensin homolog deleted on chromosome 10
RARβ2	retinoic acid receptor beta 2
R	Arginine
RAS	rat sarcoma transforming oncogene
RASSF1A	RAS association domain family 1A
RECK	reversion-inducing cysteine-rich protein with Kazal motifs repressive complex 3
RXR alpha	retinoid X receptor alpha
SAH	S-adenosyl-L-homocysteine
SAM	S-adenosyl methionine
SAMC	S-allylmercaptocysteine
SIRT1	sirtuin (silent mating type information regulation 2 homolog) 1
SLC16A1	solute carrier family 16 member 1
SNX19	sorting nexin-19
SP1	transcription Factor Sp1
TCF	multiple T-cell factor
TGFBR2	transforming growth factor beta receptor II
TGF-β	transforming growth factor beta
TIMP-2	tissue inhibitor of metalloproteinase 2
TTK	phosphotyrosine picked threonine-protein kinase
VEGF	vascular endothelial cell growth factor
ZBTB10	zinc finger and BTB domain containing 10
ZEB1	zinc finger E-box binding homeobox 1
ZNF513	zinc finger protein 513

Introduction

Epidemiological studies in humans and dietary intervention experiments using laboratory animals have provided evidence to suggest that lifestyle and environmental factors play a critical role in the development of a wide variety of neoplasms. Environmental factors including chemical carcinogens, environmental pollutants, dietary contaminants and physical carcinogens play important role in the etiology of human cancer (Kupchella 1986). Additionally, lifestyle factors, such as alcohol consumption, smoking, exposure to sunlight, increased fat consumption and chronic stress can also promote the development and progression of cancer (Stein and Colditz 2004). It has further been demonstrated that maternal nutrition imbalance and metabolic disturbances during embryonic development have a persistent effect on the health of the offspring and may be passed down to the next generation (Attig et al. 2010). These studies provide evidence that cancer is a complex disease and manifestation of both genetic and epigenetic modifications (Macaluso et al. 2003). Cancer initiation and progression are primarily driven by acquired genetic alterations however microenvironment-mediated epigenetic perturbations play an important role in neoplastic development (Cho et al. 2007). "Epigenetics" is defined as heritable changes in gene activity and expression that occur without alteration in DNA sequences and are sufficiently powerful to regulate the dynamics of gene expression (Goldberg et al. 2007). Epigenetic modifications are potentially reversible, which makes them attractive and promising avenues for catering cancer preventive and therapeutic strategies. The key processes responsible for epigenetic regulation are DNA methylation, modifications in chromatin [covalent modification of core histones], and post-transcriptional gene regulation by non-coding RNA [micro-RNAs] (Dehan et al. 2009).

DNA Methylation

DNA methylation is responsible, in part, for regulating gene expression and interacting with the nucleosomes that control DNA packaging, and can affect entire domains of DNA (Issa and Kantarjian 2009). In mammalian cells, DNA methylation occurs within CpG dinucleotides via addition of a methyl group at the 5′ position of the cytosine ring, forming 5-methyl cytosine, in a reaction catalyzed by enzymes known as DNA methyl transferases [DNMTs] (Issa and Kantarjian 2009). There are three main DNA methyltransferases: DNMT1, DNMT3a and DNMT3b. DNMT1 is the primary maintenance enzyme that preserves existing methylation patterns following DNA replication by adding methyl groups to corresponding daughter strands at the hemi-methylated CpG sites. DNMT3a and DNMT3b are methyltransferases that preferentially target unmethylated CpGs to initiate *de novo* methylation; they are highly expressed during embryogenesis but minimally expressed in adult tissues. A fourth family member, DNMT-3L, lacks intrinsic methyltransferase activity; however it facilitates methylation of retrotransposons by interaction with DNMT3a and 3b (Denis et al. 2011). DNA methylation regulates gene expression in normal tissues through genomic imprinting and female X-chromosome inactivation. Unlike normal tissues, these processes are significantly altered in cancer due to a process known as 'loss of imprinting' [LOI]. LOI is the earliest genomic lesion observed in Wilms' tumors and in stem cell populations of organs and tissues, ultimately leading to additional downstream genetic and epigenetic perturbations (Jelinic and Shaw 2007).

In addition to regulation by DNA methylation, methylated DNA binding proteins [MBD's] can bind to methylated cytosine, and sequentially form a complex with histone deacetylase [HDAC] leading to chromatin compaction and gene silencing. To date, six methyl-CpG-binding proteins, including MECP2, MBD1, MBD2, MBD3, MBD4 and Kaiso, have been identified in mammals. MECP2 binds methylated DNA *in vitro* and *in vivo*; it contains a methyl-CpG-binding domain [MBD] at its amino terminus and a transcription repression domain [TRD] in the central domain. MBDs1–4 were cloned on the basis of their sequence homology to MECP2 in the MBD, and all except MBD3 bind preferentially to the methylated CpG islands. MBD1 and MBD2 also function as transcription repressors, whereas MBD4 is a DNA glycosylase and is involved in DNA mismatch repair. Kaiso, although lacking an MBD domain, binds methylated CGCG through its zinc-finger domain. Different methyl-CpG binding proteins may recruit diverse chromatin-remodeling proteins and transcription-regulatory complexes to methylated DNA targets in the genome. Furthermore, it has been demonstrated that nucleosome remodeling complex [NuRD] can methylate DNA by interacting with DNA methylation binding protein MBD2, which directs the NuRD complex to methylate DNA (Lan et al. 2010).

In humans, 50–70% of all CpG islands are methylated, primarily in the heterochromatin i.e. tightly packed form regions of the DNA, and these methylated CpG islands are believed to be critical for the control of gene silencing and chromosomal stability. In contrast, euchromatin (relaxed region in the DNA) CpG islands remain locally unmethylated, allowing access to transcription factors and chromatin-associated proteins for the expression of housekeeping genes and other regulatory genes. In cancer cells, global hypomethylation is accompanied by the hypermethylation of localized promoter-associated CpG islands, which are usually unmethylated in normal cells. Global hypomethylation can lead to chromosomal instability, mutations and reactivation of various oncogenes. DNMT1 is responsible for the establishment of the DNA methylation pattern during DNA synthesis, its deficiency in cells may lead to global hypomethylation. Another common alternation observed in cancer cells is DNA hypermethylation of promoter-associated CpG islands of tumor suppressor genes, which could serves as a surrogate for point mutations or deletions to cause transcriptional silencing of these genes (Jones 2002). Several detailed and informative reviews on DNA methylation and cancer are available, but are beyond the scope of the chapter.

Histone Modification

Chromatin structure is influenced by various histone modifications which play important roles in gene regulation and carcinogenesis (Sawan and Herceg 2010). Chromatin proteins serve as building blocks to package eukaryotic DNA into higher order chromatin fibers. Each nucleosome encompasses ~146 bp of DNA wrapped around an octamer of histone proteins. These octamers consist of double subunits of H2A, H2B, H3 and H4 core histone proteins. The histone proteins coordinate the changes between tightly packed DNA [heterochromatin] which is inaccessible to transcription, and exposed DNA [euchromatin] which is available for binding to and regulation of transcription factors. These changes occur due to structural characteristics of the nucleosome that are known as 'histone tails', which extend from the core octamer. These tails consist of N-termini of the histone proteins and are the major sites for posttranslational modifications. The deregulation of genes has been associated with acetylation of histone proteins by histone deacetylases (HDACs) and histone acetyltransferases (HATs), the two opposing group of enzymes involved in chromatin remodeling. HATs catalyze histone acetylation on the ε-amino groups of lysine residues in the N-terminal tails of core histones, neutralizing the positive charge and facilitating the binding of transcription factors to nucleosomal DNA. In contrast, HDACs catalyze deacetylation by cleavage of acetyl groups, typically producing a compact chromatin configuration that restricts transcription factor access to DNA and repressing gene expression. HDACs and HATs comprise a large group of enzymes which are classified into several families and control various physiological functions of the cells (Sawan and Herceg 2010). Extensive literature is available on this topic, and it is impossible to sufficiently cover all classifications and modifications in depth in this chapter.

Non-coding RNAs

Non-coding RNAs were initially noted to perform catalytic functions in facilitating RNA splicing, but it was later recognized that they participate in the epigenetic phenomenon of posttranscriptional gene modification. They are also known as non-protein coding RNA or microRNA, and are 21–23 nucleotides in length. Approximately 1,000 miRNA genes have been computationally predicted in the human genome, with each miRNA targeting multiple protein coding transcripts. Although miRNA are vital to normal cell physiology their mis-expression has been linked to carcinogenesis, and miRNA profiles are now being used to classify human cancers. The influence of miRNA on the epigenetic machinery and the reciprocal epigenetic regulation of miRNA expression suggest that its deregulation during carcinogenesis has important implications for global regulation of epigenetics and cancer (Garzon et al. 2009). Several detailed and informative reviews of the association between miRNA and cancer are available, but their description is beyond the scope of this chapter.

Dietary Agents as Epigenetic Target

The most interesting and important feature of epigenetics in disease development is the fact that unlike genetic changes, epigenetic alterations can be modified by the environment, diet or pharmacological intervention. Dietary phytochemicals present in fruit, vegetables and beverages have shown to possess potential anticancer properties. There has been considerable interest in the use of naturally occurring phytochemicals for disease prevention including cancer. Previous studies have demonstrated that phytochemicals can work through number of complementary and overlapping mechanisms of action, including induction of detoxification enzymes, antioxidant effects, and inhibition of the formation of nitrosamines, binding/dilution of carcinogens in the digestive tract, alteration of hormone metabolism and modulation of carcinogenic cellular and signaling events. However, it was not more than a decade ago, studies demonstrate that phytochemicals could target the activity of various epigenetic factors, such as DNMTs and HDACs and could be useful to prevent and treat various diseases including cancer. Although several dietary agents or nutrients regulate different molecular and epigenetic targets in human cancers, here we summarize the role of some common bioactive dietary phytochemicals and their epigenetic targets in various human cancers. The agents which we discuss include tea polyphenols, genistein, curcumin, sulforaphane, phenyl isothiocyanate, lycopene, resveratrol, quercetin, indol-3-carbinol, ellagitannin and organosulfur compounds. A brief discussion includes their epigenetic targets in various human cancers leading to their multiple roles in the regulation of cancer prevention and therapy. Additionally, dietary phytochemicals, and their epigenetic targets associated with tumorigenesis are summarized in Table 19.1.

Tea Polyphenols

Tea is the most widely consumed beverage in the world [average per capita consumption ~120 mL/day] in the form of green or black tea. Epidemiological, case control and laboratory data have shown that polyphenols present in green and black tea may have potential to reduce the risk of many potential diseases including cancer. The major polyphenols present in green tea are [−]-epicatechin [EC], [−]-epicatechin-3-gallate [ECG], [−]-epigallocatechin [EGC], and [−]-epigallocatechin-3-gallate [EGCG], where EGCG constitutes more than 50% of total catechins present therein. The major polyphenols in black tea are catechins, flavanols, methylxanthines, theaflavins and thearubigens, respectively (Siddiqui et al. 2006).

EGCG was the first major polyphenol reported to have the potential to inhibit DNMT activity and reactivate methylation-silenced genes. Treatment of human esophageal cancer KYSE 510 cells with EGCG caused reversal of hypermethylation of $p16^{INK4a}$, RARβ, MGMT, and hMLH1 genes through suppression of DNMT1 activity. EGCG has been shown to bind to the catalytic pocket of DNMT1 and inhibit its enzyme activity (Fang et al. 2003). Besides, EGCG has shown its ability to inhibit dihydrofolate reductase [DHFR] leading to inhibition of DNA and RNA synthesis. Studies have further demonstrated that EGCG-mediated altered DNA methylation could be achieved by enhancing the formation of S-adenosyl-L-homocysteine

Table 19.1 Epigenetic regulation by dietary phytochemicals

Dietary agent	Epigenetic modification(s)	Epigenetic target(s)
Tea polyphenols (Fang et al. 2003; Lee et al. 2005; Kato et al. 2008; Murugan et al. 2009; Lin et al. 2006; Ran et al. 2005; Yuasa et al. 2005; Xiao et al. 2006; Navarro-Perán et al. 2007; Gu et al. 2009; Gao et al. 2009; Pandey et al. 2010; Volate et al. 2009; Berletch et al. 2008; Balasubramanian et al. 2010; Tsang and Kwok 2010; Fix et al. 2010)	DNA methylation	P16^{INK4a}, RARβ, MGMT, hMLH1, RECK1, hTERT, WIF-1, RXRα, GSTP1, CDKN2A, RXRβ, CDX2/ DNMTI, MBD1, MeCP2,
	Histone modifications	H3 and H4 acetylation, H3K27m3, NF-κB, IL-6, BMI-1, EZH2, SUZ12/HAT, HDAC, HMT
	miR-16, miR-21, miR-27, miR-330	Bcl-2, AR
Genistein (Fang et al. 2005; King-Batoon et al. 2008; Majid et al. 2008, 2009, 2010a, b; Qin et al. 2009; Hong et al. 2004; Kikuno et al. 2008; Basak et al. 2008; Parker et al. 2009; Li et al. 2009; Sun et al. 2009)	DNA methylation	p16, RARβ2, MGMT, hTERT, BTG3, GSTP1 and EPHB2, HMGNS, CDKN2A/DNMT, MBD1, MBD4, MeCP2
	Histone modifications	H3, H4,H2A and H2B acetylation, H3K4me2, H3K9me3, p21, p16, PTEN, p53, FOXA3, BTG3, RARβ, hTERT, CCLD/HAT, HDAC, SIRT1
	miR-200a-c, let-7a-f, mir-27b, miR-146a	ZEB1, ZBTB10, EGFR
Curcumin (Medina-Franco et al. 2011; Liu et al. 2005, 2009; Marcu et al. 2006; Balasubramanyam et al. 2004; Kang et al. 2005; Chen et al. 2007; Bora-Tatar et al. 2009; Sun et al. 2008; Ali et al. 2010; Zhang et al. 2010; Yang et al. 2010; Muddu uru et al. 2011; Banerjee et al. 2011)	DNA methylation	Unknown/DNMT1
	Histone modifications	H3 and H4 deacetylation, p53, GATA4, GZMB, PRF1, EOMES/ HAT, HDAC
	miR-22, miR-199*,miR-21, miR-200,	SP1, ESR1, PTEN

(continued)

Table 19.1 (continued)

Dietary agent	Epigenetic modification(s)	Epigenetic target(s)
Indole-3-carbinol (I3C) and Diindolylmethane (DIM) (Li et al. 2009, 2010a, b; Jin et al. 2010; Izzotti et al. 2010a)	Histone modifications miR-200(a–c), let-7(a–f), miR-146a	COX-2/HDAC ZEB1, EGFR
Sulforaphane (Traka et al. 2005; Meeran et al. 2010; Myzak et al. 2004, 2006a, b, 2007; Pledgie-Tracy et al. 2007)	DNA methylation Histone modifications	Unknown /DNMT1 H3 and H4 acetylation, H3K9ac, H3K9me3, HBD-2, H3K27me3, RARβ, HBD-2, p21, Bax/HDAC
Phenethyl isothiocyanate (Izzotti et al. 2010a, b; Wang et al. 2007; Lea et al. 2001)	DNA methylation Histone modifications	GSTP1/ Unknown H3 and H4 acetylation, p21, GSTP1/HDAC
Resveratrol (Stefanska et al. 2010; Wang et al. 2008; Tili et al. 2010)	DNA methylation Histone modifications	Unknown /DNMT TNFα, IL-8, RBP/SIRT1
Organosulfur compounds (Lea et al. 1999, 2002; Druesne et al. 2004)	DNA methylation Histone modifications	H3 and H4 acetylation, p21/HDAC
Lycopene (King-Batoon et al. 2008)	DNA methylation	GSTP1, RARβ, HIN-1/Unknown
Quercetin (Tan et al. 2008; Ruiz et al. 2007; Lee et al. 2011; Priyadarsini et al. 2011)	DNA methylation Histone modifications	CDKN2A/DNMT IP-10, MIP-2/HAT, SIRT1
Ellagitannins (Wen et al. 2009)	miRNA	miRNA array

[SAH], a potent inhibitor of DNMT. SAH is produced from the demethylation of S-adenosyl methionine [SAM] when catechol-O-methyltransferase [COMT] inactivates catechol molecules by introducing methyl group to the catecholamine group, donated by SAM (Lee et al. 2005).

Numerous studies have confirmed that tea polyphenols can reactivate tumor suppressor genes by promoter demethylation. Treatment of oral cancer cells with EGCG partially reversed the hypermethylation status of tumor suppressor gene RECK and enhanced the expression of RECK mRNA, which correlated with reduced expression of matrix metalloproteinases: MMP-2 and MMP-9 and suppressed the invasive ability of cancer cells (Kato et al. 2008). Administration of black tea polyphenols [Polyphenon-B] significantly reduced the incidence of DAB-induced hepatomas in male Sprague-Dawley rats, as evidenced by alterations in the expression of MMP-2, MMP-9, and TIMP-2; reversion-inducing cysteine rich protein with Kazal motifs RECK; and suppression of HIF1alpha, VEGF, and VEGFR1 which correlated with HDAC1 levels (Murugan et al. 2009).

EGCG and [-]-epigallocatechin repressed telomerase mRNA in lung, oral cavity, thyroid, and liver cancer cells may be linked to inhibition of cell growth (Lin et al. 2006). EGCG also demonstrated anti-neoplastic activity by suppressing the telomerase activity of digestive cancer cells (Ran et al. 2005). EGCG can inhibit DNMT activity and reactivate methylation silenced retinoic acid receptor β gene in human colon and prostate cancer cells (Lee et al. 2005). In another study, methylation of CDX2 and other genes involved in gastric carcinogenesis was investigated in relation to the clinico-pathologic and selected lifestyle factors of patients with gastric cancer. An inverse association of CDX2 methylation with the intake of green tea was observed in this study (Yuasa et al. 2005).

Decreased annexin-I expression is a common event in early-stage bladder cancer development. In part, green tea induced the expression of mRNA and protein levels of the actin binding protein, annexin-I, through demethylation of its promoter and actin remodeling (Xiao et al. 2006). EGCG, an efficient inhibitor of human dihydrofolate reductase, altered the p16 methylation pattern [from methylated to unmethylated] after folic acid deprivation resulting in growth inhibition of a human colon carcinoma cell line in a concentration- and time- dependent manner. The same study also demonstrated that through disruption of purine metabolism, EGCG caused adenosine release from the cells, and modulation of different signaling pathways via binding to adenosine-specific receptors (Navarro-Perán et al. 2007).

EGCG inhibits growth and induces apoptosis in renal cell carcinoma through TFPI-2 mRNA and protein overexpression (Gu et al. 2009). Promoter demethylation of WIF-1 by epigallocatechin-3-gallate in lung cancer cells was also reported (Gao et al. 2009). Epigenetic silencing of glutathione-S-transferase pi [GSTP1] by hypermethylation is recognized as being a molecular hallmark of human prostate cancer. Recently our laboratory reported that exposure of LNCaP cells to GTP concentrations as low as 1–10 μg/mL up to 7 days caused demethylation in the proximal GSTP1 promoter and regions distal to the transcription factor binding sites. This also caused a concentration- and time- dependent re-expression of GSTP1 and DNMT1 inhibition. GTP exposure also decreased mRNA and protein levels of MBD1, MBD4 and MeCP2; HDAC 1–3 whereas levels of acetylated histone H3 [LysH9/18] and H4 increased. In addition, GTP reduced MBD2 association with accessible Sp1 binding sites causing increased binding and transcriptional activation of the GSTP1 gene. Importantly, GTP treatment did not result in global hypomethylation and promoted maintenance of genomic integrity. Unlike 5-aza-2′deoxycitidine treatment, GTP exposure did not activate prometastatic gene S100P. This study demonstrates the dual potential of tea polyphenols at physiologically attainable non-toxic doses to alter DNA methylation and chromatin modeling, the two global epigenetic mechanisms of gene regulation at physiologically attainable non-toxic doses (Pandey et al. 2010). Another report showed a significant reduction in the number of newly formed tumors in the Apc [Min/+] mice treated with azoxymethane-treated after they were given a solution of green tea [0.6% W/V] as the only source of beverage for 8 weeks. RXR alpha downregulation was observed as an early event in colorectal carcinogenesis and green tea significantly increased the mRNA and protein levels of RXR alpha. Green tea treatment also significantly decreased CpG methylation in the promoter region of the RXR alpha gene (Volate et al. 2009). Recent reports demonstrated that treatment of breast cancer and promyelocytic leukemia cells with EGCG resulted in a time-dependent decrease in hTERT promoter methylation including E2F-1 binding sites and ablated histone H3Lys9 acetylation which led to increased binding of E2F-1 repressor at the hTERT promoter, and ultimately caused cell death (Berletch et al. 2008). The Polycomb Group [PcG] proteins are epigenetic repressors of gene expression and their repression is achieved via action of two multi-protein PcG complexes-PRC2 [eed] and PRC1 [Bmi-1]. These complexes increase histone methylation and reduce acetylation that leads to a closed chromatin conformation. Bmi-1 is over-expressed in breast, prostate, colon, pancreatic and non-small cell lung cancers. EGCG treatment caused suppression of two key PcG protein, Bmi-1 and Ezh2 and lead to global reduction in histone H3-K27-trimethylation. This caused reduced expression of key proteins that enhance progression through the cell cycle [cdk1, cdk2, cdk4, cyclin D1, cyclin E, cyclin A, and cyclin B1] and increased expression of proteins that inhibit cell cycle progression [p21 and p27]. EGCG treatment also enhanced apoptosis because of increased caspase 9, 8 and 3 and poly ADP-ribose polymerase [PARP] cleavage, increased Bax, and decreased Bcl-xL expression (Balasubramanian et al. 2010).

Another important epigenetic regulation occurs via modifications of microRNA [miRNA] expression. Limited studies are available in the literature that explored the influence of tea polyphenols on the expression of miRNAs in various human cancers. One recent report showed that EGCG treatment altered the expression of miRNAs in human hepatocellular carcinoma HepG2 cells. Thirteen miRNAs were upregulated and 48 were downregulated. Among the miRNAs upregulated by EGCG, some target genes include: RAS, Bcl2, E2F, TGFBR2 and c-Kit. Among those miRNAs downregulated by EGCG include the target genes comprised of HOX family proteins, including PTEN, SMAD, MCL1, SLC16A1, TTK, PRPS1, ZNF513, and SNX19 with diversified functions. Further treatment with EGCG down-regulated Bcl-2, an anti apoptotic protein, and transfection with anti-miR-16 inhibitor suppressed miR-16 expression and counteracted the EGCG effects on Bcl-2 down-regulation and induced apoptosis in these cells (Tsang and Kwok 2010). In another study, treatment with Polyphenon-60 significantly altered the expression of 23 miRNAs which includes downregulation of miR-21 and miR-27. These miRNAs have previously demonstrated to over-express in MCF-7 breast cancer cells. Furthermore, treatment of hepatocellular carcinoma HepG2 cells with EGCG resulted in the induction of apoptosis by the upregulation of miRNA-16, and downregulation of its target gene Bcl-2, an anti-apoptotic protein. Transfection of cells with anti-miR-16 inhibitor confirmed the role of miR-16 in downregulation of Bcl-2 and induction of apoptosis by EGCG. More recent studies in prostate cancer LNCaP cells demonstrated that EGCG treatment repressed the transcriptional activation of AR. EGCG inhibited AR nuclear translocation and protein expression which correlated with significant down-regulation of androgen regulated miRNA-21 and up-regulation of a tumor suppressor, miRNA-330, in in vivo tumor bearing mice with EGCG (Fix et al. 2010). The results obtained for miRNA profiling suggests that EGCG may exert its biologic functions through modulation of miRNA expression.

Genistein

Genistein is the major isoflavone derived from soy. Epidemiological studies indicate an inverse correlation between soy rich diet and risk of prostate and breast cancers. Studies indicate that genistein can target various enzymes and pathways which has relevance in cancer (Banerjee et al. 2008). Recent studies demonstrate that genistein is involved in the regulation of gene transcription by modification of epigenetic events including DNA methylation and histone modifications. Genistein and other flavonoids of soy are potent modifier of DNA methylation. Genistein, biochanin A and daidzein has shown to cause reversal of DNA hypermethylation and reactivated methylation-silenced genes including p16^{INK4a}, RARβ, and MGMT genes in human esophageal squamous KYSE 510 carcinoma cells; RARβ in human prostate cancer LNCaP and PC-3 cells which correlated with inhibition of DNMT1, 3a and 3b (Fang et al. 2005). Studies have shown that low, non-toxic concentrations of genistein partially demethylate promoter of the GSTP1 gene and its expression was restored in human breast cancer MDA-MB-468 cells (King-Batoon et al. 2008). Genistein treatment has shown to demethylate the promoter region of BTG3, a tumor suppressor gene downregulated in renal cancer by inhibiting the activity of DNMT and MBD2 in renal cell carcinoma A498, ACHN and HEK-293 cells (Majid et al. 2009). Treatment with genistein also increased HAT activity and the levels of acetylated histones 3, 4, di and trimethylated H3K 4, and RNA polymerase II at the BTG3 promoter which correlated with the inhibition of prostate cancer cell growth and cell cycle arrest (Majid et al. 2010a). Studies on DNA methylation with genistein have shown inconsistent results. Though studies in cell culture have shown that genistein treatment inhibits DNA methylation by inhibiting DNMT activity in various cancer cells, however in vivo studies have demonstrated opposite findings. For example, a randomized, double-blind trial conducted on 34 healthy premenopausal women conducted to determine the effect of 40 or 140 mg of isoflavones [including genistein, daidzein, and glycitein] taken daily through one menstrual cycle on the methylation status of p16, RASSF1A, RARb2, ER, and CCND2 genes which are known to be methylated in breast cancer. The results performed on intraductal specimens showed that RARβ2 and CCND2 methylation was increased after treatment and correlated with serum genistein levels (Qin et al. 2009).

Genistein has been shown to possess highest histone modifying activity in comparison with other isoflavones. The isoflavones genistein and daidzein and the daidzein metabolite equol have been reported to exert their effects by elevating histone acetylation through modulating HAT activity and co-activator activity of ER (Hong et al. 2004). Genistein has shown to induce the expression of p21WAF1/CIP1 and $p16^{INK4a}$ tumor suppressor genes in human prostate cancer cells by epigenetic mechanisms involving active chromatin modification including upregulation of the expression of HATs (Majid et al. 2008). Furthermore, treatment with genistein caused demethylation and acetylation of histone H3-K9 at the PTEN and the CYLD promoter and acetylation of Histone H3-K9 on p53 and FOXO3a promoter through reduction of SIRT1 activity. Increase expression of these genes reciprocally relate to attenuation of p-AKT and NF-κB binding activity (Kikuno et al. 2008). In another study, treatment of LNCaP cells with genistein exhibit increased ubiquitination of AR protein which was due to decrease in the chaperone activity and increase acetylation of Hsp90. This study also demonstrated that HDAC6, an Hsp90 deacetylase, was the target of the anti-estrogenic activity of genistein (Basak et al. 2008).

Soy isoflavones have shown the potential to modulate miRNAs. In a study using UL-3A and UL-3B cells established from an ovarian cancer patient treated with genistein. The miRNA profile of untreated and their treated counterpart cells were compared. A total of 53 genes were found to be differentially regulated after genistein treatment. Genistein resulted in the induction of ERα and ERβ mRNA and proteins and reduction in migration and invasion ability of treated cells. The study however did not characterize the involvement of miRNAs in the induction of ERα and ERβ (Parker et al. 2009). In another study, treatment with genistein of gemcitabine-resistant human pancreatic cancer cell lines viz. MiaPaCa-2, Panc-1, and Aspc-1 resulted in downregulation of miRNA-200, which positively correlated with the mesenchymal markers including ZEB1, slug, and vimentin and reversal of EMT (Li et al. 2009). In prostate cancer cells, genistein treatment caused upregulation of miRNA-1296 and accumulation of cells in the S phase of the cell cycle along with significant decrease in mRNA and protein levels of minichromosome maintenance gene [MCM-2], which is a target of miRNA-1296 (Majid et al. 2010b). Furthermore, genistein has shown to suppress growth of uveal melanoma C918 cells by inhibition of miRNA-27a and its target gene ZBTB10 (Sun et al. 2009).

Curcumin

Curcumin is a major active ingredient of the popular Indian spice turmeric which has been associated with multiple health benefits including cancer prevention. Curcumin has shown ability to modulate many components of intracellular signaling pathways implicated in inflammation, proliferation, invasion, survival, and apoptosis (Teiten et al. 2010). In-silico DNMT docking studies with curcumin and other related compounds indicate that curcumin has ability to inhibit DNMT1 activity by covalently blocking the catalytic thiol group of C1226 binding site (Medina-Franco et al. 2011). Treatment of human leukemia MV4-11 cells with curcumin has shown to cause global hypomethylation, but sequence-specific demethylation at promoter regions of epigenetically silenced genes with curcumin has not been demonstrated (Liu et al. 2009).

Curcumin is a potential modulator of histones and modulate the HATs and HDACs enzymes activity. Results obtained from computational screening algorithms demonstrate that curcumin binds covalently to HATs. Curcumin has been shown to promote proteasome-dependent degradation of p300 and other closely related CBP proteins without affecting HATs such as PCAF or GCN5. This activity effectively blocks histone hyperacetylation in prostate cancer PC3-M cells and peripheral blood lymphocytes induced by the HDAC inhibitor MS-275 (Marcu et al. 2006). Several cell culture studies using various cancer cell types have confirmed that curcumin has potential to inhibit HAT activity of p300/CBP. Inhibition of p300/CBP by curcumin suppresses histone acetylation as well as acetylation of non-histone protein like p53 (Balasubramanyam et al. 2004). In another study, exposure of human hepatoma cells to curcumin resulted in a significant decrease in histone acetylation due to inhibition of HAT activity without alterations in HDAC levels (Kang et al. 2005). A recent study has shown that curcumin represses the activity of NF-κB and Notch1 in Raji cells by inhibition of HDAC1, HDAC3 and p300/CBP resulting in inhibition of cell proliferation (Chen et al. 2007). Another study confirmed that curcumin has ability to inhibit the expression of class I HDACs [HDAC1, HDAC3, and HDAC8], and can increase the expression of Ac-histone H4 in Raji cells (Liu et al. 2005). HDAC inhibition activity of curcumin was also investigated using fluorometric assay as well by performing molecular docking for human HDAC8 enzyme and was found that curcumin is highly potent compared to well known HDAC inhibitor, sodium butyrate (Bora-Tatar et al. 2009).

Antitumor activity of curcumin has been linked to its ability to modulate miRNA expression in cancer cells. Treatment of human pancreatic carcinoma BxPC-3 cells with curcumin resulted in significant change in the expression of 29 miRNA. Further investigation confirmed curcumin induced upregulation of miRNA-22 and suppresses the expression of its target genes SP1 and ESR1 (Sun et al. 2008). In human pancreatic cancer cell lines MIAPaCa-E, MIAPaCa-M, and BxPC-3, curcumin and its derivate CFD sensitize these cells to gemcitabine by inhibiting NF-κB, COX-2, and their downstream target molecules, which is in part due to inactivation of miR-21 and reactivation of miR-200b and miR-200c (Ali et al. 2010). Curcumin promoted apoptosis in A549/DDP multidrug-resistant human lung adenocarcinoma cells by downregulation of miR-186*. Downregulation of miR-186* caused an increase in caspase-10 activity (Zhang et al. 2010). Curcumin has shown to reduce the expression of Bcl-2 in breast cancer MCF-7 cells by upregulating miR-15a and miR-16 expression (Yang et al. 2010). In another study, curcumin has shown to suppress miR-21 levels in human colon cancer RKO and HCT116 cells, which is over-expressed in several human tumors and promote invasion and metastasis. Curcumin also stabilized the expression of the tumor suppressor Pdcd4 in colorectal cancer (Mudduluru et al. 2011).

Indole-3-Carbinol [I3C] and Diindolylmethane [DIM]

Cruciferous vegetables, particularly *Brassica* genus which includes broccoli, cabbage, cauliflower, mustard, radish etc. contains glucosinolate, a phytochemical which is hydrolyzed to indole-3-carbinol by myrosinase, an enzyme present in these plants. I3C is converted to many diindolylmethane condensation products in the acidic pH of the stomach. Both I3C and DIM induced apoptosis in cancer cell lines from solid tumors of different organs by modulating various kinases and nuclear receptor mediated signaling (Banerjee et al. 2011). A recent study using various human colon cancer cell lines viz. HT-29, SW620, RKO, LS174T, and HCT-116 have shown that DIM selectively induced proteasomal degradation of class I histone deacetylases [HDAC1, HDAC2, HDAC3, and HDAC8] without affecting class II HDAC proteins both in vitro and in vivo. Significant decreases in the levels of HDAC1, HDAC2, and HDAC3 was associated with the promoters of p21 and p27 genes which led to cell cycle arrest and DNA damage in tumor cells (Li et al. 2010a).

In another study, DIM treatment of gemcitabine-resistant human pancreatic cancer cells viz. MiaPaCa-2, Panc-1, and Aspc-1 resulted in alteration in miRNA expression. DIM treatment caused upregulation of miR-let-7b, miR- let-7e, miR-200b, and miR-200c. Furthermore, treatment of pancreatic cancer cells with DIM correlated with upregulation of E-cadherin, an epithelial cell marker and downregulation of mesenchymal markers ZEB1 and vimentin (Li et al. 2009). Recent study has shown that DIM treatment influences the invasion capacity of pancreatic cells via a miRNA-regulated mechanism. Treatment of pancreatic cancer cells with DIM caused upregulation of miR-146 which correlated with reduced expression of EGFR, MTA-2 and members of the NF-κB signaling pathway (Li et al. 2010b). Another recent study with DIM on estrogen-dependent MCF-7 and estrogen receptor negative p53 mutant MDA-MB-468 human breast cancer cells resulted in upregulation of miR-21 which correlated with downregulation of CDK2, CDK 4 and Cdc25A and cell cycle arrest (Jin et al. 2010). In vivo studies demonstrate that I3C intake resulted the attenuation of symptoms of cigarette smoke in rats and altered miRNAs involved in p53 functions [miR-34b], TGF-β expression [miR-26a], ERBB2 activation [miR-125a-prec], and angiogenesis [miR-10a] in the lungs (Izzotti et al. 2010a).

Sulforaphane

Sulforaphane [SFN] is a bioactive phytochemical found in broccoli, broccoli sprouts, cabbage and kale. Sulforaphane has ability to alter anti-carcinogenic activity, enhance xenobiotic metabolism, induce cell cycle arrest and apoptosis in various human cancer cells which has relevance in cancer chemoprevention (Clarke et al. 2008). The effect of sulforaphane on methylation of DNA has not been specifically studied, whereas downregulation of DNMT1 activity has been demonstrated in human colon cancer CaCo-2 cells (Traka et al. 2005). Treatment of breast cancer MCF-7 and MDA-MB-231 cells with SFN resulted in the inhibition of human telomerase reverse transcriptase [hTERT], the catalytic regulatory subunit of telomerase. SFN-mediated decrease in DNMT1 and DNMT3a was observed after treatment and site-specific CpG demethylation occurred primarily in the first exon of the hTERT gene which facilitated CTCF binding associated with hTERT repression. SFN treatment has shown to increase acetylation of acetyl-H3, acetyl-H3K9 and acetyl-H4; and decrease in the trimethyl-H3K9 and trimethyl-H3K27, respectively. This hyperacetylation enhanced the binding of many hTERT repressor proteins such as MAD1 and CTCF to the hTERT regulatory region resulting in cellular apoptosis. SFN treatment inhibited HDAC activity and modulated histone methylation by increasing the expression of histone demethylase RBP2 (Meeran et al. 2010). Treatment of human embryonic kidney, HEK293 and human HCT116 colorectal cancer cells with SFN resulted in inhibition of HDAC activity and increase activity of multiple T-cell factor [TCF]/lymphoid enhancer factor [LEF] binding sites along with increase acetylation of histone and p21 (Myzak et al. 2004). SFN treatment of human prostate epithelial BPH-1, LNCaP and PC-3 cells exhibited inhibition of HDAC activity which was accompanied by increase in acetylated histones and their increased binding on the promoters of p21 and Bax genes. These events correlated with cell cycle arrest and induction of caspase-dependent apoptosis (Myzak et al. 2006a). In another study, SFN exposure to human breast cancer cell lines viz. MDA-MB-231, MDA-MB-468, MCF-7, and T47D resulted in HDAC inhibition and decrease in the protein expression of ER, EGFR, and HER-2 in these cancer cells which correlated with cell growth inhibition and induction of apoptosis. Specifically, SFN treatment did not cause any change in acetylation pattern of histones in this study (Pledgie-Tracy et al. 2007).

A single oral dose of 10 μM SFN in wild-type [C57BL/6 J+/+] mice caused significant inhibition in HDAC activity in the colonic mucosa and concomitant transient increase in ac-H3 and ac-H4 levels. In another study using APCMin/+ mice, SFN treatment reduced tumor formation and increased global histone acetylation and increase association of acetylated histone H3 on the promoters of p21 and Bax genes, and increase expression of Bax protein (Myzak et al. 2006b). Consumption of SFN in the diet at an average daily dose of 7.5 μM per animal for 21 days resulted in 40% reduced growth in PC-3 tumor xenograft in nude mice. These results correlated with a significant decrease in HDAC activity, increase in global histone acetylation and increase expression of Bax in the tumors and mononuclear blood cells

(Myzak et al. 2007). Furthermore, in a pilot study, 3 human subjects fed with a single dose of 68 g broccoli sprouts demonstrated significant inhibition of HDAC activity and induced acetylation of histone H3 and H4 at 3 and 6 h following intake, in their peripheral blood mononuclear cells (Myzak et al. 2007).

Phenethyl Isothiocyanate

Isothiocyanates, such as phenethyl isothiocyanate [PEITC] has shown to inhibit carcinogenic process and as such is a useful chemopreventive agent. PEITC has ability to suppress growth of various cancer cell types and induces apoptosis in cancer cells (Cheung and Kong 2010). In a recent study, treatment of human prostate cancer LNCaP cells with PEITC resulted in demethylation of GSTP1 gene promoter, inhibited the activity of HDACs, and induced selective histone acetylation and methylation (Wang et al. 2007). In another study, treatment of DS19 mouse erythroleukemia cells with allyl isothiocyanate exhibited increase acetylation of histones but had no effect on HDACs (Lea et al. 2001). Recent studies demonstrate that PEITC can modulate miRNAs expression induced by cigarette smoke. Rats were pretreated with PEITC alone or in combination with IC3 for 3 days, before been exposed to cigarette smoke for 28 days. PEITC strongly counter-regulated the expression of majority of miRNAs downregulated by cigarette smoke. Several of the miRNAs which were modified by PEITC include miR-125b, miR-26a, miR-146-pre, let-7a, let-7c, miR-192, miR-222-pre, miR-99, miR-123-pre designated for TGF-β expression, NF-κB activation, Ras activation, cell proliferation, apoptosis and angiogenesis (Izzotti et al. 2010a).

In another study, the effect of PEITC or the glucocorticoid budesonide treatment either alone or in combination was analyzed on miRNA expression in mouse liver and lungs. Treatment was started after weaning for 2 weeks or directly after birth in combination with exposure to cigarette smoke. PEITC caused modest effect on miRNA expression in the lungs, but in the liver, it significantly downregulated nine and upregulated three miRNAs. Co-treatment group significantly up-regulated 12 and downregulated 11 miRNAs in comparison to the group treated with cigarette smoke only. These differentially expressed miRNAs were shown to be associated with genes regulating stress response, protein repair, cell proliferation, and inflammation (Izzotti et al. 2010b).

Resveratrol

Resveratrol [3, 5, 4′-trihydroxy-trans-stilbene] is a stilbenoid, a type of natural phenol, and a phytoalexin produced naturally by several plants. It has been reported to have anti-cancer, anti-inflammatory and blood-sugar-lowering potential (Savouret and Quesne 2002). In breast cancer MCF7 cells, resveratrol exhibited a weak

DNMT inhibitory activity and was unable to reverse the methylation of several tumor suppressor genes. Effect of resveratrol alone and in combination with adenosine analogues: 2-chloro-2′-deoxyadenosine [2CdA] and 9-beta-d-arabinosyl-2-fluoroadenine [F-ara-A] on methylation and expression of RARbeta2 in MCF-7 breast cancer cell lines was studied. Exposure to resveratrol improved the action of adenosine analogues to inhibit methylation of the promoter of RARb2 gene which correlated with increase expression however resveratrol alone was ineffective (Stefanska et al. 2010).

Reports demonstrate that class III HDAC, sirtuin 1 [SIRT1] and p300 are targets of resveratrol. Activated SIRT1 negatively regulates survivin expression through its deacetylase activity. SIRT1 also plays critical role in the aging processes. In breast cancer, human BRCA1 is associated with lower levels of SIRT1 expression. Resveratrol has ability to increase the expression of human BRAC1 by altering H3 acetylation, which is an important strategy for targeted therapy for BRCA1-associated breast cancer (Tili et al. 2010). Studies in vivo on APC/+ mice demonstrate similar findings that SIRT1-encoded proteins are required for resveratrol-mediated tumor growth inhibition (Wang et al. 2008).

In another study, resveratrol treatment of human SW480 colon cancer cells demonstrate a decrease in the levels of several oncogenic miRNAs targeting genes encoding Dicer1, a cytoplasmic RNase III producing mature miRNAs from their immediate precursors and tumor-suppressor factors PDCD4 and PTEN. This microarray study on miRNA indicated that resveratrol treatment significantly upregulated the expression of 22 miRNA and downregulated 26 miRNA. Several of the downregulated miRNAs include miR-17, miR-21, miR-25, miR-92a-2, constitutively upregulated in colon cancer. The level of miR-663 was increased after resveratrol treatment, which possess putative tumor-suppressor functions and targets TGF1 transcript. Resveratrol treatment also upregulated components of the TGFβ signaling pathway, including TGFβ receptors type I and type II and downregulated the transcriptional activity of canonical TGFβ key effectors proteins, SMADs. These findings suggest that miR-663 is a target for resveratrol action which contributes to its anticancer properties (Tili et al. 2010).

Organosulfur Compounds

Allium vegetables, such as garlic, have been in use in traditional medicine for a long period of time and impart health benefits as hypoglycemic agent, and in improving immunity, cardiovascular health, protection from microbial, radiation and cancer. Their anticancer effects have been attributed to organosulfur compounds [OSCs] released on processing. OSCs are generated upon conversion of alliin to allicin and other alkyl alkane-thiosulfinates by the action of alliinase. These products are highly unstable and decompose to various sulfur compounds such as diallyl sulfide [DAS], diallyl disulfide [DADS] and diallyl trisulfide [DATS]. Regular consumption of Allium vegetables is inversely related to the risk of the development of stomach and colon cancers. DADS has been shown to inhibit growth of cancer cells by causing cell cycle arrest and apoptosis, inhibits angiogenesis, and suppresses metastasis (Ariga and Seki 2006). In in vivo models, DADS treatment protected against chemically-induced cancer of various organs and inhibited tumor growth in xenograft models. DADS generates its active metabolite S-allylmercaptocysteine [SAMC] and both are finally metabolized to allyl mercaptan [AM] and other metabolites (Lea et al. 1999).

Studies have shown that DADS and SAMC induces histone acetylation and cell growth inhibition in DS19 mouse erythroleukemia cells and their metabolite AM was found to be a more potent HDAC inhibitor. In silico docking studies predicted their direct binding to the HDAC active site and their HDACs inhibitory potential was confirmed by performing activity assays (Lea et al. 2002). DADS caused increased global acetylation of H3 and H4 histones and increased binding of acetylated histone H3 onto the promoter of p21 gene which correlated with upregulation of p21 and cell cycle arrest and HDAC inhibition. Induction of histone acetylation by S-allylmercaptocysteine was observed in human colon cancer Caco-2 cells and human breast cancer T47D cells, where HDAC activity was inhibited by allyl butyrate (Druesne et al. 2004). In another study, treatment of DS19 cells with S-allylmercaptocysteine or allyl isothiocyanate resulted in downregulation of HDACs and HATs. Furthermore, hyperacetylation of histones was induced in a number of cancer cell lines by DADS treatment, causing p21 upregulation, cell-cycle arrest and induction of differentiation and apoptosis. Treatment of colon cancer Caco-2 and HT-29 cells inhibited HDACs and in turn caused acetylation of histones H3 and H4 with increase in the expression of p21/Waf1, resulting in cell cycle arrest (Druesne et al. 2004).

Lycopene

Lycopene is one of the naturally occurring classes of tetra-terpenoids mainly present in tomato and tomato products. It is a potent antioxidant and has been shown to reduce oxidative DNA damage. Studies with animal cancer models exhibit that lycopene reduced tumor growth in breast, prostate and lungs whereas it was ineffective in preventing colon, kidney and liver cancers (Giovannucci 1999). In a study using a single dose of 2 μM lycopene partially demethylate GSTP1 gene and increased its mRNA expression in MDA-MB-468 breast cancer cell line but RARβ2 gene was not demethylated in either MDA-MB-468 or MCF-7 breast cancer cell lines. Lycopene treatment caused demethylation of the RARβ2 and HIN-1 genes in the non-tumorigenic MCF10A fibrocystic breast cells. This data demonstrate that lycopene might have DNA demethylating potential however further investigation is needed to understand the mechanism[s] of demethylation of gene promoter by lycopene (King-Batoon et al. 2008).

Quercetin

Quercetin is a dietary polyphenol, predominantly present in citrus fruits and buckwheat. It is a multi-potent bioflavonoid with immense potential for the prevention and treatment of cancer (Gibellini et al. 2011). Quercetin has been shown to activate NAD+ dependent histone deacetylase SIRT1 in yeast. Quercetin has been shown to inhibit the growth of colon cancer RKO cells by reversing the hypermethylation of $p16^{INK4a}$ gene (Tan et al. 2008). Quercetin has been shown to inhibit the expression of TNF-induced interferon-gamma-inducible protein 10 [IP-10] and macrophage inflammatory protein 2 [MIP-2] which were associated with inhibition of CBP/p300 activity and phosphorylation/acetylation of histone H3 on the promoter region of these genes (Ruiz et al. 2007). In another study, quercetin induced FasL-mediated apoptosis in human leukemia HL-60 cells by transactivation through activation of c-jun/AP-1 and promotion of histone H3 acetylation (Lee et al. 2011). Recent study demonstrates that administration of quercetin to DMBA-painted hamsters reduced tumor incidence and tumor burden, whereas post-treatment of quercetin resulted in a significant tumor growth delay. Quercetin administration caused cell cycle arrest and apoptosis and blocked invasion and angiogenesis which correlated with the inhibition of HDAC-1 and DNMT1 (Priyadarsini et al. 2011).

Ellagitannins

Ellagitannins are phytochemicals present in high concentrations in many fruits and nuts, such as pomegranate, raspberries, walnuts and almonds. These are polyesters of ellagic acid and a sugar moiety and upon hydrolysis release ellagic acid. Ellagitannins exhibit anti-oxidant and radical scavenging, antiviral, antimicrobial, anti-mutagenic, anti-inflammatory, anti-tumor promoting and immunomodulatory properties (Heber 2008). Ellagitannins elicit their anticancer effects by modulating transcription factors and signaling pathways which inhibit cancer cells proliferation and induces apoptosis. In particular, exposure of liver cancer cells with ellagitannin BJA3121 isolated from a plant *Balanophora japonica* resulted in cell growth inhibition and alteration in the expression of several miRNAs. BJA3121 treatment resulted in upregulation of miR-let-7e, miR-370, miR-373* and miR-526b and downregulation of let-7a, let-7c, let-7d which correlated with genes involved in cell differentiation and proliferation (Wen et al. 2009).

Other Dietary Phytochemicals

In addition to aforementioned dietary phytochemicals, a number of other natural dietary compounds are under scrutiny for their ability to exhibit chemopreventive/ therapeutic potential through epigenetic modification(s). These phytochemicals include apigenin, biacalein, cyanidins, rosmarinic acid, silibinin/silymarin, dihydrocoumarin and others which have been reported to have either direct or indirect epigenetic targets in cancer prevention and therapy. These compounds are integral part of regular food products and can be integrated in the diet on regular basis leading to reversal in epigenetic modifications.

Conclusions and Future Directions

The awareness campaign of chemoprevention has led to widespread recognition and use of bioactive phytochemicals around the globe. From the studies described herein, it is clear that dietary phytochemicals hold great promise in cancer prevention and in therapy by causing epigenetic modifications. As the importance of epigenetic modifications in cancer is well recognized, precise contribution of epigenetic mechanisms and cellular targets of epigenetic alterations by dietary phytochemicals in human cancer needs further investigation. Although recent advances in the field of cancer epigenetics has enhanced our understanding of epigenetic changes in normal cellular processes and abnormal events leading to tumorigenesis, however deeper understanding of the global patterns of epigenetic modifications by phytochemicals in cancer will lead to design better strategies to prevent and cure cancer. Moreover, sufficient preclinical and clinical data is required on the epigenetic changes induced by dietary phytochemicals which will to lead to better understanding of the epigenetic targets and pathways altered by these agents to elicit their efficacy in cancer. Additional preclinical and clinical studies are required to analyze the safety profile of doses, route of administration, organ bioavailability alone and in combination in order to obtain maximum beneficial effects. At last, systematic well-designed randomized placebo-controlled trials with adequate power and relevant clinical epigenetic endpoints are needed. Despite these challenges, research on dietary phytochemicals continues to emerge and will offer new epigenetic targets and promising agents with more opportunities for prevention, and perhaps therapy of cancer in the near future.

Acknowledgements The original work from author's laboratory outlined in this review was supported by United States Public Health Service Grants RO1CA108512, RO1CA115491 and RO1AT002709. We apologize to those investigators whose original work could not be cited owing to the space limitations.

Conflict of interest: The authors have no competing interest

Dr Sanjay Gupta is Carter Kissell Associate Professor & Research Director in the Department of Urology and holds secondary appointment in the Department of Nutrition at Case Western Reserve University and Division of General Medical Sciences at Case Comprehensive Cancer Center, Cleveland, Ohio, USA.

Dr Vijay S Thakur is Senior Research Associate in the Department of Urology at Case Western Reserve University, Cleveland, Ohio, USA.

References

Ali S, Ahmad A, Banerjee S, Padhye S et al (2010) Gemcitabine sensitivity can be induced in pancreatic cancer cells through modulation of miR-200 and miR-21 expression by curcumin or its analogue CDF. Cancer Res 70(9):3606–3617

Ariga T, Seki T (2006) Antithrombotic and anticancer effects of garlic-derived sulfur compounds: a review. Biofactors 26(2):93–103

Attig L, Gabory A, Junien C (2010) Symposium 2: modern approaches to nutritional research challenges nutritional developmental epigenomics: immediate and long-lasting effects in the conference on 'Over- and undernutrition: challenges and approaches. Proc Nutr Soc 69:221–231

Balasubramanian S, Adhikary G, Eckert RL (2010) The Bmi-1 polycomb protein antagonizes the (-)-epigallocatechin-3-gallate-dependent suppression of skin cancer cell survival. Carcinogenesis 31(3):496–503

Balasubramanyam K, Varier RA, Altaf M, Swaminathan V et al (2004) Curcumin, a novel p300/CREB-binding protein-specific inhibitor of acetyltransferase, represses the acetylation of histone/nonhistone proteins and histone acetyltransferase-dependent chromatin transcription. J Biol Chem 279(49):51163–51171

Banerjee S, Li Y, Wang Z, Sarkar FH (2008) Multi-targeted therapy of cancer by genistein. Cancer Lett 269(2):226–242

Banerjee S, Kong D, Wang Z, Bao B et al (2011) Attenuation of multi-targeted proliferation-linked signaling by 3,3′-diindolylmethane (DIM): from bench to clinic. Mutat Res 728(1–2):47–66

Basak S, Pookot D, Noonan EJ, Dahiya R (2008) Genistein down-regulates androgen receptor by modulating HDAC6-Hsp90 chaperone function. Mol Cancer Ther 7(10):3195–3202

Berletch JB, Liu C, Love WK, Andrews LG et al (2008) Epigenetic and genetic mechanisms contribute to telomerase inhibition by EGCG. J Cell Biochem 103(2):509–519

Bora-Tatar G, Dayangaç-Erden D, Demir AS, Dalkara S et al (2009) Molecular modifications on carboxylic acid derivatives as potent histone deacetylase inhibitors: activity and docking studies. Bioorg Med Chem 17(14):5219–5228

Chen Y, Shu W, Chen W, Wu Q et al (2007) Curcumin, both histone deacetylase and p300/CBP-specific inhibitor, represses the activity of nuclear factor kappa B and Notch 1 in Raji cells. Basic Clin Pharmacol Toxicol 101(6):427–433

Cheung KL, Kong AN (2010) Molecular targets of dietary phenethyl isothiocyanate and sulforaphane for cancer chemoprevention. AAPS J 12(1):87–97

Cho HS, Park JH, Kim YJ (2007) Epigenomics: novel aspect of genomic regulation. J Biochem Mol Biol 40(2):151–155

Clarke JD, Dashwood RH, Ho E (2008) Multi-targeted prevention of cancer by sulforaphane. Cancer Lett 269(2):291–304

Dehan P, Kustermans G, Guenin S, Horion J et al (2009) DNA methylation and cancer diagnosis: new methods and applications. Expert Rev Mol Diagn 9(7):651–657

Denis H, Ndlovu MN, Fuks F (2011) Regulation of mammalian DNA methyltransferases: a route to new mechanisms. EMBO rep 12(7):647–656

Druesne N, Pagniez A, Mayeur C, Thomas M et al (2004) Diallyl disulfide (DADS) increases histone acetylation and p21(waf1/cip1) expression in human colon tumor cell lines. Carcinogenesis 25(7):1227–1236

Fang MZ, Wang Y, Ai N, Hou Z et al (2003) Tea polyphenol (-)-epigallocatechin-3-gallate inhibits DNA methyltransferase and reactivates methylation-silenced genes in cancer cell lines. Cancer Res 63(22):7563–7570

Fang MZ, Chen D, Sun Y, Jin Z (2005) Reversal of hypermethylation and reactivation of p16INK4a, RARbeta, and MGMT genes by genistein and other isoflavones from soy. Clin Cancer Res 11(19 Pt 1):7033–7041

Fix LN, Shah M, Efferth T, Farwell MA et al (2010) MicroRNA expression profile of MCF-7 human breast cancer cells and the effect of green tea polyphenon-60. Cancer Genomics Proteomics 7(5):261–277

Gao Z, Xu Z, Hung MS, Lin YC et al (2009) Promoter demethylation of WIF-1 by epigallocatechin-3-gallate in lung cancer cells. Anticancer Res 29(6):2025–2030

Garzon R, Calin GA, Croce CM (2009) MicroRNAs in cancer. Annu Rev Med 60:167–179

Gibellini L, Pinti M, Nasi M, Montagna JP et al (2011) Quercetin and cancer chemoprevention. Evid Based Complement Altern Med 2011:591356

Giovannucci E (1999) Tomatoes, tomato-based products, lycopene, and cancer: review of the epidemiologic literature. J Natl Cancer Inst 91(4):317–331

Goldberg AD, Allis CD, Bernstein E (2007) Epigenetics: a landscape takes shape. Cell 128(4):635–638

Gu B, Ding Q, Xia G, Fang Z (2009) EGCG inhibits growth and induces apoptosis in renal cell carcinoma through TFPI-2 overexpression. Oncol Rep 21(3):635–640

Heber D (2008) Multi-targeted therapy of cancer by ellagitannins. Cancer Lett 269(2):262–268

Hong T, Nakagawa T, Pan W, Kim MY et al (2004) Isoflavones stimulate estrogen receptor-mediated core histone acetylation. Biochem Biophys Res Commun 317(1):259–264

Issa JP, Kantarjian HM (2009) Targeting DNA methylation. Clin Cancer Res 15(12):3938–3946

Izzotti A, Calin GA, Steele VE, Cartiglia C et al (2010a) Chemoprevention of cigarette smoke–induced alterations of microRNA expression in rat lungs. Cancer Prev Res (Phila) 3(1):62–72

Izzotti A, Larghero P, Cartiglia C, Longobardi M et al (2010b) Modulation of microRNA expression by budesonide, phenethyl isothiocyanate and cigarette smoke in mouse liver and lung. Carcinogenesis 31(5):894–901

Jelinic P, Shaw P (2007) Loss of imprinting and cancer. J Pathol 211(3):261–268

Jin Y, Zou X, Feng X (2010) 3,3′-Diindolylmethane negatively regulates Cdc25A and induces a G2/M arrest by modulation of microRNA 21 in human breast cancer cells. Anticancer Drugs 21(9):814–822

Jones PA (2002) DNA methylation and cancer. Oncogene 21(35):5358–5360

Kang J, Chen J, Shi Y, Jia J et al (2005) Curcumin-induced histone hypoacetylation: the role of reactive oxygen species. Biochem Pharmacol 69(8):1205–1213

Kato K, Long NK, Makita H, Toida M et al (2008) Effects of green tea polyphenol on methylation status of RECK gene and cancer cell invasion in oral squamous cell carcinoma cells. Br J Cancer 99(4):647–654

Kikuno N, Shiina H, Urakami S, Kawamoto K et al (2008) Genistein mediated histone acetylation and demethylation activates tumor suppressor genes in prostate cancer cells. Int J Cancer 123(3):552–560

King-Batoon A, Leszczynska JM, Klein CB (2008) Modulation of gene methylation by genistein or lycopene in breast cancer cells. Environ Mol Mutagen 49(1):36–45

Kupchella CE (1986) Environmental factors in cancer etiology. Semin Oncol Nurs 2(3):161–169

Lan J, Hua S, He X, Zhang Y (2010) DNA methyltransferases and methyl-binding proteins of mammals. Acta Biochim Biophys Sin 42(4):243–252

Lea MA, Randolph VM, Patel M (1999) Increased acetylation of histones induced by diallyl disulfide and structurally related molecules. Int J Oncol 15(2):347–352

Lea MA, Randolph VM, Lee JE, des Bordes C (2001) Induction of histone acetylation in mouse erythroleukemia cells by some organosulfur compounds including allyl isothiocyanate. Int J Cancer 92(6):784–789

Lea MA, Rasheed M, Randolph VM, Khan F et al (2002) Induction of histone acetylation and inhibition of growth of mouse erythroleukemia cells by S-allylmercaptocysteine. Nutr Cancer 43(1):90–102

Lee WJ, Shim JY, Zhu BT (2005) Mechanisms for the inhibition of DNA methyltransferases by tea catechins and bioflavonoids. Mol Pharmacol 68(4):1018–1030

Lee WJ, Chen YR, Tseng TH (2011) Quercetin induces FasL-related apoptosis, in part, through promotion of histone H3 acetylation in human leukemia HL-60 cells. Oncol Rep 25(2):583–591

Li Y, VandenBoom TG 2nd, Kong D, Wang Z et al (2009) Up-regulation of miR-200 and let-7 by natural agents leads to the reversal of epithelial-to-mesenchymal transition in gemcitabine-resistant pancreatic cancer cells. Cancer Res 69(16):6704–6712

Li Y, Li X, Guo B (2010a) Chemopreventive agent 3,3′-diindolylmethane selectively induces proteasomal degradation of class I histone deacetylases. Cancer Res 70(2):646–654

Li Y, Vandenboom TG 2nd, Wang Z, Kong D et al (2010b) miR-146a suppresses invasion of pancreatic cancer cells. Cancer Res 70(4):1486–1495

Lin SC, Li WC, Shih JW, Hong KF et al (2006) The tea polyphenols EGCG and EGC repress mRNA expression of human telomerase reverse transcriptase (hTERT) in carcinoma cells. Cancer Lett 236(1):80–88

Liu HL, Chen Y, Cui GH, Zhou JF (2005) Curcumin, a potent anti-tumor reagent, is a novel histone deacetylase inhibitor regulating B-NHL cell line Raji proliferation. Acta Pharmacol Sin 26(5):603–609

Liu Z, Xie Z, Jones W, Pavlovicz RE et al (2009) Curcumin is a potent DNA hypomethylation agent. Bioorg Med Chem Lett 19(3):706–709

Macaluso M, Paggi MG, Giordano A (2003) Genetic and epigenetic alterations as hallmarks of the intricate road to cancer. Oncogene 22(42):6472–6478

Majid S, Kikuno N, Nelles J, Noonan E et al (2008) Genistein induces the p21WAF1/CIP1 and p16INK4a tumor suppressor genes in prostate cancer cells by epigenetic mechanisms involving active chromatin modification. Cancer Res 68(8):2736–2744

Majid S, Dar AA, Ahmad AE, Hirata H et al (2009) BTG3 tumor suppressor gene promoter demethylation, histone modification and cell cycle arrest by genistein in renal cancer. Carcinogenesis 30(4):662–670

Majid S, Dar AA, Shahryari V, Hirata H et al (2010a) Genistein reverses hypermethylation and induces active histone modifications in tumor suppressor gene B-Cell translocation gene 3 in prostate cancer. Cancer 116(1):66–76

Majid S, Dar AA, Saini S, Chen Y et al (2010b) Regulation of minichromosome maintenance gene family by microRNA-1296 and genistein in prostate cancer. Cancer Res 70(7):2809–2818

Marcu MG, Jung YJ, Lee S, Chung EJ et al (2006) Curcumin is an inhibitor of p300 histone acetylatransferase. Med Chem 2(2):169–174

Medina-Franco JL, López-Vallejo F, Kuck D, Lyko F (2011) Natural products as DNA methyltransferase inhibitors: a computer-aided discovery approach. Mol Divers 15(2):293–304

Meeran SM, Patel SN, Tollefsbol TO (2010) Sulforaphane causes epigenetic repression of hTERT expression in human breast cancer cell lines. PLoS One 5(7):e11457

Mudduluru G, George-William JN, Muppala S, Asangani IA et al (2011) Curcumin regulates miR-21 expression and inhibits invasion and metastasis in colorectal cancer. Biosci Rep 31(3):185–197

Murugan RS, Vinothini G, Hara Y, Nagini S (2009) Black tea polyphenols target matrix metalloproteinases, RECK, proangiogenic molecules and histone deacetylase in a rat hepatocarcinogenesis model. Anticancer Res 29(6):2301–2305

Myzak MC, Karplus PA, Chung FL, Dashwood RH (2004) A novel mechanism of chemoprotection by sulforaphane: inhibition of histone deacetylase. Cancer Res 64(16):5767–5774

Myzak MC, Hardin K, Wang R, Dashwood RH et al (2006a) Sulforaphane inhibits histone deacetylase activity in BPH-1, LnCaP and PC-3 prostate epithelial cells. Carcinogenesis 27(4):811–819

Myzak MC, Dashwood WM, Orner GA, Ho E et al (2006b) Sulforaphane inhibits histone deacetylase in vivo and suppresses tumorigenesis in Apc-minus mice. FASEB J 20(3):506–508

Myzak MC, Tong P, Dashwood WM, Dashwood RH et al (2007) Sulforaphane retards the growth of human PC-3 xenografts and inhibits HDAC activity in human subjects. Exp Biol Med (Maywood) 232(2):227–234

Navarro-Perán E, Cabezas-Herrera J, del Campo LS, Rodríguez-López JN (2007) Effects of folate cycle disruption by the green tea polyphenol epigallocatechin-3-gallate. Int J Biochem Cell Biol 39(12):2215–2225

Pandey M, Shukla S, Gupta S (2010) Promoter demethylation and chromatin remodeling by green tea polyphenols leads to re-expression of GSTP1 in human prostate cancer cells. Int J Cancer 126(11):2520–2533

Parker LP, Taylor DD, Kesterson J, Metzinger DS et al (2009) Modulation of microRNA associated with ovarian cancer cells by genistein. Eur J Gynaecol Oncol 30(6):616–621

Pledgie-Tracy A, Sobolewski MD, Davidson NE (2007) Sulforaphane induces cell type-specific apoptosis in human breast cancer cell lines. Mol Cancer Ther 6(3):1013–1021

Priyadarsini RV, Vinothini G, Murugan RS, Manikandan P et al (2011) The flavonoid quercetin modulates the hallmark capabilities of hamster buccal pouch tumors. Nutr Cancer 63(2):218–226

Qin W, Zhu W, Shi H, Hewett JE et al (2009) Soy isoflavones have an anti-estrogenic effect and alter mammary promoter hypermethylation in healthy premenopausal women. Nutr Cancer 61(2):238–244

Ran ZH, Zou J, Xiao SD (2005) Experimental study on anti-neoplastic activity of epigallocatechin-3-gallate to digestive tract carcinomas. Chin Med J (Engl) 118(16):1330–1337

Ruiz PA, Braune A, Hölzlwimmer G, Quintanilla-Fend L et al (2007) Quercetin inhibits TNF-induced NF-kappaB transcription factor recruitment to proinflammatory gene promoters in murine intestinal epithelial cells. J Nutr 137(5):1208–1215

Savouret JF, Quesne M (2002) Resveratrol and cancer: a review. Biomed Pharmacother 56(2):84–87

Sawan C, Herceg Z (2010) Histone modifications and cancer. Adv Genet 70:57–85

Siddiqui IA, Adhami VM, Saleem M, Mukhtar H (2006) Beneficial effects of tea and its polyphenols against prostate cancer. Mol Nutr Food Res 50(2):130–143

Stefanska B, Rudnicka K, Bednarek A, Fabianowska-Majewska K (2010) Hypomethylation and induction of retinoic acid receptor beta 2 by concurrent action of adenosine analogues and natural compounds in breast cancer cells. Eur J Pharmacol 638(1–3):47–53

Stein CJ, Colditz GA (2004) Modifiable risk factors for cancer. Br J Cancer 90(2):299–303

Sun M, Estrov Z, Ji Y, Coombes KR et al (2008) Curcumin (diferuloylmethane) alters the expression profiles of microRNAs in human pancreatic cancer cells. Mol Cancer Ther 7(3):464–473

Sun Q, Cong R, Yan H, Gu H et al (2009) Genistein inhibits growth of human uveal melanoma cells and affects microRNA-27a and target gene expression. Oncol Rep 22(3):563–567

Tan S, Wang C, Lu C, Zhao B et al (2008) Quercetin is able to demethylate the p16INK4a gene promoter. Chemotherapy 55(1):6–10

Teiten MH, Eifes S, Dicato M, Diederich M (2010) Curcumin-the paradigm of a multi-target natural compound with applications in cancer prevention and treatment. Toxins 2(1):128–162

Tili E, Michaille JJ, Alder H, Volinia S et al (2010) Resveratrol modulates the levels of microRNAs targeting genes encoding tumor-suppressors and effectors of TGFβ signaling pathway in SW480 cells. Biochem Pharmacol 80(12):2057–2065

Traka M, Gasper AV, Smith JA, Hawkey CJ et al (2005) Transcriptome analysis of human colon Caco-2 cells exposed to sulforaphane. J Nutr 135(8):1865–1872

Tsang WP, Kwok TT (2010) Epigallocatechin gallate up-regulation of miR-16 and induction of apoptosis in human cancer cells. J Nutr Biochem 21(2):140–146

Volate SR, Muga SJ, Issa AY, Nitcheva D et al (2009) Epigenetic modulation of the retinoid X receptor alpha by green tea in the azoxymethane-Apc Min/+ mouse model of intestinal cancer. Mol Carcinog 48(10):920–933

Wang LG, Beklemisheva A, Liu XM, Ferrari AC et al (2007) Dual action on promoter demethylation and chromatin by an isothiocyanate restored GSTP1 silenced in prostate cancer. Mol Carcinog 46(1):24–31

Wang RH, Zheng Y, Kim HS, Xu X et al (2008) Interplay among BRCA1, SIRT1, and survivin during BRCA1-associated tumorigenesis. Mol Cell 32(1):11–20

Wen XY, Wu SY, Li ZQ, Liu ZQ et al (2009) Ellagitannin (BJA3121), an anti-proliferative natural polyphenol compound, can regulate the expression of miRNAs in HepG2 cancer cells. Phytother Res 23(6):778–784

Xiao GS, Jin YS, Lu QY, Zhang ZF et al (2006) Annexin-I as a potential target for green tea extract induced actin remodeling. Int J Cancer 120(1):111–120

Yang J, Cao Y, Sun J, Zhang Y (2010) Curcumin reduces the expression of Bcl-2 by upregulating miR-15a and miR-16 in MCF-7 cells. Med Oncol 27(4):1114–1118

Yuasa Y, Nagasaki H, Akiyama Y, Sakai H et al (2005) Relationship between CDX2 gene methylation and dietary factors in gastric cancer patients. Carcinogenesis 26(1):193–200

Zhang J, Zhang T, Ti X, Shi J et al (2010) Curcumin promotes apoptosis in A549/DDP multidrug-resistant human lung adenocarcinoma cells through an miRNA signaling pathway. Biochem Biophys Res Commun 399(1):1–6

Chapter 20
Modulation of the Nrf2 Signaling Pathway by Chemopreventive Dietary Phytoconstituents

Altaf S. Darvesh M.Pharm., Ph.D. and Anupam Bishayee

Contents

Abstract Epidemiological studies have revealed the healing power of a diet rich in fruits and vegetables in both the prevention and amelioration of chronic illness. Chemoprevention, utilizing dietary agents, has been suggested as a fascinating strategy in the fight against cancer. Dietary phytoconstituents, such as carotenoids, polyphenols and organosulfur compounds, present in a multitude of dietary sources have been shown to possess potent antioxidant and anti-inflammatory properties as well as the ability to modulate a multitude of signaling mechanisms. Oxidative stress is a key element of the pathogenesis of neoplastic diseases and its attenuation is a vital step in the chemopreventive strategy. The nuclear factor-erythroid 2-related factor 2 (Nrf2)-mediated signaling pathway is the primary antioxidant mechanism in nature and thus an extremely critical element of the chemopreventive strategy. This chapter highlights the Nrf2-modulating property of dietary phytoconstituents in their ability to afford chemoprevention against a multitude of neoplastic diseases. This article provides a brief explanation of the Nrf-2 signaling pathway, its

A.S. Darvesh M.Pharm., Ph.D.
Department of Pharmaceutical Sciences, College of Pharmacy, Northeast Ohio Medical University, Rootstown, OH 44272, USA
e-mail: adarvesh@neomed.edu

A. Bishayee (✉)
Department of Pharmaceutical and Administrative Sciences, School of Pharmacy, American University of Health Sciences, 1600 East Hill Street, Signal Hill, CA 90755, USA
e-mail: abishayee@auhs.edu

S. Shankar and R.K. Srivastava (eds.), *Nutrition, Diet and Cancer*,
DOI 10.1007/978-94-007-2923-0_20,

antioxidant effects and its role in the chemoprevention as well as amelioration of neoplastic disorders. Essentially reviewed are studies which elucidate pharmacological effects of select dietary phytochemicals in pre-clinical models of cancer with special emphasis on their Nrf2 modulating properties. The article also highlights the current status of progress entailed in the development of the Nrf2 modulation pathway using dietary phytonutrients as a robust chemopreventive strategy with practical significance in the clinic.

Introduction

Epidemiological evidence presents a strong indication that a diet rich in the consumption of fruits, vegetables, nuts and spices has tremendous potential in the prevention of chronic illnesses, such as cardiovascular, endocrine, neurodegenerative and neoplastic diseases (Eussen et al. 2011). Cancer chemoprevention utilizing dietary intervention has been suggested as an extremely safe, effective and clinically relevant strategy in the battle against cancer (Ross 2010; Johnson and de Meija 2011; Schmid et al. 2011). Dietary agents are a rich source of phytochemicals which possess potent antioxidant and anti-inflammatory properties as well as the ability to modulate pleotropic signaling mechanisms most of which regulate the aforementioned properties (Eggler et al. 2008; Khor et al. 2008; Kang et al. 2011).

Oxidative stress has been strongly implicated in the pathogenesis of neoplastic progression. Cancer cells have been shown to have a significantly higher redox imbalance as compared to normal cells. Although oxidative damage to lipids, proteins and nucleic acids all contribute to the process of carcinogenesis, it is the oxidation of both the nuclear and mitochondrial DNA, which leads to DNA mutation, has been shown to be the primary contributor to the process of carcinogenesis (Klaunig and Kamendulis 2004; Valko et al. 2004, 2006). Lipid peroxidation results in the formation of both DNA-DNA interstrand crosslinks as well as DNA-protein crosslinks. DNA oxidation leads to formation of a variety of modified bases and sugars, strand breaks and DNA-replication crosslinks. These changes lead to genomic instability with accompanying errors in transcription and replication as well as modulation of several signal pathways which contribute to the process of carcinogenesis (Cooke et al. 2003; Treuba et al. 2004). Although free radicals are implicated in oxidative damage to biomolecules, they have also been shown to influence varied aspects of cell signal regulation and gene expression (Palmer and Paulson 1997).

Carcinogenesis is a complex process consisting of three distinct, but closely linked stages, namely initiation, promotion and progression. The initial stage is the rapid and irreversible uptake of the carcinogen, its distribution, metabolic activation ultimately leading to genotoxic damage. Tumor promotion is a rather lengthy process in which there is accumulation of preneoplastic cells. This leads to the final stage of tumor progression with invasive and metastatic potential (Moolgavkar 1978). The inhibition, reversal or delay of the biochemical actions which lead to neoplastic transformation provides an effective means to control cancer. The strategy to block the development of carcinogenic events rather than to merely treat neoplastic growth after its formation has been a forceful strategy especially in the past two decades for the control of cancer (Kelloff et al. 1999; Sporn and Suh 2002).

Michael Sporn pioneered the concept of *'chemoprevention'* about three decades ago and advocated the use of potentially safe and relatively non-toxic compounds, either of natural or synthetic origin, to arrest the process of carcinogenesis in its earliest stage (Sporn 1991). The Wattenberg classification categorizes chemopreventive agents into blocking agents and suppressing agents (Wattenberg 1985). Blocking agents prevent the access and metabolic activation of carcinogens and its interaction with biomolecules such as cellular proteins and DNA. Suppressing agents on the other hand prevent both pre-malignant and malignant transformation of carcinogens. This process is achieved by modulation of several biochemical processes such as activation of tumor suppressor genes and inactivation of oncogenes (Manson et al. 2000).

One of the most promising mechanisms to ensure chemoprevention is by activation of the signaling pathway mediated by nuclear transcription factor erythroid-2 related factor (Nrf2) which leads to the induction of a multitude of detoxifying antioxidant enzymes. Several chemopreventive agents, either synthetic or natural in origin, possess the potent ability to activate the Nrf2 signal cascade and induce expression of antioxidant enzymes (Manson et al. 2000; Kong et al. 2001; Hayes and McMahon 2001; Hayes et al. 2010). In this succinct review, we describe the role of Nrf2 modulation in the chemopreventive effects of several popular compounds of dietary origin.

The NRF2 Pathway

The biological system has developed an efficient mechanism to protect itself from environmental insult, such as exposure to toxins and carcinogens. This is primarily achieved by either inhibiting the formation of the xenobiotic reactive species or by detoxification mechanisms. Xenobiotic metabolism primarily occurs by phase 1 and 2 biotransformation. Phase 1 reactions by cytochrome P450 enzymes such as oxidation and reduction increase the carcinogenic activation and enhance xenobiotic reactivity. Phase 2 metabolism leading to the conjugation of carcinogenic compounds with endogenous ligands, such as glucuronic acid and glutathione, leads to a reduction in electrophilicity and a resulting loss of carcinogen reactivity (Wattenberg 1975). The induction of phase 2 detoxifying enzymes and the resulting inactivation of the carcinogenic moiety remains key to effective chemoprevention (Lee and Surh 2005; Kundu and Surh 2010). Chemopreventive agents with blocking effects have been shown to induce the expression and resulting activity of a myriad spectrum of phase 2 enzymes, such as glutathione *S*-transferase (GST) (Benson et al. 1978), NAD(P)H:quinone oxidoreductase 1 (NQO1) (Benson et al. 1980), UDP-glucuronosyltransferase (UGT) (Cha and Heine 1982) and hemeoxygenase-1 (HO-1) (Primiano et al. 1996).

The antioxidant-response element (ARE) is a specific DNA-promoter-binding region present in the 5′ region of the genes encoding for phase enzymes such as GST, UGT, NQO1, HO-1 as well as several others. ARE transcription occurs due to presence of toxic electrophiles such as carcinogens as well as various antioxidant compounds (Nguyen et al. 2009). ARE transcription and the resulting expression of detoxifying phase 2 enzymes are regulated in part by Nrf2, a member of the helix-loop-helix basic leucine zipper family of transcription factors. Under basal conditions, in the absence of stressful stimuli or lack of exposure to antioxidants, Nrf2 remains sequestered in the cytoplasm by Kelch-like ECH-associated protein 1 (Keap1). ARE inducers, either carcinogenic toxins or antioxidants, lead to the dissociation and nuclear translocation of Nrf2 from Keap1. In the nucleus, the unbound Nrf2 then undergoes heterodimerization with the small Maf protein and subsequently binds to ARE. The final result of these molecular events is the transcription of antioxidant genes and expression of phase 2 enzymes. The Keap1-Nrf2-ARE signaling pathway is also modulated by several upstream kinases, such as the family of mitogen-activated protein kinases. The Nrf2 signaling cascade has been cited as the most important antioxidant process with potent chemopreventive properties. Several excellent reviews have been published which describe, in effective detail, the molecular events involved in the Nrf2 signaling cascade (Hayes et al. 2010; Lee and Surh 2005; Kundu and Surh 2010; Nguyen et al. 2009; Li and Kong 2009; Hu et al. 2010; Kensler and Wakabayashi 2010; Klaassen and Reisman 2010; Maher and Yamamoto 2010; Slocum and Kensler 2011).

Dietary Phytoconstituents and Chemoprevention: The Role of NRF2

A multitude of potent chemopreventive agents owe their anticancer properties due to their Nrf2 modulatory effects. Synthetic Nrf2 activating chemopreventive agents such as oltipraz have received considerable attention for their chemopreventive potential in neoplastic diseases, such as liver cancer (Zhang and Munday 2008). Besides synthetics, the classes of agents that have shown tremendous chemopreventive potential due to their potent modulatory effects of the Keap1-Nrf2-ARE cascade are phytochemicals of dietary origin. Dietary phytoconstituents from varied sources and diverse chemical structures have been shown to possess the ability to cause activation of the Nrf2 signaling mechanisms. Dietary polyphenols, such as catechins obtained from tea leaves, curcumin from the curry spice turmeric, resveratrol from grapes as well as organosulfur compounds from garlic and onions have been shown to possess Nrf2 modulatory properties (Eggler et al. 2008; Khor et al. 2008; Surh 2008; Surh et al. 2008; Tao et al. 2008; Zhao et al. 2010; Scapagnini et al. 2011). In Tables 20.1 and 20.2, we have presented several studies which have investigated the

Table 20.1 Biological effects of dietary phytoconstituents on the Nrf2 pathway in *in vitro* models of cancer

Model system	Biological effect	Mechanism	Reference
Allyl isothiocyanate			
HepG2 cells *(Liver cancer)*		↑ARE, ↑Nrf2, ↑HO-1	Jeong et al. (2005)
Coffee			
HepG2 cells *(Liver cancer)*		↑UGT genes, ↑UGT1A mRNA	Kalthoff et al. (2010)
Caco-2 cells *(Colon cancer)*			
KYSE70 cells *(Esophageal cancer)*			
Capsaicin			
HepG2 cells *(Liver cancer)*		↑ARE, ↑Nrf2, ↑HO-1, ↑NQO1	Joung et al. (2007)
β-Damascenone, 3-hydroxy-β-damascone			
Hepa1c1c7 cells *(Liver cancer)*		↑QR, iNOS, ↑Nrf2	Gerhäuser et al. (2009)
Epicatechin			
HepG2 cells *(Liver cancer)*		↑IKK, ↑NF-κB,↑AP-1, ↑Nrf2, ↑PI3K/AKT, ↑ERK	Granado-Serrano et al. (2010)
Epigallocatechin-3-gallate			
Caco-2 cells *(Colon cancer)*		↑Nrf2, ↑UGT1A	Zhang et al. (2009)
Gallic acid			
HepG2 cells *(Liver cancer)*		↑PST-P, ↑MAPK	Yeh and Yen (2006)
Hydroxytyrosol			
HepG2 cells *(Liver cancer)*	Protected cells against *t*-BOOTH-induced cytotoxicity	↑GPx, ↑GR, ↑GST, ↑Nrf2, ↑PI3K/AKT, ↑ERK	Martín et al. (2010)
Organosulfur garlic compounds-DAS, DADS, DATS			
HepG2 cells *(Liver cancer)*		↑ARE, ↑Nrf2, ↑HO-1, ↑NQO1, ↑MAPK	Chen et al. (2004)
Lycopene			
HepG2 cells *(Liver cancer)*		↑NQO1, ↑NQO1 mRNA, ↑GCS	Ben-Dor et al. (2005)

(continued)

Table 20.1 (continued)

Model system	Biological effect	Mechanism	Reference
MCF-7 cells *(Breast cancer)*			
BEAS-2B cells *(Lung cancer)*	Reduced the H_2O_2-induced oxidative damage	↑Nrf2, ↑HO-1, ↑NQO1, ↑GCL, ↑GST ↓ROS	Lian and Wang (2008)
Parthenolide			
HepG2 cells *(Liver cancer)*		↑ARE, ↑Nrf2, ↑HO-1	Jeong et al. (2005)
Phenethyl isothiocyanate			
HeLa cells *(Cervical cancer)*		↑Nrf2, ↑JNK	Keum et al. (2003)
PC-3 cells *(Prostate cancer)*		↑Nrf2 translocation, ↑ARE activity, ↑ERK1/2, ↑JNK, ↑HO-1	Xu et al. (2006)
Quercetin			
HepG2 cells *(Liver cancer)*		↑ARE, ↑Nrf2, ↓Keap1	Tanigawa et al. (2007)
Caco-2 cells *(Colon cancer)*		↑Nrf2, ↑NQO1, ↑GCLC, ↑GST-A1,P1	Niestroy et al. (2011)
Quercitrin			
Mouse JB6 cells *(Skin cancer)*	Prevented the UVB/TPA-induced neoplastic transformation	↑ARE, ↑Nrf2, ↓p-MAPK	Ding et al. (2010)
Resveratrol			
PC12 cells *(Tumor of adrenal medulla)*	Prevented H_2O_2-induced cell death	↑HO-1, ↑Nrf2, ↑Akt/PKB, ↑ERK1/2, ↑GCL mRNA	Chen et al. (2005)
K562 cells *(Leukemia)*		↑NQO1 protein, ↑NQO1 mRNA, ↑NQO1 enzyme activity, ↑p-Nrf2	Hsieh et al. (2006)

A549 epithelial cells	Protected against CSE-induced toxicity	↑GSH, ↑GCL, ↑Nrf2, ↑Keap1, ↓ROS, ↓4-HNE, ↓3-NT	Kode et al. (2008)
SAEC cells *(Lung cancer)*			
Rat hepatocytes *(Liver cancer)*	Protected against tBHP-induced oxidative damage	↑Nrf2 mRNA, ↑CAT, ↑SOD, ↑GPx, ↑GST	Rubiolo et al. (2008)
Quail hepatocytes *(Liver cancer)*	Protected against heat stress-induced toxicity	↑Nrf2, ↑CAT, ↑SOD, ↑GPx, ↓HSP70, ↓HSP90, ↓NF-κB	Sahin et al. (2011)
HUH7 human hepatoma cells *(Liver cancer)*	Slightly decreased the cell viability	↑Nrf2, ↑HO-1, ↑PON-1	Wagner et al. (2011)
Sulforaphane			
HepG2 cells *(Liver cancer)*		↑Nrf2, ↑HO-1	Jeong et al. (2005)
HepG2 cells *(Liver cancer)*		↑MT-I mRNA, ↑MT-II mRNA, ↑ERK, ↑p38, ↑JNK	Yeh and Yen (2005)
Tigloylgomisin			
HepG2 cells *(Liver cancer)*		↑QR, ↑ARE, ↑Nrf2	Lee et al. (2009)
Zerumbone			
RL34 cells		↑GST, ↑GCS, ↑GPx, ↑OH-1	Nakamura et al. (2004)

Abbreviations: *AP-1* activator protein-1, *ARE* antioxidant responsive element, *CAT* catalase, *CSE DAS* diallyl sulfide, *DADS* diallyl disulfide, *DATS* diallyl trisulfide; cigarette smoke extract, *ERK1/2* extracellular signal-regulated protein kinase, *GCL* glutamate-cysteine ligase, *GCLC* glutamate-cysteine ligase catalytic subunit, *GCS* γ-glutamylcysteine synthetase, *GSH* glutathione, *GST* glutathione-*S*-transferase, *GPx* glutathione peroxidase, *GR* glutathione reductase, *4-HNE* 4-hydroxy-2-nonenal, H_2O_2 hydrogen peroxide, *HO-1* heme oxygenase-1, *HSP70* heat shock protein 70, *HSP90* heat shock protein 90, *IKK* IκB kinase, *iNOS* inducible nitric oxide synthase, *JNK* c-Jun N-terminal kinase, *Keap1* Kelch-like ECH-associated protein 1, *MAPK* mitogen-activated protein kinase, *MT* metallothionein, *NF-κB* nuclear factor-κB, *Nrf2* nuclear factor-erythroid 2-related factor 2, *NQO1* NAD(P)H dehydrogenase (quinone 1), *PI3K/AKT* phosphatidyl inositol 3-kinase/ protein kinase B, *PKB* protein kinase B, *PON-1* paraoxonase-1, *PST-P* phenol sulfotransferase, *p-MAPK* phosphorylated mitogen activated protein kinase, *p-Nrf2* phosphorylated nuclear factor-Erythroid2-related factor 2, *3-NT* 3-nitrotyrosine, *QR* NAD(P)H: quinone reductase, *ROS* reactive oxygen species, *SAEC* small airway epithelial cells, *SOD* superoxide dismutase, *tBHP tert*-butyl hydroperoxide, *t-BOOTH tert*-butyl hydroperoxide, *TPA* 12-*O*-tetradecanoylphorbol-13-acetate, *UGT1A* uridine 5′-diphosphate-glucuronosyltransferase 1A, *UVB* ultraviolet B

Table 20.2 Biological effects of dietary phytoconstituents on the Nrf2 pathway in *in vivo* models of cancer

Model system	Biological effect	Mechanism	Reference
Astaxanthin			
Male Sprague-Dawley rats exposed to cyclophosphamide *(Liver cancer)*	Reduced the size and number of hepatic GST-positive foci	↑NQO-1, ↑HO-1, ↑Nrf2	Tripathi and Jena (2010)
Auraptene			
Female Nrf2 KO and WT mice treated with DMBA *(Breast cancer)*	Did not attenuate the formation of mammary tumors		Becks et al. (2010)
Citrus coumarins			
Nrf2 KO mice		↑ARE, ↑GST, ↑NQO1	Prince et al. (2009)
Coffee			
Humanized UGT1A transgenic mice		↑UGT1A, ↑UGT1A mRNA	Kalthoff et al. (2010)
Curcumin			
C57BL/6J Nrf2 WT and KO mice		Modulation of Nrf2-dependent genes	Shen et al. (2006)
Male Swiss albino mice treated with B[*a*]P *(Lung cancer)*		↑ARE, ↑Nrf2, ↑GST, ↑NQO1, ↓8-OH-dG	Garg et al. (2008)
Male Wistar rats treated with DMN *(Liver cancer)*	Protected the liver against DMN toxicity and possibly carcinogenicity	↑GSH, ↓MDA, ↑HO-1, ↑Nrf2	Farombi et al. (2008)
Epigallocatechin-3-gallate			
BALBcA nude mice injected with HT-29 cells *(Colon cancer)*	Inhibited the metastases of orthotopic colon cancer	↑Nrf2, ↑Nrf mRNA, ↑UGT1A, ↑UGT1A mRNA	Yuan et al. (2007)
BALB/cA nude mice treated with IQ *(Colon cancer)*	Reduced the formation of IQ-induced aberrant crypt foci and atypical hyperplasia	↑Nrf2, ↑Nrf mRNA, ↑UGT1A mRNA	Yuan et al. (2008)
BALB/c mice		↑Nrf2, ↑Nrf mRNA, ↑UGT1A	Zhang et al. (2009)

Phenethyl isothiocyanate			
C57BL/SV129 Nrf (−/−) mice		↑Nrf-regulated genes	Hu et al. (2006a)
Male C57BL/6 mice treated with AOM *(Colon cancer)*	Prevented the AOM-induced polyps and tumor incidence and multiplicity	↑Nrf2, ↑HO-1, ↑NQO1, ↑GST	Cheung et al. (2010)
Pomegranate phytochemicals			
Male Sprague-Dawley rats treated with DENA *(Liver cancer)*	Suppressed the formation and size of GGT-positive hepatic foci and reduced the incidence, total number, multiplicity, size and volume of hepatocyte nodules	↓TBARS, ↓PC, ↑NQO1, ↑GSTA2, ↑GSTA5, ↑GSTM1, ↑GSTM7, ↑GSTT1, ↑UGT1A1, ↑UGT2B17, ↑Nrf2	Bishayee et al. (2011)
Pterostilbene			
Male BALB/c mice treated with AOM *(Colon cancer)*	Reduced the formation of AOM-induced aberrant crypt foci, lymphoid nodules and tumors	↑HO-1, ↑GR, ↑Nrf2	Chiou et al. (2011)
Resveratrol			
Male BALB/c mice treated with AOM *(Colon cancer)*	Reduced the formation of AOM-induced aberrant crypt foci, lymphoid nodules and tumors	↑HO-1, ↑GR, ↑Nrf2	Chiou et al. (2011)
Female Sprague-Dawley rats treated with DENA *(Liver cancer)*	Inhibited the incidence, total number, multiplicity, size and volume of hepatic nodules	↓HSP70, ↓COX-2, ↓iNOS, ↓3-NT, ↓TBARS, ↓PC, ↓NF-κB, ↑Nrf2	Bishayee and Dhir (2009), Bishayee et al. (2010a, b)
Sulforaphane			
Male C57BL/6J/Nrf2 (−/−) mice		↑expression of genes through the Nrf2 signaling pathway	Hu et al. (2006b)
Female Swiss albino mice treated with B[*a*]P *(Lung cancer)*		↑Nrf2	Priya et al. (2011)

Abbreviations: *AOM* azoxymethane, *B[a]P* benzo[*a*]pyrene, *COX-2* cyclooxygenase-2, *DENA* diethylnitrosamine, *DMBA* 7,12-demethylbenz[*a*]anthracene, *DMN* dimethylnitrosamine, *GGT* γ-glutamyl transpeptidase, *GR* glutathione reductase, *GST* glutathione *S*-transferase, *HO-1* heme oxygenase-1, *HSP70* heat shock protein70, *iNOS* inducible nitric oxide, *IQ* 2-amino-3-methylimidazo[4,5-f]quinolone, *KO* knockout, *MDA* malondialdehyde, *NF-κB* nuclear factor-kappaB, *NQO1* NAD(P)H dehydrogenase (quinone 1), *Nrf2* nuclear factor-erythroid 2-related factor 2, *3-NT* 3-nitrotyrosine, *8-OH-dG* 8-hydroxy-2′-deoxyguanosine, *PC* protein carbonyls, *TBARS* thiobarbituric acid-reactive substances, *UGT* uridine 5′-diphosphate-glucuronosyltransferase, *WT* wild type

chemopreventive potential of several compounds of dietary agents in pre-clinical *in vitro* and *in vivo* models of various cancers, respectively, in relation to their effects on the Nrf2 antioxidant system. Oxidative stress and inflammatory insult are intimately connected to each other in multi-stage carcinogenesis with potential cross-talk between Nrf2 and nuclear factor-kappaB (NF-κB) pathways (Surh 2008; Li et al. 2008). Hence, an agent with anti-inflammatory property is expected to inhibit oxidative stress and *vice versa*. Indeed, several studies as presented in Tables 20.1 and 20.2 provide evidence that Nrf2-mediated chemopreventive effects of several dietary constituents could be achieved by simultaneous activation of antioxidant pathway and inhibition of inflammatory cascade regulated by NF-κB.

Our laboratory has shown that several dietary phytoconstituents prevent chemically-induced rat liver carcinogenesis by antioxidant mechanisms through modulation of the Nrf2 pathway. In one of these studies, resveratrol (a grape polyphenol that is also found in berries, plums and peanuts) has been found to reduce the incidence, total number and average number/liver (multiplicity) of visible hepatocyte nodules (precursors of hepatocellular carcinoma) in a two-stage rat liver tumorigenesis model initiated with potent hepatocarcinogen diethylnitrosamine (DENA) and promoted by phenobarbital (PB) (Bishayee and Dhir 2009). Ancillary studies reveal that resveratrol suppressed DENA-induced elevated expressions of hepatic preneoplastic and inflammatory markers, such as heat shock protein 70, cyclooxygenase and nuclear factor-kappaB (NF-κB) p65 and blocked the translocation of NF-κB p65 from the cytoplasm to the nucleus by stabilizing the inhibitor of κB (Bishayee et al. 2010a). Resveratrol also manifested a potent antioxidant effect during hepatocarcinogenesis as evidenced from the inhibition of DENA-induced hepatic lipid peroxidation, protein oxidation (protein carbonyl formation), inducible nitric oxide synthase and 3-nitrotyrosine (Bishayee et al. 2010b). Mechanistically, resveratrol elevated hepatic protein and mRNA expression of Nrf2 in DENA-exposed animals (Bishayee et al. 2010b). All these results provide conclusive evidence that resveratrol exerts chemoprevention of experimentally-induced hepatocarcinogenesis possibly by suppressing the inflammatory cascades and abrogating oxidative stress through the modulation of Nrf2 and NF-κB signaling pathways (Fig. 20.1).

The *'superfruit'* pomegranate is gaining incredible importance because of its potent antioxidant properties (Gil et al. 2000; Faria et al. 2007) attributed largely to polyphenolic constituents, such as anthocyanins, hydrolysable tannins (ellagitannins and gallotannins) and condensed tannins (proanthocyanidins) (Gil et al. 2000; Seeram et al. 2005; Lansky and Newman 2007). Our laboratory has investigated the mechanism-based chemopreventive potential of a formulation (emulsion) containing pomegranate phytochemicals against DENA-initiated hepatocarcinogenesis in rats. Pomegranate emulsion significantly attenuated the number and area of γ-glutamyl transpeptidase-positive hepatic foci (preneoplastic lesion linked to oxidative stress) as well as reduced the incidence, number, multiplicity, size and volume of hepatic nodule compared to the DENA control animals (Bishayee et al. 2011). Mechanistic studies revealed that the pomegranate-derived product under investigation elevated gene expression of an array of hepatic antioxidant and

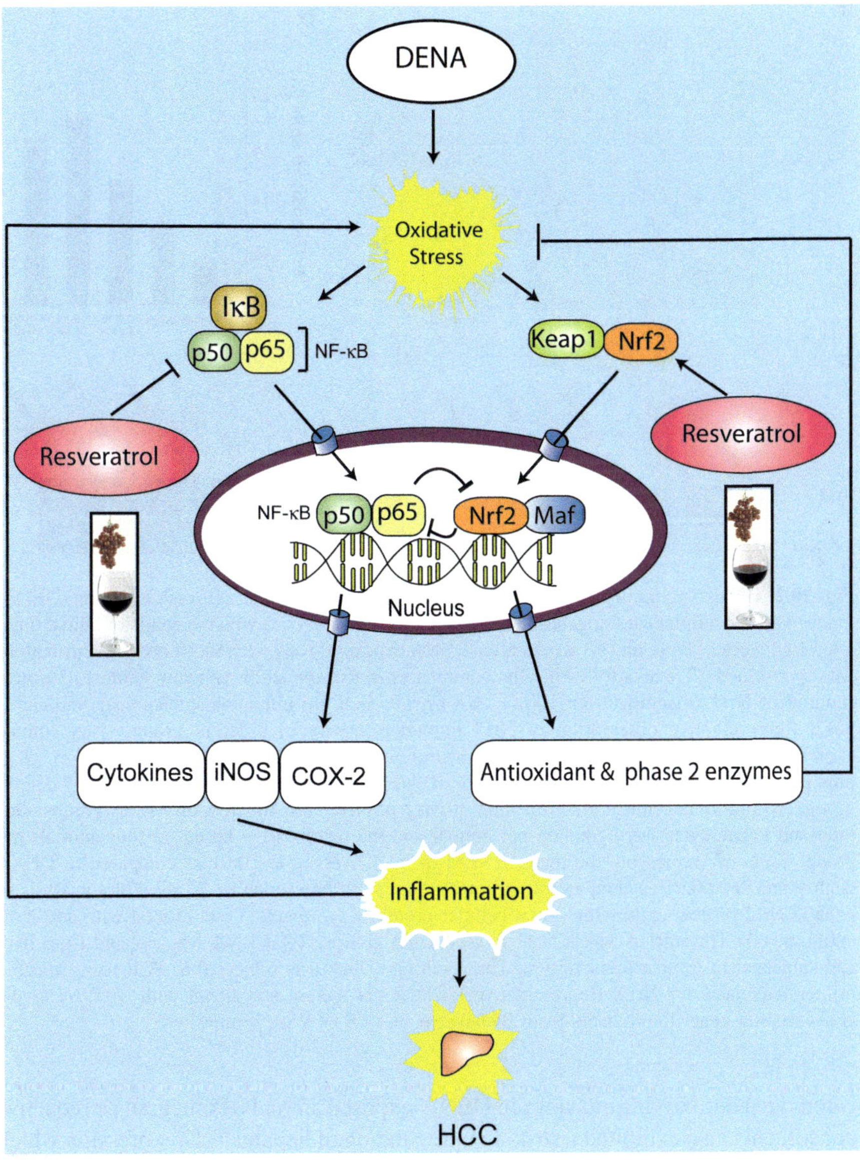

Fig. 20.1 Schematic representation of the possible molecular mechanisms of resveratrol chemoprevention during DENA hepatocarcinogenesis. Elevated oxidative stress concomitant with chronic inflammatory insult through activation of NF-κB results in hepatic neoplasia. Resveratrol activates Nrf2-regulated antioxidant and phase 2 enzymes in liver to combat oxidative stress and inhibit NF-κB-mediated inflammatory cascades resulting in protection against inflammation and subsequent HCC. A possible cross-talk between Nrf2 and NF-κB may be involved in resveratrol action

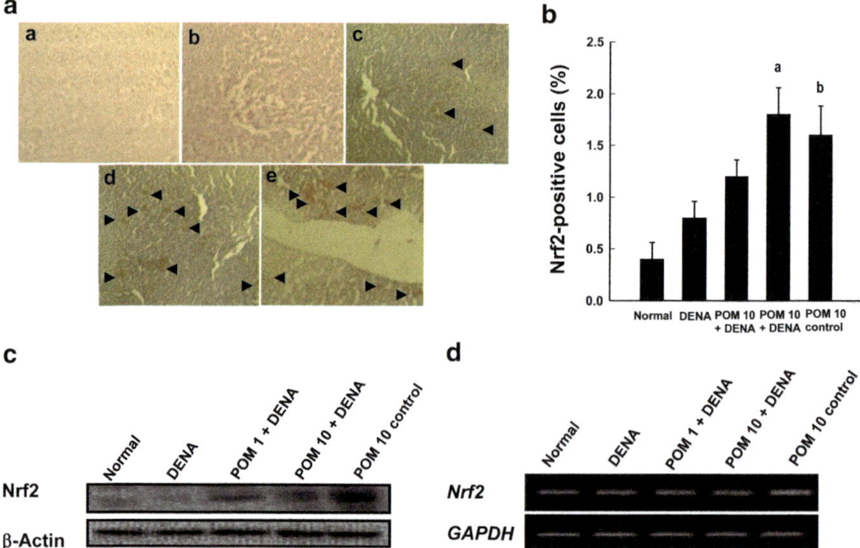

Fig. 20.2 Effects of pomegranate emulsion (*PE*) on hepatic Nrf2 expression during DENA-induced hepatocellular carcinogenesis in rats. Rats were fed (*per os*) with the emulsion (three times a week) 4 weeks before and 18 weeks after DENA exposure. Rats were sacrificed and estimations were performed 22 weeks following the commencement of the study. (**A**) Immunohistochemical staining of Nrf2 (magnification: 100×). *Arrowheads* indicate immunohistochemical staining of Nrf2. Representative observation of Nrf2 immunoreactivity in different groups: very limited expression in (**a**) normal and (**b**) DENA control liver; (**c**) moderate induction in PE (1 g/kg) plus DENA; (**d**) substantial induction in PE (10 g/kg) plus DENA and (**e**) PE (10 g/kg) control group. (**B**) Immunochemical quantification of Nrf2-positive cells in livers of various groups. One thousand hepatocytes were counted per animal and the results were based on four animals per group. Each *bar* represents the mean ± SEM (n = 4 livers). $^{a}P < 0.01$ as compared to DENA control and $^{b}P < 0.01$ as compared to normal group. (**C**) Representative Western blot analysis of hepatic Nrf2 protein expression. Total cellular protein was separated and blotted with anti-Nrf2 antibody. (**D**) The mRNA levels Nrf2 in several rat groups. Total RNA was isolated from liver and subjected to reverse transcription. The resulting cDNA was subjected to PCR using specific primer sequences for Nrf2. Representative RT-PCR gel picture are shown with *GAPDH* as the housekeeping gene (Reproduced from Bishayee et al. (2011). With permission)

carcinogen detoxifying enzymes in DENA-exposed animals. Pomegranate bioactive constituents also exhibited a striking upregulation of hepatic Nrf2 expression which could be a cardinal mechanism of liver cancer chemoprevention by this fruit (Fig. 20.2) (Bishayee et al. 2011).

Since oxidative stress play an extremely crucial role in the development and progression of human liver cancer (Kawanishi et al. 2006; Ha et al. 2010; Lawless et al. 2010), our aforementioned findings underscore the potential of diminishing oxidative insult through the modulation of Nrf2 signaling as a viable strategy for achieving liver cancer chemoprevention by non-toxic dietary phytochemicals.

Conclusion

The current article highlights the importance and the significant benefit that the use of phytochemicals, of dietary origin, offer in modulation of the Nrf2 pathway – a key factor of the chemopreventive design against neoplastic diseases. The diverse array of phytoconstituents present in the human diet with their proven ability to enhance the Nrf2 pathway leading to increased expression of the phase 2 detoxifying and antioxidant enzymes and consequently the overall antioxidant portfolio represents one of the most effective measures of affording chemoprevention (Zhao et al. 2010). The Nrf2 modulating phytoconstituents being of dietary origin are essentially safe and carry a minimal burden of toxicity. Also, a large number of bioactive phytochemicals are available as regular part of the diet throughout the world and thus offer a practical means to enhance the detoxifying and antioxidant profile. This dietary chemopreventive strategy is especially useful in locations where there is a high environmental exposure to potent carcinogens.

Although the chemopreventive use of dietary phytochemicals by enhancing the Nrf2 signal holds considerable promise significant efforts are required to translate it into an effective, robust and practical means to prevent the onset of the carcinogenesis process. As evident from the studies listed in Tables 20.1 and 20.2 only a select number of dietary phytochemicals have been studied for their role in activating the Nrf2 pathway and thus afford chemoprevention in both *in vitro* and *in vivo* pre-clinical models of cancer (Eggler et al. 2008; Kwon et al. 2007; Cheung and Kong 2010). It is extremely critical that studies be initiated which systematically elucidate the Nrf2 modulating potential of prominent members of the major classes of phytochemicals found in the human diet. Even though chemoprevention has shown potential benefit in human intervention trials the chemopreventive potential of dietary agents especially due to their Nrf2 modulatory property need rigorous clinical examination (Sporn and Suh 2000, 2002; Manson et al. 2000; Goodman et al. 2011).

A major aspect of dietary phytotherapy research is the elucidation of safe and effective dosing regimens in order to achieve the required molecular concentrations needed to activate the signaling pathways. An effective means is to conduct correlative studies which compare the serum concentrations achieved after oral administration of dietary phytoconstituents. *In vitro* studies evaluating the effect of dietary phytochemicals on molecular targets of the Nrf2 signaling pathway offer a clear benchmark of the molecular concentrations required to initiate the biochemical processes. Dietary phytochemicals, due to their poor absorption and rapid metabolism, shown poor bioavailability and thus their oral administration may not achieve the molecular concentrations critical to initiate the Nrf2 antioxidant cascade (Del Rio et al. 2010; Shehzad et al. 2010; Darvesh et al. 2012). Formulations of dietary phytoconstituents utilizing novel drug delivery systems such as nanoparticles, liposomes, miceller preparations as well as phospholipid complexes are under investigation for their potential to enhance the bioavailability (Nair et al. 2010; Bansal et al. 2011). The role of synergy in utilizing the potential of complex mixtures can also be elucidated with '*head-to-head*' comparison, such as curcumin with curcuminoid-rich turmeric extract and EGCG with total green tea polyphenols, for their role in enhancing the Nrf2 signaling mechanisms also needs systematic pre-clinical and clinical investigation (Liu 2004).

In conclusion, dietary intervention using select phytochemicals with the proven ability to modulate the Nrf2 signaling pathway is an effective means to achieve chemoprevention and enhance the antioxidant and detoxification portfolio of humans. This strategy is especially effective and has tremendous usefulness in high-risk populations with significant exposure to environmental carcinogens.

Acknowledgments Our research on chemoprevention of liver cancer by modulation of Nrf2 pathway by several dietary phytoconstituents as described in this chapter was carried out at the Northeast Ohio Medical University (Rootstown, OH) supported by Research Incentive Grant from the Ohio Board of Regents and a New Faculty Start-Up Research Grant to A.B. The authors sincerely thank Animesh Mandal, Ph.D., for assistance with the bibliographic work and Werner J. Geldenhuys, Ph.D., for technical assistance with the illustration (Fig. 20.1).

References

Bansal SS, Goel M, Aqil F, Vadhanam MV et al (2011) Advanced drug delivery systems of curcumin for cancer chemoprevention. Cancer Prev Res 8:1158–1171

Becks L, Prince M, Burson H, Christophe C et al (2010) Aggressive mammary carcinoma progression in Nrf2 knockout mice treated with 7,12-dimethylbenz[a]anthracene. BMC Cancer 10:540

Ben-Dor A, Steiner M, Gheber L, Danilenko M et al (2005) Carotenoids activate the antioxidant response element transcription system. Mol Cancer Ther 4:177–186

Benson AM, Batzinger RP, Ou SY, Bueding E et al (1978) Elevation of hepatic glutathione S-transferase activities and protection against mutagenic metabolites of benzo(a)pyrene by dietary antioxidants. Cancer Res 38:4486–4495

Benson AM, Hunkeler MJ, Talalay P (1980) Increase of NAD(P)H:quinone reductase by dietary antioxidants: possible role in protection against carcinogenesis and toxicity. Proc Natl Acad Sci U S A 77:5216–5220

Bishayee A, Dhir N (2009) Resveratrol-mediated chemoprevention of diethylnitrosamine-initiated hepatocarcinogenesis: inhibition of cell proliferation and induction of apoptosis. Chem Biol Interact 179:131–144

Bishayee A, Waghray A, Barnes KF, Mbimba T et al (2010a) Suppression of the inflammatory cascade is implicated in resveratrol chemoprevention of experimental hepatocarcinogenesis. Pharm Res 27:1080–1091

Bishayee A, Barnes KF, Bhatia D, Darvesh AS et al (2010b) Resveratrol suppresses oxidative stress and inflammatory response in diethylnitrosamine-initiated rat hepatocarcinogenesis. Cancer Prev Res 3:753–763

Bishayee A, Bhatia D, Thoppil RJ, Darvesh AS et al (2011) Pomegranate-mediated chemoprevention of experimental hepatocarcinogenesis involves Nrf2-regulated mechanisms. Carcinogenesis 32:888–896

Cha YN, Heine S (1982) Comparative effects of dietary administration of 2(3)-*tert*-butyl-4-hydroxyanisole and 3,5-di-tert-butyl-4-hydroxytoluene on several hepatic enzyme activities in mice and rats. Cancer Res 42:2609–2615

Chen C, Pung D, Leong V, Hebber V et al (2004) Induction of detoxifying enzymes by garlic organosulfur compounds through transcription factor Nrf2: effect of chemical structure and stress signals. Free Radic Biol Med 37:1578–1590

Chen CY, Jang JH, Li MH, Surh YJ (2005) Resveratrol upregulates heme oxygenase-1 expression via activation of NF-E2-related factor in PC12 cells. Biochem Biophys Res Commun 331: 993–1000

Cheung KL, Kong AL (2010) Molecular targets of dietary phenethyl isothiocyanate and sulforaphane for cancer chemoprevention. AAPS J 12:87–97

Cheung KL, Khor TO, Huang MT, Kong AH (2010) Differential in vivo mechanism of chemoprevention of tumor formation in azoxymethane/dextran sodium sulfate mice by PEITC and DBM. Carcinogenesis 31:880–885

Chiou YS, Tsai ML, Nagabhushanam K, Wang YJ et al (2011) Pterostilbene is more potent that resveratrol in preventing azoxymethane (AOM)-induced colon tumorigenesis via activation of the NF-E2-related factor (Nrf2)-mediated antioxidant signaling pathway. J Agric Food Chem 59:2725–2733

Cooke MS, Evans MD, Evans M, Dizdaroglu M et al (2003) Oxidative DNA damage: mechanisms, mutation, and disease. FASEB J 17:1195–1214

Darvesh AS, Aggarwal BB, Bishayee A (2012) Curcumin and liver cancer: a review. Curr Pharm Biotechnol 13:218–228

Del Rio D, Borges G, Crozier A (2010) Berry flavonoids and phenolics: bioavailability and evidence of protective effects. Br J Nutr 104:S67–S90

Ding M, Zhao J, Bowman L, Lu Y et al (2010) Inhibition of AP-1 and MAPK signaling and activation of Nrf2/ARE pathway by quercitrin. Int J Oncol 36:59–67

Eggler AL, Gay KA, Mesecar AD (2008) Molecular mechanisms of natural products in chemoprevention: induction of cytoprotective enzymes by Nrf2. Mol Nutr Food Res 52:S84–S94

Eussen SR, Verhagen H, Klungel OH et al (2011) Functional foods and dietary supplements: products at the interface between pharma and nutrition. Eur J Pharmacol 668:S2–S9

Faria A, Monteiro R, Mateus N, Azevedo I et al (2007) Effect of pomegranate (*Punica granatum*) juice intake on hepatic oxidative stress. Eur J Nutr 46:271–278

Farombi EO, Shrotriya S, Na HK, Kim SH et al (2008) Curcumin attenuates dimethylnitrosamine-induced liver injury in rats through Nrf2-mediated induction of heme oxygenase-1. Food Chem Toxicol 46:1279–1287

Garg R, Gupta S, Maru GB (2008) Dietary curcumin modulates transcriptional regulators of phase I and phase II enzymes in benzo[*a*]pyrene-treated mice: mechanism of its anti-initiating action. Carcinogenesis 29:1022–1032

Gerhäuser C, Klimo K, Hümmer W, Hölzer J et al (2009) Identification of 3-hydroxy-beta-damascone and related carotenoid-derived aroma compounds as novel potent inducers of Nrf2-mediated phase 2 response with concomitant anti-inflammatory activity. Mol Nutr Food Res 53:1237–1244

Gil MI, Tomas-Barberan FA, Hess-Pierce B, Holcroft DM et al (2000) Antioxidant activity of pomegranate juice and its relationship with phenolic composition and processing. J Agric Food Chem 48:4581–4589

Goodman M, Bostick RM, Kucuk O, Jones DP (2011) Clinical trials of antioxidants as cancer prevention agents. Free Radic Biol Med 51:1068–1084

Granado-Serrano AB, Martín MA, Haegeman G, Goya L et al (2010) Epicatechin induces NF-kappaB, activator protein-1 (AP-1) and nuclear transcription factor erythroid 2p45-related factor-2 (Nrf2) via phosphatidylinositol-3-kinase/protein kinase B (PI3K/AKT) and extracellular regulated kinase (ERK) signalling in HepG2 cells. Br J Nutr 103:168–179

Ha HL, Shin HJ, Feitelson MA, Yu DY (2010) Oxidative stress and antioxidants in hepatic pathogenesis. World J Gastroenterol 16:6035–6043

Hayes JD, McMahon M (2001) Molecular basis for the contribution of the antioxidant response element to cancer chemoprevention. Cancer Lett 174:103–113

Hayes JD, McMahon M, Chowdhry S, Dinkova-Kostova AT (2010) Cancer chemoprevention mechanisms mediated through the Keap1-Nrf2 pathway. Antioxid Redox Signal 13:1713–1748

Hsieh TC, Lu X, Wang Z, Wu JM (2006) Induction of quinone reductase NQO1 by resveratrol in human K562 cells involves the antioxidant response element ARE and is accompanied by nuclear translocation of transcription factor Nrf2. Med Chem 2:275–285

Hu R, Xu SG, Jain MR et al (2006a) Identification of Nrf2-regulated genes induced by chemopreventive isothiocyanate PETIC by oligonucleotide microarray. Life Sci 79:1944–1955

Hu R, Xu C, Shen G, Jain MR et al (2006b) Gene expression profiles induced by cancer chemopreventive isothiocyanate sulforaphane in the liver of C57BL/6J mice and C57BL/gJ/Nrf2 (-/-) mice. Cancer Lett 243:170–192

Hu R, Constance LS, Yu R, Kong AT (2010) Regulation of NF-E2-related factor 2 signaling for cancer chemoprevention: antioxidant coupled with anti-inflammatory. Antioxid Redox Signal 13:1679–1698

Jeong WS, Keum YS, Chen C, Jain MR et al (2005) Differential expression and stability of endogenous nuclear factor E2-related factor 2 (Nrf2) by natural chemopreventive compounds in HepG2 human hepatoma cells. J Biochem Mol Biol 38:167–176

Johnson J, de Meija EG (2011) Dietary factors and pancreatic cancer: the role of food bioactive compounds. Mol Nutr Food Res 55:58–73

Joung EJ, Li MH, Lee HG, Somparn N et al (2007) Capsaicin induces heme oxygenase-1 expression in HepG2 cells via activation of PI3K-Nrf2 signaling: NAD(P)H:Quinone oxidoreductase as a potential target. Antioxid Redox Signal 9:2087–2098

Kalthoff S, Ehmer U, Freiberg N, Manns MP et al (2010) Coffee induces expression of glucuronosyltransferases by the aryl hydrocarbon receptor and Nrf2 in liver and stomach. Gastroenterology 139:1699–1710

Kang NJ, Shin SH, Lee HJ, Lee KW (2011) Polyphenols as small molecular inhibitors of signaling cascades in carcinogenesis. Pharmacol Ther 130:310–324

Kawanishi S, Hiraku Y, Pinlaor S, Ma N (2006) Oxidative and nitrative DNA damage in animals and patients with inflammatory diseases in relation to inflammation-related carcinogenesis. Biol Chem 387:365–372

Kelloff GJ, Sigman CC, Greenwald P (1999) Cancer chemoprevention: progress and promise. Eur J Cancer 35:1755–1762

Kensler TW, Wakabayashi N (2010) Nrf2: friend or foe of chemoprevention? Carcinogenesis 31:90–99

Keum YS, Owner ED, Kim BR, Hu R et al (2003) Involvement of Nrf2 and JNK1 in the activation of antioxidant responsive element (ARE) by chemopreventive agent phenethyl isothiocyanate (PETIC). Pharm Res 20:1351–1356

Khor TO, Yu S, Kong AH (2008) Dietary cancer chemopreventive agents – targeting inflammation and Nrf2 signaling pathway. Planta Med 74:1540–1547

Klaassen CD, Reisman SA (2010) Nrf2 the rescue: effects of the antioxidative/electrophilic response on the liver. Toxicol Appl Pharmacol 244:57–65

Klaunig JE, Kamendulis LM (2004) The role of oxidative stress in carcinogenesis. Annu Rev Pharmacol Toxicol 44:239–267

Kode A, Rajendrasozhan S, Caito S, Yang SR et al (2008) Resveratrol induces glutathione synthesis by activation of Nrf2 and protects against cigarette smoke-mediated oxidative stress in human lung epithelial cells. Am J Physiol Lung Cell Mol Physiol 294:L478–L488

Kong AN, Yu R, Hebbar V, Chen C et al (2001) Signal transduction events elicited by cancer prevention compounds. Mutat Res 480–481:231–241

Kundu JK, Surh YJ (2010) Nrf2-Keap1 signaling as a potential target for chemoprevention of inflammation-associated carcinogenesis. Pharm Res 27:999–1013

Kwon KH, Barve A, Yu S et al (2007) Cancer chemoprevention by phytochemicals: potential molecular targets, biomarkers and animal models. Acta Pharmacol Sin 28:1409–1421

Lansky EP, Newman RA (2007) *Punica granatum* (pomegranate) and its potential for prevention and treatment of inflammation and cancer. J Ethnopharmacol 109:177–206

Lawless MW, O'Byrne KJ, Gray SG (2010) Targeting oxidative stress in cancer. Expert Opin Ther Targets 14:1225–1245

Lee JS, Surh YJ (2005) Nrf2 as a novel molecular target for chemoprevention. Cancer Lett 224:171–184

Lee SB, Kim CY, Lee HJ, Yun JH et al (2009) Induction of the phase II detoxification enzyme NQO1 in hepatocarcinoma cells by lignans from the fruit of *Schisandra chinensis* through nuclear accumulation of Nrf2. Planta Med 75:1314–1318

Li W, Kong AN (2009) Molecular mechanisms of Nrf2-mediated antioxidant response. Mol Carcinog 48:91–104

Li W, Khor TO, Xu C, Shen G et al (2008) Activation of Nrf2-antioxidant signaling attenuates NF-κB-inflammatory response and elicits apoptosis. Biochem Pharmacol 76:1485–1489

Lian F, Wang XD (2008) Enzymatic metabolites of lycopene induce Nrf2-mediated expression of phase II detoxifying/antioxidant enzymes in human bronchial epithelial cells. Int J Cancer 123:1262–1268

Liu RH (2004) Potential synergy of phytochemicals in cancer prevention: mechanism of action. J Nutr 134:3479S–3485S

Maher J, Yamamoto M (2010) The rise of antioxidant signaling-the evolution and hormetic actions of Nrf2. Toxicol Appl Pharmacol 244:4–15

Manson MM, Gescher A, Hudson EA et al (2000) Blocking and suppressing mechanisms of chemoprevention by dietary constituents. Toxicol Lett 112:499–505

Martín MA, Ramos S, Granado-Serrano AB, Rodríguez-Ramiro I et al (2010) Hydroxytyrosol induces antioxidant/detoxificant enzymes and Nrf2 translocation via extracellular regulated kinases and phosphatidylinositol-3-kinase/protein kinase B pathways in HepG2 cells. Mol Nutr Food Res 54:956–966

Moolgavkar SH (1978) The multistage theory of carcinogenesis and the age distribution of cancer in man. J Natl Cancer Inst 61:49–52

Nair HB, Sung B, Yadav VR et al (2010) Delivery of antiinflammatory nutraceuticals by nanoparticles for the prevention and treatment of cancer. Biochem Pharmacol 80:1833–1843

Nakamura Y, Yoshida C, Murakami A, Ohigashi H et al (2004) Zerumbone, a tropical ginger sesquiterpene, activates phase II drug metabolizing enzymes. FEBS Lett 572:245–250

Nguyen T, Nioi P, Pickett CB (2009) The Nrf2-antioxidant response element signaling pathway and its activation by oxidative stress. J Biol Chem 284:13291–13295

Niestroy J, Barbara A, Herbst K, Rode S et al (2011) Single and concerted effects of benzo[a]pyrene and flavonoids on the AhR and Nrf2-pathway in the human colon carcinoma cell line Caco-2. Toxicol In Vitro 25:671–683

Palmer HJ, Paulson KE (1997) Reactive oxygen species and antioxidants in signal transduction and gene expression. Nutr Rev 55:479–489

Primiano T, Kensler TW, Kuppusamy P, Zweier JL et al (1996) Induction of hepatic hemeoxygenase-1 ferritin in rats by cancer chemopreventive dithiolethiones. Carcinogenesis 17:2291–2296

Prince M, Li Y, Childers A, Itoh K et al (2009) Comparison of citrus coumarins on carcinogen-detoxifying enzymes in Nrf2 knockout mice. Toxicol Lett 185:180–186

Priya DKD, Gayathri R, Sakthisekaran D (2011) Role of sulforaphane in the anti-initiating mechanism of lung carcinogenesis in vivo by modulating the metabolic activation and detoxification of benzo(a)pyrene. Biomed Pharmacother 65:9–16

Ross SA (2010) Evidence for the relationship between diet and cancer. Exp Oncol 32:137–142

Rubiolo JA, Mithieux G, Vega FV (2008) Resveratrol protects primary rat hepatocytes against oxidative stress damage: activation of the Nrf2 transcription factor and augmented activities of antioxidant enzymes. Eur J Pharmacol 591:66–72

Sahin K, Orhan C, Akdemir F, Tuzcu M et al (2011) Resveratrol protects quail hepatocytes against heat stress: modulation of the Nrf2 transcription factor and hear shock proteins. J Anim Physiol Anim Nutr. doi:10.1111/j.1439-0396.2010.01123.x, PMID: 21244525

Scapagnini G, Vasto S, Abraham NG, Caruso C et al (2011) Modulation of Nrf2/ARE pathway by food polyphenols: a nutritional neuroprotective strategy for cognitive and neurodegenerative disorders. Mol Neurobiol 44:192–201

Schmid HP, Fischer C, Engeler DS, Bendhack ML et al (2011) Nutritional aspects of primary prostate cancer prevention. Recent Results Cancer Res 188:101–107

Seeram NP, Adams LS, Henning SM, Niu Y et al (2005) *In vitro* antiproliferative, apoptotic and antioxidant activities of punicalagin, ellagic acid and a total pomegranate tannin extract are enhanced in combination with other polyphenols as found in pomegranate juice. J Nutr Biochem 16:360–367

Shehzad A, Wahid F, Lee YS (2010) Curcumin in cancer chemoprevention: molecular targets, pharmacokinetics, bioavailability and clinical trials. Arch Pharm 343:489–499

Shen G, Xu C, Hu R, Jain MR et al (2006) Modulation of nuclear factor E2-related factor 2-mediated gene expression in mice liver and small intestine by cancer chemopreventive agent curcumin. Mol Cancer Ther 5:39–51

Slocum SL, Kensler TW (2011) Nrf2: control of sensitivity to carcinogens. Arch Toxicol 85: 273–284

Sporn MB (1991) Carcinogenesis and cancer: different perspectives on the same disease. Cancer Res 51:6215–6218

Sporn MB, Suh N (2000) Chemoprevention of cancer. Carcinogenesis 21:525–530

Sporn MB, Suh N (2002) Chemoprevention: an essential approach to controlling cancer. Nat Rev Cancer 2:527–543

Surh YJ (2008) NF-κB and Nrf2 as potential chemopreventive targets of some anti-inflammatory and antioxidative phytonutrients with anti-inflammatory and antioxidative activities. Asia Pac J Clin Nutr 17:269–272

Surh YJ, Kundu JK, Na HK (2008) Nrf2 as a master redox switch in turning on the cellular signaling involved in the induction of cytoprotective genes by some chemopreventive phytochemicals. Planta Med 74:1526–1539

Tanigawa S, Fujii M, Hou DX (2007) Action of Nrf2 and Keap1 in ARE-mediated *NQO1* expression by quercetin. Free Radic Biol Med 42:1690–1703

Tao KS, Wang W, Wang L, Cao DY et al (2008) The multifaceted mechanisms for coffee's anti-tumorigenic effect on liver. Med Hypotheses 71:730–736

Treuba GP, Sanchez GM, Giuliani A (2004) Oxygen free radical and antioxidant defense mechanism in cancer. Front Biosci 9:2029–2044

Tripathi DN, Jena GB (2010) Astaxanthin intervention ameliorates cyclophosphamide-induced oxidative stress, DNA damage and early hepatocarcinogenesis in rat: role of Nrf2, p53, p38 and phase-II enzymes. Mutat Res 696:69–80

Valko M, Izakovic M, Mazur M, Rhodes CJ (2004) Role of oxygen radicals in DNA damage and cancer incidence. Mol Cell Biochem 266:37–56

Valko M, Rhodes CJ, Moncol J, Izaokovic M et al (2006) Free radicals, metals and antioxidants in oxidative stress-induced cancer. Chem Biol Interact 160:1–40

Wagner AE, Boesch-Saadatmandi C, Breckwoldt D, Schrader C et al (2011) Ascorbic acid partly antagonizes resveratrol mediated heme oxygenase-1 but not paraoxo-nase-1 induction in cultured hepatocytes – role of the redox-regulated transcription factor Nrf2. BMC Complement Altern Med 11:1–8

Wattenberg LW (1975) Effects of dietary constituents on the metabolism of chemical carcinogens. Cancer Res 35:3326–3331

Wattenberg LW (1985) Chemoprevention of cancer: different perspectives on the same disease. Cancer Res 45:1–8

Xu C, Yuan X, Pan Z, Shen G et al (2006) Mechanism of action of isothiocyanates: the induction of ARE-regulated genes is associated with activation of ERK and JNK and the phosphorylation and nuclear translocation of Nrf2. Mol Cancer Ther 5:1918–1926

Yeh CT, Yen GC (2005) Effect of sulforaphane on metallothionein expression and induction of apoptosis in human hepatoma HepG2 cells. Carcinogenesis 26:2138–2148

Yeh CT, Yen GC (2006) Involvement of p38 MAPK and Nrf2 in phenolic acid-induced P-form phenol sulfotransferase expression in human hepatoma $HepG_2$ cells. Carcinogenesis 27: 1008–1017

Yuan JH, Li YQ, Yang XY (2007) Inhibition of epigallocatechin gallate on orthotopic colon cancer by unregulating the Nrf2-UGT1A signal pathway in nude mice. Pharmacology 80:269–278

Yuan JH, Li YQ, Yang XY (2008) Protective effects of epigallocatechin gallate on colon preneoplastic lesions induced by 2-amino-3-methylimidazo[4,5-*f*]quinolone in mice. Mol Med 14:590–598

Zhang Y, Munday R (2008) Dithiolethiones for cancer chemoprevention: where do we stand? Mol Cancer Ther 7:3470–3479

Zhang Z, Yang X, Yuan J, Zi S et al (2009) Modulation of Nrf2 and UGT1A expression by epigallocatechin-3-gallate in colon cancer cells and BALB/c mice. Chin Med J 122:1660–1665

Zhao CR, Gao ZH, Qu XJ (2010) Nrf2-ARE signaling pathway and natural products for cancer chemoprevention. Cancer Epidemiol 34:523–533

Chapter 21
Role of Fish Oil from Gene Expression to Pharmacological Effect in Cancer Prevention

Malay Chatterjee, Subhadeep Das, Mary Chatterjee, and Kaushik Roy

Contents

Abstract Cancer is the most common cause of death worldwide. Several dietary supplements have been found to be potential for cancer prevention. Anti-inflammatory, apoptotic, cell growth inhibitory role of fish oil and its bioactive forms (EPA & DHA) have been studied extensively. Synergistic effect of fish oil has been established with several other chemopreventive agents. A voluminous number of clinical trials and epidemiological study was performed which supports for its beneficiary role.

M. Chatterjee (✉) • S. Das • M. Chatterjee • K. Roy
Department of Pharmaceutical Technology, Jadavpur University, PO Box: 17028, Kolkata 700032, West Bengal, India
e-mail: mcbiochem@yahoo.com

S. Shankar and R.K. Srivastava (eds.), *Nutrition, Diet and Cancer*,
DOI 10.1007/978-94-007-2923-0_21,

Background

Now-a-days nutritionalresearch got its interests in the treatment of chronic diseases (vel Szic et al. 2010). Several epidemiological studies have shown that environmental changes/conditions, life style, diet/food habits/nutrients are responsible for any mutagenic alteration causing neurodegenerative diseases including cancer (Wu et al. 2011). Recent studies have furnished several information indicating that many dietary supplements interfere with early cancer development (Weinstein 1991). Resveratrol, green tea, soya proteins, fish oil are some of those dietary supplements which have been evidenced to have potentials in cancer treatment, though the mechanism is yet to be explored. Most of the people consume dietary supplements with least awareness of their benefits or risk factors (Satia et al. 2009). Fish oil, an ideal enriched source of n-3 polyunsaturated fatty acids, is very common in diet worldwide (Simopoulos 1991). Polyunsaturated fatty acids are major players engaged in modulation of cancer symptoms. α-linolenic acid is a member of n-3 PUFA family and is a precursor of EPA & DHA which have been successfully exploited in the treatment of cancer. On the other hand, the members of n-6 PUFA family, like arachidonic acid, linoleic acid are the precursors of 5-HETE (5-Hydroxyeicosatetraenoic acid), leukotrienes which lead to worsening of cancer symptoms by their overproduction. Eicosapentaenoic acid (EPA) & docosahexaenoic acid (DHA) are the most bioactive form of n-3 polyunsaturated fatty acids available in fish oil. EPA & DHA cannot be synthesized in mammals which make them so important in our diet due to their contributory role in maintaining healthy life. Suppression of mutation,cell growth inhibition and induction of apoptosis have been evidenced in fish oil supplemented rodents (Fernandez et al. 1999; Karmali 1989; Rose and Connolly 1999). Coincubation of various cancer cell lines with n-3 FAs leads to a reduction in cell number in a time and dose-dependent manner (Be'gin et al. 1986; Jordan and Stein 2003; Sharma et al. 2005). In this review, we have discussed and analyzed the potential role of fish oil or its bioactive forms in cancer prevention in a comprehensive manner.

Fish Oil and Gene Expression

Life cycle of any living organism is comprised of different physiological processes. The complex patterns of these physiological processes are regulated by expressions of several proteins. Cell-growth and cell-death mechanisms are essential to maintain life processes. Upregulation and downregulation of various genes modulate these mechanisms (Weinstein 1991). Fish oil as a dietary chemopreventive, can be used as suppressing agent (arrest or reverse the promotion and progression of cancer) by influencing cell proliferation, apoptosis, cell differentiation (Chen and Kong 2005; Michael 1999). Dietary fish oil modulates transcription of several genes either positively or negatively.

Kramer et al. (2009) investigated the impact of soya-derived isoflavonoids and n-3 fatty acids from fish oil, both individually and in combination, on apoptosis, cell proliferation and oestrogen receptor (ER) expression in the colon and mammary gland of the rat. Fish oil significantly increased apoptosis and decreased mitosis in both tissues, an effect associated with a decrease in the expressions of ERα and ERβ. Their result provided a novel mechanism by which n-3 fatty acids could reduce cancer risk.

Davidson et al. (2004) conducted a DNA microarray analysis containing approximately 9,000 genes to trace the global changes in colonocyte gene expression profiles in carcinogen-injected Sprague Dawley rats. Animals were assigned to three dietary treatments differing only in the type of fat (corn oil/n-6 PUFA, fish oil/n-3 PUFA, or olive oil/n-9 monounsaturated fatty acid), two treatments (injection with the carcinogen azoxymethane or with saline), and two time points (12 h and 10 weeks after first injection). At the initiation (DNA adduct formation) and promotional (aberrant crypt foci) stages only the consumption of n-3 PUFA exerted a protective effect. Dietary fat composition not only alters the molecular portrait of gene expression profiles in the colonic epithelium at both the initiation and promotional stages of tumor development but these findings also indicate that the chemopreventive effect of fish oil is due to the direct action of n-3 PUFA and not to a reduction in the content of n-6 PUFA.

The growth factor receptor protein HER-2/neu (Human Epidermal growth factor Receptor 2) overexpression is an indicative of advanced metastatic stage. Ki-67 is a cell proliferation marker while c-myc overexpression causes genomic instability. In our laboratory we have reported earlier that fish oil supplementation causes substantial reduction in HER-2/neu, Ki-67 and c-myc expressions in contrast to their carcinogen counterparts (Chatterjee et al. 2010a, b).In another study from our laboratory, influence of fish oil on suppression of neoplastic transformation has been documented. The success of the process was evidenced through reduction in cell proliferation, DPCs (DNA protein crosslink) with subsequent increase in p53 tumor suppressor protein leading to apoptosis (Chatterjee et al. 2007).

Fish Oil and Cell Growth Inhibition

One of the recently proposed strategies for tumor growth reduction is selective knock down of fatty acid synthases gene (FAS) by n-3 polyunsaturated fatty acids (Mashima et al. 2009; Menendez and Lupu 2006). Both of the genes CPT-1 (Carnitine palmitoyltransferase I), the regulatory enzyme of mitochondrial β-oxidation and PEPCK-C (Phosphoenolpyruvate carboxykinase-C), the major enzyme in adipocyte glyceroneogenesis, i.e., glycerol-3 phosphate synthesis from non-carbohydrate substrates (pyruvate, amino acids), are induced by DHA treatment. The expression of these genes increases at confluence of the cells when the proliferation rate decreases. So DHA mediated induction of these genes can be well correlated with the reported anti-proliferative action of DHA (Blouin et al. 2010).

Ectopic expression of polo-like kinase-3 (PLK3) is reflected in cell cycle arrest. Expression of PLK3 was downregulated significantly in quantitative polymerase chain reaction studies of azoxymethane-induced rat colon tumors in comparison to their uninvolved normal colonic mucosa. No significant changes in PLK3 mRNA expression was detected in the normal mucosa isolated from rats fed on diets with various levels of fat (low fat diet with corn oil, LFCO, or high fat diet with corn oil, HFCO, or high fat supplemented with fish oil, HFFO). Rats fed with HFCO diet contained a very low level of PLK3 mRNA expression as observed from the isolated tumors. Surprisingly, tumors from rats fed with HFFO diet did not exhibit as dramatic downregulation of PLK3 as the HFCO diet supplemented animals. (Dai et al. 2002).

Fish oil supplementation was found to inhibit NNK (Nicotine-derived nitrosamine ketone)-induced lung carcinogenesis in the A/J mouse. The inhibitory effect of fish oil on lung tumor prevalence was accompanied with upregulation of cell cycle inhibitor p21Cip1 and lipoxygenase isoform 15-LOX (15-lipoxygenase) in the lungs. This study suggests that fish oil with a low ratio of n-6/n-3 PUFA may be promising in the prevention of lung carcinogenesis partially by inhibiting cell cycle progression (Mernitz et al. 2009).

In a study by Han et al. (2009), fish oil was shown to inhibit non-small cell lung carcinoma (NSCLC) cell growth by affecting PPARγ (peroxisome proliferator-activated receptor γ) followed by inhibition of integrin-linked kinase (ILK) expression. Silencing ILK expression enhanced the inhibitory effect of fish oil on cell growth. SB239023, the p38 mitogen-activated protein kinase inhibitor, abrogated the inhibitory effect of fish oil on ILK expression. Results showed that fish oil inhibits ILK expression through activation of PPARγ-mediated and p38 mitogen-activated protein kinase-mediated induction of AP-2α that ultimately leads to inhibition of NSCLC cell proliferation .

Fish Oil an Apoptosis

Using the xenograft model in nude mice, Ghosh-Choudhury et al. (2009) reported for the first time that the fish oil diet significantly increased the level of PTEN (Phosphatase and tensin homolog) protein in the breast tumors. Moreover, the fish oil diet attenuated Akt kinase and PI 3 kinase activities in tumors leading to significant inhibition of NF-κB (nuclear factor kappa-light-chain-enhancer of activated B cells) activation. Fish oil constituents, DHA and EPA treatment inhibited the phosphorylation of p65 subunit of NF-κB and increased PTEN mRNA and protein expression in MDA MB-231 cells. Furthermore, DHA and EPA reduced expression of Bcl-2 and Bcl-XL with concomitant increase in caspase 3 activity. NF-κB DNA binding activity and NF-κB -dependent Bcl-2 (B-cell lymphoma 2) and Bcl-XL (B-cell lymphoma-extra large) gene transcription were also prevented by DHA and EPA treatment. They showed that PTEN expression significantly inhibited NF-κB-dependent transcription of Bcl-2 and Bcl-XL genes. Their data revealed a novel signaling pathway which correlates fish oil diet to increase PTEN expression that attenuates growth promoting signal and augments the apoptotic signal, resulting in breast tumor regression. This finding is well corroborated with the data from our laboratory (Chatterjee et al. 2008). It showed that the fish oil-treated group exhibited a substantial increase in Bax immunolabelling and a reduction of Bcl-2 immunopositivity, and increased TUNEL-positive apoptotic cells; however, corn oil treatment did not show these beneficial effects toward mammary preneoplasia. It has been evidenced from other laboratory that bioactive components of fish oil actually triggers an oxidation-reduction imbalance in the intestine, which in turn enhanced apoptosis and reduced colonic cancer risks (Sanders et al. 2004; Chapkin et al. 2002; Latham et al. 1999). Actually, when the level of ROS is so severely elevated that mitochondria becomes unable to detoxify, resulting chronic oxidative stress activates/sets off the release of proapoptotic factors (Bayir et al. 2006).

Omega-3 PUFA enriched diet inhibit colon carcinogenesis through the regulation of cyclooxygenase-2 (COX-2), colonic ras-p21 (Ras GTPase activating protein) and inducible nitric oxide synthase (iNOS) activities and apoptosis. Gene expression analysis using DNA microarrays by Reddy (Reddy 2002) indicated that DHA on one hand activates cyclin-dependent kinase (CDK) inhibitors such as p19, p21, p27, p57. On the other hand, it inactivates prostaglandin family of genes and antiapoptotic Bcl-2 family of genes as it was observed in previously mentioned reports. Potential of n-3 PUFAs, particularly EPA and DHA of being promising major components of colon cancer control have been established from these results.

Fish Oil and Inflammation

Inflammation being linked to carcinogenesis acts as a driving force in premalignant and malignant transformation of cells (Maeda and Omata 2008). Suppression of the biosynthesis of proinflammatory molecules is one of the important mechanisms of fish oil, responsible for its chemopreventive nature. Suppression of interleukin 1beta (IL-1β), tumor necrosis factor-alpha (TNFα) interleukin-6 (IL-6) reflect anti-inflammatory role of omega-3 fatty acids (Simopoulos 2006). It has been evidenced from various studies that EPA pretreatment causes inhibition of TNFα-induced MMP-9 (matrix metalloproteinase-9) expression through blocking of p38, NFκB and Akt activation (Kim et al. 2008). The enzyme, cyclooxygenase-2 (COX-2) catalyzes the production of arachidonic acid metabolites PGE_2 which is directly associated with inflammation (Hardman 2002, 2004). Earlier studies on global gene expression with cDNA microarrays, revealed that DHA treatment of CaCo-2 colon cancer cells down-regulated the prostaglandin family of genes, as well as COX-2 expression(Narayanan et al. 2003). Synergistic action of genistein and fish oil downregulate COX-2 expression to lower PGE_2 expression in MDA-MB-231 human breast cancer cells (Horia and Watkins 2007). In a recent study, omega-3 fatty acids were observed to be beneficial in the prevention of oxidative stress-induced inflammation by suppressing inflammatory cytokine expression through inhibition of AP-1 in rat pancreatic AR42J cells (Park et al. 2009).

Fish oil has been shown to downregulate inflammation and upregulate apoptosis targeted at damaged rat colonocyte cells. Authors showed that fish oil can protect rat intestine against 8-oxodG formation during dextran sodium sulfate- (DSS-) induced inflammation. Fish oil fed rats had lower levels of 8-oxodG and increased apoptosis was found in the upper crypt region. Results of their study suggest that fish oil protects intestinal cells against oxidative DNA damage in part via deletion mechanisms (Bancroft et al. 2003).

Fish Oil and Inhibition of Tumor Growth

The potentiality of fish oil in tumor growth inhibition has been studied in several preclinical models. Its antiproliferative, apoptotic nature has been attempted in cancer prevention in experimental models with pre-malignant lesions, or delaying on set of it. Even in some translational study fish oil with other supplements have substantially accelerated postoperative recovery of the cancer patients (Faber et al. 2008; van Norren et al. 2009).

The tumor growth inhibitory effect of dietary fish oil has been studied extensively. In an in vivo study male buffalo rats implanted with rat hepatoma 7288CTC cell lines were fed with dietary fish oil and rate of tumor growth was analyzed. Fish oil fed rats was observed with reduced tumor growth, fatty acid uptake, cAMP (cyclic adenosine monophosphate) content, 13-hydroxyoctadecadienoic acid formation in compare to the control ones. Suppression of tumor growth followed a specific linoleic acid-dependent, inhibitory G protein-coupled, growth-promoting signaling pathway (Smith et al. 2006). Some contradictory findings were reported by Griffini et al. who have inferred that ω-3 fatty acids available from fish oil are capable of reducing the growth of primary tumors. But in the advanced metastatic stage of colon cancer, they promote tumor growth (Griffini et al. 1998). Later, a team led by Gutt using CC 531 cell line (the same cell line used by Griffini et al.) has explained that a diet extremely rich in fats impose an artificial situation which is possibly not reflected in physiology of the concerned group. Moreover, the time of feeding of ω-3 fatty acids before cancer cell administration differs greatly with Griffini et al. They concluded that ω-3 fatty acid is sufficiently capable of inhibiting tumor growth at metastatic stage of colon cancer and their effect is time and concentration dependent (Gutt et al. 2007). In an in vitro study, cell cycle arrest at G_2/M phase was observed in ω-3 PUFA treated human colon cancer cell line, SW620. Downregulation of the nuclear form of sterol regulatory element-binding protein 1 (nSREBP1) possibly responsible for cell cycle arrest and disturbances in lipid homeostasis (Schonberg et al. 2006). This finding from in vitro study was further confirmed by in vivo experimentation. Xenografts were initiated in nude mice by subcutaneous administration of SW620 cells. From the observations it was inferred that increased ω-3 fatty acid levels with subsequent decrease in phosphocholine leads to tumor suppression (Bathen et al. 2008). The inhibitory effect of EPA, on tumorigenic growth of COX-2 (cyclooxygenase-2) positive and COX-2 negative PaCa cells has been studied by Funahashi et al. Binding of PGE_2 (prostaglandin E_2) to its receptors (EP2 and EP4) regulates its COX-2 dependent mechanism. Thus, it is confirmed that ω-3 PUFA enriched diet is significantly capable of lowering pancreatic cancerous growth in a xenograft model (Funahashi et al. 2008). In an experimental study, fish oil consuming rats exhibited significant reduction in DMH (dimethyl hydrazine)-induced ACF. Thus, fish oil ingestion can impart its protective effect against preneoplastic lesions and adenoma development in rat colon (Moreira et al. 2009).

Pharmacological potentiality of fish oil has been observed to be retained in lipid-emulsive form in several experimental data. The anti-invasive property of fish oil-based emulsion in a dose dependent-manner was observed in AH109A cells when pretreated for 48 h (Hagi et al. 2007). Some previous data confirmed that PGE_2 stimulates tumor cell invasion while PGE_3 suppresses the invasion (Denkins et al. 2005).In FO-based emulsion pretreated AH109A cells, EPA replaces AA (arachidonic acid) at the C2 position resulting in lowering of PGE_2 production with concomitant increase in PGE_3 production(Hagi et al. 2007). Similar type of results were obtained in MCF-7 cancer cell lines being treated with lipid emulsions prepared with fish oil and egg-yolk phosphatides. PGE_3 derived from n-3 fatty acids by COX-mediated pathway, is believed to have suppressive role against tumor cell growth. Thus, lipid emulsions incorporating triglycerides of n-3 FAs becomes capable to exhibit anti-tumor activity (Ueda et al. 2008). In an *in vitro* culture the growth inhibitory effect of a lipid emulsion based on fish oil was established on human colon adenocarcinoma cell line HT-29. The percentage of apoptotic cells did not significantly altered upon FO emulsion and as such apoptosis induction was not responsible for this growth inhibitory effect. 5-FU is a chemopreventive agent which arrests cell cycle of tumor cells by halting S-phase. This effect of 5-FU (5-fluorouracil) was found to be potentiated in FO emulsion treated rats (Sala-Vila et al. 2010).

According to Cho et al. fish oil and pectin-containing (FO/P) diets protect against colon cancer compared with corn oil and cellulose (CO/C) by upregulating apoptosis and suppressing proliferation. The mechanism by which FO/P containing diets induce apoptosis and suppress proliferation during tumorigenic process was elucidated by analyzing the temporal gene expression profiles from exfoliated rat colonocytes. They used a noninvasive methodology to monitor gene expression at three biologically important time points during colon tumorigenesis; initiation, aberrant crypt foci (ACF) formation, and tumor stage. The expression of 11 genes (Slc8a1, Dupd1, Ppp1r7, Mfn1, Stx1a, Smoc1, Snip, Nrn1, Il23a, Il6ra, and Pthr2) involved in several signal transduction pathways was downregulated in FO/P rats compared with CO/C rats which suggests that FO/P is capable of attenuating multiple signaling pathways at the tumor stage. At the ACF stage, the expression of genes involved in cell cycle regulation was modulated by FO/P and the zone of proliferation was reduced in FO/P rats compared with CO/C rats. FO/P also increased apoptosis and the expression of genes that promote apoptosis at the tumor endpoint compared with CO/C. (Cho et al. 2011).

Fish oil with a highly fermented product like pectin has shown significant pharmacological implications. In an in vivo study, fish oil-pectin fed rats were subjected to radiation prior to AOM (azoxymeyhane) administration. Suppression of COX and Wnt/β-catenin pathways was responsible for partial induction of apoptosis in rat colonocytes. Furthermore, concurrent suppression of the nuclear transcription factor PPARδ is also associated with suppression of above mentioned pathways. It was inferred from the current study that fish oil-pectin diet has its ability to be exploited against radiation enhanced colon carcinogenesis (Vanamala et al. 2008). Kolar et al. examined the combined effect of fish oil (enriched in DHA) with butyrate on mitochondrial Ca^{2+} accumulation in human colonocyte tumor HCT-116 cell lines. They have observed that apoptosis is enhanced by mitochondrial Ca^{2+} accumulation in a p53 independent pathway. Ca^{2+} accumulation activates mitochondrial transition pore (MTP) to trigger a series of events leading to cellular apoptosis. The cotreatment with DHA and butyrate enhances apoptosis in an oxidation sensitive, mitochondrial Ca^{2+} dependent pathway. The physiological relevancy of this observation was further supported by an in vivo proof-of-principle experiment. Colonic crypts were collected as intact from rats fed with DHA. DHA enriched crypt cultures were found to undergo apoptosis more readily upon ex vivo incubation with butyrate (Hong et al. 2002; Kolar et al. 2007).

Loss of adipose tissue and lean body mass due to metabolic alterations affect physical performance and life style quality of cancer patients suffering from cachexia. In male CD2F1 mice subcutaneously inoculated with murine adenocarcinoma cells (C26) cachetic symptoms were observed to be improved on treatment with the nutritional mixture of fish oil, high protein, leucin. The nutritional mixture supplemented mice exhibited reduced loss of carcass, muscle and fat mass which support the synergistic effect of the constituents (van Norren et al. 2009). To investigate the role of fish oil in lowering cancer cachexia peritoneal carcinosis (PC) was inoculated in BDIX rats. There is a hypermetabolism state in PC rats which is reflected in their lower body weight gain. Fish oil diet delayed anorexia occurrence in PC rats (Dumas et al. 2010). Impaired immune competence is a significant problem in advanced cancer patients. Faber et al. (2008) conducted a translational study with an aim to improve immune response in tumor bearing patients. They employed a specific nutritional combination comprising of fish oil, specific oligosaccharide mixture, high protein content and leucine to lessen severity and frequency (infectious) of complications in cancer patients. The nutritional mixture improved Th1 immune response in tumour-affected mice prior to weight loss. In mice already suffering from cachexia, the mixture improved several physiological and immune parameters, with lowering inflammatory state, less wasting of protein and lipid stores, better immune responses leading to less severe cachexia. Thus, an improved health status can be attained. Clinical studies with human patients are required to extrapolate these results.

Pharmacological Intervention

The chemopreventive effects of several other therapeutics when applied in combination with fish oil have been observed to be substantially elevated. It has been evidenced that a high fat diet with combination of fish oil and (-)epigallocatechin-3-gallate (EGCG) is able to reduce intestinal tumorigenesis in AOM treated $Apc^{Min/+}$ mouse model. This combination treatment is considered to be a better one than single agent. Apoptosis is significantly enhanced with substantial decrease in cell proliferation. Moreover, phosphorylated Akt, PGE_2 levels in small intestinal tumors were reduced significantly. The additive effects of these chemopreventive agents contribute to the lowering of tumorigenesis (Bose et al. 2007).

The side effects of some chemotherapeutic agents have been found to be almost eliminated when treated with fish oil. Vitamin D_3 is a well known therapeutic in the treatment of hepatocellular carcinoma. But at high concentration it causes hypercalcemia. It has been evidenced that in presence of PUFA as fish oil, lower concentration of vitamin D_3 can effectively inhibit HepG2 cell proliferation and eliminates the possibility of hypercalcemia (Chiang et al. 2009). The combinatorial effect of fish oil with vitamin D_3 is well being studied from our laboratory, too. The beneficiary role of combined supplementation is reflected in the inhibition of mammary 7-methylguanine DNA adducts formation, which is associated with reduced mRNA expression of iNOS and suppression of cell proliferation (Chatterjee et al. 2010a, b).

Cisplatin, the chemopreventive agent causes cellular damage and necrosis in malignant cells through generation of reactive oxygen species. But excessive free radical generation may appear fatal as because it can affect normal tissue. To get rid of this complication fish oil is suggested to use during chemotherapy. Fish oil acts as antioxidant, so protects normal cells from free radical damage and thus improves therapeutic efficacy of cisplatin (Ma et al. 2009).

Celecoxib, a non steroidal anti-inflammatory drug, follows a COX-2 inhibitory pathway. But, there are some side effects which add limitations in its usage. Fish oil which also followed COX -2 inhibitory pathway may be exploited along with celecoxib. It has been observed that pretreatment with fish oil and celecoxib in DMBA-induced rats resulted in normal histology, increase in DNA fragmentation with subsequent decrease in total sialic acid (TSA), lipid-associated sialic acid (LASA) followed by reduced oxidative stress (Kansal et al. 2011).

Tamoxifen is a FDA (Food and Drug Administration) approved chemopreventive agent employed in the treatment of breast cancer at the high risk of estrogen-receptor- positive tumors (Fisher et al. 1998).But it is incapable against hormone independent tumor. Manni et al. reported for the first time that fish oil supplementation during tamoxifen treatment of N-methyl-N-nitrosourea-induced rat mammary carcinogenesis reduces tumor volume and multiplicity to a significant amount in contrast to the individual ones. Lowering in oxidative stress by n-3 PUFA-rich diet probably potentiated the chemopreventive efficacy of tamoxifen (Manni et al. 2010).

Clinical Trials

There was lacking of clinical trials using parenteral fish oil in the diet of cancer patients in postoperative stage. A study was conducted with colorectal cancer patients staging TNM I-III (cancer staging system) and they have undergone/gone through radical resection. Serum levels of IL-6 and TNF-α were observed to be significantly depressed after 8 days of FO treatment. Elevation of $CD4^+/CD8^+$ ratio, $CD3^+$ and $CD4^+$ lymphocyte percentage were also observed as a result of ω-3 fatty acid supplementation. Thus modulation of immune responses and reduction of inflammatory responses together lessens postoperative hospital stay for colorectal cancer patients (Liang et al. 2008). Systemic inflammatory response syndrome (SIRS) is a very common symptom appeared in cancer patients in postoperative stage. Fish oil as an immunonutrient may reduce such postoperative complications. In a clinical trial, 206 patients with colon or gastrointestinal cancer received either soyabean oil or soyabean plus fish oil supplementation for 7 days after surgery. Fish oil emulsion-supplementation substantially reduced SIRS and thus shortens hospital stay (Jiang et al. 2010).

Epidemiological Study

In an epidemiological study, fish oil supplementation was found to be capable 35% reduction colorectal cancer risk (Satia et al. 2009). This is because of the availability of n-3 PUFAs in fish oil (EPA & DHA), precursors of eicosanoids that reduce inflammation (Reddy 2004; Calviello et al. 2007). In a case-control study performed in Japan, it is shown that dietary intake of n-3PUFA is inversely related to colon cancer risk. But, this relation is statistically significant only for distal colon cancer (Kimura et al. 2007). Similar trend was also observed in Scotland (Theodoratou et al. 2007). In another study, similar inverse relationship was established in between prostate cancer risk and long chain n-3 fatty acid intake through the measurement of blood fatty acid levels (Chavarro et al. 2007). The weight loss of cancer patients with cachexia has substantially been checked upon dietary intake of n-3 PUFA (Wigmore et al. 2000; Gogos et al. 1998; Burns et al. 1999; Mantovani et al. 2006). Bougnoux et al. (2006) reported that dietary intake of DHA (high incorporation) with anthracyclin as a chemotherapeutic agent for the treatment of breast cancer patients appeared beneficiary regarding overall survival and tolerance of side effects (Mantovani et al. 2006). In a VITAL (VITamin And Life style) cohort female members of western Washington State, aged 50–76 years, in their postmenopausal stage received fish oil as specialty supplement. An inverse relationship between fish oil uptake and breast cancer risk was observed in participants (Brasky et al. 2010). In a double-blind, randomized, placebo-controlled study, n-3 PUFA as oral nutritional supplement was given to stage III NSCLC patients (2 cans/day) undergoing multimodality treatment. The beneficiary effect was reflected in preservation of body weight and fat free mass (FFM). In addition, clinically relevant reduced resting energy expenditure (REE) was associated with high energy and protein intake in fish oil supplemented group. Altogether, fish oil intake by the lung cancer patients with cachexia resulted in improved physical functioning and quality of life (van der Meij et al. 2010).

Concluding Remarks

Chemoprevention by natural dietary compounds has been focused on the reduction of cancer incidence by modulation of development pathways in tumor cells which promote growth and metastases. Bioactive forms of fish oil influences functions of diverse array of proteins, which in turn affect cellular processes that affect cancer development, progression. Extensive research is required to understand the mechanism that counteracts genetic insult responsible for tumorigenesis.

Before applying to human subjects, fish oil has to be passed through epidemiological study, basic laboratory experiments (in vivo and *in vitro*), followed by stepwise clinical trials (Kakizoe 2003; Tsao et al. 2004). Furthermore, it is now essential to bridge the gap between basic laboratory experiments (in vivo and in vitro), clinical trials and epidemiological study to improve public health.

Further studies are needed to provide a complete picture of the present scenario of cancer treatment with fish oil which will hopefully help the future scientists, clinicians to choose avenues in order to establish fish oil as a safe, effective therapeutics in cancer.

References

Bancroft LK, Lupton JR, Davidson LA et al (2003) Dietary fish oil reduces oxidative DNA damage in rat colonocytes. Free Radic Biol Med 35(2):149–159

Bathen TF, Holmgren K, Lundemo AG et al (2008) Omega-3 fatty acids suppress growth of SW620 human colon cancer xenografts in nude mice. Anticancer Res 28(6A):3717–3723

Bayir H, Fadeel B, Palladino MJ et al (2006) Apoptotic interactions of cytochrome c: redox flirting with anionic phospholipids within and outside of mitochondria. Biochim Biophys Acta 1757:648–659

Be'gin ME, Ells G, Das UN et al (1986) Differential killing of human carcinoma cells supplemented with n-3 and n-6 polyunsaturated fatty acids. J Natl Cancer Inst 77(5):1053–1062

Blouin JM, Bortoli S, Nacfer M et al (2010) Down-regulation of the phosphoenolpyruvate carboxykinase gene in human colon tumors and induction by omega-3 fatty acids. Biochimie 92(12):1772–1777

Bose M, Hao X, Ju J et al (2007) Inhibition of tumorigenesis in ApcMin/+ mice by a combination of (-)-epigallocatechin-3-gallate and fish oil. J Agric Food Chem 55(19):7695–7700

Bougnoux P, Hajjaju N, Baucher MA et al (2006) Docosahexaenoic acid (DHA) intake during first line chemotherapy improves survival in metastatic breast cancer. Proc Am Assoc Cancer Res 47:1237

Brasky TM, Lampe JW, Potter JD et al (2010) Specialty supplements and breast cancer risk in the VITamins And Lifestyle (VITAL) cohort. Cancer Epidemiol Biomarkers Prev 19(7):1696–1708
Burns CP, Halabi S, Clamon GH et al (1999) Phase I clinical study of fish oil fatty acid capsules for patients with cancer cachexia: cancer and leukemia group B study 9473. Clin Cancer Res 5:3942–3947
Calviello G, Serini S, Piccioni E (2007) n-3 polyunsaturated fatty acids and the prevention of colorectal cancer: molecular mechanisms involved. Curr Med Chem 14:3059–3069
Chapkin RS, Hong MY, Fan YY et al (2002) Dietary n-3 PUFA alter colonocyte mitochondrial membrane composition and function. Lipids 37:193–199
Chatterjee M, Manna S, Chakraborty T (2007) Protective role of **fish oil** (Maxepa) on early events of rat mammary carcinogenesis by modulation of DNA-protein crosslinks, cell proliferation and p53 expression. Cancer Cell Int 7:6
Chatterjee M, Manna S, Chakraborty T (2008) Dietary fish oil associated with increased apoptosis and modulated expression of Bax and Bcl-2 during 7,12-dimethylbenz(alpha)anthracene-induced mammary carcinogenesis in rats. Prostaglandins Leukot Essent Fatty Acids 79 (1–2):5–14
Chatterjee M, Manna S, Janarthan M et al (2010a) Fish oil regulates cell proliferation, protect DNA damages and decrease HER-2/neu and c-Myc protein expression in rat mammary carcinogenesis. Clin Nutr 29(4):531–537
Chatterjee M, Chatterjee M, Janarthan M (2010b) Combinatorial effect of fish oil (Maxepa) and 1alpha,25-dihydroxyvitamin D(3) in the chemoprevention of DMBA-induced mammary carcinogenesis in rats. Chem Biol Interact 188(1):102–110
Chavarro JE, Stampfer MJ, Li H et al (2007) A prospective study of polyunsaturated fatty acid levels in blood and prostate cancer risk. Cancer Epidemiol Biomarkers Prev 16:1364–1370
Chen C, Kong AN (2005) Dietary cancer-chemopreventive compounds: from signaling and gene expression to pharmacological effects. Trends Pharmacol Sci 26:318–326
Chiang KC, Persons KS, Istfan NW et al (2009) Fish oil enhances the antiproliferative effect of 1alpha,25-dihydroxyvitamin D3 on liver cancer cells. Anticancer Res 29(9):3591–3596
Cho Y, Kim H, Turner ND et al (2011)A chemoprotective fish oil- and pectin-containing diet temporally alters gene expression profiles in exfoliated rat colonocytes throughout oncogenesis. J Nutr 141(6):1029–1035
Dai W, Liu T, Wang Q et al (2002) Down-regulation of PLK3 gene expression by types and amount of dietary fat in rat colon tumors. Int J Oncol 20(1):121–126
Davidson LA, Nguyen DV, Hokanson RM et al (2004) Chemopreventive n-3 polyunsaturated fatty acids reprogram genetic signatures during colon cancer initiation and progression in the rat. Cancer Res 64(18):6797–6804
Denkins Y, Kempf D, Ferniz M et al (2005) Role of ω-3 polyunsaturated fatty acids on cyclooxygenase-2 metabolism in brain-metastatic melanoma. J Lipid Res 46:1278–1284
Dumas JF, Goupille C, Pinault M et al (2010) n-3 PUFA-enriched diet delays the occurrence of cancer cachexia in rat with peritoneal carcinosis. Nutr Cancer 62(3):343–350
Faber J, Vos P, Kegler D et al (2008) Beneficial immune modulatory effects of a specific nutritional combination in a murine model for cancer cachexia. Br J Cancer 99(12):2029–2036
Fernandez E, Chatenoud L, La Vecchia C et al (1999) Fish consumption and cancer risk. Am J Clin Nutr 70:85–90
Fisher B, Costantino JP, Wickerham DL et al (1998) Tamoxifen for prevention of breast cancer: report of the National Surgical Adjuvant Breast and Bowel Project P-1 Study. J Natl Cancer Inst 90:1371–1388
Funahashi H, Satake M, Hasan S et al (2008) Opposing effects of n-6 and n-3 polyunsaturated fatty acids on pancreatic cancer growth. Pancreas 36(4):353–362
Ghosh-Choudhury T, Mandal CC, Woodruff K et al (2009) Fish oil targets PTEN to regulate NFkappaB for downregulation of anti-apoptotic genes in breast tumor growth. Breast Cancer Res Treat 118(1):213–228

Gogos CA, Ginopoulos P, Salsa B et al (1998) Dietary omega-3 polyunsaturated fatty acids plus vitamin E restore immunodeficiency and prolong survival for severely ill patients with generalized malignancy: a randomized control trial. Cancer 82:395–402

Griffini P, Fehres O, Klieverik L et al (1998) Dietary omega-3 polyunsaturated fatty acids promote colon carcinoma metastasis in rat liver. Cancer Res 58:3312–3319

Gutt CN, Brinkmann L, Mehrabi A et al (2007) Dietary omega-3-polyunsaturated fatty acids prevent the development of metastases of colon carcinoma in rat liver. Eur J Nutr 46(5):279–285

Hagi A, Nakayama M, Miura Y et al (2007) Effects of a fish oil-based emulsion on rat hepatoma cell invasion in culture. Nutrition 23(11–12):871–877

Han S, Sun X, Ritzenthaler JD et al (2009) Fish oil inhibits human lung carcinoma cell growth by suppressing integrin-linked kinase. Mol Cancer Res 7(1):108–117

Hardman WE (2002) Omega-3 FA to augment cancer therapy. J Nutr 132:3508S–3512S

Hardman WE (2004) N – 3 fatty acids and cancer therapy. J Nutr 134:3427S–3430S

Hong MY, Chapkin RS, Barhoumi R et al (2002) Fish oil increases mitochondrial phospholipid unsaturation, upregulating reactive oxygen species and apoptosis in rat colonocytes. Carcinogenesis 23:1919–1925

Horia E, Watkins BA (2007) Complementary actions of docosahexaenoic acid and genistein on COX-2, PGE2 and invasiveness in MDA-MB-231 breast cancer cells. Carcinogenesis 28(4):809–815

Jiang ZM, Wilmore DW, Wang XR et al (2010) Randomized clinical trial of intravenous soybean oil alone versus soybean oil plus fish oil emulsion after gastrointestinal cancer surgery. Br J Surg 97(6):804–809

Jordan A, Stein J (2003) Effect of an omega-3 fatty acid containing lipid emulsion alone and in combination with 5-fluorouracil (5-FU) on growth of the colon cancer cell line Caco-2. Eur J Nutr 42(6):324–331

Kakizoe T (2003) Chemoprevention of cancer – focusing on clinical trials. Jpn J Clin Oncol 33:421–442

Kansal S, Negi AK, Kaur R et al (2011) Evaluation of the role of oxidative stress in chemopreventive action of fish oil and celecoxib in the initiation phase of 7,12-dimethyl benz(α)anthracene-induced mammary carcinogenesis. Tumour Biol 32(1):167–177

Karmali RA (1989) n-3 Fatty acids and cancer. J Intern Med Suppl 225:197–200

Kim HH, Lee Y, Eun HC et al (2008) Eicosapentaenoic acid inhibits TNF-alpha-induced matrix metalloproteinase-9 expression in human keratinocytes, HaCaT cells. Biochem Biophys Res Commun 368(2):343–349

Kimura Y, Kono S, Toyomura K et al (2007) Meat, fish and fat intake in relation to subsitespecific risk of colorectal cancer: the Fukuoka Colorectal Cancer Study. Cancer Sci 98:590–597

Kolar SS, Barhoumi R, Callaway ES et al (2007) Synergy between docosahexaenoic acid and butyrate elicits p53-independent apoptosis via mitochondrial Ca(2+) accumulation in colonocytes. Am J Physiol Gastrointest Liver Physiol 293(5):G935–G943

Kramer F, Johnson IT, Doleman JF et al (2009) A comparison of the effects of soya isoflavonoids and fish oil on cell proliferation, apoptosis and the expression of oestrogen receptors alpha and beta in the mammary gland and colon of the rat. Br J Nutr 102(1):29–36

Latham P, Lund EK, Johnson IT (1999) Dietary n-3 PUFA increases the apoptotic response to 1,2-dimethylhydrazine, reduces mitosis and suppresses the induction of carcinogenesis in the rat colon. Carcinogenesis 20:645–650

Liang B, Wang S, Ye YJ et al (2008) Impact of postoperative omega-3 fatty acid-supplemented parenteral nutrition on clinical outcomes and immunomodulations in colorectal cancer patients. World J Gastroenterol 14(15):2434–2439

Ma H, Das T, Pereira S et al (2009) Efficacy of dietary antioxidants combined with a chemotherapeutic agent on human colon cancer progression in a fluorescent orthotopic mouse model. Anticancer Res 29(7):2421–2426

Maeda S, Omata M (2008) Inflammation and cancer: role of nuclear factor-kappaB activation. Cancer Sci 99(5):836–842

Manni A, Xu H, Washington S et al (2010) The impact of fish oil on the chemopreventive efficacy of tamoxifen against development of N-methyl-N-nitrosourea-induced rat mammary carcinogenesis. Cancer Prev Res (Phila) 3(3):322–330

Mantovani G, Maccio A, Madeddu C et al (2006) A phase II study with antioxidants, both in the diet and supplemented, pharmaconutritional support, progestagen, and anti-cyclooxygenase-2 showing efficacy and safety in patients with cancer-related anorexia/cachexia and oxidative stress. Cancer Epidemiol Biomarkers Prev 15:1030–1034

Mashima T, Seimiya H, Tsuruo T (2009) De novo fatty-acid synthesis and related pathways as molecular targets for cancer therapy. Br J Cancer 100(9):1369–1372

Menendez JA, Lupu R (2006) Oncogenic properties of the endogenous fatty acid metabolism: molecular pathology of fatty acid synthase in cancer cells. Curr Opin Clin Nutr Metab Care 9(4):346–357

Mernitz H, Lian F, Smith DE et al (2009) Fish oil supplementation inhibits NNK-induced lung carcinogenesis in the A/J mouse. Nutr Cancer 61(5):663–669

Michael B (1999) Prevention of cancer in the next millennium: report of the chemoprevention working group to the American Association for Cancer Research. Cancer Res 59:4743–4758

Moreira AP, Sabarense CM, Dias CM et al (2009) Fish oil ingestion reduces the number of aberrant crypt foci and adenoma in 1,2-dimethylhydrazine-induced colon cancer in rats. Braz J Med Biol Res 42(12):1167–1172

Narayanan BA, Narayanan NK, Simi B et al (2003) Modulation of inducible nitric oxide synthase and related proinflammatory genes by the omega-3 fatty acid docosahexaenoic acid in human colon cancer cells. Cancer Res 63(5):972–979

Park KS, Lim JW, Kim H (2009) Inhibitory mechanism of omega-3 fatty acids in pancreatic inflammation and apoptosis. Ann N Y Acad Sci 1171:421–427

Reddy BS (2002) Types and amount of dietary fat and colon cancer risk: prevention by omega-3 fatty acid-rich diets. Environ Health Prev Med 7(3):95–102

Reddy BS (2004) Omega-3 fatty acids in colorectal cancer prevention. Int J Cancer 112:1–7

Rose DP, Connolly JM (1999) Omega-3 fatty acids as cancer chemopreventive agents. Pharmacol Ther 83:217–244

Sala-Vila A, Folkes J, Calder PC (2010) The effect of three lipid emulsions differing in fatty acid composition on growth, apoptosis and cell cycle arrest in the HT-29 colorectal cancer cell line. Clin Nutr 29(4):519–524

Sanders LM, Henderson CE, Hong MY et al (2004) Enhancement of reactive oxygen species by dietary fish oil and attenuation of antioxidant defenses by dietary pectin coordinately heightens apoptosis in rat. J Nutr 134:3233–3238

Satia JA, Littman A, Slatore CG et al (2009) Associations of herbal and specialty supplements with lung and colorectal cancer risk in the VITamins and Lifestyle study. Cancer Epidemiol Biomarkers Prev 18(5):1419–1428

Schonberg SA, Lundemo AG, Fladvad T et al (2006) Closely related colon cancer cell lines display different sensitivity to polyunsaturated fatty acids, accumulate different lipid classes and downregulate sterol regulatory element binding protein 1. FEBS J 273:2749–2765

Sharma A, Belna J, Logan J et al (2005) The effects of ω-3 fatty acids on growth regulation of epithelial ovarian cancer cell lines. Gynecol Oncol 99(1):58–64

Simopoulos AP (1991) Omega-3 fatty acids in health and disease and in growth and development. Am J Clin Nutr 54:438–463

Simopoulos AP (2006) Evolutionary aspects of diet, the omega-6/omega-3 ratio and genetic variation: nutritional implications for chronic diseases. Biomed Pharmacother 60(9):502–507

Smith LC, Dauchy EM, Dauchy RT et al (2006) Dietary fish oil deactivates a growth-promoting signaling pathway in hepatoma 7288CTC in buffalo rats. Nutr Cancer 56(2):204–213

Theodoratou E, McNeill G, Cetnarskyj R et al (2007) Dietary fatty acids and colorectal cancer: a casecontrol study. Am J Epidemiol 166:181–195

Tsao AS, Kim ES, Hong WK (2004) Chemoprevention of cancer. CA Cancer J Clin 54:150–180

Ueda K, Asai Y, Yoshimura Y et al (2008) Effect of oil-in-water lipid emulsions prepared with fish oil or soybean oil on the growth of MCF-7 cells and HepG2 cells. J Pharm Pharmacol 60(8):1069–1075

van der Meij BS, Langius JA, Smit EF et al (2010) Oral nutritional supplements containing (n-3) polyunsaturated fatty acids affect the nutritional status of patients with stage III non-small cell lung cancer during multimodality treatment. J Nutr 140(10):1774–1780

van Norren K, Kegler D, Argilés JM et al (2009) Dietary supplementation with a specific combination of high protein, leucine, and fish oil improves muscle function and daily activity in tumour-bearing cachectic mice. Br J Cancer 100(5):713–722

Vanamala J, Glagolenko A, Yang P et al (2008) Dietary fish oil and pectin enhance colonocyte apoptosis in part through suppression of PPARdelta/PGE2 and elevation of PGE3. Carcinogenesis 29(4):790–796

vel Szic KS, Ndlovu MN, Haegeman G et al (2010) Nature or nurture: let food be your epigenetic medicine in chronic inflammatory disorders. Biochem Pharmacol 80(12):1816–1832

Weinstein IB (1991) Cancer prevention: recent progress and future opportunities. Cancer Res 51:5080s–5085s

Wigmore SJ, Barber MD, Ross MJ et al (2000) Effect of oral eicosapentaenoic acid on weight loss in patients with pancreatic cancer. Nutr Cancer 36:177–184

Wu S, Liang J, Zhang L et al (2011) Fish consumption and the risk of gastric cancer: systematic review and meta-analysis. BMC Cancer 11:26

Chapter 22
Antioxidant Supplements: An Evidence-Based Approach to Health Benefits and Risks

Goran Bjelakovic, Dimitrinka Nikolova, and Christian Gluud

Contents

The major issues of the modern medicine in high-income countries are how to prevent chronic diseases including cancer and cardiovascular diseases in order to prolong life span. It has been speculated that the aging process and development of chronic diseases are consequences of oxidative damage to cells and tissues. Oxidative stress defined as an imbalance between oxidants and antioxidants in our body in favour of the former (Sies 1985) is thought to cause a spectrum of diseases. During human life, an antioxidant network counteracts the deleterious action of reactive oxygen species. Our cells synthesize some antioxidants, while other are obtained from diet. The beneficial influence of diet on health has been known since Ancient Greeks (Jones 1923). It has been suggested that specific diet like high intake of fruits and vegetables is associated with a lower cancer incidence and lower risk of death. The protective effect of dietary fruits and vegetables has been ascribed to the antioxidant vitamins and trace elements. The question whether antioxidant supplements may protect against chronic diseases and cancer and prolong life span has drawn much attention. Some researchers have even hypothesized that long-living animal species have more efficient antioxidant systems than shorter-living species (Cutler 1991).

G. Bjelakovic (✉) • D. Nikolova • C. Gluud
Department of Internal Medicine – Gastroenterology and Hepatology, Medical Faculty, University of Nis, Boulevard Dr Zorana Djindjica 81, 18000 Nis, Serbia

G. Bjelakovic • D. Nikolova • C. Gluud
The Cochrane Hepato-Biliary Group, Copenhagen Trial Unit, Centre for Clinical Intervention Research, Rigshospitalet, Copenhagen University Hospital, 2100 Copenhagen, Denmark
e-mail: G.Bjelakovic@ctu.rh.dk

S. Shankar and R.K. Srivastava (eds.), *Nutrition, Diet and Cancer*,
DOI 10.1007/978-94-007-2923-0_22,

Many studies have been conducted in order to verify the assumed beneficial effects of antioxidant supplements. While the results of epidemiological studies were almost uniformly positive, the results of clinical trials undertaken to corroborate this hypothesis, remained largely inconclusive. Even though a healthy diet provides a sufficient amount of antioxidants, a number of people regularly take antioxidant supplements hoping to improve their health and prevent diseases. More than one third of adults in high-income countries ingest antioxidant pills (Millen et al. 2004).

Gastrointestinal cancers are among the most common cancers and are a leading cause of cancer death worldwide (Ferlay et al. 2004). The poor prognosis of patients with gastrointestinal cancers has focused interest on prevention and especially chemoprevention. Chemoprevention is defined as use of agents that can inhibit, delay, or reverse carcinogenesis (Sporn et al. 1976). Many classes of agents including antioxidants have shown promise in chemoprevention. However, the evidence on whether antioxidants are effective in decreasing the incidence of gastrointestinal cancers is contradictory.

Vitamin A is essential for growth. Since cancer involves disturbances in normal tissue growth and differentiation, it was one of the first vitamins to be evaluated with respect to carcinogenesis. Later studies indicated that protective effects were only observed for dietary vitamin A from plant sources (beta-carotene) (Peto et al. 1981; Ziegler 1989). Vitamin C has antioxidative properties with possible cancer preventive potential (Hanck 1988). Vitamin E acts as a free radical scavenger to prevent lipid peroxidation of polyunsaturated fatty acids and block nitrosamine formation (Oshima and Berezial 1982; Poppel and Berg 1997). Vitamin E supplementation can increase production of humoral antibodies and may have antitumour proliferation capacities, possibly by modulating gene expression (Knekt 1994). Selenium, a trace element, is also important for antioxidant defences of the body as an integral component of metalloprotein enzymes. It is a component of selenoproteins, which have important enzymatic functions (Hughes 2000; Rayman 2000). Observational studies found an inverse relationship between selenium intake and cancer mortality (Schrauzer et al. 1977). Cancer mortality rates are significantly higher in regions with low selenium content in diet (Clark et al. 1991).

A large number of primary or secondary prevention randomised trials have been conducted to assess the benefits and harms of antioxidant supplements versus placebo or no intervention. With our research, we aimed to assess the beneficial and harmful effects of antioxidant supplements, namely beta-carotene, vitamins A, C, E and selenium in preventing gastrointestinal cancers (i.e., oesophageal, gastric, small intestine, colorectal, pancreatic, liver, and biliary tract cancers) (Bjelakovic et al. 2004a, b). We reviewed all randomised trials comparing antioxidant supplements with placebo or no intervention for prevention of gastrointestinal cancers. We could not find evidence that the studied antioxidant supplements prevent gastrointestinal cancers. More importantly, we observed that antioxidant supplements seem to increase overall mortality (Bjelakovic et al. 2004a, b).

During our research we identified eight randomised trials that assessed antioxidant supplements in the primary or secondary prevention of colorectal adenomas, considered as an intermediate step towards colorectal cancer. The pooled effect of all trials on colorectal adenomas was not statistically significant (Bjelakovic et al. 2006).

The Cochrane approach to systematic reviews is to look at the whole evidence for the effects of an intervention (Higgins and Green 2008). Therefore, we decided to assess the beneficial and harmful effects of antioxidant supplementation on mortality in all randomised trials involving all potential healthy participants and patient groups, i.e., primary and secondary prevention. We excluded tertiary prevention trials, i.e., randomised trials in which antioxidant supplements were used to treat a specific disease or nutritional defect, like trials in patients with acute, infectious, or malignant diseases (except non-melanoma skin cancer), and trials including children and pregnant women since the latter groups may be in need of certain antioxidant supplements.

Our analyses showed that antioxidant supplements, namely beta-carotene, vitamins A, C, E, and selenium given singly or combined significantly increased mortality (Bjelakovic et al. 2007, 2008) Specifically, our analyses showed that beta-carotene, vitamin A, and vitamin E given singly or combined with other antioxidant supplements significantly increased mortality with 7%, 16%, and 4%, respectively. We found no evidence that vitamin C may increase longevity. Selenium tended to reduce mortality, but these observations were hampered by the risk of bias in a large proportion of these trials (Bjelakovic et al. 2007, 2008). Recently, two randomised trials and one observational study have shown that selenium might carry health risks(Stranges et al. 2007; Lippman et al. 2009; Bleys et al. 2007).

Free radicals have been shown to play dual biological function, both harmful and beneficial. In moderate concentrations they are essential mediators of reactions by which unwanted cells are eliminated from our body. By decreasing free radicals from our organism we may interfere with some essential defensive mechanisms like apoptosis, phagocytosis, and detoxification. Consequently, it may be dangerous to interfere with the delicate balance between oxidative stress and antioxidants in our cells (Salganik 2001).

The randomised trials we identified were mainly conducted in high-income countries among populations already well saturated with vitamins and trace elements through their diet. Western diet provides more than sufficient amount of the recommended dietary allowances for beta-carotene, vitamin A, C and E (Herbert et al. 1990). A balanced diet typically contains safe levels of antioxidant vitamins and trace elements (Camire and Kantor 1999). The majority of the trials included in our review have neither taken into account the recommended daily allowances of antioxidant vitamins nor the recommended relative amounts in case of combination of two or more antioxidants. This might be a cause for the detrimental effects of antioxidant supplements (Panel on Micronutrients et al. 2000; Panel on Dietary Antioxidants and Related Compounds et al. 2000).

There are still many gaps in our knowledge of the mechanisms of bioavailability, biotransformation, and action of antioxidant supplements (Bast and Haenen 2002). Antioxidant supplements also possess pro-oxidant effects (Vertuani et al. 2004; Podmore et al. 1998; Paolini et al. 2003).

The available data on adverse effects of antioxidant supplements are limited (Mulholland and Benford 2007) and often underreported (Woo 2007). It is estimated that less than 1% of all adverse effects associated with antioxidant supplements are notified. Consumers presume antioxidant supplements to be safe and use them without supervision of their doctors. We find it is high time that antioxidant supplements are moved from the free 'over the counter' market to the prescription medicine market regulated by physicians.

It should be emphasized that our review examined only the influence of the factory- produced antioxidant supplements. Therefore the results cannot be translated to all antioxidant supplements nor fruits and vegetables. Some antioxidant supplements may have protective effects and they should also be studied.

We cannot recommend the use of antioxidant supplements as a primary or secondary preventive measure in the population groups studied in our reviews. According to our evidence, antioxidant supplements cause unwanted consequences to our health. The optimal source of antioxidant supplements seems to come from our diet, not from antioxidant supplements in pills or tablets. While we await a better understanding of mechanisms involved in metabolism of antioxidant supplements, consumption of a varied 'healthy' diet seems a prudent preventive strategy.

References

Bast A, Haenen GR (2002) The toxicity of antioxidants and their metabolites. Environ Toxicol Pharmacol 11:251–258

Bjelakovic G, Nikolova D, Simonetti RG, Gluud C (2004a) Antioxidant supplements for preventing gastrointestinal cancers. Cochrane Database Syst Rev, Issue 4, Art. No.: CD004183.pub2. doi: 10.1002/14651858.CD004183.pub2

Bjelakovic G, Nikolova D, Simonetti RG, Gluud C (2004b) Antioxidant supplements for prevention of gastrointestinal cancers: a systematic review and meta–analysis. Lancet 364:1219–1228

Bjelakovic G, Nagorni A, Nikolova D, Simonetti RG, Bjelakovic M, Gluud C (2006) Meta-analysis: antioxidant supplements for primary and secondary prevention of colorectal adenoma. Aliment Pharmacol Ther 24:281–291

Bjelakovic G, Nikolova D, Gluud LL, Simonetti RG, Gluud C (2007) Mortality in randomized trials of antioxidant supplements for primary and secondary prevention: systematic review and meta–analysis. JAMA 297:842–857

Bjelakovic G, Nikolova D, Gluud LL, Simonetti RG, Gluud C (2008) Antioxidant supplements for prevention of mortality in healthy participants and patients with various diseases. Cochrane Database Syst Rev (2):CD007176

Bleys J, Navas-Acien A, Guallar E (2007) Serum selenium and diabetes in U.S. adults. Diabetes Care 30:829–834

Camire ME, Kantor MA (1999) Dietary supplements: nutritional and legal considerations. Food Technol 53:87–95

Clark LC, Cantor KP, Allaway WH (1991) Selenium in forage crops and cancer mortality in U.S. counties. Arch Environ Health 46:37–42

Cutler RG (1991) Antioxidants and aging. Am J Clin Nutr 53:373S–379S

Ferlay J, Bray F, Pisani P, Parkin DM (2004) GLOBOCAN 2002: cancer incidence. Mortality and prevalence worldwide. IARC cancer base no. 5, version 2.0. IARC Press, Lyon

Hanck AB (1988) Vitamin C and cancer. Prog Clin Biol Res 259:307–320

Herbert V, Subak-Sharpe GJ, Hammock D (eds) (1990) The Mount Sinai School of Medicine complete book of nutrition. St Martin's Press, New York

Higgins JPT, Green S (eds) (2008) Cochrane handbook for systematic reviews of interventions version 5.0.0 [updated Feb 2008]. The Cochrane Collaboration. Available from www.cochrane-handbook.org

Hughes D (2000) Dietary antioxidants and human immune function. Nutr Bull 25:35–41

Jones WHS (ed) (1923) Hippocrates. Nutriment 351

Knekt P (1994) Vitamin E and cancer prevention. In: Frei B (ed) Natural antioxidants in human health and disease. Academic Press, San Diego, pp 199–239

Lippman SM, Klein EA, Goodman PJ et al (2009)Effect of selenium and vitamin E on risk of prostate cancer and other cancers: the selenium and vitamin E effect of selenium and vitamin E on risk of prostate cancer prevention trial (SELECT). JAMA 301(1):39–51

Millen AE, Dodd KW, Subar AF (2004) Use of vitamin, mineral, nonvitamin, and nonmineral supplements in the United States: the 1987, 1992, and 2000 National Health Interview Survey results. J Am Diet Assoc 104:942–950

Mulholland CA, Benford DJ (2007) What is known about the safety of multivitamin-multimineral supplements for the generally healthy population? Theoretical basis for harm. Am J Clin Nutr 85:318S–322S

Oshima H, Berezial J (1982) Monitoring N-nitrosamino acids excreted in the urine and feces of rats as an index of endogenous nitrozation. Carcinogenesis 3:115–120

Panel on Dietary Antioxidants and Related Compounds, Subcommittees on Upper Reference Levels of Nutrients, Interpretation and Uses of DRIs, Standing Committee on the Scientific Evaluation of Dietary Reference Intakes, Food and Nutrition Board, Institute of Medicine (2000) Dietary reference intakes for vitamin C, vitamin E, selenium, and carotenoids. National Academy Press, Washington, DC, pp 1–529

Panel on Micronutrients, Subcommittees on Upper Reference Levels of Nutrients, Interpretation and Use of Dietary Reference Intakes, Standing Committee on the Scientific Evaluation of Dietary Reference Intakes, Institute of Medicine, Food and Nutrition Board (2000) Dietary reference intakes for vitamin A, vitamin K, arsenic, boron, chromium, copper, iodine, iron, manganese, molybdenum, nickel, silicon, vanadium, and zinc. National Academy Press, Washington, DC, pp 1–800

Paolini M, Abdel-Rahman SZ, Sapone A, Pedulli GF, Perocco P, Cantelli-Forti G et al (2003) Beta-carotene: a cancer chemopreventive agent or a co-carcinogen? Mutat Res 7719:1–6

Peto R, Doll R, Buckley JD, Sporn MB (1981) A dietary carotene materially reduces human cancer rates? Nature 290:201–208

Podmore ID, Griffiths HR, Herbert KE, Mistry N, Mistry P, Lunec J (1998) Vitamin C exhibits pro-oxidant properties. Nature 392:559

Poppel G, Berg H (1997) Vitamins and cancer. Cancer Lett 114:195–202

Rayman M (2000) The importance of selenium to human health. Lancet 356:233–241

Salganik RI (2001) The benefits and hazards of antioxidants: controlling apoptosis and other protective mechanisms in cancer patients and the human population. J Am Coll Nutr 20: 464S–472S

Schrauzer GN, White DA, Schneider CJ (1977) Cancer mortality correlation studies. III. Statistical association with dietary selenium intakes. Bioinorg Chem 7:35–56

Sies H (1985) Introductory remarks. In: Sies H (ed) Oxidative stress. Academic, Orlando, pp 1–7

Sporn MB, Dunlop NM, Newton DL, Smith JM (1976) Prevention of chemical carcinogenesis by vitamin A and its synthetic analogs (retinoids). Fed Proc 35:1332–1338

Stranges S, Marshall JR, Natarajan R, Donahue RP, Trevisan M, Combs GF et al (2007) Effects of long-term selenium supplementation on the incidence of type 2 diabetes: a randomized trial. Ann Intern Med 147:217–223

Vertuani S, Angusti A, Manfredini S (2004) The antioxidants and pro-antioxidants network: an overview. Curr Pharm Des 10:1677–1694

Woo JJ (2007) Adverse event monitoring and multivitamin-multimineral dietary supplements. Am J Clin Nutr 85:323S–324S

Ziegler RG (1989) A review of epidemiologic evidence that carotenoids reduce the risk of cancer. J Nutr 119:116–122

Chapter 23
Natural Antioxidants and Their Role in Cancer Prevention

Akanksha Singh, Akansha Jain, Birinchi Kumar Sarma, Alok Jha, and H.B. Singh

Contents

A. Singh • A. Jain
Centre of Advanced Studies, Faculty of Sciences, Banaras Hindu University, Varanasi 221 005, Uttar Pradesh, India
e-mail: bhuaks29@gmail.com; akansha007@rediffmail.com

B.K. Sarma • H.B. Singh (✉)
Department of Mycology & Plant Pathology, Institute of Agricultural Sciences, Banaras Hindu University, Varanasi 221 005, Uttar Pradesh, India
e-mail: birinchi_ks@yahoo.com; hbs1@rediffmail.com

A. Jha
Department of Food Science and Technology, Institute of Agricultural Sciences, Banaras Hindu University, Varanasi 221 005, Uttar Pradesh, India
e-mail: alok_ndri@rediffmail.com

S. Shankar and R.K. Srivastava (eds.), *Nutrition, Diet and Cancer*,
DOI 10.1007/978-94-007-2923-0_23,

Abstract We often credit antioxidants because of their ability to protect cells from the oxidative/electrophilic damage that makes them turn cancerous. A number of antioxidants have shown to inhibit the induction of cancer by a wide variety of chemical carcinogens and/or radiation at many target sites in mice, rats, and hamsters. Epidemiological studies suggest that a diet rich in plant products containing natural antioxidants may be a deterrent to carcinogenicity. Many antioxidants were tested to determine if they would inhibit tumor initiation, promotion, and/or progression. Use of a number of important antioxidants can be helpful in the treatment of cancer, either as sole agents or as adjuncts to standard radiation and chemotherapy protocols. Our knowledge of antioxidants in a cancer setting is still at its infancy stage. In order to understand antioxidants and their role in cancer prevention, we must know what exactly antioxidants are and how they help our bodies. The interactions between antioxidant and cancer prevention cannot be decided solely on the basis of presumed mechanism of action when used concurrently. Numerous natural antioxidants appear to have beneficial health effects. There is sufficient evidence to recommend consuming food sources rich in antioxidants but still much scientific research needs to be carried out before we can begin to make dietary recommendations. This chapter summarizes the current knowledge on the occurrence, types and antioxidative properties of natural antioxidants, underlying the necessity of further research.

Introduction

Cancer is still a mystery disease for the oncologists across the world till date. It could be described as an uncontrolled growth invasion and sometimes metastasis. Cancers are mostly caused by abnormalities in the genetic material of the transformed cells which may be due to the effects of carcinogens, such as tobacco smoke, radiation, chemicals, or infectious agents. In lay man terminology, cancer is an atypical growth of harmful cells called free radicals (Halliwell 2007). These types of cells start to grow uncontrollably and threaten normal cells and cancer like an uncontrolled monster does not discriminate where it grows or who it chooses, and every part of the body can be at risk. If the cancer is of the malignant type it could lead to death. There is no clear cause why one person gets cancer and another does not. Cancer develops over time when certain normal genes start mutating. These gene mutations occur due to multiple factors related to lifestyle, heredity and environment (Bendich 1996). Potential catalysts of cancer are tobacco, certain diets, alcohol, exposure to ultraviolet (UV) radiation, and to a lesser extent, exposure to cancer causing agents (carcinogens) in the environment and the workplace (Rietjens et al. 2002).

Information on certain foods contain potential harmful elements in low amounts have been identified which does not show immediate effects but over a period of time its amount accumulates in the body putting people at risk of becoming cancer patients. The treatment plan depends mainly on the type of cancer, stage of the disease, patient's age and general health. The goal of the treatment is to cure the disease but till date full proof cure has still not been achieved. Most treatment plans include surgery, radiation therapy, or chemotherapy, hormone therapy or biological therapy (Willcox et al. 2004). In addition, these days stem cell transplantation is being used so that a patient can receive very high doses of chemotherapy or radiation therapy. However, these treatments come with many side effects (Halliwell 2007). Therefore, an alternative remedy for curing is being searched out for which natural antioxidants seem to show promising results. Fresh green vegetables, plants, fruits and juices have been shown to be rich source of anti-oxidants that prevents as well as cures cancer. Green foods produce antioxidants that attack and replace free radical cells which are finally morphed into healthy cells of the body.

The oxidative deterioration of fats and oils in foods is responsible for rancid odours and favours, with a consequent decrease in nutritional quality and safety caused by the formation of secondary, potentially toxic, compounds. The addition of antioxidants is required to preserve flavour and colour and to avoid vitamin destruction. Among the synthetic types, the most frequently used to preserve food are butylated hydroxyanisole (BHA), butylated hydroxytoluene (BHT), propyl gallate (PG) and tert-butyl hydroquinone (TBHQ). Tocopherols are also used as antioxidants for food. Reports revealing that BHA and BHT could be toxic, and the higher manufacturing costs and lower efficiency of natural antioxidants such as tocopherols, together with the increasing consciousness of consumers with regard to food additive safety, created a need for identifying alternative natural and probably safer sources of food antioxidants (Bendich 1996). The replacement of synthetic antioxidants by natural ones may have benefits due to health implications and functionality such as solubility in both oil and water, of interest for emulsions, in food systems. Natural antioxidant has been repeatedly advised, since the fact than an antioxidant comes from a natural source does not prove its assumed safety. Carotenoids, tocopherols, ascorbates and polyphenols are strong natural antioxidants generally found in plants and foods. Vegetables, fruits, herbs, spices and other plants contain many compounds with cancer preventive potentials (Bendich 1996; Halliwell 2007). Several plants have been studied as sources of potentially safe natural antioxidants for the food industry; various compounds have been isolated, many of them being polyphenols. A large range of low and high molecular weight plant polyphenolics presenting antioxidant properties have been studied and proposed for protection against different types of human cancer (Moure et al. 2003).

Reactive Oxygen Species (ROS)

The recent growth in knowledge of free radicals and reactive oxygen species (ROS) in biology is producing a medical revolution that promises a new age of health. Reactive oxygen species (ROS) and reactive nitrogen species (RNS) are the terms collectively described free radicals and other non-radical reactive derivatives also called oxidants. Radicals are more unstable and generally more reactive than non-radical species which are formed from molecules via the breakage of a chemical

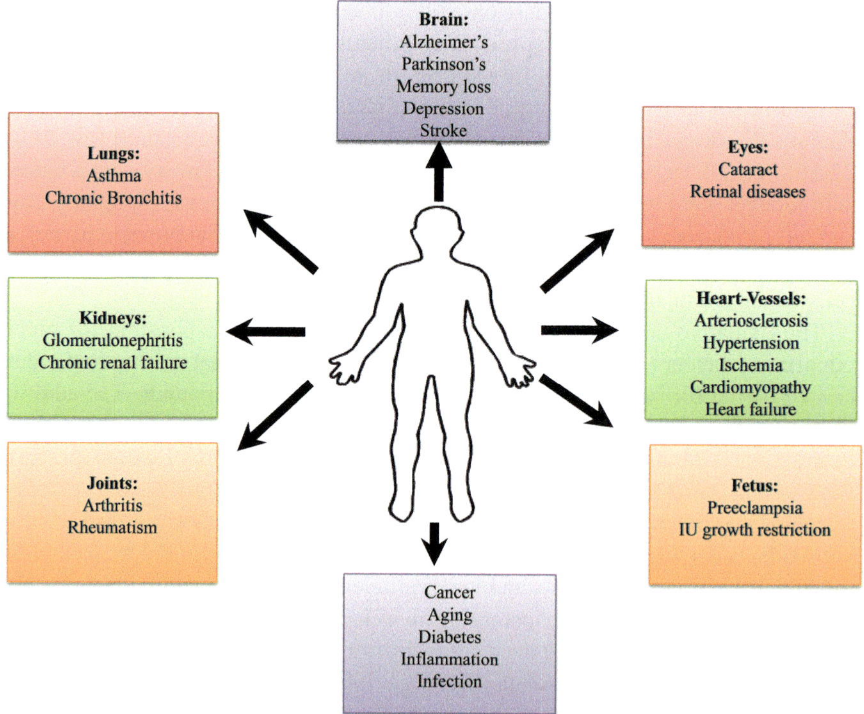

Fig. 23.1 Different types of human diseases caused by oxidative stress

bond such that each fragment keeps one electron, by cleavage of a radical to give another radical and, also via redox reactions (Bahorun et al. 2004; Halliwell and Gutteridge 2007). Reactive oxygen species (ROS) include free radicals such as superoxide ($O_2^{\bullet-}$), peroxyl ($ROO^{\bullet}$), alkoxyl ($RO^{\bullet}$), hydroxyl ($HO^{\bullet}$), nitric oxide ($NO^{\bullet}$), nitrogen dioxide ($NO_2^{\bullet}$), peroxyl ($ROO^{\bullet}$) and lipid peroxyl ($LOO^{\bullet}$), hydrogen peroxide (H_2O_2), ozone (O_3), singlet oxygen ($^1O_2$), hypochlorous acid (HOCl), nitrous acid (HNO_2), peroxynitrite ($ONOO^-$), dinitrogen trioxide (N_2O_3), lipid peroxide (LOOH) are not actually free radicals but oxidants which easily lead to free radical reactions in living organisms. Exogenous sources of ROS include tobacco smoke, certain pollutants, organic solvents, exposure to sunlight, X-rays, ozone, auto-exhaust and pesticides. ROS are known to induce some oxidative damage to biomolecules like lipids, DNA, RNA, proteins and carbohydrates, leading to mutations, faulty repair mechanism, altering enzymes, surface receptor and other essential functions ROS have been implicated in more than 100 diseases, including malaria, ageing, acquired immunodeficiency syndrome, cardiovascular diseases, diabetes, cancer, etc. (Fig. 23.1) (Bendich 1996; Bingham et al. 2003).

Formation of ROS and RNS can occur in the cells by two ways:

(i) enzymatic and
(ii) non-enzymatic reactions.

Enzymatic reactions generating free radicals include those involved in the respiratory chain, the phagocytosis, the prostaglandin synthesis and the cytochrome P450 system (Pacher et al. 2007; Genestra 2007; Halliwell 2007).

DNA Damage

ROS can cause oxidative damages to DNA: both nuclear and mitochondrial. The damages are done mainly by base modification, deoxyribose oxidation, strand breakage, and DNA–protein cross-links. Among the various ROS generated, $OH^{\cdot}$ produces various products from the DNA bases which mainly include C-8 hydroxylation of guanine to form 8-oxo-7,8 dehydro-2'-deoxyguanosine, a ring-opened product; 2,6-Diamino-4-hydroxy-5-formamimodipyrimidine, 8-OH-adenine, 2-OH-adenine, thymine glycol, cytosine glycol, etc. ROS-induced DNA damages include various mutagenic alterations as well. The action of 8-oxo-deoxy-guanosine as a promutagen, as well as in altering the binding of methylase to the oligomer so as to inhibit methylation of adjacent cytosine has been reported in cases of cancer development. Besides, ROS may interfere with normal cell signalling, resulting thereby in alteration of the gene expression, and development of cancer by redox regulation of transcriptional factors/activator and/or by oxidatively modulating the protein kinase cascades. ROS have also been shown to activate mutations in human *C-Ha-ras-1* protooncogene, and to induce mutation in the *p53* tumour-suppressor gene. Activation of the early-response protooncogenes plays a vital role in signal transduction, leading to cell proliferation and transformation. The oxidative damage of mitochondrial DNA leads to formation of abnormal components of the electron transport chain which results in the generation of more ROS through increased leakage of electrons, and therefore further cell damage. Oxidative damage to mitochondrial DNA may promote cancer and aging, eventually (Bandopadhyay et al. 2001).

Carcinogenesis

A large number of investigators have proposed participation of free radicals in carcinogenesis, mutation and transformation, particularly in the past 20 years. Although there is no definitive evidence that free radicals involvement is obligatory in these processes, it is clear that their presence in biosystem could lead to mutation, transformation and ultimately cancer. Induction of mutagenesis, the best known of the biological effect of radiation, occurs mainly through damage of DNA by the HO· radical and other species produced by radiolysis of water, and also by direct radiation effect on DNA. These effects can cause cell mutagenesis and carcinogenesis. Lipid peroxides are also suspected of being responsible for the activation of benzo (a) pyrene and other carcinogens, as well as for the production of some types of promoter (Hertog et al. 1992, 1993a, b).

Antioxidant Defence Enzyme Network

'Antioxidants' are substances that neutralize free radicals or their actions (Stahl and Sies 1996). Human's have evolved with time various antioxidant systems to protect themselves against the hazardous effects of free radicals. These systems include some antioxidants produced in the body (endogenous) and the others obtained from the diet (exogenous). (a) Enzymatic defenses, such as *Se*-glutathione peroxidase, catalase, and superoxide dismutase, which metabolize superoxide, hydrogen peroxide, and lipid peroxides, thus preventing most of the formation of the toxic HO, and (b) Non enzymatic defenses, such as glutathione, histidine-peptides, the iron-binding proteins transferring and ferritin, dihydrolipoic acid, reduced CoQ10, melatonin, urate, and plasma protein thiols, with the last two accounting for the major contribution to the radical-trapping capacity of plasma.

The various defense responses are complementary to each other, as they act against different species at different cellular compartments. However, despite these defense antioxidants some ROS still escape and cause damage. Thus, at this stage repair antioxidant system (able to repair damage, and based on proteases, lipases, transferases, and DNA repair enzymes) comes into action (Varma et al. 1995).

Epidemiological and animal studies suggest that the regular consumption of fruits, vegetables and whole grains, reduces the risk of chronic diseases associated with oxidative damages. Carotenoids, tocopherols, ascorbates, lipoic acids and polyphenols are strong natural antioxidants with free radical scavenging activity. To protect the cells and organ systems of the body against reactive oxygen species, humans have evolved a highly sophisticated and complex antioxidant protection system (Fig. 23.2) It involves a variety of components, both endogenous and exogenous in origin, that function interactively and synergistically to neutralize free radicals (Table 23.1). Antioxidant defense system against oxidative stress is composed of several lines, and the antioxidants are classified into four categories based on function (Fig. 23.3)

Natural Antioxidants and Chemoprevention

All the living forms inhabiting the Earth's atmosphere must be equipped with systems to deal with the action of oxygen in living matter. Plants are especially susceptible to damage by active oxygen because of which plants have developed

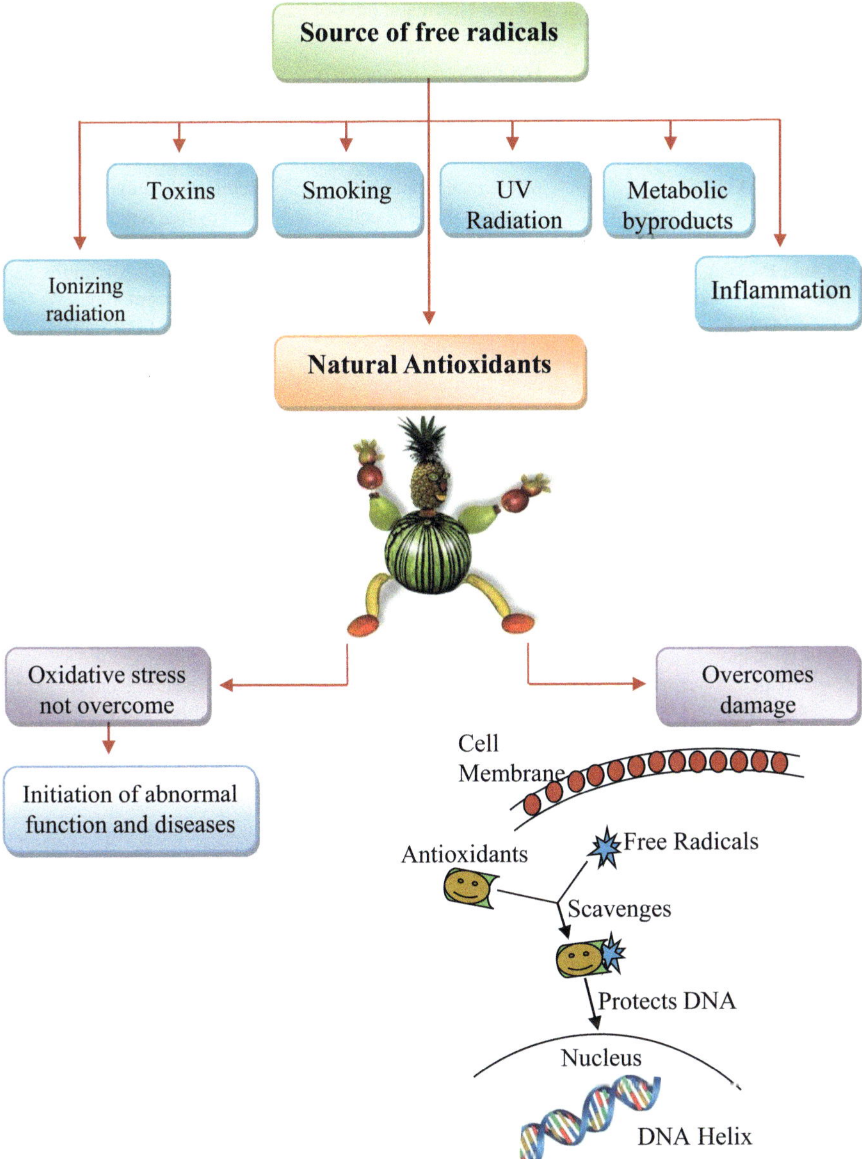

Fig. 23.2 Model representing mechanism of quenching of free radicals

numerous antioxidant defense systems that results in certain numbers of very potent antioxidants. Besides plants many of microbial and animal products such as fermented products, seaweeds, protein hydrolisates were found to be powerful antioxidants. Daily foods contain a wide variety of free radicals scavenging molecules, thus vegetables, fruit, tea, wine are product rich in natural antioxidant

Table 23.1 Important enzymatic and non-enzymatic physiological antioxidants

Enzymatic and non-enzymatic antioxidants	Location	Properties
Superoxide dismutase (SOD)	Mitochondria and cytosol	Dismutase superoxide radicals
Glutathione peroxidase (GSH)	Mitochondria and cytosol	Removes hydrogen peroxide and organic hydroperoxide
Catalase (CAT)	Mitochondria and cytosol	Removes hydrogen peroxide
Vitamin C	Aqueous phase of cell	Acts as free radical scavenger and recycles vitamin E
Vitamin E	Cell membrane	Major chain-break antioxidant in cell membrane
Uric acid	Product of purine metabolism	Scavenger of OH radicals
Glutathione	Nonprotein thiol in cell	Serves multiple roles in the cellular antioxidant defense
α-lipoic acid	Endogenous thiol	Effective in recycling vitamin C, may also be an effective glutathione substitute
Carotenoids	Lipid soluble antioxidants, located in membrane tissue	Scavengers of reactive oxygen species, singlet oxygen quencher
Metals ions sequestration: transferrin, ferritin, lactoferrin,	–	Chelating of metals ions, responsible for Fenton reactions
Nitric oxide	–	Free radical scavenger, inhibitor of LP

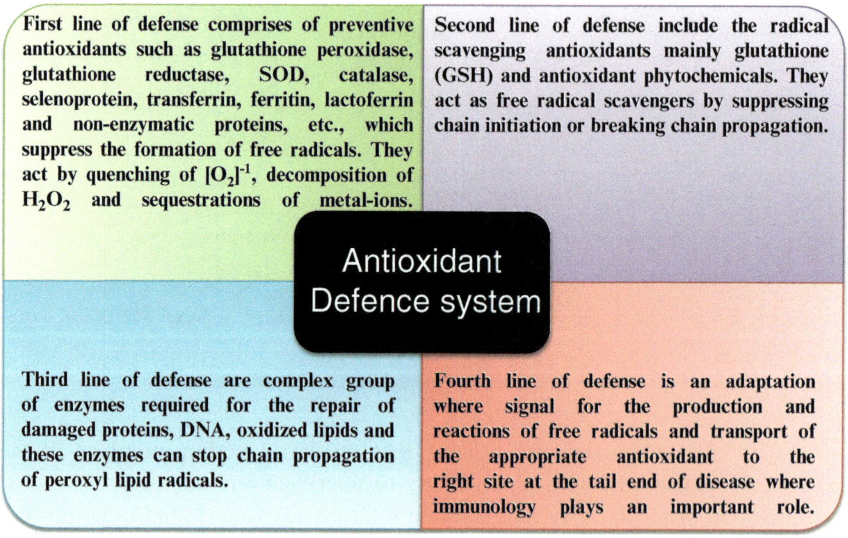

First line of defense comprises of preventive antioxidants such as glutathione peroxidase, glutathione reductase, SOD, catalase, selenoprotein, transferrin, ferritin, lactoferrin and non-enzymatic proteins, etc., which suppress the formation of free radicals. They act by quenching of $[O_2]^{-1}$, decomposition of H_2O_2 and sequestrations of metal-ions.

Second line of defense include the radical scavenging antioxidants mainly glutathione (GSH) and antioxidant phytochemicals. They act as free radical scavengers by suppressing chain initiation or breaking chain propagation.

Antioxidant Defence system

Third line of defense are complex group of enzymes required for the repair of damaged proteins, DNA, oxidized lipids and these enzymes can stop chain propagation of peroxyl lipid radicals.

Fourth line of defense is an adaptation where signal for the production and reactions of free radicals and transport of the appropriate antioxidant to the right site at the tail end of disease where immunology plays an important role.

Fig. 23.3 Various types of antioxidants based on their functions

compounds. Among numerous antioxidants following plant secondary products are of particular interest (Bendich 1996):

- Plant phenolics: phenylpropanoids, coumarines, flavonoids
- Polyphenolic: tannins, proanthocyanidins
- Nitrogen containing compounds: alkaloids, nonproteins amino acids, isocyanate, indoles
- Phytosterols
- Carotenoids
- Chlorophyll derivatives

Polyphenols are the most widely distributed groups of phytochemicals which range from simple phenolics to highly polymerized complex tannins. Their consumption is beneficial to human beings because of their outstanding feature of blocking specific enzymes that cause inflammation. They also modify the prostaglandin pathways and thereby protect platelets from clumping. The flavonoids in particular, act as antioxidant, anti-allergic, anti-inflammatory, immuno-stimulant, anti-hepatotoxic and hypoglycemic along with numerous other actions including stabilizing capillary permeability. Specifically phenols may help in lowering the risk of cancer, cardiovascular diseases, Alzheimer's disease, Parkinson's disease, age related vision disorders, asthma and reduce inflammation (Escarpa and Gonzalez 2001; Nichenametla et al. 2006). Therefore, there is a strong potential in the study of phytochemicals with free radical scavenging capacity and their role in human health care system as nutraceuticals and functional foods (Rowan-Robinson et al. 1997) which are discussed below.

Polyphenols

Polyphenolics are benzene ringed phytochemicals ubiquitous in plants, which function in various protective roles. There is a recent evidence that polyphenolics also have 'indirect' antioxidant effects through induction of endogenous protective enzymes. There is also an increasing evidence for many potential benefits through polyphenolic mediated regulation of cellular processes such as inflammation and cancer. Flavonoids and phenolic acids also have antioxidative and anticarcinogenic effects. Inverse relationships between the intake of flavonoids (flavonols and flavones) and the risk of coronary heart disease and stomach cancer have been shown in epidemiological studies. Many so-called secondary products can act as potent bio-antimutagens. Antimutagen action of green tea extract has been studied, for which epigallocatecin gallate seems to be most responsible (Wang et al. 1989, 1994).

They are the most abundantly occurring polyphenols in plants, of which flavonoids and phenolic acids accounts for about 60% and 30% of total dietary phenols respectively (Escarpa and Gonzalez 2001; Nichenametla et al. 2006). Antioxidant activity and biological properties of polyphenols from berries, red wine, ginkgo, onions, apples, grapes, chamomile, citrus, dandelion, green tea, hawthorn, licorice, rosemary, thyme, fruits, vegetables and beverages have been studied which have been found to be rich source of phenols that can enhance the efficacy of vitamin C, reduce the risk of cancer, act against allergies, ulcers, tumors, platelet aggregation and are also effective in controlling hypertension (Kondratyuk and Pezzuto 2004).

Flavonoids and their relatives are derived biosynthetically from the Shikimate pathway which has been classified into flavones, flavonols, flavanones, flavanols, isoflavones, anthocyanidins and proanthocyanidins. Flavonoids possess ideal structure for free radicals scavenging activity and have been found to be more effective antioxidants *in vitro* than tocopherols and ascorbates (Amić et al. 2003). They are efficient reducing agents that can stabilize the polyphenols derived radicals and delocalise the unpaired electrons. Flavonoids can also generate H_2O_2 by donating a hydrogen atom from their pyrogallol or catechol structure to oxygen, through a superoxide anion radical (Andjelković et al. 2006). The pyrogallol-type compounds generate more H_2O_2 than that of catechol. H_2O_2 has been reported to raise levels of intracellular Ca^{2+}, activate transcription factors, repress expression of certain genes, promote or inhibit cell proliferation, be cytotoxic, activate or suppress certain signal transduction pathways, promote or suppress apoptosis (Rietjens et al. 2002).

Carotenoids

Carotenoids are plant pigments that are present in the human diet as microcomponents of fruits and vegetables. There are more than 700 naturally occurring carotenoids that act as biological antioxidants and protect cells and tissues from the damaging effects of free radicals. Carotenoids are present in many human foodstuffs, of both plant and animal origin, but are majorly found in fruits and vegetables. The major carotenoids are α-carotene, β-carotene, β-cryptoxanthin, lutein and lycopene. Among the carotenes, only alpha, beta and epsilon carotenes possess vitamin A activity and out of them β-carotene is the most active. Natural β-carotene is the precursor of vitamin A and has preventive action against eye diseases and cancer. Lycopene gives tomatoes their red color and is particularly effective at quenching the destructive singlet oxygen. Along with carotene and lutein, it provides protection against lung, breast, uterus and prostate cancers. Limonoids, the second major subclass of terpenoids, are the biologically active phytochemicals present in citrus which act as antioxidant and protect lung tissues from free oxygen radicals. In vitro studies show that limonin, nomilin and limonoid glycosides have significant ability to inhibit proliferation of human breast cancer (Ortuño et al. 2006; Sun et al. 2005).

Epidemiologic studies suggest that dietary intake of carotenoids influences the risk for certain types of cancer, cardiovascular disease and other chronic diseases. Although it would be ideal to use humans directly to answer critical questions regarding carotenoid absorption, metabolism and effects on disease progression, appropriate animal models offer many advantages. Each potential model has strengths and weaknesses (Willcox et al. 2004; Kris-Etherton et al. 2002; Papas 1999). However, mice, rats and ferrets can be used to study cancer, whereas primates and gerbils are probably more appropriate for studies on biomarkers of heart disease (Papas 1999).

Epidemiologic studies indicate that an increased intake of fruits and vegetables that contain carotenoids is associated with a decreased risk of many types of cancer including lung, breast and those affecting the gastrointestinal tract (Kornsteiner et al. 2006), a decreased risk of cardiovascular disease (Park and Pezzuto 2002). Consumption of certain fruits and vegetables has also been associated with a decreased risk of prostate cancer (Lee et al. 2001), and β-carotene supplementation has been shown to enhance natural killer cell activity in elderly men (Lee et al. 2001). In contrast, it has been reported that supplementation of bC either with or without VA to high risk populations may increase the risk of lung cancer (Lutsenko et al. 2002). Many clinical studies indicate a protective effect. Inhibitory effects were reported in two studies using aberrant crypt foci, an intermediate lesion leading to colon cancer, as an end point and in two mammary tumor studies, one using the dimethylbenz(a)anthracene model, and the other the spontaneous mouse model. Inhibitory effects were also reported in mouse lung and rat hepatocarcinoma and bladder cancer models. However, a report from the author's laboratory found no effect in the *N*-nitrosomethylurea-induced mammary tumor model when crystalline lycopene or a lycopene-rich tomato carotenoid oleoresin was administered in the diet. Several retrospective and prospective epidemiological studies indicate that tomato consumption (Lee et al. 2001), lycopene intake (Izzo et al. 2002), and serum lycopene levels are associated with decreased risk of cancers, most notably prostate and lung cancer.

In addition, positive results have been reported in rat aberrant colon crypt formation (Cai et al. 2004) and the rat hepatic preneoplasia model (Ferguson et al. 2004). However, with regard to mammary tumorigenesis, results have proven ambiguous. Kushi et al. (1996) recently showed no association between intake of fruits and vegetables and breast cancer risk.

Vitamin E (Tocopherols and Tocotrienols)

Vitamin E refers to a family of eight molecules having a chromanol ring (chroman ring with an alcoholic hydroxyl group) and a 12-carbon aliphatic side chain containing two methyl groups in the middle and two more methyl groups at the end. Tocopherols and tocotrienols are non-polar constituents of biological membranes that exist in nature in lipid phase. Vitamin E is a natural antioxidant which fights damaging natural substances known as free radicals. Mode of action of Vitamin E is by working in lipids (fats and oils), making it complementary to vitamin C, which finally fights free radicals dissolved in water. As an antioxidant, vitamin E has been widely advocated for preventing heart disease and cancer. α-tocopherol is the most abundant form, with high vitamin E activity and singlet oxygen quenching ability than other forms of tocopherols (Rietjens et al. 2002). The anti-carcinogenic activity of vitamin E is attributed largely to its potent antioxidant activity where the major hydrophobic chain-breaking antioxidant protects membrane lipids from oxidation. Vitamin E has also been reported to interfere with hormone signaling, which is particularly relevant to prostate carcinogenesis. Data from mechanistic studies show that vitamin E acts synergistically with other antioxidant nutrients *in vitro*. For example, vitamin C and various flavonoids have been reported to regenerate α- tocopherol from α-tocopheroxyl radicals, which are formed when the parent molecule reduces free radicals (May 1999; Pedrielli and Skibsted 2002; Zhu et al. 1999). In addition, α-tocopherol has been shown to regulate the expression of several genes involved in growth, apoptosis, and inflammation, including (AP-1), cyclin D1, p53, a-tropomyosin, collagenase, cytokine interleukin-1-b (IL-1b), glycoprotein IIB, and intercellular adhesion molecule 1 (ICAM-1), as well as several antioxidant defense genes (Azzi et al. 2004). Synergy between antioxidants has also been observed in human prostate cancer cell lines, although the resulting effects may not be attributable to their antioxidant activity per se. Some, preclinical, epidemiological, and phase III data from randomized, placebo-controlled clinical trials suggest that both selenium and vitamin E have potential efficacy in prostate cancer prevention. *In vitro* evidence suggests that selenium and vitamin E work synergistically to cause cell-cycle arrest, induce caspase-mediated apoptosis, and act as antiandrogens in arresting clonal expansion of nascent tumors (Klein 2006). A recent study showed that people consuming the highest amounts of vitamin E had the greatest benefit. When they compared persons taking the most vitamin E with those taking the least, there was a 61% reduction in lung cancer risk. (Mahabir et al. 2008). Similarily, another study was done on patients with colon cancer who received a daily dose of 750 mg of vitamin E during a period of 2 weeks which showed that short-term supplementation with high doses of dietary vitamin E lead to increased CD4:CD8 ratios and to enhanced capacity by their T cells to produce the T helper 1 cytokines interleukin 2 and IFN-gamma. Thus, conclusion was drawn that vitamin E may be used to improve the immune functions in patients with advanced cancer (Malmberg et al. 2002). The role of vitamin E in cancer prevention is ambiguous. Some data from observational studies suggest a positive association between consumption of foods high in vitamin E and reduced risk of cancer while in others, supplementation with vitamins E, C, and beta carotene did not prevent cancer incidence in randomized clinical trials (Bjelakovic et al. 2004) nor did it affect cancer mortality (Lin et al. 2009). Similarily, in another study Vitamin E supplementation (VES) was not associated with a reduction in total mortality, cancer incidence, or cancer mortality, but it was associated with a statistically significant reduction in the incidence of prostate cancer. However, it was concluded that Vitamin E can be used in the prevention of prostate cancer in men who are at high risk of prostate cancer (Alkhenizan and Hafez 2007). In human prostate carcinoma cell lines, VES has also been found to inhibit prostate cancer cell invasiveness through reduction of secreted matrix metallo- proteinase 9 (MMP-9) (Jiang et al. 2000). Some studies also reported that common SNPs in genes encoding for proteins are responsible for uptake, transport, and delivery of tocopherols and tocotrienols to the prostate which may impact upon prostate cancer risk but, the theory has not been examined and warrants future research (Margarete and Leitzmann 2005).

Ascorbic Acid

Ascorbic acid (vitamin C) is a powerful natural antioxidant that neutralizes damaging natural substances called free radicals. It has been reported to scavenge ROS and has anticarcinogenic effects (Kim and Lee 2004; Lee et al. 2001). Vitamin C is the single most popular vitamin supplement in the United States. Two-time Nobel Prize winner Dr. Linus Pauling in 1960s claimed that vitamin C could effectively treat both cancer and the common cold. The antioxidant mechanism of ascorbic acid is based on hydrogen atom donation to lipid radicals, quenching of singlet oxygen and removal of molecular oxygen. Oxidation of ascorbic acid is highly influenced by heat, light, water, pH, oxygen concentration and metal ions like Cu^{+2} and Fe^{+3}. It may be related to the prevention of some forms of cancer and heart diseases. Ascorbic acid and tocopherol supplementation can substantially reduce oxidative damage. In light of the favorable initial response to intravenous (IV) vitamin C, ascorbic acid was investigated. Vitamin C is preferentially toxic to tumor cells, that is, it kills tumor cells but not normal cells. In low doses, vitamin C assumes the nature of an antioxidant; in high dosages, vitamin C changes roles and becomes a prooxidant, inducing peroxide production.

Vitamin C usage for cancer treatment is safe compared to standard chemotherapeutics and has an ability to preserve immune function. Many patients die not because of cancer, but rather from a post-chemotherapeutic toxicity, resulting from a damaged and weak immune system. Vitamin C is preferentially toxic to many types of cancer cells, including 20 different melanoma cell lines. Ovarian cell lines are more susceptible to vitamin C-induced toxicity than pancreatic cells while breast cancer appears to be one of the most responsive cancers to IV vitamin C. Concentrations greater than 600 mg/dL are required to kill cancer cells. Vitamin C in combination with lipoic acid acts in a better way for treating cancer.

Lipoic Acid

Some sulphur containing compounds like glutathione (GSH), lipoic acid (1, 2-dithilane-3-pentanoic acid) and dihydrolipoic acid present in meat, liver and heart show antioxidant activities. They prevent oxidative damage of proteins; regenerate GSH in liver, kidney and lung tissues. Lipoic acid occurs in three different forms: R-Lipoic Acid (the R (+) enantiomer) is the pure form found in each and every cell of the body from the simplest organisms up to humans. S-Lipoic acid (The S (-) enantiomer) is a by-product from chemical synthesis and may interfere with some of the beneficial properties of the R-form, especially in interactions with proteins and enzymes. Some group of researchers believe that lipoic acid may inhibit genes that trigger cancer cells to grow, and some recommend it as one component of an alternative anti-cancer regimen or as a complementary therapy to prevent or relieve some side effects of conventional cancer treatments. The antioxidant α-lipoic acid (ALA) has been shown to affect a variety of biological processes associated with oxidative stress including cancer. In recent years, LA has gained considerable attention in the cancer field as an anticancer agent. Results from antiproliferation studies on cancerous cell-based models have suggested that the tumor-suppressive effect of LA corresponds with apoptosis induction, a critical parameter impaired in cancer cells, and this induction is selectively exerted in cancer and transformed cell lines, while being less active toward normal non transformed cells (Pack et al. 2002; Wenzel et al. 2005). A recent study conducted showed that ALA and DHLA can effectively induce apoptosis in human colon cancer cells by a prooxidant mechanism that is initiated by an increased uptake of oxidizable substrates into mitochondria (Wenzel et al. 2005). ALA has been reported to have beneficial effects in patients with advanced cancers by increasing the glutathione peroxidise activity and by reducing oxidative stress (Mantovani et al. 2003). ALA was shown to trigger apoptosis in human cancer cell lines while inducing a reversible cell-cycle arrest but failed to induce apoptosis in non-transformed cell lines. A group of researchers investigated that LA elicited its anti-tumor effects by inducing cell cycle arrest and cell death in human promyelocytic HL-60 cells which was achieved by inhibition of both cell growth and viability in a time- and dose-dependent manner. Disruption of the G1/S and G2/M phases of cell cycle progression accompanied by the induction of apoptosis was also observed following LA treatment (Selvakumar and Hsieh 2008). In human leukemic T cells, LA has been reported to potentiate Fas-mediated apoptosis through redox regulation without affecting peripheral blood monocytes from healthy humans (Sen et al. 1999). Similarily, in experiments using antioxidant response element (ARE) reporter assays, LA has also been shown to induce phase II protective genes which are involved in the prevention of carcinogenesis, in non-cancerous animal- and cell-based studies (Flier et al. 2002; Cao et al. 2003)

A study using a 10:1 ratio of vitamin C to lipoic acid showed a synergistic effect as the mixture killed 50% of all cancer cells at a concentration of only 4.5 mM. The researchers concluded that it would be feasible to obtain this concentration by intravenous infusion and urge further work to investigate the use of a combination of vitamin C and lipoic acid as an anti-cancer agent in humans (Casciari et al. 2001). A recent indicate a novel pro-oxidant role of LA in apoptosis induction and its regulation by Bcl-2, which may be exploited for the treatment of cancer and related apoptosis disorders (Moungjaroen et al. 2006).

Selenium (Se)

Se is a trace mineral found in soil, water, vegetables (garlic, onion, grains, nuts, soybean), sea food, meat, liver, yeast (Willcox et al. 2004). At low dose, Se has many health benefits like that of antioxidant, anti-carcinogenic and immunomodulator (Pham-Huy et al. 2001). The role of Se in cancer prevention has been the subject of recent study and debate. Numerous mechanisms have been explored to explain the modulation of carcinogenesis by selenium (Medina and Morrison 1988; El-Bayoumy 1991). Se has been reported to have a significant anti-cancer effect on breast, lung, liver and small intestinal tumour cells. The best explained function of selenium in mammalian cells is its being a component of the seleno-enzyme, glutathione peroxidase which is localized in the cytosol and mitochondrial matrix, and it eliminates organic peroxides from the cell (Medina and Morrison 1988). However, some other available evidence suggests that the prevention of carcinogenesis by selenium is not related to its function in glutathione peroxidise but because of certain seleno proteins whose impact on carcinogenesis is not defined (Medina and Morrison 1988). There are also some reports that selenium may alter the metabolism of carcinogens or the interaction of chemical carcinogens with DNA (Medina and Morrison 1988). Additional mechanistic studies suggest that selenium may alter cell proliferation and/or immunologic responses (Medina and Morrison 1988; El-Bayoumy 1991). Many researchers have demonstrated that application or intakes of Se at higher levels than required for normal metabolism inhibited carcinogenesis/tumorigenesis (El-Bayoumy 1991; Combs and Gray 1998). A study of 34,000 men found that men with low baseline Se levels were three times more likely to develop advanced prostate cancer than men with high Se levels (Yoshizawa et al. 1998). Another study proved that women who are born with mutations of the *BRCA1* gene had a high risk of breast and ovarian cancer and Se supplementation for 1–3 months reduced chromosome breaks in those women to normal levels (Kowalska et al. 2005). In a study a co-relation was established between smokers, their blood selenium levels and cancer risk as the male smokers in Finland who entered the trial early (when Se levels were quite low) and had blood Se levels in the lowest quarter had a five-fold higher risk of lung cancer than those men in the highest quarter of blood Se level (Hartman et al. 2002). Cancer risk in men has been shown in a number of studies to be more profoundly influenced by Se status than in women. Factors contributing to the apparent difference in the effects of Se on cancer incidence in men and women may include sex-based differences in the metabolism and/or tissue distribution of Se, as well as sex-related factors that influence tumour biology (Waters et al. 2004). Some of the most impressive data suggest that exposure to Se-methylselenocysteine (SeMC), a naturally occurring selenium compound blocks clonal expansion of premalignant lesions at an early stage which is achieved by simultaneously modulating certain molecular pathways that are responsible for inhibiting cell proliferation and enhancing apoptosis (Clement et al. 2000). Unlike selenomethionine, which is incorporated into protein in place of methionine, SeMC is not incorporated into any protein, thereby offering a completely bioavailable compound for preventing cancer.

Results from clinical and cohort studies about cancer prevention, especially lung, colorectal, and prostate cancers are mixed (Higdon et al. 2007). Recently many animal studies have been conducted to evaluate the effects of super nutritional levels of selenium on experimental carcinogenesis using chemical, viral, and transplantable tumor models. Two thirds of these studies conducted showed that high levels of selenium reduced the development of tumors at least moderately (14–35% compared to controls) and, in most cases, significantly (by more than 35%) (Whanger 2004). A group of researchers showed the impact of selenium supplementation on basal cell carcinoma by conducting the study on 1,312 subjects. Within 6–9 months, the group receiving 200 mcg a day of selenium realized about a 67% increase in plasma selenium levels. The non-supplemented group, although judged "normal" in regard to plasma selenium levels, experienced twice the rate of cancer as those receiving selenium. Thus, researchers concluded that higher amounts of dietary selenium than the amount recommended by the FDA are needed to prevent cancer. The overall reduction in cancer incidence was 37% in the selenium-supplemented group; a 50% reduction in cancer mortality was observed over a 10-year period (Clark et al. 1996). It was deduced by a group of workers that as the male population ages selenium levels decrease, paralleling an increase in prostate cancer (Brooks et al. 2001).

There are numerous reports on the usefullness and protective action of selenium as shown by Whanger (1998) who deduced that selenium addition to salt reduced cancer incidence. Similarly, a significant increase in apoptosis and a decrease in DNA synthesis in breast cancers cells (MCF-7 and SKBR-3) occurred with selenium supplementation. The selenium benefit was just as impressive in cancers of the lung (RH2), small intestine (HCF8), colon (Caco-2), and liver (HepG2). Prostate cancers (PC-3 and LNCaP) as well as colon cancer (T-84), although initially less affected by supplementation, became responsive when selenium was coadministered with Adriamycin or Taxol (Vadgama et al. 2000). This study suggested that selenium potentiates the anti-cancer effects of chemotherapy. Selenium supplementation in patients undergoing radiation therapy for rectal cancer improved life quality and simultaneously also reduced the occurence of secondary cancers (Hehr et al. 1997). However, further clinical trials are needed to understand the exact mechanisms whereby selenium prevents cancer.

Sources of Natural Antioxidants

Antioxidants act as radical scavenger, hydrogen donors, electron donor, peroxide decomposer, singlet oxygen quencher, enzyme inhibitor, synergist, and metal-chelating agents (Aruoma 1994). Polyphenols are considered to be the most effective antioxidants, and they can also intensify the activity of other antioxidants. The most popular polyphenols are flavonoids, among which quercetin, kaempferol and apigenin glycosides dominate. Some antioxidants are made in our cells and include enzymes and the small molecules glutathione, uric acid, coenzyme Q-10 and lipoic acid (Halliwell 1996). Other essential antioxidants such as phenolics, vitamin C, E, and selenium must be obtained from our diet. A whole variety of phenolic compounds, in addition to flavonoids, are widely distributed in grains, fruits, vegetables and herbs (Table 23.2). An extensive research on food having

Table 23.2 Polyphenolic content in some natural sources

Class and subclass	Foods or beverages
Flavonoids Anthocyanidins	**Fruits**: blackberries, black currant, blueberries, black grape, elderberries, strawberries, cherries, pomegranate juice, raspberry
	Others: red wine
Anthoxanthins Flavonols	**Vegetables**: capers, celery, chives, onions, red onions, dock leaves, fennel, hot peppers, cherry tomatoes, spinach, lettuce, celery, broccoli
	Cereal: buckwheat, beans (green/yellow)
	Fruits: apples, apricots, grapes, plums, bilberries, blackberries, cherries, black currant juice, apple juice, ginkgo biloba
	Others: red wine, tea (green, black), tea (black beverage), cocoa powder, turnip (green), endive, leek
Flavanones	**Citrus fruits and juices**: lemon, lemon juice, lime juice, orange, tangerine juice
Flavones	**Fruits**: celery, olives
	Vegetables: hot peppers, celery hearts, fresh parsley
Phenolic acids Hydroxycinnamic acids	**Fruits**: blueberry, cranberry, pear, cherry(sweet), apple, orange, grapefruit, cherry juice, apple juice, lemon, peach
	Vegetables: potato, lettuce, spinach
	Others: coffee beans, tea, coffee, cider
Trihydroxystilbenes	**Fruits**: grapes, peanuts
	Others: red wine
Tannins	**Fruits**: grapes, apple juice, strawberries, longan, raspberries, pomegranate, walnuts, peach, blackberry, olive, plum
	Vegetables: chick pea, black-eyed peas, lentils
	Cereal: haricot bean
	Others: wine, cocoa, chocolate, tea, cider, tea, coffee

anticancerous properties is being done to search for an alternative remedy to deal with the cancer. We are what we eat is a very true saying. Therefore, right eating habits are expected to reduce the risk of cancer to a good extent.

Conclusion

Increasing evidences from the recent studies suggests that oxidative stress mediated diseases like cardiovascular diseases and cancer-causing oxidation of the DNA molecule can be counteracted by natural antioxidants such as flavonoids, antioxidative vitamins, antioxidative trace elements, plant phenolic compounds or combinations of these ingredients. Conventional therapies are well known to cause serious side effects. Thus, there is the need to utilise alternative concepts or approaches like usage of natural food for the prevention of cancer. Compelling data suggest that various natural antioxidants contribute to cancer prevention; however, further and detailed molecular cellular mechanism studies in animals and humans will be required to clarify the nature of the impact and interactions between these bioactive constituents and other dietary components. Also, many plant materials and foods have not yet received much attention as sources of antioxidant phenols due to limited popularity or lack of commercial applications which needs to be explored for the promotion of human health.

References

Alkhenizan A, Hafez K (2007) The role of vitamin E in the prevention of cancer: a meta-analysis of randomized controlled trials. Ann Saudi Med 27:409–414

Amić D, Davidović-amić D, Bešlo D, Trinajstić N (2003) Structure-radical scavenging activity relationships of flavonoids. Croat Chemica Acta 76:55–61

Andjelković M, Camp JV, Meulenaer BD, Depaemelaere G, Socaciu C, Verloo M, Verhe R (2006) Iron-chelation properties of phenolic acids bearing catechol and galloyl groups. Food Chem 98:23–31

Aruoma OI (1994) Nutrition and health aspect of free radicals and antioxidants. Food Chem Toxicol 62:671–683

Azzi A, Gysin R, Kempna P (2004) Regulation of gene expression by alpha-tocopherol. Biol Chem 385:585–591

Bahorun T, Luximon-Ramma A, Crozier A, Aruoma O (2004) Total phenol, flavonoid, proanthocyanidin and vitamin C levels and antioxidant activities of Mauritian vegetables. J Sci Food Agric 84:1553–1561

Bandopadhyay D, Biswas K, Bhattacharyya M, Reiter RJ, Banerjee RK (2001) Gastric toxicity and mucosal ulceration induced by oxygen-derived reactive species: protection by melatonin. Curr Mol Med 1:501–513

Bendich A (1996) Antioxidants, vitamins and immune response. In: Litwack G (ed) Vitamins and harmones, vol 52. Elsevier Science, New York, pp 35–62

Bingham M, Gibson G, Gottstein N, Pascual-Teresa SD, Minihane AM, Rimbach G (2003) Gut metabolism and cardio protective effects of dietary isoflavones. Curr Top Nutr Res 1:31–48

Bjelakovic G, Dimitrinka N, Simonetti RG, Gluud C (2004) Antioxidant supplements for prevention of gastrointestinal cancers: a systematic review and meta-analysis. Lancet 364:1219–1228

Brooks JD, Metter EJ, Chan DW, Sokoll LJ, Landis P, Nelson WG, Muller D, Andre R, Carter HB (2001) Plasma selenium level before diagnosis and the risk of prostate cancer development. J Urol 166:2034–2038

Cai Y, Luo Q, Sun M, Corke H (2004) Antioxidant activity and phenolic compounds of 112 traditional medicinal plants associated with anticancer. Life Sci 74:2157–2184

Cao Z, Tsang M, Zhao H, Li Y (2003) Induction of endogenous antioxidants and phase 2 enzymes by alpha-lipoic acid in rat cardiac H_9C_2 cells: protection against oxidative injury. Biochem Biophys Res Commun 310:979–985

Casciari JJ, Riordan NH, Schmidt TL, Meng XL, Jackson JA, Riordan HD (2001) Cytotoxic of ascorbate, lipoic acid and other antioxidants in hollow fiber in vitro tumors. Br J Cancer 84:1544–1550

Clark LC, Combs GF Jr, Turnbull BW, Slate EH, Chalker DK, Chow J, Davis LS, Glover RA, Graham GF, Gross EG, Krongrad A, Lesher JL Jr, Park HK, Sanders BB Jr, Smith CL, Taylor JR (1996) Effects of selenium supplementation for cancer prevention in patients with carcinoma of the skin. A randomized controlled trial. Nutr Prev Cancer Study Group 276:1957–1963

Clement IP, Thompson J, Zhu Z, Ganther HE (2000) *In vitro* and *in vivo* studies of methylseleninic acid: evidence that a monomethylated selenium metabolite is critical for cancer chemoprevention. Cancer Res 60:2882–2886

Combs GF, Gray WP (1998) Chemopreventive agents: selenium. Pharmacol Ther 79:179–192

El-Bayoumy K (1991) The role of selenium in cancer prevention. In: Practice of oncology, 4th edn. Lippincott, Philadelphia, pp 1–15

Escarpa A, Gonzalez MC (2001) An overview of analytical chemistry of phenolic compounds in foods. Crit Rev Anal Chem 31:57–139

Ferguson RL, Philpott M, Karunasinghe N (2004) Dietary cancer and prevention using antimutagens. Toxicology 198:147–159

Flier J, Van Muiswinkel FL, Jongenelen CA, Drukarch B (2002) The neuroprotective antioxidant alpha-lipoic acid induces detoxication enzymes in cultured astroglial cells. Free Radic Res 36:695–699

Genestra M (2007) Oxyl radicals, redox-sensitive signalling cascades and antioxidants. Cell Signal 19:1807–1819

Halliwell B (2007) Biochemistry of oxidative stress. Biochem Soc Trans 35:1147–1150

Halliwell B, Gutteridge JMC (2007) Free radicals in biology and medicine, 4th edn. Clarendon, Oxford

Hartman TJ, Taylor PR, Alfthan G, Fagerstrom R, Virtamo J, Mark SD, Virtanen M, Barrett MJ, Albanes D (2002) Toenail selenium concentration and lung cancer in male smokers (Finland). Cancer Causes Control 13:923–928

Hehr T, Hoffman W, Bamberg M (1997) Role of sodium selenite as an adjuvant in radiotherapy of rectal carcinoma. Med Clin 92:48–49

Hertog MGL, Hollman PCH, Venema DP (1992) Optimization of a quantitative HPLC determination of potentially anticarcinogenic flavonoids in vegetables and fruits. J Agric Food Chem 40:1591–1598

Hertog MGL, Feskens EJM, Hollman PCH, Katan MB, Kromhout D (1993a) Dietary antioxidant flavonoids and risk of coronary heart disease: the Zuthpen elderly study. Lancet 342:1007–1011

Hertog MGL, Hollman PCH, van de Putte B (1993b) Content of potentially anticarcinogenic flavonoids of tea infusions, wines, and fruit juices. J Agric Food Chem 41:1242–1246

Higdon J, Drake VJ, Whanger PD (2007) Selenium. Linus Pauling Institute, Oregon State University, Micronutrient Information Center. http://lpi.oregonstate.edu/infocenter/minerals/selenium/

Izzo FN, Quartacci MF, Sgherri C (2002) Lipoic acid: a unique antioxidant in the detoxification of activated oxygen species. Plant Physiol Biochem 40:463–470

Jiang Q, Elson-Schwab I, Courtemanche C, Ames BN (2000) Gamma- tocopherol and its major metabolite, in contrast to alpha- tocopherol, inhibit cyclooxygenase activity in macrophages and epithelial cells. Proc Natl Acad Sci U S A 97:11494–11499

Kim DO, Lee CY (2004) Comprehensive study on vitamin C equivalent antioxidant capacity (VCEAC) of various polyphenolics in scavenging a free radical and its structural relationship. Crit Rev Food Sci Nutr 44:253–273

Klein E (2006) Selenium and vitamin E cancer prevention trial. Ann NY Acad Sci 1031:234–241

Kondratyuk T, Pezzuto J (2004) Natural product polyphenols of relevance to human health. Pharm Biol 42:46–63

Kornsteiner M, Wagner KH, Elmadfa I (2006) Tocopherols and total phenolics in 10 different nut types. Food Chem 98:381–387

Kowalska E, Narod SA, Huzarski T, Zajaczek S, Huzarska J, Gorski B, Lubinski J (2005) Increased rates of chromosome breakage in BRCA1 carriers are normalized by oral selenium supplementation. Cancer Epidemiol Biomarkers Prev 14:1302–1306

Kris-Etherton P, Hecker K, Bonanome A, Coval S, Binkoski A, Hilpert K (2002) Bioactive compounds in foods: their role in the prevention of cardiovascular disease and cancer. Am J Med 113:71S–78S

Kushi LHRM, Sellers TA, Zheng W, Folsom AR (1996) Intake of vitamins A, C, and E and postmenopausal breast cancer. The Iowa Women's Health Study. Am J Epidemiol 144:165–174

Lee SH, Oe T, Blair IA (2001) Vitamin C induced decomposition of lipid hydroperoxides to endogenous genotoxins. Science 292:2083–2086

Lin J, Cook NR, Albert C, Zaharris E, Gaziano M, Denburgh MV, BuringJE MJE (2009) Vitamins C and E and beta carotene supplementation and cancer risk: a randomized controlled trial. J Natl Cancer Inst 101:14–23

Lutsenko EA, Carcamo JM, Golde DW (2002) Vitamin C prevents DNA mutation induced by oxidative stress. J Biol Chem 277:16895–16899

Mahabir S, Schendel K, Dong YQ, Barrera SL, Spitz MR, Forman MR (2008) Dietary alpha, beta, gamma and delta tocopherols in lung cancer risk. Int J Cancer 123:1173–1180

Malmberg KJ, Lenkei R, Petersson M, Ohlum T, Ichihara F, Glimelius B, Frodin JE, Masucci G, Kiessling R (2002) A short-term dietary supplementation of high doses of vitamin E increases T helper 1 cytokine production in patients with advanced colorectal cancer. Clin Cancer Res 8:1772–1778

Mantovani G, Maccio A, Madeddu C (2003) The impact of different antioxidant agents alone or in combination on reactive oxygen species, antioxidant enzymes and cytokines in a series of advanced cancer patients at different sites: correlation with disease progression. Free Radic Res 37:213–223

May JM (1999) Is ascorbic acid an antioxidant for the plasma membrane? FASEB J 13:995–1006

Medina D, Morrison DG (1988) Current ideas on selenium as a chemopreventive agent. Pathol Immunopathol Res 7:187–189

Moungjaroen J, Nimmannit U, Callery PS, Wang L, Azad N, Lipipun V, Chanvorachote P, Rojanasakul Y (2006) Reactive oxygen species mediate caspase activation and apoptosis induced by lipoic acid in human lung epithelial cancer cells through Bcl-2 downregulation. J Pharmacol Ther 319:1062–1069

Moure A, Jose CM, Franco D, Manuel JD, Sineiro J, Dominguez H, Nunez MJ, Parajo JC (2003) Natural antioxidants from residual sources. Food Chem 72:145–171

Nichenametla SN, Taruscio TG, Barney DL, Exon JH (2006) A review of the effects and mechanism of polyphenolics in cancer. Crit Rev Food Sci Nutr 46:161–183

Ortuño A, Báidez A, Gómez P, Arcas MC, Porras I, García-lidón A, Rìo JAD (2006) *Citrus paradisi* and *Citrus sinensis* flavonoids: their influence in the defence mechanism against *Penicillium digitatum*. Food Chem 98:351–358

Pacher P, Beckman JS, Liaudet L (2007) Nitric oxide and peroxynitrite in health and disease. Physiol Rev 87:315–424

Pack RA, Hardy K, Madigan MC, Hunt NH (2002) Differential effects of the antioxidant alpha-lipoic acid on the proliferation of mitogen-stimulated peripheral blood lymphocytes and leukaemic T cells. Mol Immunol 38:733–745

Papas AM (1999) Antioxidants status, diet, nutrition and health. CRC Press, Boca Raton/London/New York/Washington, DC, pp 189–210

Park EJ, Pezzuto JM (2002) Encyclopedia of pharmaceutical technology, 2nd edn. Marcel Decker, New York, pp 97–113

Pedrielli P, Skibsted LH (2002) Antioxidant synergy and regeneration effect of quercetin, (-) epicatechin, and (+) catechin on alpha tocopherol in homogeneous solutions of peroxidating methyl linoleate. J Agric Food Chem 50:7138–7144

Pham-Huy C, Nguyen P, Marchand V et al (2001) Selenium and tobacco smoke tars: in vitro effects on different immunocompetent cells. Toxicology 164:111–112, Presented in International Congress of Toxicology XI, Brisbane (Australia)

Rietjens IMCM, Boersma MG, de Haan L, Spenkelink B, Awad HM, Cnubben NHP, van Zanden JJ, van der Woude H, Alink GM, Koeman JH (2002) The pro-oxidant chemistry of the natural antioxidants vitamin C, vitamin E, carotenoids and flavonoids. Environ Toxicol Pharmacol 11:321–333

Rowan-Robinson M, Mann R, Oliver S, Efstathiou A (1997) Observations of the Hubble Deep Field with ISO V: spectral energy distributions and star formation history. Mon Not R Assoc Soc 289:490

Sen CK, Sashwati R, Packer L (1999) Fas mediated apoptosis of human Jurkat T-cells: intracellular events and potentiation by redox active alpha lipoic acid. Cell Death Differ 6:481–491

Stahl W, Sies H (1996) Perspectives in biochemistry and biophysics. Lycopene: a biologically important carotenoid in humans? Arch Biochem Biophys 336:1–9

Sun DC, Chen KS, Chen Y, Chen Q (2005) Content and antioxidant capacity of limonin and nomilin in different tissues of citrus fruit of four cultivars during fruit growth and maturation. Food Chem 93:599–605

Vadgama JV, Wu Y, Shen D, Hsia S, Block J (2000) Effect of selenium in combination with adriamycin or taxol on several different cancer cells. Anticancer Res 20:1391–1414

Varma SD, Devamanoharan PS, Morris SM (1995) Prevention of cataracts by nutritional and metabolic antioxidants. Crit Rev Food Sci Nutr 35:111–129

Wang ZY, Cheng SJ, Zhou ZC, Athar M, Khan WA, Bickers DR, Mukhtar H (1989) Antimutagenic activity of green tea polyphenols. Mutat Res/Gen Toxicol 223:273–285

Wang ZY, Huang MT, Lou YR, Xie JG, Reuhl KR, Newmark HL, Ho CT, Yang CS, Conney AH (1994) Inhibitory effects of black tea, green tea, decaffeinated black tea, and decaffeinated green tea on ultraviolet B light-induced skin carcinogenesis in 7,12-dimethylbenz[*a*] anthracene-initiated SKH-1 mice. Cancer Res 54:3428–3435

Waters DJ, Chiang CDM, Morris JS (2004) Making sense of sex and supplements: differences in the anticarcinogenic effects of selenium in men and women. Mutat Res 551:91–107

Wenzel U, Nickel A, Daniel H (2005) Alpha-Lipoic acid induces apoptosis in human colon cancer cells by increasing mitochondrial respiration with a concomitant O^{2-}generation. Apoptosis 10:359–368

Whanger PD (2004) Selenium and its relationship to cancer: an update. Br J Nutr 91:11–28

Willcox JK, Ash SL, Catignani GL (2004) Antioxidants and prevention of chronic disease. Crit Rev Food Sci Nutr 44:275–295

Yoshizawa K, Willett WC, Morris SJ, Stampfer MJ, Spiegelman D, Rimm EB, Giovannucci E (1998) Study of prediagnostic selenium level in toenails and the risk of advanced prostate cancer. J Natl Cancer Inst 90:1219–1224

Zhu QY, Huang Y, Tsang D, Chen ZY (1999) Regeneration of alpha- tocopherol in human low-density lipoprotein by green tea catechin. J Agric Food Chem 47:2020–2050

Chapter 24
Dietary and Non-dietary Phytochemicals in Cancer Control

Dhanir Tailor and Rana P. Singh

Contents

D. Tailor • R.P. Singh
School of Life Sciences, Central University of Gujarat, Sector-30,
Gandhinagar 382030, Gujarat, India

R.P. Singh (✉)
Cancer Biology Laboratory, School of Life Sciences, Jawaharlal Nehru University,
New Delhi, India
e-mail: ranaps@hotmail.com; rana_singh@mail.jnu.ac.in

S. Shankar and R.K. Srivastava (eds.), *Nutrition, Diet and Cancer*,
DOI 10.1007/978-94-007-2923-0_24,

Abstract Cancer is the constantly increasing and a life threatening disease condition that contributes approximately 13% in total death per year throughout the world. Constant efforts are being made to explore the existing therapies as well as to understand the disease processes. However, due to the ineffectiveness or limitation of present therapeutics, a new strategy, cancer chemoprevention has been come up which mainly involves the use of phytochemicals present in regular dietary system or non-dietary plants. Studies with phytochemicals suggest their potency with comparatively low toxicity or more effectiveness than chemically synthesized drugs. Phytochemicals like EGCG, silibinin, IP6, curcumin, genistein, luteolin and resveratrol which are present in normal diet in variable amount have shown cancer anticancer efficacy. Non-dietary phytochemicals like carnosol, 5-deoxykaempferol, rooibos tea, deguelin have also shown their abilities to act as both therapeutic and preventive agents. Their chemopreventive mechanisms have also been shown in many cancer models, however, more studies are needed to for its clear understanding as well as for their clinical significance. Herein, we have discussed the chemopreventive activities and mechanisms of action of selected phytochemicals. Overall, novel phytochemicals with chemopreventive activity are expected to play an important role in cancer control.

Introduction

Thirteen million individuals lost their life around the world in 2008 due to cancer (Jemal et al. 2011). In developed country like United States of America (USA) every year 22% of total deaths occur due to the different types of cancers (Fig. 24.1). According to National Cancer Institute (NCI) "Cancer is a term used for diseases in which abnormal cells divide without control and are able to invade other tissues. Cancer cells can spread to other parts of the body through the blood and lymph systems". It cannot be claimed as a single disease but is a group of diseases and common terminology used for a range of symptoms and complications. There are wide varieties of cancer causing agents like some chemicals and viruses present in food and environment, hormonal and physiological conditions and radiation. Cancer cases are also contributed through hereditary mechanisms. Currently, there is availability of various treatment options; however, each methodology has its own merits and demerits.

Surgery is oldest methodology used for cancer treatment and plays important role in both diagnostics as well as therapeutics. During the course of time, many advancements in procedures and its applications have given chance to surgeons to treat constantly increasing number of cancer patients. The types of surgery can be listed as preventive, diagnostic, staging, curative, debulking, palliative, supportive and restorative. Inspite of advancements in surgical techniques, the success ratio is different for all cancers. According to world cancer report 2008, after surgery followed by radio- or chemotherapy, the 5-year relative survival rate is approximately 85% for breast cancer but in case of lung cancer it is only 14%

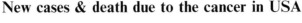

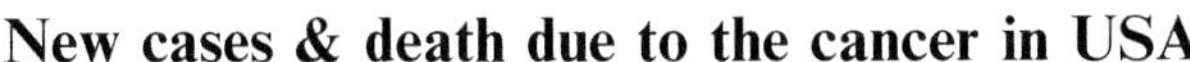

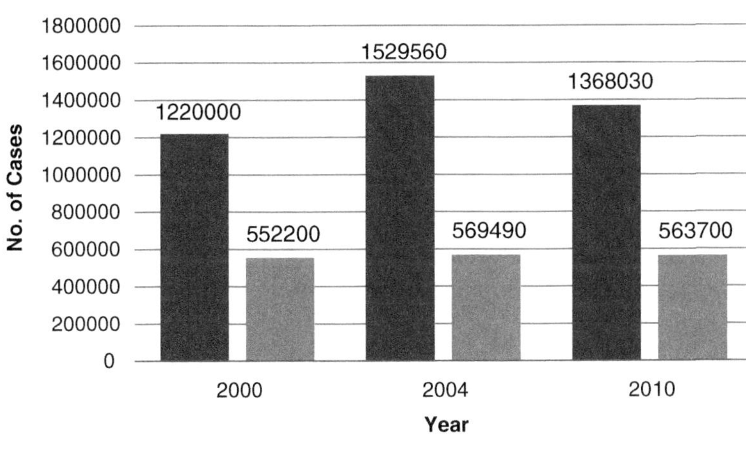

Fig. 24.1 New cases and death due to the cancer in USA. (Data source: Mathews and MacDorman 2007; Miniño et al. 2002)

(Boyle and Levin 2008; Minna and Schiller 2008). The surgical procedures are limited when cancer has reached to the stage of metastasis. This area needs more sophisticated technology at micro to nano level to improve its efficiency and least damage to normal cells.

Cancer drugs market is increasing with 12.3% growth rate in previous decade and is expected to reach 78 billion US$ by 2012 (RNCOS 2008), and in that stream US FDA has approved 129 drugs for the oncology category till 2011. They mainly target different molecules implicated in cancer growth and progression, for example tamoxifen, the famous breast cancer drug, targets to all stages of estrogen-receptor-positive breast cancer, and therefore, World Health Organization (WHO) has put tamoxifen in the list of essential drug for the treatment and control of breast cancer (Jordan 2003). The demerits of various chemotherapies include multiple side effects like immunosuppression, myelosuppression, vomiting, nausea and hair loss (Coates et al. 1983), emotional distress (Love et al. 1989) and motion sickness (Morrow 1985). However, cancer chemotherapies have only ~2.2% success rate in developed countries (Mileshkin et al. 2005). In future, viable applications depend on development of broad range of drugs with less systemic toxicity.

The high-energy radiation is clinically used to kill cancer cells or lead to shrinkage of tumors (Lawrence 2008). Use of either photons or charged particle causing DNA damage can lead to the death of cancer cells. The global market of equipments for cancer radiation therapy is predicted to cross 3.6 billion US$ by 2015 (Jose 2010). This methodology can be classified in two types, the external-beam radiation therapy and internal radiation therapy. These methodologies are applicable to the limited cancerous conditions and show acute and chronic side effects like the damage of salivary glands, hair loss and urinary problems. In rare cases, there are chances to develop second cancer to the individual by radiation exposure. This field requires more attention to make radiation therapy more effective *via* creating drugs like radiosensitizers and radioprotectors to make it more safe and effective.

Immunotherapy or biologic therapy is used to adjust or optimize the host immune system, and to divert or utilize components of the immune system for cancer treatment (Dillman 2011). They induce cancer cells to apoptosis, block growth factor receptors, arrest tumor cells proliferation and anti-idiotype antibody formation. Till date approximately 17 immunological therapeutic agents got approval which are the nonspecific immune stimulants BCG and levamisole, the cytokines interferon-α and interleukin 2, the monoclonal antibodies rituximab (1997, re-approved in 2010), ofatumumab (2009), alemtuzumab (2001), trastuzumab (1998, re-approved in 2010), bevacizumab (2004–2009, revised every year), cetuximab (2004, re-approved in 2006), panitumumab (2006), the radiolabeled antibodies Y-90 ibritumomab tiuxetan (2002), I-131 tositumomab (2003), the immunotoxins denileukin diftitox, gemtuzumab ozogamicin (2000, approval withdrawn in October 2010), non-myeloablative allogeneic transplants with donor lymphocyte infusions and the anti-prostate cancer cell-based therapy sipuleucel-T(2009) (Dillman 2011). Its global market is expected to reach 37.2 billion US$ by 2012 (Immunotherapy of Cancer 2007). Main limitation of immune-based therapy is circumventing immune responses created by the tumor cells (Prins and Liau 2004). Even after 25 years, only 17 drugs are available in the market and thus more extensive research is needed to develop more safe monoclonal antibodies, cancer vaccines and immunotherapeutics.

Other than the therapeutic strategies discussed above, gene therapy, bone marrow transplantation and high-intensity light laser based cancer treatment are presently being employed to treat or control few type of cancers. But still due to the ineffectiveness or long list of limitations of all the post cancer therapies, Sporn and Wattenberg gave the concept of cancer chemoprevention, in which rather to fight against cancer they emphasized to avoid its courses of development and prevent its occurrence (Sporn 1976; Wattenberg 1985). In chemoprevention, the use of non-toxic phytochemicals could be a relevant strategy in the present situation, and has been discussed in detail in the following sections.

Dietary Phytochemicals in Cancer Chemoprevention

Many phytochemicals are used conventionally in the house hold practices for many purposes. In 2009, WHO stated that one third life can be save out of total cancer deaths by changing the dietary habits (Bode 2009). The results from population based studies show that macronutrients and micronutrients from vegetables and fruits have potential to reduce the risk of cancer (Surh 2003). Food items like vegetables, fruits, cereals, beans, and plant-based beverages such as tea and wine are the rich sources of different phytochemicals (Arts 2005). These phytochemicals based

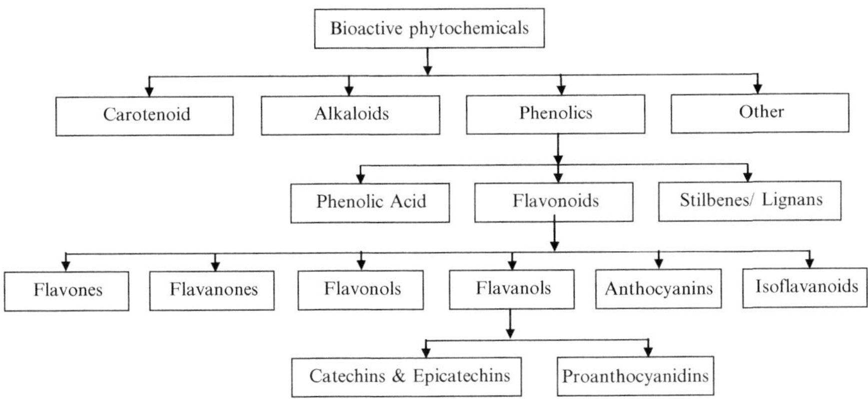

Fig. 24.2 Bioactive phytochemicals having cancer chemopreventive activities. These phytochemicals belong to both dietary as well as non-dietary plants. These phytochemicals are found in various classes of chemicals as shown in the figure

on their structure are divided into four groups: carotenoids, phenolics, alkaloids and others (Fig. 24.2). Phenolics comprise the major group of phytochemicals which have been studied for the chemopreventive properties. The dietary phytochemicals which are extensively investigated for various cancer chemopreventive studies are discussed below.

Epigallocatechin-3-gallate (EGCG)

A tea plant (*Camellia sinensis)* has been used and cultivated in Asia for a long period of time and two-third population consumes it in different forms of beverages. This plant has polyphenolic compounds, (–)-epigallocatechin-3-gallate (EGCG), (–)-epigallocatechin (EGC), (–)-epicatechin-3-gallate (ECG) and (–)-epicatechin (EC) (Khan and Mukhtar 2008). EGCG is degraded in the colon, and its metabolites appear in urine and plasma after ingestion (Schantz et al. 2010). EGCG which is a catechin that shows antioxidant and inhibitory effects in different types of cancer and cancer survival pathways (Dou 2009, Table 1).

Inositol Hexaphosphate (IP6)

IP6 is a naturally available polyphosphorylated carbohydrate (Fig. 24.2), present in many plants like beans, corn, brown rice, wheat bran, sesame seeds, and other high-fiber foods. It is also present in mammalian cells, where it regulates essential cellular functions like cell proliferation, signal transduction, and differentiation (Bacić et al. 2010). IP6 shows its effectiveness as both preventive as well as chemotherapeutic agent for cancer control. Other than its efficacy against cancer, IP6 also shows the beneficial effects against cardiovascular disease, diabetes and kidney stone formation (Eiseman et al. 2011). The effectiveness of IP6 as preventive and therapeutic agents against various cancers has been summarized in Table 24.1, which includes, prostate cancer, colon cancer, skin cancer etc.

Silibinin

Silibinin is a flavonol compound present in the extract of milk thistle plant (*Silybum marianum*) and artichoke (*Cynara scolymus*). Originally, it was isolated from the flavonolignan complex called silymarin, which shows strong antioxidant activity (Singh and Agarwal 2009; Fig. 2). This was being used from the ancient time, and in last three to four decades there are records for its extensive use by the Europeans to treat various liver ailments (Wellington and Jarwis 2001). Silibinin is also known as silybin or silibin in literature, having different isomers, that is silybin A, silybin B, isosilibinin A and isosilibinin B (Davis-Searles et al. 2005). Due to the identification of anticancer activity of silibinin in beginning, now it is being explored for broad spectrum efficacy against various cancers. It targets several biological events including proliferation, inflammation, apoptosis, angiogenesis, and metabolism of cancerous cells (Table 24.1).

Genistein

Genistein (4′,5,7-Trihydroxyisoflavone) is an isoflavone present in number of plants like soybeans, fava beans, lupin, kudzu, psoralea, coffee and many medicinal plants including *Flemingia vestita* (Fig. 24.2). It was first isolated from soybeans by Perkin and Newbury in 1899 (Walter 1941). It is an estrogen-like chemical compound and known as phytoestrogen. Since it mimics the estrogen and have antioxidant activity, it is able to act as anti-cancer agent and is also helpful against some metabolic syndromes (Leclerq and Heuson 1979; Hughes 1998). It inhibits the carcinogenesis *in vitro* as well as *in vivo* and it is under clinical studies for different cancer conditions (Table 24.1). Other than cancer, genistein is also reported to play an important role in prevention of cardiovascular diseases and osteoporosis, and attenuation of post-menopausal problems (Banerjee et al. 2008).

Curcumin

Curcumin in mainly isolated from the roots of *Curcuma longa,* and is a widely used spice and coloring agent in food since the time of Ayurveda (1900 BC) in India and

Table 24.1 Summary of the anticancer efficacy of dietary phytochemicals against various cancers

Phytochemicals, structure, source	Effective against	*In vitro* studies	*In vivo* studies	Clinical studies	References
Epigallocatechingallate (EGCG) ($C_{22}H_{18}O_{11}$)	Prostate cancer	+	TRAMP mice, C57BL/6 mice	In phase II trial	Khan et al. (2009) and Johnson et al. (2010a)
Molar mass:458.37 g mol^{-1}	Skin cancer	+	SKH-1 Mouse	–	Filip et al. (2011)
Major source: tea	Lung cancer	+	NCr nu/nu mice with H1299 xenograft	–	Li et al. (2010a) and Tan et al. (2010)
IUPAC name:	Colon cancer	+	Xenograft model	In phase I trial	Kumar et al. (2007)
[(2*R*,3*R*)-5,7-dihydroxy-2-(3,4,5-trihydroxyphenyl)chroman-3-yl] 3,4,5-trihydroxybenzoate	Breast cancer	+	C3H/OuJ mice	–	Meeran et al. (2011) and Sakata et al. (2011)

(continued)

Table 24.1 (continued)

Phytochemicals, structure, source	Effective against	*In vitro* studies	*In vivo* studies	Clinical studies	References
	Glioblastoma cancer	+	Glioblastoma model with human U87/U251	–	Chen et al. (2011c)
Soluble in water	Hepatic cancer	+	Hepatoma growth in a xenograft mouse model	–	Liang et al. (2010)
	Ovarian cancer	+	–	–	Huh et al. (2004) and Yan et al. (2011)
	Urinary bladder cancer	+	–	–	Coyle et al. (2008)
	Leukemia	+	Xenograft model	In phase I trial	Shanafelt et al. (2009)
	Cervical cancer	+	–	–	Noguchi et al. (2006) and Tudoran et al. (2011)
	Kidney cancer	+	–	–	Gu et al. (2009a)
	Laryngeal cancer	+	–	–	Lee et al. (2010c)
	Osteosarcoma cancer	+	–	–	Ji et al. (2006)
	Oral cancer	+	SCC-9 xenograft in nude mice, C3H/HeJ syngeneic mice	–	Chen et al. (2011a, b, c) and Koh et al. (2011)
	Gastric cancer	+	–	–	Zhu et al. (2007, 2011)
	Anaplastic thyroid carcinoma	+	–	–	Lim and Cha (2011)
Inositol hexaphosphate	Prostate cancer	+	Athymic (nu/nu) male nude mice with PC-3 xenograft	–	Singh and Agarwal (2005), Gu et al. (2009a, b), and Roy et al. (2009)

(IP6) $(C_6H_{18}O_{24}P_6)$ Molar mass: 660.04 g mol^{-1}	Skin cancer	+	SKH1 hairless mice	–	Kolappaswamy et al. (2009)
Major source: nuts, Legumes	Colon cancer	+	Male Sprague-Dawley rats	–	Weglarz et al. (2006) and Norazalina et al. (2010)
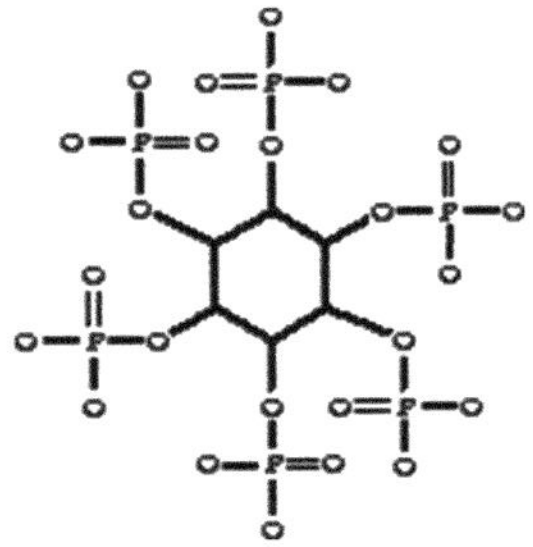 IUPAC name: (1*r*,2*R*,3*S*,4*s*,5*R*,6*S*)-cyclohexane-1,2,3,4,5,6-hexayl hexakis[dihydrogen (phosphate)]					
Miscible in water	Breast cancer	+	C.B17 SCID mice and MDA-MB-231 xenograft	–	Eiseman et al. (2011)

(continued)

Table 24.1 (continued)

Phytochemicals, structure, source	Effective against	*In vitro* studies	*In vivo* studies	Clinical studies	References
	Glioblastoma cancer	+	–	–	Karmakar et al. (2007)
	Hepatic cancer	+	Nude mice with HepG2 xenograft	–	Vucenik et al. (1998a, b)
	Leukemia	+	–	–	Deliliers et al. (2002)
	Laryngeal cancer	+	–	–	Dorsey et al. (2005)
	Oral cancer	+	–	–	Janus et al. (2007)
	Gastric cancer	+	–	–	Wang et al. (2010)
Silibinin ($C_{25}H_{22}O_{10}$) Molar mass:482.44 g mol^{-1}	Prostate cancer	+	Xenografts and TRAMP mice model	In phase II trial	Flaig et al. (2007), Raina et al. (2009), and Flaig et al. (2010)
Major source: milk thistle plant	Skin cancer	+	Chemical- and UVB-induced skin carcino-genesis models	–	Gu et al. (2005, 2007)

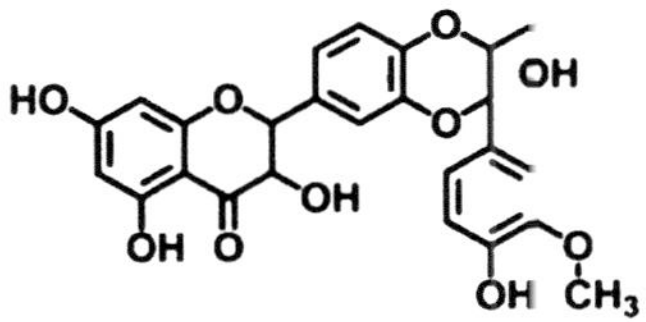 IUPAC name: (2*R*,3*R*)-3,5,7-trihydroxy-2-[(2*R*,3*R*)-3-(4-hydroxy-3-methoxyphenyl)-2-(hydroxymethyl)-2,3-dihydrobenzo[*b*][1,4]dioxin-6-yl]chroman-4-one	Lung cancer	+	Xenografts and urethane-induced lung carcinogenesis model	–	Mateen et al. (2010)
	Colon cancer	+	Xenografts, AOM-induced colon carcinogenesis model, Apc^{min} transgenic mice model	In phase I trial	Hoh et al. (2006) and Rajamanickam et al. (2010)
Poorly water soluble	Breast cancer	+	HER-2/neu and C3(1) SV40 T, t antigen transgenic mouse model	–	Verschoyle et al. (2008) and Tiwari et al. (2011)
	Glioblastoma cancer	+	Xenograft model	–	Kim et al. (2009a) and Momeny et al. (2010)

(continued)

Table 24.1 (continued)

Phytochemicals, structure, source	Effective against	*In vitro* studies	*In vivo* studies	Clinical studies	References
	Hepatic cancer	+	Xenograft model	–	Cui et al. (2009)
	Ovarian cancer	+	Xenograft model	–	Zhou et al. (2008)
	Urinary bladder cancer	+	Nitrosamine-induced urinary bladder carcinogenesis	–	Singh et al. (2008)
	Leukemia	+	–	–	Zhang et al. (2010b)
	Cervical cancer	+	–	–	García-Maceira and Mateo (2009)
	Kidney cancer	+	Xenograft model	–	Cheung et al. (2007)
	Laryngeal cancer	+	–	–	Bang et al. (2008)
	Osteosarcoma cancer	+	–	–	Hsieh et al. (2007)
	Oral cancer	+	–	–	Chen et al. (2006)
	Gastric cancer	+	–	–	Kim et al. (2009b)
Genistein ($C_{15}H_{10}O_5$) Molar mass: 270.24 g mol^{-1}	Prostate cancer	+	Xenograft model	In phase II trial	Lazarevic et al. (2011) and Nakamura et al. (2011)
Major source: soya bean	Skin cancer	+	Hairless mouse model	–	Lee et al. (2011)

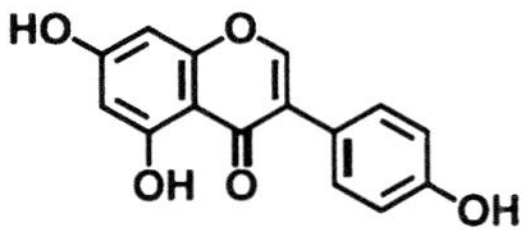 IUPAC name:	Lung cancer	+	–	–	Han et al. (2010)
	Colon cancer	+	–	–	Qi et al. (2011)
5,7-Dihydroxy-3-(4-hydroxyphenyl)chromen-4-one	Breast cancer	+	MCF-7 xenograft athymic mice	Plasma Level study	Verheus et al. (2007)
Insoluble in water	Glioblastoma cancer	+	–	–	Das et al. (2010)
	Hepatic cancer	+	Swiss Webster mice	–	Froyen et al. (2009)
	Ovarian cancer	+	–	–	Ouyang et al. (2009)
	Urinary bladder cancer	+	–	–	Wu et al. (2007b)
	Leukemia cancer	+	–	–	Yamasaki et al. (2010)
	Cervical cancer	+	–	–	Xiao et al. (2011)
	Osteosarcoma cancer	+	–	–	Zhang et al. (2010a)
	Oral cancer	+	–	–	Park et al. (2010)
	Gastric cancer	+	–	–	Ko et al. (2010)
Curcumin	Prostate cancer	+	PC3/DU145 xenograft mice	–	Weng and Yen (2011)

(continued)

Table 24.1 (continued)

Phytochemicals, structure, source	Effective against	*In vitro* studies	*In vivo* studies	Clinical studies	References
($C_{21}H_{20}O_6$) Molar mass: 368.38 g mol^{-1} Major source: turmeric	Skin cancer	+	SCID xenograft mice	–	Phillips et al. (2011)
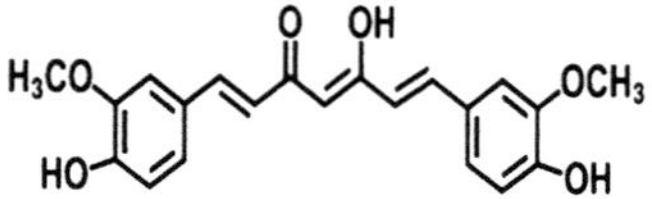	Lung cancer	+	CBO140C12 mice	–	Weng and Yen (2011)
IUPAC name: (1*E*,6*E*)-1,7-bis (4-hydroxy-3-methoxyphenyl) -1,6-heptadiene-3,5-dione	Colon cancer	+	Xenograft model	In Phase II trial	Carroll et al. (2011)
	Breast cancer	+	MDA-MB-435 xenograft mice		Weng and Yen (2011)
Insoluble in water	Glioblastoma cancer	+	–	–	Senft et al. 2010
	Hepatic cancer	+	–	–	Weng and Yen (2011)
	Ovarian cancer	+	–	–	Saunders et al. (2010)
	Urinary bladder cancer	+	C57BL/6 mice	–	Leite et al. (2009)
	Leukemia	+	–	–	Rao et al. 2011

	Cervical cancer	+	Xenograft model of human cervical cancer	–	Sreekanth et al. (2011)
	Laryngeal cancer	+	–	–	Mitra et al. (2006)
	Osteosarcoma cancer	+	–	–	Fossey et al. (2011)
	Oral cancer	+	–	–	Weng and Yen (2011)
	Gastric cancer	+	–	–	Weng and Yen (2011)
Luteolin ($C_{15}H_{10}O_6$) Molar mass: 286.24 g mol^{-1}	Prostate cancer	+	Xenograft in nude mice	–	Tsai et al. (2009) and Markaverich et al. (2010)
Major source: plant leaves 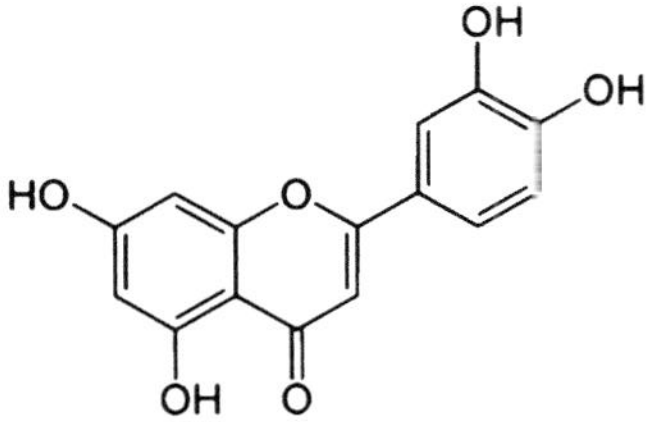	Skin cancer	+	–	–	Seelinger et al. (2008)
IUPAC name: 2-(3,4-Dihydroxyphenyl)-5,7-dihydroxy-4-chromenone	Lung cancer	+	Xenograft in athymic mice	–	Attoub et al. (2011) and Cai et al. (2011)
	Colon cancer	+	LNM35 tumor xenograft in athymic mice	–	Attoub et al. (2011)

(continued)

Table 24.1 (continued)

Phytochemicals, structure, source	Effective against	*In vitro* studies	*In vivo* studies	Clinical studies	References
Poorly water soluble	Breast cancer	+	–	–	Markaverich et al. (2011)
	Glioblastoma cancer	+	–	–	Lin et al. (2010)
	Hepatic cancer	+	–	–	Loa et al. (2009)
	Ovarian cancer	+	–	–	Wang et al. (2009)
	Leukemia	+	–	–	Cheng et al. (2005)
	Cervical cancer	+	–	–	Horinaka et al. (2005)
	Oral cancer	+	–	–	Yang et al. (2008)
	Gastric cancer	+	–	–	Zhang et al. (2009)
Resveratrol ($C_{14}H_{12}O_3$)	Prostate cancer	+	Xenograft model	–	Ganapathy et al. (2010)
	Skin cancer	+	SKH-1 mice, female CD-1 mice, SENCAR mice	–	Kowalczyk et al. (2010)
Molar mass: 228.24 g mol^{-1} Major source: wine					

IUPAC name: (*E*)-5-(*p*-Hydroxystyryl)resorcinol (*E*)-5-(4-hydroxystyryl)benzene-1,3-diol	Lung cancer	+	A/J mice, HER-2/neu transgenic mice	–	Berge et al. (2004) and Provinciali et al. (2005)
	Colon cancer	+	SCID mice	In phase I trial	Nguyen et al. (2009) and Paul et al. (2010)
Poorly water soluble	Breast cancer	+	Xenograft in female athymic nude mice	–	Fukui et al. (2010)
	Glioblastoma cancer	+	–	–	Castino et al. (2011)
	Hepatic cancer	+	C57BL/6 J mice		Salado et al. (2011)
	Ovarian cancer	+	Xenograft in nude mice	–	Guo et al. (2010)
	Urinary bladder cancer	+	Xenograft model	–	Bai et al. (2010)
	Leukemia	+	Xenograft in Kasumi-1-bearing mice	–	Kartal et al. 2011 and Li et al. (2010a, b)
	Cervical cancer	+	–	–	Hsu et al. (2009)
	Laryngeal cancer	+	–	–	Li et al. (2007)
	Osteosarcoma cancer	+	–	–	Rusin et al. (2009)
	Oral cancer	+	–	–	Cardile et al. (2007)
	Gastric cancer	+	–	–	Mitruţ et al. (2009)

Asian sub-continent. It shows abundant therapeutic actions performed by turmeric to diseases of skin, pulmonary, liver, gastrointestinal systems, and against aches, pains, wounds and sprains (Aggarwal et al. 2007). Curcumin (diferuloylmethane) is a polyphenolic compound present in *Curcuma longa* and mainly responsible for the yellow pigment in turmeric (Fig. 24.2). It shows anti-inflammatory, antioxidant, antifungal, antibacterial, antiviral, and anticancer activities. Large number of reports (*in vitro*, *in vivo* and clinical) has shown the potential of curcumin as an antimetastatic and anti-invasive on different cancer types (Table 24.1).

Luteolin

Luteolin (3′,4′,5,7-tetrahydroxyflavone) is a flavone compound which is common in many edible plants (Fig. 24.2). This is widely distributed throughout plant kingdom including many plant families like Bryophyta, Pteridophyta, Pinophyta and Magnoliophyta. Its dietary sources are peppers, carrots, celery, peppermint, olive oil, thyme, rosemary and oregano (López-Lázaro 2009). It is quite heat stable and its loss due to cooking is reported to be less (Marchand 2002). Plants extract which have luteolin are commonly used as traditional medicine in China for treating diseases such as hypertension, inflammatory disorders as well as cancer (Lin et al. 2008; Table 24.1).

Resveratrol

Resveratrol (3,4′,5-trihydroxy-*trans*-stilbene) belongs to the group of stilbenes/lignans, which are dietary polyphenol compounds found in the plant products like grapes, berries and peanuts (Fig. 24.2). Resveratrol is produced by the enzyme stilbene synthase in environmental stress condition (Athar et al. 2009). It had been traditionally used as an antiviral, antiinflammatory, antioxidative, anticoagulant and anticancer agent (Pace-Asciak et al. 1996). In 1997, it was recognized to have anticancer activity, by blocking initiation, promotion, and progression of cancer (Jang et al. 1997). Studies show the potential of resveratrol as cancer chemopreventive agent in various cellular as well as animal and human studies (Table 24.1).

Other than above phytochemicals, several other phytochemicals have also shown the potential as a chemopreventive agent like procyanidin B3 (Veluri et al. 2006), cyanidin from anthocyanins (Cvorovic et al. 2010), many alkaloids such as camptothecin (Botella et al. 2011), vincristine (Souza et al. 2011) and vinblastine (Jakacki et al. 2011), and carotenoids such as lutein (Reynoso-Camacho et al. 2011). This long list of phytochemicals indicates the richness of nature for therapeutic and preventive agents for various ailments including cancer.

Mechanisms of Cancer Chemopreventive Effects of Phytochemicals

Mainly three steps are involved in cancer development and its progression, that can be summarized as first DNA damage due to carcinogenic agent or genetic inheritance; second accumulation of DNA damage by escaping regulation, and the last one includes the progression and survival which lead to uncontrolled growth of the abnormal cells, and to survive by invasion, metastasis, and angiogenesis (Ramos 2008). The control strategies developed by the cell includes cell cycle arrest, apoptosis induction, inhibition of proliferation and inflammation, inhibition of angiogenesis and metastasis, epigenetic regulation, and regulation of biochemical pathways. These regulatory mechanisms can be modulated by phytochemicals to reduce the risk of cancer. Here some of the dietary phytochemicals which help in regulation and control of cancer growth and development are discussed.

EGCG Inhibits Cancer Cell Proliferation and Survival

EGCG has been studied extensively for its anticancer potential. It is shown to affect gene expression, growth factor-mediated pathways including the mitogen activated protein kinase (MAPK)-dependent pathway, multiple cytokine-mediated pathways and the ubiquitin/proteasome degradation pathway in cancer cells (Chen et al. 2011a). EGCG induces the expression of Cip1/p21 and Kip1/p27 (cyclin-dependent kinase inhibitors, CDKI), inhibits the activity of CDK2 and CDK4 leading to Rb hypophosphorylation. In prostate cancer cells, EGCG increases the expression of p16, p18, p21, and p53, which are associated with negative regulation of cell cycle progression. EGCG induces apoptosis and cell cycle arrest at the concentration of 40–80 μM within 24–72 h by releasing cytochrome c in cytosol, apoptotic protease-activating factor 1 (Apaf-1), endonuclease G, apoptosis-inducing factor and activation of pro-caspase-3, -8, -9 (Green 2000). EGCG is observed to regulate apoptosis related mitochondrial proteins (Siddiqui et al. 2011), decrease the level of nuclear factor kappa B (NF-κB) by decreasing level of p65 and/or p50 subunits, through activation of inhibitor of κB (IκB) and inactivation of IκB kinase (IKK) in different types of cancer (Ramos 2008; Sen et al. 2006). EGCG targets 5′-AMP-activated protein kinase (AMPK) pathway (Hwang et al. 2005), and androgen and estrogen receptors (Shenouda et al. 2004) for inhibition. EGCG is a competitive inhibitor of ATP for phosphoinositide-3-kinase (PI3K) and mammalian target of rapamycin (mTOR). It strongly binds to active site of PI3K kinase domain and inhibits the phosphorylation of Akt at Ser473 in MDA-MB-231 and A549 cells (Aller et al. 2011). A study with NMR spectroscopy showed the direct binding of tea polyphenols to the BH3 pocket of anti-apoptotic Bcl-2 family proteins, suggesting a mechanism for EGCG to inhibit the anti-apoptotic function of Bcl-2 proteins, and thus BH3 domain has been recognized as one of the binding sites of tea polyphenols (Leone et al. 2003). Orally administered EGCG inhibits the activity of matrix metalloproteinase (MMP)-2 and MMP-9 in transgenic adenocarcinoma of the mouse prostate (TRAMP) model, also inhibits the invasion and migration of human oral cancer cells through decrease in level of MMP-2, MMP-9, and urokinase type plasminogen activator (uPA) productions (Khan and Mukhtar 2008). EGCG inhibits the epidermal growth factor receptor (EGFR) mediated pathways by binding to a 67-kDa laminin metastasis associated receptor, and also suppresses the gene expression of EGFR *in vitro* as well as *in vivo* condition which is mediated by reduction of trans activation of Egr-1 activity (Khan and Mukhtar 2008). EGCG also inhibits EGF-dependent activation of EGFR, ERK1/2 and Akt activity in cancer cells (Sah et al. 2004).

IP6 Inhibits Cancer Cell Proliferation and Cell Cycle Progression

A prominent action of IP6 as anticancer agents has been confirmed in different experimental models and conditions. It is shown to reduce cell proliferation, enhance immunity, antioxidant properties and help in tumor cell destruction. Administration of IP6 externally leads to its rapid absorption by cells which further dephosphorylated into lower inositol phosphates and affects signal transduction pathways for cell cycle arrest (Vucenik and Shamsuddin 2006). IP6 shows dose-dependent increase in levels of Kip1/p27 and Cip1/p21 but independent to p53, and induces G1 arrest in prostate cancer cells. It increases the hypophosphorylation of Rb/p110, Rb/p107 and Rb2/p130, leading to the increased interaction of pRb/p107 and pRb2/p130 with E2F4, and a decrease in the level of transcriptionally active free E2Fs leading to growth inhibition of prostate cancer cells *via* G1 arrest (Singh et al. 2003). IP6 increases the ratio of Bax:Bcl-2 in LNCaP cells, which is associated with increased apoptosis (Singh and Agarwal 2006a). IP6 restricts to endocytosis of activated EGFR by inhibiting its binding to AP-2, and it also inhibits the down-stream phosphorylation of Shc. Further, it has been also observed to strongly inhibit TGF-induced activation of ERK1/2 and AP-1, and activation of PI3K-Akt pathway in prostate cancer cells (Singh and Agarwal 2005).

Silibinin Inhibits Various Attributes of Cancer Growth and Progression

Several reports have shown cancer chemopreventive efficacy of silibinin in both *in vivo* and *in vitro* models. Silibinin modulates difference between cell survival and apoptosis by interfering with the expressions of cell cycle regulators and proteins involved in apoptosis. It shows anti-inflammatory and anti-metastatic activity in many experimental models. In addition studies at cellular and tissue levels suggest that it can be applicable for clinical application in different cancers and prevent toxicity induced through chemotherapy and radiotherapy (Ramasamy and Agarwal 2008; Table 24.2). Silibinin induces G1 arrest by inhibiting kinase activity of CDK4, CDK6, and CDK2 through increase in protein expression of Cip1/p21 and Kip1/p27. It also decreases the expression of Cdc2 and cyclin B1 and associated kinase activity leading to a G2–M arrest in prostate cancer cells (Singh and Agarwal 2006a). Silibinin enhanced Chk2 phosphorylation at Thr68/Ser19 site, which was responsible for Cdc25C phosphorylation which has been confirmed by the use of Chk2 siRNA. It also hypophosphorylated Rb/p110 and decreased Rb/p110 phosphorylation at Ser780, Ser795, Ser807/811 and Ser249/Thr252 sites in androgen-dependent prostate cancer cells. Silibinin strongly decreases the levels of E2F1, E2F2, E2F3, E2F4 and E2F5 (Agarwal et al. 2004; Singh and Agarwal 2006a). Silibinin inhibits IKKα kinase activity accompanied by an inhibition in IkBα phosphorylation and NF-κB transcriptional activity in androgen-independent cells (Dhanalakshmi et al. 2002). Silibinin also showed a decrease in nuclear translocation of p65 and p50 with a concomitant increase in their cytoplasmic levels, and increases TNFα-induced apoptosis human prostate cancer cells. Silibinin caused phosphorylation of ATM(Ser1981) which lead cell-cycle arrest and apoptosis *via* Chk2 activation in keratinocytes. Silibinin decreases survivin protein expression concomitant with an increase in caspase activity and causes apoptosis in many types of cancer cells. It also inhibits mitogenic signaling and decreases expression of VEGF and COX-2 and/or iNOS expression (Singh and Agarwal 2006a). By using 100 μM of silibinin, it is shown to inhibit invasion and motility in SCC-4 tongue cancer in A459 lung cancer cells. It involves down-regulation of MMP-2 and uPA through inhibition of ERK1/2 and Akt phosphorylation and an increase in tissue inhibitor of metalloproteinase-2 (TIMP-2) and PAI-1 expressions (Chen et al. 2006). Silibinin also inhibits the PMA-induced invasion of MCF-7 cells by decreasing AP-1-dependent MMP-9 gene expression. At present, it has entered to phase II clinical trials for human prostate cancer patients (Deep and Agarwal 2010).

Genistein Inhibits Various Signaling Pathways in Cancer Cells

Genistein is shown to modulate the expression of many genes which are related with the control of cell cycle and apoptosis. It shows the inhibitory effect on activation of NF-κB and Akt signaling pathways which is known to maintain a homeostatic balance between cell survival and apoptosis. It is reported to act on estrogen and androgen-mediated signaling pathways of carcinogenesis. In addition, it has strong antioxidant properties, and potential to inhibit angiogenesis and metastasis (Banerjee et al. 2008; Table 24.2). It blocks cell cycle in cancer cells by down-regulation of cyclin B leading to G2-M arrest. It up-regulates Cip1/p21 expression

Table 24.2 Molecular mechanisms of dietary phytochemicals for cancer chemoprevention

Phytochemicals	Cell cycle arrest	Apoptosis induction	Proliferation and inflammation inhibition	Inhibition of angiogenesis and metastasis	Genetic and epigenetic expression	References
EGCG	↓CDK6; ↓PCNA; ↑p16; ↑p18; ↑p21; ↑p27; ↑pRb; ↑p53; ↓Cyclin E; ↓CDK1; ↓CDK2; ↓CDK4; ↓Cyclin D	↑ROS; ↑Caspase-3; ↑Caspase-8; ↑Caspase-9; ↑Cytochrome c; ↑Smac/DIABLO; ↑↓ Bax; ↑Bak; ↑Cleaved PPAR; ↑↓ Bcl-2; ↓Bcl-xL; ↓Bid; ↓c-myc; ↓c-IAP2; ↓Mcl-1; ↓Survivin; ↓XIAP	↓PI3K; ↓↑AKT; ↑↓ERK; ↓p90RSK; ↓FKHR; ↓PDGF; ↓PDGFRβ; ↓EGFR; ↓↑c-fos; ↓egr-1; ↓AP-1; ↓NF-κB; ↓IKK; ↓COX-2; ↑JNK; ↑Ras; ↑MEKK1; ↑MEK3; ↑↓ p38; ↑IκB; ↑AMPK; ↑PGE2; ↑TNF-α	↓HIF-1a; ↓VEGF; ↓VEGFR1; ↓VEGFR2, ↓MMP-2; ↓MMP-9; ↓FAK; ↓ProMMP-2; ↓MRLC; ↓Vimentin; ↓Laminin; ↓Integrina2b1; ↓uPA; ↓HuR; ↑proMMP-7	↑Methylation of ESR1; ↑Methylation of p16(INK)[4] ; ↑Methylation of p15(INK)[4] ; ↓hTERT transcription	Ramos (2008), Berner et al. (2010), and Meeran et al. (2011)
Curcumin	↓Cyclin A; ↓CDK1; ↑p21; ↑Cdc2	↑Caspase-3; ↑Caspase-7; ↑Caspase-8; ↑Caspase-9; ↑AIF; ↑Cleaved PPAR; ↓m; ↓Bcl-xL	↓AKT; ↓mTOR; ↓p70S6K1; ↓4E-BP-1; ↓IGF-I; ↓NF-κB; ↓IKK; ↓IκB; ↓COX-2; ↓PGE2	↓MMP-1; ↓MMP-2	–	Ramos (2008)
Genistein	↓Cyclin B1; ↓Cdc25C; ↓Cdc2;↑p21; ↓PCNA ; ↑p53; ↓Cyclin E; ↓CDK2; ↑pRb	↑Caspase-9; ↑Caspase-3; ↑Caspase-7; ↓c-IAP1; ↑↓ Bcl-2	↓AKT; ↓ERK; ↓NF-κB; ↓AP-1; ↓COX-2; ↓PGE2; ↑p38	↓VEGF; ↓FGF; ↓uPA; ↓uPAR; ↑PAI	↑p21(WAF1/CIP1); ↑p16(INK)[4a]; ↓hTERT transcription; ↑BRAC1; ↑RARb; ↑MGMT	Ramos (2008), Yu et al. (2008), Meeran et al. (2010), Li et al. (2011), and Seo et al. (2011)

IP6	↑p21; ↑p27; ↑p53; ↓CDK4; ↓Cyclin D; ↑pRb; ↓PCNA	↓Bcl-2; ↑Caspase-3; ↑Bax	↓NF-κB; ↓IGF-I	↓VEGF; ↓bFGF	–	Agarwal et al. (2004), Singh and Agarwal (2006a), and Tian and Song (2006)
Silibinin	↓Cyclin E; ↓Cyclin D; ↓CDK2; ↓CDK4; ↑p21; ↑p27; ↓CDK2; ↓CDK6; ↓Cyclin E; ↑p53; ↓PCNA	↑Bax; ↓PARP; ↑Caspase-9; ↑Caspase-3; ↑Caspase-2	↓ NF-κB; ↓TNF-α; ↓JNK; ↓PI3K; ↓COX-2	↓VEGF; ↓MMP-2; ↓MMP-9; ↓CD34	–	Ramasamy and Agarwal (2008), Ramos (2008), and Vaid and Katiyar (2010)
Luteolin	↑p21; ↑p27; ↑p53; ↓CDK2	↑Bax; ↑DR5; ↑Fas; ↑Caspase-2; ↑Caspase-3; ↑Caspase-9; ↓Bcl-xL; ↓XIAP	↓PI3K; ↓AKT; ↓NF-κB; ↑JNK	↓VEGF;↓VEGFR1; ↓MMP-9; ↓MMP-1; ↓TNF-α; ↓ERK	–	Lin et al. (2008) and Cai et al. (2011)
Resveratrol	↑p21; ↑p27; ↑pRb; ↑p27; ↓Cyclin B; ↓Cyclin D; ↓Cyclin E; ↓CDK4	↑Caspase-3; ↑Caspase-8; ↑Caspase-9; ↑Cytochrome c; ↓Smac/DIABLO; ↑Bax; ↓Bcl-2; ↓Mcl-1; ↓Survivin	↓PI3K; ↓AKT; ↓ERK; ↓COX-1; ↓COX-2; ↓NF-κB; ↑AMPK; ↑JNK	↓HIF-1a; ↓VEGF; ↓MMP-2; ↓MMP-9; ↓ERK	–	Athar et al. (2009) and Bishayee (2009)

The arrow indicates an increase (↑) or decrease (↓) in the levels of protein expression/activation, genetic and epigenetic expression in a dose-dependent manner in breast cancer cells, such as MDA-MB-231, MDA-MB-435 and MCF-7 cancer cells. Genistein induces apoptosis in cancer cells *via* activation of caspase-3 and down-regulation of Bcl-2, Bcl-xL, and HER-2/neu (Li et al. 1999; Sakla et al. 2007). It inhibits IκB phosphorylation and NF-κB translocation to the nucleus, which does not allow binding of NF-κB to target DNA and inhibit the NF-κB-dependent transcription of downstream genes. Genistein induced apoptosis is also shown to involve proteosome inhibition and induction of KIP1/p27, IκBα, and Bax. In hepatocellular carcinoma, it induces apoptosis by endoplasmic reticulum (ER) stress-relevant regulators activation like GADD153 transcription factor, *m*-calpain, GRP78 and caspase-12. In human prostate epithelial cells, genistein inhibits the activation of p38MAP kinase and MMP-2, and cell invasion mediated by TGF-β, and also prevents cytokine-induced ERK1/2 activation and promotes apoptotic cell death. It is also reported to inhibit insulin-like growth factor-1 receptor (IGF-1R) signaling leading to inhibition of cell proliferation and induction of apoptosis. It is reported to enhance radiotherapy index in prostate cancer through the down-regulation of the expression of apurinic apyrimidine endonuclease 1/redox factor-1 (Banerjee et al. 2008).

Curcumin Suppresses Several Inflammatory and Pro-cancerous Mechanisms

Many *in vitro* and *in vivo* studies have provided the evidence for the potential of curcumin as anti-invasive and/or antimetastatic agent for variety of cancers. Curcumin is shown to inhibit several cell signaling pathways at multiple levels, such as receptor, transcription factors and enzymes, and leads to cell cycle arrest, and decreased survival through down-regulation of anti-apoptotic genes (Shehzad et al. 2010; Table 24.2). Curcumin induces apoptosis and cell cycle arrest *via* up-regulating the expression of p53 gene followed by induction of Cip1/p21, Kip1/p27. It inhibits association of cyclin D1 with CDK4/CDK6 and pRb phosphorylation as a result blocks cell cycle in G1 phase. It also blocks cell cycle in G1 or G2-M phase in umbilical vein endothelial (ECV304) cells *via* up-regulation of CDKI and down-regulation of cyclin B1 and Cdc2. Curcumin inhibits IKK responsible for IκB phosphorylation, and suppresses NF-κB activation and induces apoptosis. In human colon cancer cells, it induces apoptosis and cytotoxicity *via* caspase-3 activation, increase in Bax expression, cytochrome c release, and increase in p53, together with the decrease in the expression of Bcl-2 and Bcl-xL. Curcumin suppresses the TPA-induced activation of ERK as well as transcriptional activation of NF-κB leading to decreased expression of MMPs in human breast cancer epithelial cells. In brain tumors, curcumin down-regulated the expression of MMP-9 through inhibition of NF-κB and AP-1 binding to the DNA promoter region (Shehzad et al. 2010). Hence, curcumin targets multiple pathways in cancer cells.

Luteolin Inhibits Cell Proliferation and Survival of Cancer Cells

Luteolin is also shown to have cancer chemopreventive effects in various experimental models. It is observed to induce apoptosis in response to redox regulation and DNA damage. It inhibits the activation of many protein kinases leading to suppression of cancer cell proliferation, metastasis and angiogenesis. It induces cytotoxicity by suppressing cell survival pathways and activating apoptotic pathways (Lin et al. 2008). Some part of this compound gets converted in to glucuronides while passing through intestinal mucosa (Shimoi et al. 1998). Remarkably, it is permeable to blood-brain barrier (Wruck et al. 2007). Luteolin shows preventive effect against carcinogenesis *in vivo*, and reduces tumor growth *via* cytotoxic effects (Table 24.2). Luteolin induces G1 arrest by up regulation of Kip1/p27 and Cip1/p21, and inhibition of CDK2 activity in OCM-1 melanoma and HT-29 colorectal cancer cells. It inhibits IGF-1R and Akt induced by IGF-1, and leads to inhibition of phosphorylation of p70S6K1, GSK-3β, and FKHR/FKHRL1, the Akt targets, which is associated with suppression of cyclin D1 and amplification of Cip1/p21 expression. In human hepatoma cells, luteolin enhances Fas expression and induces apoptosis *via* triggering the STAT3 degradation, as well as through the induction of DNA damage and activation of p53. Luteolin inhibits the expression of apoptosis inhibitors and anti-apoptotic Bcl-2 family proteins. It inhibits PKC activity, which decrease XIAP by ubiquitination and proteasomal degradation. In hepatocellular carcinoma cells, luteolin decreases the level of Bcl-xL, and increases the ratio of Bax/Bcl-xL to induce apoptosis. Further, luteolin shows inhibition to MMP, in some cases through suppression of NF-κB signaling (Lin et al. 2008). Thus luteolin targets multiple molecules in imparting its cancer chemopreventive activity.

Resveratrol Inhibits Various Attributes of Cancer Growth and Progression

Resveratrol acts on many cell signaling pathways in cancer cells that lead to arrest in cell cycle progression, induction of apoptosis, and reduction of inflammation, angiogenesis and metastasis. In addition to these, resveratrol shows pro oxidant activity which causes oxidative DNA damage that also leads to cell cycle arrest and apoptosis (Athar et al. 2009; Table 24.2). Resveratrol regulates cell cycle through Rb, CDKs, cyclins and c-myc regulation. It induces apoptosis *via* p53 up-regulation and down-regulation of anti-apoptotic Bcl-2, Bcl-xL, XIAP, survivin and TRAF2. Resveratrol activates SIRT1 related to apoptosis. Resveratrol also inhibits angiogenesis and metastasis pathways *via* regulating the expression of MMPs, VEGF, cathepsin D, ICAM-1 and E-selectin. It also shows antioxidant effects, which are mediated through induction of antioxidant enzymes like glutathione peroxidase, hemoxygenase, catalase and superoxide dismutase. Its anti-inflammatory effects are mediated *via* down-regulation of various biomarkers like TNF, COX-2, iNOS, CRP, interferon-γ and interleukines (Harikumar and Aggarwal 2008). Thus like other dietary phytochemicals discussed above, resveratrol has potential for multi-targeting to halt the growth and development of cancer.

Non-dietary Phytochemicals in Cancer Chemoprevention

There are several phytochemicals which are present in non-dietary plants have shown preventive and therapeutic values. Traditionally, many plants have used for medicinal purposes and some of them have shown their effect as anticancer agents. There is a wealth of medicinal herbs and plants which are yet to be explored scientifically for their medicinal values. In India, it is anticipated that more than 90% of such medicinal plants require attention of the scientists for their scientific validation. However, many of these plants are already in use in the form of Ayurvedic medicine for various ailments. Studies with some plants have shown their anticancer activity in laboratory experiments, and active principles have been identified. Below we have discussed the cancer chemopreventive efficacy and associated mechanisms of some active phytochemicals and plants against various cancers.

Carnosol

Carnosol is the polyphenolic compound found in rosemary (*Rosmarinus officinalis*) and sage (*Salvia carnosa*) and has been used for food processing and medicinal purposes in Europe. It was first isolated from sage in 1942 and its chemical structure was given by Brieskorn et al. in 1964 (Johnson 2011; Brieskorn et al. 1964). It shows anti-cancer activity in prostate (Johnson et al. 2008, 2010a, b), breast (Hussein et al. 2007), skin (Mengoni et al. 2011; Huang et al. 1994), leukemia (Zunino and Storms 2009; Dörrie et al. 2001), and colon cancer (Cheng et al. 2011). These studies show the potential of carnosol to target pathways which are associated with cancer like apoptosis related proteins (Cheng et al. 2011), NF-κB (Lian et al. 2010), AMPK pathway (Johnson et al. 2008), androgen and estrogen receptors (Johnson et al. 2010b) and PI3K/Akt (Martin et al. 2004). These all results are mainly based on the studies in cell culture and animal models, and therefore, studies are warranted in animal models to prove its activity as a cancer chemopreventive agent.

5-Deoxykaempferol

It is a natural flavonol isolated from the leaves of *Astragalus beckari* (Hasan et al. 2010). It was found to target Src, PI3K and ribosomal S6 kinase (RSK2) in *in vitro* as well as mice study for skin cancer (Lee et al. 2010c). It shows chemopreventive effect for UVB-induced two stage skin carcinogenesis as well as inhibits UVB-induced COX-2 and VEGF expression (Lee et al. 2010c). These data are based on laboratory experiments of one type of condition; it needs further studies to assess its efficacy and toxicity, if any, in various cancer models. Nevertheless, 5-deoxykaempferol has the potential of a chemopreventive agent.

Deguelin

Deguelin is the derivative of rotenoid found in *Mundulea sericea*, and its anticancer activity is being assessed since 1997 by different research groups. Deguelin shows anticancer activity against different types of cancers like gastric (Lee et al. 2010c), breast (Chu et al. 2011), prostate (Thamilselvan et al. 2011), lung (Hu et al. 2010) and leukemia (Wu et al. 2007a, b). Studies have provided evidence that deguelin targets multiple pathways associated with cancer that include PI3K/Akt (Chu et al. 2011), glycogen synthase kinase-3 β/β-catenin pathway (Thamilselvan et al. 2011), heat shock protein 90 (Kim et al. 2009c), NF-κB (Dat et al. 2008), antiangiogenesis and apoptosis induction (Lee et al. 2008). However, more studies are needed in future for its efficacy and safety in animal models in order to prove it a useful cancer chemopreventive agent.

Rooibos Tea

Rooibos (*Aspalathus linearis*) is plant of legume family found in the South Africa. It is used as herbal tea and called as red tea or African red tea. It was used in combination with bush (*Sutherlandia frutescens*), Devil's claw (*Harpagophytum procumbens*) and Bambara groundnut (*Vignea subterranean*) to treat some malignancies and inflammatory disorders in Africa (Na et al. 2004). It shows inhibitory effect on NF-κB in dose-dependent manner and also inhibits TPA-induced COX-2 expression (Na et al. 2004). Studies related to the rooibos tea are in infancy stage and need more research to prove its applicability at clinical level.

Conclusions

All the phytochemicals discussed above have multi-ring chemical structures so they are large in size and are less water soluble which does create the problems of bioavailability (Table 24.1). This can be improved by using drug carriers like polyamidoamine dendrimers which enhances the aqueous solubility and oral bioavailability of silibinin (Huang et al. 2011). Further studies require potential carrier of delivery system like Nanocurc^{Tm} for curcumin delivery with nanoparticles (Bisht et al. 2010), and identification of mechanisms at epigenetic level.

The current therapeutic methods like chemotherapy, radiation therapy, surgery, immunotherapy and gene therapy have many limitations, side effects and are expensive and more toxic in comparison to phytochemicals. Dietary and non-dietary phytochemicals have shown their potentials for cancer therapy and many of them are at clinical trials for few cancers. Since many of them are the part of normal diets, WHO suggests that by using regular healthy diets we can save several lives from cancer to greater extent or may provide shelter either complete or incomplete from cancer. Thus better advancement in bioactive phytochemicals research and public awareness for such compounds will certainly help to improve public health.

Acknowledgement The authors acknowledge the fellowship support to D. Tailor from University Grant Commission (UGC), through Central University of Gujarat (CUG), India.

References

Agarwal C, Dhanalakshmi S, Singh RP, Agarwal R (2004) Inositol hexaphosphate inhibits growth and induces G1 arrest and apoptotic death of androgen-dependent human prostate carcinoma LNCaP cells. Neoplasia 6(5):646–659

Aggarwal B, Sundaram C, Malani N, Ichikawa H (2007) Curcumin: the Indian solid gold. Adv Exp Med Biol 595:1–75

Aller GV, Carson J, Tang W, Peng H, Zhao L, Copeland R et al (2011) Epigallocatechin gallate (EGCG), a major component of green tea, is a dual phosphoinositide-3-kinase/mTOR inhibitor. Biochem Biophys Res Commun 406(2):194–199

Arts IA (2005) Polyphenols and disease risk in epidemiologic studies. Am J Clin Nutr 81: 317S–325S

Athar M, Back JH, Kopelovich L, Bickers DR, Kim AL (2009) Multiple molecular targets of resveratrol: anti-carcinogenic mechanisms. Arch Biochem Biophys 486(2):95–102

Attoub S, Hassan AH, Vanhoecke B, Iratni R, Takahashi T, Gaben AM et al (2011) Inhibition of cell survival, invasion, tumor growth and histone deacetylase activity by the dietary flavonoid luteolin in human epithelioid cancer cells. Eur J Pharmacol 651(1–3):18–25

Bacić I, Druzijanić N, Karlo R, Skifić I, Jagić S (2010) Efficacy of IP6 + inositol in the treatment of breast cancer patients receiving chemotherapy: prospective, randomized, pilot clinical study. J Exp Clin Cancer Res 29(1):1–5

Bai Y, Mao QQ, Qin J, Zheng XY, Wang YB, Yang K et al (2010) Resveratrol induces apoptosis and cell cycle arrest of human T24 bladder cancer cells in vitro and inhibits tumor growth *in vivo*. Cancer Sci 101(2):488–493

Banerjee S, Li Y, Wang Z, Sarkar F (2008) Multi-targeted therapy of cancer by genistein. Cancer Lett 269(2):226–242

Bang CI, Paik SY, Sun DI, Joo YH, Kim MS (2008) Cell growth inhibition and down-regulation of survivin by silibinin in a laryngeal squamous cell carcinoma cell line. Ann Otol Rhinol Laryngol 117(10):781–785

Berge G, Øvrebø S, Eilertsen E, Haugen A, Mollerup S (2004) Analysis of resveratrol as a lung cancer chemopreventive agent in A/J mice exposed to benzo[a]pyrene. Br J Cancer 91(7): 1380–1383

Berner C, Aumüller E, Gnauck A, Nestelberger M, Just A, Haslberger A (2010) Epigenetic control of estrogen receptor expression and tumor suppressor genes is modulated by bioactive food compounds. Ann Nutr Metab 57(3–4):183–189

Bishayee A (2009) Cancer prevention and treatment with resveratrol: from rodent studies to clinical trials. Cancer Prev Res (Phila) 2(5):409–418

Bisht S, Mizuma M, Feldmann G, Ottenhof NA, Hong SM, Pramanik D et al (2010) Systemic administration of polymeric nanoparticle-encapsulated curcumin (NanoCurc) blocks tumor growth and metastases in preclinical models of pancreatic cancer. Mol Cancer Ther 9(8): 2255–2264

Bode AM (2009) Cancer prevention research—then and now. Nature Rev Cancer 9:508–516

Botella P, Abasolo I, Fernández Y, Muniesa C, Miranda S, Quesada M et al (2011) Surface-modified silica nanoparticles for tumor-targeted delivery of camptothecin and its biological evaluation. J Control Release. doi:10.1016/j.jconrel.2011.06.039

Boyle P, Levin B (2008) World Cancer Report 2008. World Health Organization

Brieskorn C, Fuchs A, Bredenberg J-s, McChesney J, Wenkert E (1964) The structure of carnosol. J Org Chem 29(8):2293–2298

Cai X, Ye T, Liu C, Lu W, Lu M, Zhang J et al (2011) Luteolin induced G2 phase cell cycle arrest and apoptosis on non-small cell lung cancer cells. Toxicol In Vitro. doi:10.1016/j.tiv.2011.05.009

Cardile V, Chillemi R, Lombardo L, Sciuto S, Spatafora C, Tringali C (2007) Antiproliferative activity of methylated analogues of E- and Z-resveratrol. Z Naturforsch C 62(3–4):189–195

Carroll R, Benya R, Turgeon D, Vareed S, Neuman M, Rodriguez L et al (2011) Phase IIa clinical trial of curcumin for the prevention of colorectal neoplasia. Cancer Prev Res (Phila) 4(3): 354–364

Castino R, Pucer A, Veneroni R, Morani F, Peracchio C, Lah TT et al (2011) Resveratrol reduces the invasive growth and promotes the acquisition of a long-lasting differentiated phenotype in human glioblastoma cells. J Agric Food Chem 59(8):4264–4272

Chen PN, Hsieh YS, Chiang CL, Chiou HL, Yang SF, Chu SC (2006) Silibinin inhibits invasion of oral cancer cells by suppressing the MAPK pathway. J Dent Res 85(3):220–225

Chen D, Wan S, Yang H, Yuan J, Chan T, Dou Q (2011a) EGCG, green tea polyphenols and their synthetic analogs and prodrugs for human cancer prevention and treatment. Adv Clin Chem 53:155–177

Chen P, Chu S, Kuo W, Chou M, Lin J, Hsieh Y (2011b) Epigallocatechin-3 gallate inhibits invasion, epithelial-mesenchymal transition, and tumor growth in oral cancer cells. J Agric Food Chem 59(8):3836–3844

Chen T, Wang W, Golden E, Thomas S, Sivakumar W, Hofman F et al (2011c) Green tea epigallocatechin gallate enhances therapeutic efficacy of temozolomide in orthotopic mouse glioblastoma models. Cancer Lett 302(2):100–108

Cheng AC, Huang TC, Lai CS, Pan MH (2005) Induction of apoptosis by luteolin through cleavage of Bcl-2 family in human leukemia HL-60 cells. Eur J Pharmacol 509(1):1–10

Cheng A, Lee M, Tsai M, Lai C, Lee J, Ho C et al (2011) Rosmanol potently induces apoptosis through both the mitochondrial apoptotic pathway and death receptor pathway in human colon adenocarcinoma COLO 205 cells. Food Chem Toxicol 49(2):485–493

Cheung CW, Taylor PJ, Kirkpatrick CM, Vesey DA, Gobe GC, Winterford C et al (2007) Therapeutic value of orally administered silibinin in renal cell carcinoma: manipulation of insulin-like growth factor binding protein-3 levels. BJU Int 100(2):438–444

Chu Z, Liang X, Zhou X, Huang R, Zhan Q, Jiang J (2011) Effects of deguelin on proliferation and apoptosis of MCF-7 breast cancer cells by phosphatidylinositol 3-kinase/Akt signaling pathway. Zhong Xi Yi Jie He Xue Bao 9(5):533–538

Coates A, Abraham S, Kaye S, Sowerbutts T, Frewin C, Fox R et al (1983) On the receiving end—patient perception of the side-effects of cancer chemotherapy. Eur J Cancer Clin Oncol 19(2):203–208

Coyle C, Philips B, Morrisroe S, Chancellor M, Yoshimura N (2008) Antioxidant effects of green tea and its polyphenols on bladder cells. Life Sci 83(1–2):12–18

Cui W, Gu F, Hu KQ (2009) Effects and mechanisms of silibinin on human hepatocellular carcinoma xenografts in nude mice. World J Gastroenterol 15(16):1943–1950

Cvorovic J, Tramer F, Granzotto M, Candussio L, Decorti G, Passamonti S (2010) Oxidative stress-based cytotoxicity of delphinidin and cyanidin in colon cancer cells. Arch Biochem Biophys 501(1):151–157

Das A, Banik N, Ray S (2010) Flavonoids activated caspases for apoptosis in human glioblastoma T98G and U87MG cells but not in human normal astrocytes. Cancer 116(1):164–176

Dat N, Lee J, Lee K, Hong Y, Kim Y, Lee J (2008) Phenolic constituents of Amorpha fruticosa that inhibit NF-kappaB activation and related gene expression. J Nat Prod 71(10):1696–1700

Davis-Searles P, Nakanishi Y, Kim N (2005) Milk thistle and prostate cancer: differential effects of pure flavonolignans from Silybum marianum on antiproliferative end points in human prostate carcinoma cells. Cancer Res 65:4448–4457

Deep G, Agarwal R (2010) Antimetastatic efficacy of silibinin: molecular mechanisms and therapeutic potential against cancer. Cancer Metastasis Rev 29:447–463

Deliliers G, Servida F, Fracchiolla N, Ricci C, Borsotti C, Colombo G et al (2002) Effect of inositol hexaphosphate (IP(6)) on human normal and leukaemic haematopoietic cells. Br J Haematol 117(3):577–587

Dhanalakshmi S, Singh RP, Agarwal C, Agarwal R (2002) Silibinin inhibits constitutive and TNFalpha-induced activation of NF-kappaB and sensitizes human prostate carcinoma DU145 cells to TNFalpha-induced apoptosis. Oncogene 21:1759–1767

Dillman R (2011) Cancer immunotherapy. Cancer Biother Radiopharm 26(1):1–64

Dörrie J, Sapala K, Zunino S (2001) Carnosol-induced apoptosis and downregulation of Bcl-2 in B-lineage leukemia cells. Cancer Lett 170(1):33–39

Dorsey M, Benghuzzi H, Tucci M, Cason Z (2005) Growth and cell viability of estradiol and IP-6 treated Hep-2 laryngeal carcinoma cells. Biomed Sci Instrum 41:205–210

Dou Q (2009) Molecular mechanisms of green tea polyphenols. Nutr Cancer 61(6):827–835

Eiseman J, Lan J, Guo J, Joseph E, Vucenik I (2011) Pharmacokinetics and tissue distribution of inositol hexaphosphate in C.B17 SCID mice bearing human breast cancer xenografts. Metabolism. doi:10.1016/Jmetabol.2011.015

Filip A, Daicoviciu D, Clichici S, Mocan T, Muresan A, Postescu I (2011) Photoprotective effects of 2 natural products on ultraviolet B-induced oxidative stress and apoptosis in SKH-1 mouse skin. J Med Food 14(7–8):761–766

Flaig TW, Gustafson DL, Su LJ, Zirrolli JA, Crighton F, Harrison GS et al (2007) A phase I and pharmacokinetic study of silybin-phytosome in prostate cancer patients. Invest New Drugs 25(2):139–146

Flaig TW, Glodé M, Gustafson D, Bokhoven AV, Tao Y, Wilson S et al (2010) A study of high-dose oral silybin-phytosome followed by prostatectomy in patients with localized prostate cancer. Prostate 70(8):848–855

Fossey S, Bear M, Lin J, Li C, Schwartz E, Li P et al (2011) The novel curcumin analog FLLL32 decreases STAT3 DNA binding activity and expression, and induces apoptosis in osteosarcoma cell lines. BMC Cancer 11:112

Froyen E, Reeves J, Mitchell A, Steinberg F (2009) Regulation of phase II enzymes by genistein and daidzein in male and female Swiss Webster mice. J Med Food 12(6):1227–1237

Fukui M, Yamabe N, Zhu BT (2010) Resveratrol attenuates the anticancer efficacy of paclitaxel in human breast cancer cells in vitro and in vivo. Eur J Cancer 46(10):1882–1891

Ganapathy S, Chen Q, Singh KP, Shankar S, Srivastava RK (2010) Resveratrol enhances antitumor activity of TRAIL in prostate cancer xenografts through activation of FOXO transcription factor. PLoS One 5(12):e15627

García-Maceira P, Mateo J (2009) Silibinin inhibits hypoxia-inducible factor-1alpha and mTOR/p70S6K/4E-BP1 signalling pathway in human cervical and hepatoma cancer cells: implications for anticancer therapy. Oncogene 28(3):313–324

Green D (2000) Apoptotic pathways: paper wraps stone blunts scissors. Cell 102(1):1–4

Gu M, Dhanalakshmi S, Mohan S, Singh RP, Agarwal R (2005) Silibinin inhibits ultraviolet B radiation-induced mitogenic and survival signaling, and associated biological responses in SKH-1 mouse skin. Carcinogenesis 26(8):1404–1413

Gu M, Singh RP, Dhanalakshmi S, Agarwal C, Agarwal R (2007) Silibinin inhibits inflammatory and angiogenic attributes in photocarcinogenesis in SKH-1 hairless mice. Cancer Res 67(7):3483–3491

Gu B, Ding Q, Xia G, Fang Z (2009a) EGCG inhibits growth and induces apoptosis in renal cell carcinoma through TFPI-2 overexpression. Oncol Rep 21(3):635–640

Gu M, Roy S, Raina K, Agarwal C, Agarwal R (2009b) Inositol hexaphosphate suppresses growth and induces apoptosis in prostate carcinoma cells in culture and nude mouse xenograft: PI3K-Akt pathway as potential target. Cancer Res 69(24):9465–9472

Guo L, Peng Y, Yao J, Sui L, Gu A, Wang J (2010) Anticancer activity and molecular mechanism of resveratrol-bovine serum albumin nanoparticles on subcutaneously implanted human primary ovarian carcinoma cells in nude mice. Cancer Biother Radiopharm 25(4):471–477

Han H, Zhong C, Zhang X, Liu R, Pan M, Tan L et al (2010) Genistein induces growth inhibition and G2/M arrest in nasopharyngeal carcinoma cells. Nutr Cancer 62(5):641–647

Harikumar KB, Aggarwal BB (2008) Resveratrol: a multitargeted agent for age-associated chronic diseases. Cell Cycle 7(8):1020–1035

Hasan A, Sadiq A, Abbas A, Mughal E, Khan K, Ali M (2010) Isolation and synthesis of flavonols and comparison of their antioxidant activity. Nat Prod Res 24(11):995–1003

Hoh C, Boocock D, Marczylo T, Singh RP, Berry DP, Dennison AR et al (2006) Pilot study of oral silibinin, a putative chemopreventive agent, in colorectal cancer patients: silibinin levels in plasma, colorectum, and liver and their pharmacodynamic consequences. Clin Cancer Res 12(9):2944–2950

Horinaka M, Yoshida T, Shiraishi T, Nakata S, Wakada M, Nakanishi R et al (2005) The combination of TRAIL and luteolin enhances apoptosis in human cervical cancer HeLa cells. Biochem Biophys Res Commun 333(3):833–838

Hsieh YS, Chu SC, Yang SF, Chen PN, Liu YC, Lu KH (2007) Silibinin suppresses human osteosarcoma MG-63 cell invasion by inhibiting the ERK-dependent c-Jun/AP-1 induction of MMP-2. Carcinogenesis 28(5):977–987

Hsu KF, Wu CL, Huang SC, Wu CM, Rhsiao J, Yo YT et al (2009) Cathepsin L mediates resveratrol-induced autophagy and apoptotic cell death in cervical cancer cells. Autophagy 5(4):451–460

Hu J, Ye H, Fu A, Chen X, Wang Y, Chen X et al (2010) Deguelin–an inhibitor to tumor lymphangiogenesis and lymphatic metastasis by downregulation of vascular endothelial cell growth factor-D in lung tumor model. Int J Cancer 127(10):2455–2466

Huang M, Ho C, Wang Z, Ferraro T, Lou Y, Stauber K et al (1994) Inhibition of skin tumorigenesis by rosemary and its constituents carnosol and ursolic acid. Cancer Res 54(3):701–708

Huang X, Wu Z, Gao W, Chen Q, Yu B (2011) Polyamidoamine dendrimers as potential drug carriers for enhanced aqueous solubility and oral bioavailability of silybin. Drug Dev Ind Pharm 37(4):419–427

Hughes C (1998) Phytochemical mimicry of reproductive hormones and modulation of herbivore fertility by phytoestrogens. Environ Health Perspect 78:171–174

Huh S, Bae S, Kim Y, Lee J, Namkoong S, Lee I et al (2004) Anticancer effects of (-)-epigallocatechin-3-gallate on ovarian carcinoma cell lines. Gynecol Oncol 94(3):760–768

Hussein A, Meyer J, Jimeno M, Rodríguez B (2007) Bioactive diterpenes from Orthosiphon labiatus and Salvia africana-lutea. J Nat Prod 70(2):293–295

Hwang J, Park I, Shin J, Lee Y, Lee S, Baik H et al (2005) Genistein, EGCG, and capsaicin inhibit adipocyte differentiation process via activating AMP-activated protein kinase. Biochem Biophys Res Commun 338(2):694–699

Immunotherapy of Cancer (2007). BCC Research, 30 Mar 2007

Jakacki RI, Bouffet E, Adamson PC, Pollack IF, Ingle AM, Voss SD et al (2011) A phase 1 study of vinblastine in combination with carboplatin for children with low-grade gliomas: a Children's Oncology Group phase 1 consortium study. Neuro Oncol. doi:10.1093/neuonc/nor090

Jang M, Cai L, Udeani GO, Slowing KV, Thomas CF, Beecher CW et al (1997) Cancer chemopreventive activity of resveratrol, a natural product derived from grapes. Science 275:218–220

Janus S, Weurtz B, Ondrey F (2007) Inositol hexaphosphate and paclitaxel: symbiotic treatment of oral cavity squamous cell carcinoma. Laryngoscope 117(8):1381–1388

Jemal A, Bray F, Center MM, Ferlay J, Ward E, Forman D (2011) Global cancer statistics. CA Cancer J Clin, pp 69–90

Ji S, Han D, Kim J (2006) Inhibition of proliferation and induction of apoptosis by EGCG in human osteogenic sarcoma (HOS) cells. Arch Pharm Res 29(5):363–368

Johnson J (2011) Carnosol: a promising anti-cancer and anti-inflammatory agent. Cancer Lett 305(1):1–7

Johnson J, Syed D, Heren C, Suh Y, Adhami V, Mukhtar H (2008) Carnosol, a dietary diterpene, displays growth inhibitory effects in human prostate cancer PC3 cells leading to G2-phase cell cycle arrest and targets the 5′-AMP-activated protein kinase (AMPK) pathway. Pharm Res 25(9):2125–2134

Johnson J, Bailey H, Mukhtar H (2010a) Green tea polyphenols for prostate cancer chemoprevention: a translational perspective. Phytomedicine 17(1):3–13

Johnson J, Syed D, Suh Y, Heren C, Saleem M, Siddiqui I et al (2010b) Disruption of androgen and estrogen receptor activity in prostate cancer by a novel dietary diterpene carnosol: implications for chemoprevention. Cancer Prev Res (Phila) 3(9):1112–1123

Jordan VC (2003) Tamoxifen: a most unlikely pioneering medicine. Nat Rev Drug Disc 2:205–213

Jose S (2010) A global strategic business report. Global Industry Analysts, Inc., San Jose

Karmakar S, Banik N, Ray S (2007) Molecular mechanism of inositol hexaphosphate-mediated apoptosis in human malignant glioblastoma T98G cells. Neurochem Res 32(12):2094–2102

Kartal M, Saydam G, Sahin F, Baran Y (2011) Resveratrol triggers apoptosis through regulating ceramide metabolizing genes in human K562 chronic myeloid leukemia cells. Nutr Cancer 63(4):637–644

Khan N, Mukhtar H (2008) Multitargeted therapy of cancer by green tea polyphenols. Cancer Lett 269(2):269–280

Khan N, Adhami VM, Mukhtar H (2009) Green tea polyphenols in chemoprevention of prostate cancer: preclinical and clinical studies. Nutr Cancer 61(6):836–841

Kim KW, Choi CH, Kim TH, Kwon CH, Woo JS, Kim YK (2009a) Silibinin inhibits glioma cell proliferation via Ca2+/ROS/MAPK-dependent mechanism in vitro and glioma tumor growth in vivo. Neurochem Res 34(8):1479–1490

Kim S, Choi MG, Lee HS, Lee SK, Kim SH, Kim WW et al (2009b) Silibinin suppresses TNF-alpha-induced MMP-9 expression in gastric cancer cells through inhibition of the MAPK pathway. Molecules 14(11):4300–4311

Kim W, Oh S, Woo J, Hong W, Lee H (2009c) Targeting heat shock protein 90 overrides the resistance of lung cancer cells by blocking radiation-induced stabilization of hypoxia-inducible factor-1alpha. Cancer Res 69(4):1624–1632

Ko K, Park S, Park B, Yang J, Cho L, Kang C et al (2010) Isoflavones from phytoestrogens and gastric cancer risk: a nested case-control study within the Korean multicenter cancer cohort. Cancer Epidemiol Biomarkers Prev 19(5):1292–1300

Koh Y, Choi E, Kang S, Hwang H, Lee M, Pyun J et al (2011) Green tea (-)-epigallocatechin-3-gallate inhibits HGF-induced progression in oral cavity cancer through suppression of HGF/c-Met. J Nutr Biochem. doi:10.1016/j.jnutbio.2010.09.005

Kolappaswamy K, Williams K, Benazzi C, Sarli G, McLeod CG Jr, Vucenik I et al (2009) Effect of inositol hexaphosphate on the development of UVB-induced skin tumors in SKH1 hairless mice. Comp Med 59(2):147–152

Kowalczyk MC, Kowalczyk P, Tolstykh O, Hanausek M, Walaszek Z, Slaga TJ (2010) Synergistic effects of combined phytochemicals and skin cancer prevention in SENCAR mice. Cancer Prev Res (Phila) 3(2):170–178

Kumar N, Shibata D, Helm J, Coppola D, Malafa M (2007) Green tea polyphenols in the prevention of colon cancer. Front Biosci 12:2309–2315

Lawrence TS (2008) Cancer: principles and practice of oncology, 8th edn. Lippincott Williams and Wilkins, Philadelphia
Lazarevic B, Boezelijn G, Diep L, Kvernrod K, Ogren O, Ramberg H et al (2011) Efficacy and safety of short-term genistein intervention in patients with localized prostate cancer prior to radical prostatectomy: a randomized, placebo-controlled, double-blind phase 2 clinical trial. Nutr Cancer. doi:10.1080/01635581.2011.582221
Leclerq G, Heuson J (1979) Physiological and pharmacological effects of estrogens in breast cancer. Biochim Biophys Acta 560:427–455
Lee J, Lee D, Lee H, Choi J, Kim K, Hong S (2008) Deguelin inhibits human hepatocellular carcinoma by antiangiogenesis and apoptosis. Oncol Rep 20(1):129–134
Lee H, Lee J, Jung K, Hong S (2010a) Deguelin promotes apoptosis and inhibits angiogenesis of gastric cancer. Oncol Rep 24(4):957–963
Lee J, Jeong Y, Lee S, Kim D, Oh S, Lim H et al (2010b) EGCG induces apoptosis in human laryngeal epidermoid carcinoma Hep2 cells via mitochondria with the release of apoptosis-inducing factor and endonuclease G. Cancer Lett 290(1):68–75
Lee K, Lee K, Byun S, Jung S, Seo S, Heo Y et al (2010c) 5-deoxykaempferol plays a potential therapeutic role by targeting multiple signaling pathways in skin cancer. Cancer Prev Res (Phila) 3(4):454–465
Lee D, Lee K, Byun S, Jung S, Song N, Lim S et al (2011) 7,3′,4′-Trihydroxyisoflavone, a metabolite of the soy isoflavone daidzein, suppresses ultraviolet B-induced skin cancer by targeting Cot and MKK4. J Biol Chem 286(16):14246–14256
Leite K, Chade D, Sanudo A, Sakiyama B, Batocchio G, Srougi M (2009) Effects of curcumin in an orthotopic murine bladder tumor model. Int Braz J Urol 35(5):599–607
Leone M, Zhai D, Sareth S, Kitada S, Reed JC, Pellecchia M (2003) Cancer prevention by tea polyphenols is linked to their direct inhibition of antiapoptotic Bcl-2-family proteins. Cancer Res 63(23):8118–8121
Li Y, Upadhyay S, Bhuiyan M, Sarkar F (1999) Induction of apoptosis in breast cancer cells MDA-MB-231 by genistein. Oncogene 18(20):3166–3172
Li Y, Xu Y, Huang D, Jiang L, Li K (2007) Inhibit affection of resveratrol on the growth of Hep-2 cell line. Lin Chung Er Bi Yan Hou Tou Jing Wai Ke Za Zhi 21(24):1129–1131
Li G, Chen Y, Hou Z, Xiao H, Jin H, Lu G et al (2010a) Pro-oxidative activities and dose-response relationship of (-)-epigallocatechin-3-gallate in the inhibition of lung cancer cell growth: a comparative study in vivo and in vitro. Carcinogenesis 31(5):902–910
Li T, Wang W, Chen H, Li T, Ye L (2010b) Evaluation of anti-leukemia effect of resveratrol by modulating STAT3 signaling. Int Immunopharmacol 10(1):18–25
Li W, Frame L, Hoo K, Li Y, D'Cunha N, Cobos E (2011) Genistein inhibited proliferation and induced apoptosis in acute lymphoblastic leukemia, lymphoma and multiple myeloma cells in vitro. Leuk Lymphoma. doi:10.3109/10428194.2011.598251
Lian K, Chuang J, Hsieh C, Wung B, Huang G, Jian T et al (2010) Dual mechanisms of NF-kappaB inhibition in carnosol-treated endothelial cells. Toxicol Appl Pharmacol 245(1):21–35
Liang G, Tang A, Lin X, Li L, Zhang S, Huang Z et al (2010) Green tea catechins augment the antitumor activity of doxorubicin in an in vivo mouse model for chemoresistant liver cancer. Int J Oncol 37(1):111–123
Lim YC, Cha YY (2011) Epigallocatechin-3-gallate induces growth inhibition and apoptosis of human anaplastic thyroid carcinoma cells through suppression of EGFR/ERK pathway and cyclin B1/CDK1 complex. J Surg Oncol. doi:10.1002/jso.21999
Lin Y, Shi R, Wang X, Shen H (2008) Luteolin, a flavonoid with potential for cancer prevention and therapy. Curr Cancer Drug Targets 8(7):634–646
Lin CW, Shen SC, Chien CC, Yang LY, Shia LT, Chen YC (2010) 12-O-tetradecanoylphorbol-13-acetate-induced invasion/migration of glioblastoma cells through activating PKCalpha/ERK/NF-kappaB-dependent MMP-9 expression. J Cell Physiol 225(2):472–481
Loa J, Chow P, Zhang K (2009) Studies of structure-activity relationship on plant polyphenol-induced suppression of human liver cancer cells. Cancer Chemother Pharmacol 63(6): 1007–1016

López-Lázaro M (2009) Distribution and biological activities of the flavonoid luteolin. Mini Rev Med Chem 9(1):31–59

Love R, Leventhal H, Easterling D, Nerenz D (1989) Side effects and emotional distress during cancer chemotherapy. Cancer 63(3):604–612

Marchand LL (2002) Cancer preventive effects of flavonoids–a review. Biomed Pharmacother 56(6):296–301

Markaverich BM, Vijjeswarapu M, Shoulars K, Rodriguez M (2010) Luteolin and gefitinib regulation of EGF signaling pathway and cell cycle pathway genes in PC-3 human prostate cancer cells. J Steroid Biochem Mol Biol 122(4):219–231

Markaverich BM, Shoulars K, Rodriguez MA (2011) Luteolin regulation of estrogen signaling and cell cycle pathway genes in MCF-7 human breast cancer cells. Int J Biomed Sci 7(2):101–111

Martin D, Rojo A, Salinas M, Diaz R, Gallardo G, Alam J et al (2004) Regulation of heme oxygenase-1 expression through the phosphatidylinositol 3-kinase/Akt pathway and the Nrf2 transcription factor in response to the antioxidant phytochemical carnosol. J Biol Chem 279(10):8919–8929

Mateen S, Tyagi A, Agarwal C, Singh RP, Agarwal R (2010) Silibinin inhibits human nonsmall cell lung cancer cell growth through cell-cycle arrest by modulating expression and function of key cell-cycle regulators. Mol Carcinog 49(3):247–258

Mathews T, MacDorman MF (2007) Infant Mortality Statistics from the 2004 Period Linked Birth/Infant Death Data Set. National Center for Health Statistics, U.S. department of health & human services. Maryland: DHHS Publication

Meeran S, Ahmed A, Tollefsbol T (2010) Epigenetic targets of bioactive dietary components for cancer prevention and therapy. Clin Epigenetics 1(3–4):101–116

Meeran S, Patel S, Chan T, Tollefsbol T (2011) A novel prodrug of epigallocatechin-3-gallate: differential epigenetic hTERT repression in human breast cancer cells. Cancer Prev Res (Phila). doi:10.1158/1940-6207

Mengoni E, Vichera G, Rigano L, Rodriguez-Puebla M, Galliano S, Cafferata E et al (2011) Suppression of COX-2, IL-1β and TNF-α expression and leukocyte infiltration in inflamed skin by bioactive compounds from Rosmarinus officinalis L. Fitoterapia 82(3):414–421

Mileshkin L, Rischin D, Prince H, Zalcberg J (2005) The contribution of cytotoxic chemotherapy to the management of cancer. Clin Oncol (R Coll Radiol) 17(4):294

Miniño AM, Arias E, Kochanek KD, Murphy SL, Smith BL (2002) Deaths: Final Data for 2000. National center for health statistics, Department of health and human services. Maryland: DHHS Publication

Minna J, Schiller J (2008) Harrison's principles of internal medicine, 17th edn. McGraw-Hill, New York

Mitra A, Chakrabarti J, Banerji A, Chatterjee A, Das B (2006) Curcumin, a potential inhibitor of MMP-2 in human laryngeal squamous carcinoma cells HEp2. J Environ Pathol Toxicol Oncol 25(4):679–690

Mitruţ P, Burada F, Enescu A, Scorei R, Badea D, Genunche-Dumitrescu A et al (2009) The genotoxicity study of resveratrol in primary gastric adenocarcinoma cell cultures. Rom J Morphol Embryol 50(3):429–433

Momeny M, Malehmir M, Zakidizaji M, Ghasemi R, Ghadimi H, Shokrgozar MA et al (2010) Silibinin inhibits invasive properties of human glioblastoma U87MG cells through suppression of cathepsin B and nuclear factor kappa B-mediated induction of matrix metalloproteinase 9. Anticancer Drugs 21(3):252–260

Morrow GR (1985) The effect of a susceptibility to motion sickness on the side effects of cancer chemotherapy. Ccancer 55:2766–2770

Na H, Mossanda K, Lee J, Surh Y (2004) Inhibition of phorbol ester-induced COX-2 expression by some edible African plants. Biofactors 21(1–4):149–153

Nakamura H, Wang Y, Kurita T, Adomat H, Cunha G, Wang Y (2011) Genistein increases epidermal growth factor receptor signaling and promotes tumor progression in advanced human prostate cancer. PLoS One 6(5):e20034

Nguyen AV, Martinez M, Stamos MJ, Moyer MP, Planutis K, Hope C et al (2009) Results of a phase I pilot clinical trial examining the effect of plant-derived resveratrol and grape powder on Wnt pathway target gene expression in colonic mucosa and colon cancer. Cancer Manag Res 1:25–37

Noguchi M, Yokoyama M, Watanabe S, Uchiyama M, Nakao Y, Hara K et al (2006) Inhibitory effect of the tea polyphenol, (-)-epigallocatechin gallate, on growth of cervical adenocarcinoma cell lines. Cancer Lett 234(2):135–142

Norazalina S, Norhaizan M, Hairuszah I, Norashareena M (2010) Anticarcinogenic efficacy of phytic acid extracted from rice bran on azoxymethane-induced colon carcinogenesis in rats. Exp Toxicol Pathol 62(3):259–268

Ouyang G, Yao L, Ruan K, Song G, Mao Y, Bao S (2009) Genistein induces G2/M cell cycle arrest and apoptosis of human ovarian cancer cells via activation of DNA damage checkpoint pathways. Cell Biol Int 33(12):1237–1244

Pace-Asciak CR, Rounova O, Hahn SE, Diamandis EP, Goldberg DM (1996) Wines and grape juices as modulators of platelet aggregation in healthy human subjects. Clin Chim Acta 246(1–2):163–182

Park S, Kim M, Kim Y, Kim S, Park J, Myoung H (2010) Combined cetuximab and genistein treatment shows additive anti-cancer effect on oral squamous cell carcinoma. Cancer Lett 292(1):54–63

Paul S, Mizuno CS, Lee H, Zheng X, Chajkowisk S, Rimoldi JM et al (2010) In vitro and in vivo studies on stilbene analogs as potential treatment agents for colon cancer. Eur J Med Chem 45(9):3702–3708

Phillips JM, Clark C, Herman FL, Moore-Medlin T, Rong X, Gill J, Clifford J, Abreo F et al (2011) Curcumin inhibits skin squamous cell carcinoma tumor growth in vivo. Otolaryngol Head Neck Surg. doi:10.1177/0194599811400711

Prins RM, Liau LM (2004) Cancer immunotherapy at the crossroads: how tumors evade immunity and what can be done. Neuro Oncol 6(3):265–266

Provinciali M, Re F, Donnini A, Orlando F, Bartozzi B, Stasio GD et al (2005) Effect of resveratrol on the development of spontaneous mammary tumors in HER-2/neu transgenic mice. Int J Cancer 115(1):36–45

Qi W, Weber C, Wasland K, Savkovic S (2011) Genistein inhibits proliferation of colon cancer cells by attenuating a negative effect of epidermal growth factor on tumor suppressor FOXO3 activity. BMC Cancer 11:219

Raina K, Serkova NJ, Agarwal R (2009) Silibinin feeding alters the metabolic profile in TRAMP prostatic tumors: 1H-NMRS-based metabolomics study. Cancer Res 69(9):3731–3735

Rajamanickam S, Velmurugan B, Kaur M, Singh RP, Agarwal R (2010) Chemoprevention of intestinal tumorigenesis in APCmin/+ mice by silibinin. Cancer Res 70(6):2368–2378

Ramasamy K, Agarwal R (2008) Multitargeted therapy of cancer by silymarin. Cancer Lett 269(2):352–362

Ramos S (2008) Cancer chemoprevention and chemotherapy: dietary polyphenols and signalling pathways. Mol Nutr Food Res 52:507–526

Rao J, Xu D, Zheng F, Long Z, Huang S, Wu X et al (2011) Curcumin reduces expression of Bcl-2, leading to apoptosis in daunorubicin-insensitive CD34+ acute myeloid leukemia cell lines and primary sorted CD34+ acute myeloid leukemia cells. J Transl Med 9:71

Reynoso-Camacho R, González-Jasso E, Ferriz-Martínez R, Villalón-Corona B, Loarca-Piña GF, Salgado LM et al (2011) Dietary supplementation of lutein reduces colon carcinogenesis in DMH-treated rats by modulating K-ras, PKB, and β-catenin proteins. Nutr Cancer 63(1):39–45

RNCOS (2008) Global cancer treatment forecast to 2012. RNCOS, Noida. http://www.rncos.com/Report/IM130.htm

Roy S, Gu M, Ramasamy K, Singh R, Agarwal C, Siriwardana S et al (2009) p21/Cip1 and p27/Kip1 Are essential molecular targets of inositol hexaphosphate for its antitumor efficacy against prostate cancer. Cancer Res 69(3):1166–1173

Rusin M, Zajkowicz A, Butkiewicz D (2009) Resveratrol induces senescence-like growth inhibition of U-2 OS cells associated with the instability of telomeric DNA and upregulation of BRCA1. Mech Ageing Dev 130(8):528–537

Sah JF, Balasubramanian S, Eckert RL, Rorke EA (2004) Epigallocatechin-3-gallate inhibits epidermal growth factor receptor signaling pathway. Evidence for direct inhibition of ERK1/2 and Akt kinases. J Biol Chem 279(13):12755–12762

Sakata M, Ikeda T, Imoto S, Jinno H, Kitagawa Y (2011) Prevention of mammary carcinogenesis in C3H/OuJ mice by green tea and tamoxifen. Asian Pac J Cancer Prev 12(2):567–571

Sakla M, Shenouda N, Ansell P, Macdonald R, Lubahn D (2007) Genistein affects HER2 protein concentration, activation, and promoter regulation in BT-474 human breast cancer cells. Endocrine 32(1):69–78

Salado C, Olaso E, Gallot N, Valcarcel M, Egilegor E, Mendoza L et al (2011) Resveratrol prevents inflammation-dependent hepatic melanoma metastasis by inhibiting the secretion and effects of interleukin-18. J Transl Med 9:59

Saunders J, Rogers L, Klomsiri C, Poole L, Daniel L (2010) Reactive oxygen species mediate lysophosphatidic acid induced signaling in ovarian cancer cells. Free Radic Biol Med 49(12):2058–2067

Schantz M, Erk T, Richling E (2010) Metabolism of green tea catechins by the human small intestine. Biotechnol J 5(10):1050–1059

Seelinger G, Merfort I, Wölfle U, Schempp CM (2008) Anti-carcinogenic effects of the flavonoid luteolin. Molecules 13(10):2628–2651

Sen P, Chakraborty P, Raha S (2006) Tea polyphenol epigallocatechin 3-gallate impedes the anti-apoptotic effects of low-grade repetitive stress through inhibition of Akt and NF-kappaB survival pathways. FEBS Lett 580(1):278–284

Senft C, Polacin M, Priester M, Seifert V, Kögel D, Weissenberger J (2010) The nontoxic natural compound curcumin exerts anti-proliferative, anti-migratory, and anti-invasive properties against malignant gliomas. BMC Cancer 10:e491

Seo H, Ju J, Jang K, Shin I (2011) Induction of apoptotic cell death by phytoestrogens by up-regulating the levels of phospho-p53 and p21 in normal and malignant estrogen receptor α-negative breast cells. Nutr Res 31(2):139–146

Shanafelt T, Call T, Zent C, LaPlant B, Bowen D, Roos M et al (2009) Phase I trial of daily oral polyphenon E in patients with asymptomatic Rai stage 0 to II chronic lymphocytic leukemia. J Clin Oncol 27(23):3808–3814

Shehzad A, Wahid F, Lee Y (2010) Curcumin in cancer chemoprevention: molecular targets, pharmacokinetics, bioavailability, and clinical trials. Arch Pharm (Weinheim) 9:489–499

Shenouda N, Zhou C, Browning J, Ansell P, Sakla M, Lubahn D et al (2004) Phytoestrogens in common herbs regulate prostate cancer cell growth *in vitro*. Nutr Cancer 49(2):200–208

Shimoi K, Okada H, Furugori M, Goda T, Takase S, Suzuki M et al (1998) Intestinal absorption of luteolin and luteolin 7-O-beta-glucoside in rats and humans. FEBS Lett 438(3):220–224

Siddiqui FA, Naim M, Islam N (2011) Apoptotic effect of green tea polyphenol (EGCG) on cervical carcinoma cells. Diagn Cytopathol 39(7):482–488

Singh RP, Agarwal R (2005) Prostate cancer and inositol hexaphosphate: efficacy and mechanisms. Anticancer Res 25(4):2891–2903

Singh RP, Agarwal R (2006a) Mechanisms of action of novel agents for prostate cancer chemoprevention. Endocr Relat Cancer 13(3):751–778

Singh RP, Agarwal R (2006b) Prostate cancer chemoprevention by silibinin: bench to bedside. Mol Carcinog 45(6):436–442

Singh RP, Agarwal R (2009) Cosmeceuticals and silibinin. Clin Dermatol 27(5):479–484

Singh RP, Agarwal C, Agarwal R (2003) a Inositol hexaphosphate inhibits growth, and induces G1 arrest and apoptotic death of prostate carcinoma DU145 cells: modulation of CDKI–CDK–cyclin and pRb-related protein-E2F complexes. Carcinogenesis 24:555–563

Singh RP, Tyagi A, Sharma G, Mohan S, Agarwal R (2008) Oral silibinin inhibits in vivo human bladder tumor xenograft growth involving down-regulation of survivin. Clin Cancer Res 14(1):300–308

Souza PS, Vasconcelos FC, Reis FR, Moraes GN, Maia RC (2011) P-glycoprotein and survivin simultaneously regulate vincristine-induced apoptosis in chronic myeloid leukemia cells. Int J Oncol. doi:10.3892/ijo.2011.1103

Sporn M (1976) Approaches to prevention of epithelial cancer during the preneoplastic period. Cancer Res 36:2699–2702

Sreekanth C, Bava S, Sreekumar E, Anto R (2011) Molecular evidences for the chemosensitizing efficacy of liposomal curcumin in paclitaxel chemotherapy in mouse models of cervical cancer. Oncogene 30(28):3139–3152

Surh Y (2003) Cancer chemoprevention with dietary phytochemicals. Nat Rev Cancer 3(10): 768–780

Tan X, Shi M, Tang H, Han W, Spivack S (2010) Candidate dietary phytochemicals modulate expression of phase II enzymes GSTP1 and NQO1 in human lung cells. J Nutr 140(8): 1404–1410

Thamilselvan V, Menon M, Thamilselvan S (2011) Anticancer efficacy of deguelin in human prostate cancer cells targeting glycogen synthase kinase-3 β/β-catenin pathway. Int J Cancer. doi:10.1002/ijc.25949

Tian Y, Song Y (2006) Effects of inositol hexaphosphate on proliferation of HT-29 human colon carcinoma cell line. World J Gastroenterol 12(26):4137–4142

Tiwari P, Kumar A, Balakrishnan S, Kushwaha HS, Mishra KP (2011) Silibinin-induced apoptosis in MCF7 and T47D human breast carcinoma cells involves caspase-8 activation and mitochondrial pathway. Cancer Invest 29(1):12–20

Tsai CH, Lin FM, Yang YC, Lee MT, Cha TL, Wu G et al (2009) Herbal extract of Wedelia chinensis attenuates androgen receptor activity and orthotopic growth of prostate cancer in nude mice. Clin Cancer Res 15(17):5435–5444

Tudoran O, Soritau O, Balacescu O, Balacescu L, Braicu C, Rus M et al (2011) Early transcriptional pattern of angiogenesis induced by EGCG treatment in cervical tumor cells. J Cell Mol Med. doi:10.1111/j.1582-4934

Vaid M, Katiyar S (2010) Molecular mechanisms of inhibition of photocarcinogenesis by silymarin, a phytochemical from milk thistle (*Silybum marianum* L. Gaertn.). Int J Oncol 36(5):1053–1060

Veluri R, Singh RP, Liu Z, Thompson JA, Agarwal R, Agarwal C (2006) Fractionation of grape seed extract and identification of gallic acid as one of the major active constituents causing growth inhibition and apoptotic death of DU145 human prostate carcinoma cells. Carcinogenesis 27(7):1445–1453

Verheus M, van Gils C, Keinan-Boker L, Grace P, Bingham S, Peeters P (2007) Plasma phytoestrogens and subsequent breast cancer risk. J Clin Oncol 25(6):648–655

Verschoyle RD, Brown K, Steward WP, Gescher AJ (2008) Consumption of silibinin, a flavonolignan from milk thistle, and mammary cancer development in the C3(1) SV40 T, t antigen transgenic multiple mammary adenocarcinoma (TAg) mouse. Cancer Chemother Pharmacol 62(2):369–372

Vucenik I, Shamsuddin A (2006) Protection against cancer by dietary IP6 and inositol. Nutr Cancer 55(2):109–125

Vucenik I, Tantivejkul K, Zhang Z, Cole K, Saied I, Shamsuddin A (1998a) IP6 in treatment of liver cancer. I. IP6 inhibits growth and reverses transformed phenotype in HepG2 human liver cancer cell line. Anticancer Res 18(6A):4083–4090

Vucenik I, Zhang Z, Shamsuddin A (1998b) IP6 in treatment of liver cancer. II. Intra-tumoral injection of IP6 regresses pre existing human liver cancer xenotransplanted in nude mice. Anticancer Res 18(6A):4091–4096

Walter ED (1941) Genistin (an isoflavone glucoside) and its aglucone, genistein, from soybeans. J Am Chem Soc 63(12):3273–3276

Wang L, Lee IM, Zhang SM, Blumberg J, Buring JE, Sesso HD (2009) Dietary intake of selected flavonols, flavones, and flavonoid-rich foods and risk of cancer in middle-aged and older women. Am J Clin Nutr 89(3):905–912

Wang L, Cheng C, Zhao H, Yang Z, Wei H, Cui H (2010) Growth inhibition and apoptosis-inducing effects of phytic acid in human gastric carcinoma cells. Wei Sheng Yan Jiu 39(1):39–41

Wattenberg L (1985) Chemoprevention of cancer Ccancer Rres 45:1–8

Weglarz L, Molin I, Orchel A, Parfiniewicz B, Dzierzewicz Z (2006) Quantitative analysis of the level of p53 and p21(WAF1) mRNA in human colon cancer HT-29 cells treated with inositol hexaphosphate. Acta Biochim Pol 53(2):349–356

Wellington K, Jarwis B (2001) Silymarin: a review of its clinical properties in the management of hepatic disorders. BioDrugs 15:465–489

Weng C, Yen G (2011) Chemopreventive effects of dietary phytochemicals against cancer invasion and metastasis: phenolic acids, monophenol, polyphenol, and their derivatives. Cancer Treat Rev. doi:10.1016/j.ctrv.2011.03.001

Wruck CJ, Claussen M, Fuhrmann G, Römer L, Schulz A, Pufe T et al (2007) Luteolin protects rat PC12 and C6 cells against MPP+ induced toxicity via an ERK dependent Keap1-Nrf2-ARE pathway. J Neural Transm Suppl 72:57–67

Wu Q, Chen Y, Liu H, He J (2007a) Anti-cancer effects of deguelin on human leukemia K562 and K562/ADM cells in vitro. J Huazhong Univ Sci Technolog Med Sci 27(2):149–152

Wu T, Wu H, Wang Y, Chang T, Chan S, Lin Y et al (2007b) Prohibitin in the pathogenesis of transitional cell bladder cancer. Anticancer Res 27(2):895–900

Xiao J, Huang G, Geng X, Qiu H (2011) Soy-derived isoflavones inhibit HeLa cell growth by inducing apoptosis. Plant Foods Hum Nutr 66(2):122–128

Yamasaki M, Mukai A, Ohba M, Mine Y, Sakakibara Y, Suiko M et al (2010) Genistein induced apoptotic cell death in adult T-cell leukemia cells through estrogen receptors. Biosci Biotechnol Biochem 74(10):2113–2115

Yan C, Yang J, Shen L, Chen X (2011) Inhibitory effect of epigallocatechin gallate on ovarian cancer cell proliferation associated with aquaporin 5 expression. Arch Gynecol Obstet. doi:10.1007/s00404-011-1942-6

Yang SF, Yang WE, Chang HR, Chu SC, Hsieh YS (2008) Luteolin induces apoptosis in oral squamous cancer cells. J Dent Res 87(4):401–406

Yu J, Lee J, Lim Y, Kim T, Jin Y, Sheen Y et al (2008) Genistein inhibits rat aortic smooth muscle cell proliferation through the induction of p27kip1. J Pharmacol Sci 107(1):90–98

Zhang Q, Wan L, Guo Y, Cheng N, Cheng W, Sun Q et al (2009) Radiosensitization effect of luteolin on human gastric cancer SGC-7901 cells. J Biol Regul Homeost Agents 23(2):71–78

Zhang B, Shi Z, Liu B, Yan X, Feng J, Tao H (2010a) Enhanced anticancer effect of gemcitabine by genistein in osteosarcoma: the role of Akt and nuclear factor-kappaB. Anticancer Drugs 21(3):288–296

Zhang J, Harrison JS, Uskokovic M, Danilenko M, Studzinski GP (2010b) Silibinin can induce differentiation as well as enhance vitamin D3-induced differentiation of human AML cells ex vivo and regulates the levels of differentiation-related transcription factors. Hematol Oncol 28(3):124–132

Zhou L, Liu P, Chen B, Wang Y, Wang X, Internati MC et al (2008) Silibinin restores paclitaxel sensitivity to paclitaxel-resistant human ovarian carcinoma cells. Anticancer Res 28(2A): 1119–1127

Zhu B, Zhan W, Li Z, Wang Z, He Y, Peng J et al (2007) (-)-Epigallocatechin-3-gallate inhibits growth of gastric cancer by reducing VEGF production and angiogenesis. World J Gastroenterol 13(8):1162–1169

Zhu B, Chen H, Zhan W, Wang C, Cai S, Wang Z et al (2011) (-)-Epigallocatechin-3-gallate inhibits VEGF expression induced by IL-6 via Stat3 in gastric cancer. World J Gastroenterol 17(18):2315–2325

Zunino S, Storms D (2009) Carnosol delays chemotherapy-induced DNA fragmentation and morphological changes associated with apoptosis in leukemic cells. Nutr Cancer 61(1):94–102

Nutrition, Diet and Cancer

Edited by Sharmila Shankar and Rakesh K. Srivastava

Chemoprevention of cancer has been the focus of intensive research for more than two decades. Epidemiological evidence has shown a small, but significant association between fruit and vegetable intake and a reduction in cancer risk. Diet may account for about 35% of cancer. Large claims have been made for the effectiveness of particular diets in determining one's risk of developing cancer, ranging from protection against cancer initiation, progression and metastasis. A wide array of dietary components has been demonstrated to be as effective in fighting off cancer. Towards an increased understanding of the nutrition, exercise and diet in preventing cancer or inhibiting its progression has led to the discovery and development of novel and effective drugs that regulate intracellular signaling network in the body. This information will be very useful to explore novel and highly effective chemopreventive strategies for reducing the health burden of cancer.

Hippocrates, who proclaimed 25 centuries ago, 'Let food be thy medicine and medicine be thy food'. They estimated that one third of all cancer cases could be prevented by a healthier diet; statements which are widely accepted in the scientific literature. This book covers the current state-of-the art knowledge on the impact of nutrition and diet with nutrigenetics, nutritional epigenomics, nutritional transcriptomics, proteomics, and metabolomics approach in cancer prevention and therapy.

Features:

- Role of aberrant cellular signaling network in cancer biology and prime chemotherapy target of dietary agents.
- Nutritional compounds as chemopreventive agents by regulation of epigenetic alterations and proteasome inhibition.
- Modulation of transcription factors by dietary phytomolecules.
- Effects of dietary agents on gene expression and pharmacological events in cancer prevention and therapy.
- Use of natural antioxidants, fiber, micronutrients, and fish oil in treating several human cancers.

S. Shankar and R.K. Srivastava (eds.), *Nutrition, Diet and Cancer*,
DOI 10.1007/978-94-007-2923-0, © Springer Science+Business Media B.V. 2012

Index

S. Shankar and R.K. Srivastava (eds.), *Nutrition, Diet and Cancer*,
DOI 10.1007/978-94-007-2923-0, © Springer Science+Business Media B.V. 2012

P

Q

R

S

T

V

W

Z

9789400729223